Advance Praise for *101 Global Leadership Lessons for Nurses*

"Through the thoughtful and intentional sharing by international colleagues in nursing, we have been given living examples of mentoring to develop aspiring nurse leaders. These examples can serve as benchmarks for our own on-going work in expanding the leadership talents of all nurses."

—Karen S. Haase-Herrick, RN, MN
American Organization of Nurse Executives Past President

"Through the voice of leaders and emerging leaders from around the world, this book embodies the best of nursing professionalism and gives hope for an even brighter future as a result of the mentoring relationships undertaken."

—Joyce Clifford, PhD, RN, FAAN
President and Chief Executive Officer
The Institute for Nursing Healthcare Leadership

"This book was developed by a multi-generational, culturally diverse, world-wide network of nurses, all creating a vision of excellence in health care. With the ease of communications today, we must aim toward contributing meaningful change, positive outcomes, and hopeful futures to the global population of our planet. This book is a literary contribution to that effort."

—Joan Trofino, EdD, RN, NEA-BC, FAAN
Magnet Appraiser, Author, Speaker.
Faculty, and Former Chief Nursing Officer

"Being a mentor is a gift and a challenge. The role of mentor provides both parties with new knowledge and causes for recommitment. The reciprocal sharing of the pride and passion is always rewarding. To be a mentor is one of the highest honors and carries responsibility that should not be taken lightly!"

—Betty Noyes, RN, MA
President, Noyes & Associates, Ltd.

"As nurse leaders, the best investment any of us can make in our own profession is to ensure that the mantle of leadership is gently but securely placed into the hands and the hearts of those who will follow us. This book reflects on this important gift of leadership we have received and that we will, in turn, pass along to the next generation of nurses."

—Carol Bradley MSN, RN CENP
Regional Chief Nursing Officer, Tenet Healthcare, Inc.
American Organization of Nurse Executives Past President

"The breadth and depth of nursing guarantees that nurses can find a passion to pursue. That pursuit is made richer by engaging the experiences of others who have valuable lessons to share with those who are in search of trusted counsel. This compendium of wisdom is a gift from and to mentors and mentees that will serve to anchor new practices through shared experiences rich in expertise and courage."

—Katherine W. Vestal, RN, PhD, FACHE, FAAN
President, Work Innovations, LLC

"Preparation of the next wave of nursing leaders requires commitment to provide expert mentoring. The accrued benefits enrich health care organizations as well the mentors' professional journeys."

—Judy Spinella, RN, MSN, MBA, FACHE
Principal Consultant, Houston Healthcare Operations
Interim Chief Operating Officer, St. Mary's Hospital Caroldelet

"This book offers a special blend for understanding new views of leadership in relation to authenticity and personal/professional mentoring. The approach of pairing leaders with their mentees captures a level of dynamic excitement and interest and inspiration. This combined work of leaders and their mentees . . . opens new horizons for leadership legacies and serves as a model for all future mentee-leaders in the making."

—Jean Watson, PhD, RN, AHN-BC, FAAN
Distinguished Professor of Nursing
Murchinson-Scoville Endowed Chair in Caring Science
University of Colorado Denver, College of Nursing
Founding Director, Watson Caring Science Institute

"Great leaders . . . actively reach out to less experienced colleagues, share their knowledge, and leverage their own power to assist others in their career progression. Dr. Rollins Gantz has compiled this collection of experiences from outstanding nurse leaders and those they have mentored. These stories will inspire all of us to touch the lives of tomorrow's caregivers and patients through the mentoring of our evolving leaders."

—Kathleen D. Sanford, DBA, RN, FACHE
Senior Vice President and Chief Nursing Officer
Catholic Health Initiatives
Author, Leading With Love

"The unique aspect of this book is the co-authoring of the chapters by the mentors and mentees. A distinct value of this is that the mentor is demonstrating a large degree of fearlessness in meeting professional objectives. Too many men and women in all fields are afraid of the growth of leadership in colleagues. I cherish this growth and have been personally and professionally enhanced by it. This collateral growth is well exemplified in this book."

—Claire M. Fagin, PHD, RN, FAAN
Dean Emerita, Leadership Professor Emerita
University of Pennsylvania, School of Nursing

"The current and projected nursing shortage has created a significant need for nurse leaders to place a much greater commitment to mentor the new generation of nurse leaders. This book provides examples of successful mentoring strategies from nurse leaders around the globe. The urgent need for mentoring is not an activity for those only in the United States, but is a priority for nurse leaders around the world. The future of our profession depends on it."

—Peter I. Buerhaus, PhD, RN, FAAN
Valere Potter Distinguished Professor of Nursing
Director, Center for Interdisciplinary Health Workforce Studies
Institute for Medicine and Public Health
Vanderbilt University Medical Center

"Historically, mentoring has been described as a single, sustained hierarchical relationship occurring during the school years or shortly thereafter as a work career takes shape. These days, more emphasis is being placed on a person having multiple relationships of various lengths that are important to advancement and which collectively constitute an evolving network of support. Now that the concept of mentoring no longer has a narrow meaning, the time is ripe for this new book, which has mentors and their mentees tackling a broad array of leadership topics from A to Z."

—Angela Barron McBride, PhD, RN, FAAN
Distinguished Professor-University Dean Emerita
Indiana University School of Nursing
The Honor Society of Nursing, Sigma Theta Tau International Past President

"As illustrated in this book, nurses reach across cultural, national, and generational boundaries to sustain and enhance cherished values. Senior nurse leaders pass on knowledge, practice wisdom, and proven nursing strategies to junior nurses who are aspiring leaders. Junior colleagues offer new insights, challenges, and affirmation as they take our profession in new directions. My hope is that readers of this book will join the process."

—Madeline Wake, PhD, RN, FAAN
Professor of Nursing and John P. Raynor, SJ University Professor
Marquette University

"Most of us have been well mentored in our professional lives, so 'giving back' is an expectation, a way of saying 'thank you' to those who have invested in you. This ambitious compilation effectively illustrates that process on a broad national and international basis—a most impressive span of topics is presented by these 101-plus global learning duos—mentor and mentee. This book is indeed a first for the nursing literature and a source of pride for professional nursing everywhere."

—Maryann F. Fralic, RN, DrPH, FAAN
Professor and Director, Corporate and Foundation Relations
School of Nursing
Johns Hopkins University
Executive Advisor, The Nursing Executive Center

"Looking at the list of authors who have published in this book is looking at a list of accomplished leaders and soon-to-be leaders from all over the world. These authors demonstrate the art of mentoring or being a mentee from their viewpoint of country, position, and experience. This book is abundant in information for the apprentice or the teacher and will serve as an easy to read reference, guide, or compendium of experiences valuable for a world-wide audience."

—Billye Brown, EdD, FAAN
The Honor Society of Nursing, Sigma Theta Tau International Past President
Retired Dean and Professor Emerita, School of Nursing
The University of Texas at Austin

"The importance of mentorship at the beginning stage of a career is well recognized and often celebrated. Less well recognized, however, is the ongoing need for mentorship as an individual assumes new responsibilities or new roles. In this text, a number of talented and generous authors reflect on their unique experiences in nursing and provide a unique and useful compendium of wisdom for us all."

—Kathleen Dracup, RN, FNP, DNSc
Dean and Professor, School of Nursing
University of California, San Francisco

101

GLOBAL
LEADERSHIP
LESSONS
FOR NURSES

SHARED LEGACIES
FROM LEADERS AND
THEIR MENTORS

Edited by Nancy Rollins Gantz, MSN, RN,
PhD, MBA, NE-BC, MRCNA

Sigma Theta Tau International
Honor Society of Nursing®

Sigma Theta Tau International
550 West North Street
Indianapolis, IN 46202

To order additional books, buy in bulk, order for corporate use, or request a review copy for course adoption, contact Nursing Knowledge International at 888.NKI.4YOU (888.654.4968/US and Canada) or +1.317.634.8171 (outside US and Canada) or via email at solutions@nursingknowledge.org.

To request author information, or for speaker or other media requests, contact Rachael McLaughlin of the Honor Society of Nursing, Sigma Theta Tau International at 888.634.7575 (US and Canada) or +1.317.634.8171 (outside US and Canada).

ISBN-13: 978-1-930538-79-5

Library of Congress Cataloging-in-Publication Data

101 global leadership lessons for nurses : shared legacies from leaders and their mentors / edited by Nancy Rollins Gantz.
    p. ; cm.
  Includes bibliographical references and index.
  ISBN-13: 978-1-930538-79-5 (alk. paper)
  ISBN-10: 1-930538-79-0 (alk. paper)
1. Nursing services--Administration. 2. Leadership. I. Gantz, Nancy Rollins, 1949- II. Sigma Theta Tau International. III. Title: One hundred and one global leadership lessons for nurses.
  [DNLM: 1. Nursing--organization & administration--Personal Narratives. 2. Leadership--Personal Narratives. 3. Mentors--Personal Narratives. 4. Nurse Administrators--Personal Narratives. 5. Nursing, Supervisory--Personal Narratives. WY 105 Z999 2010]
  RT89.3.A15 2010
  362.17'3068--dc22
                        2009038586

First Printing, 2009

Publisher: Renee Wilmeth

Acquisitions Editor: Cynthia Saver, RN, MS

Editorial Coordinator: Paula Jeffers

Cover Design by: Gary Adair

Interior Design and Typesetting by: Rebecca Harmon

Development Editor: Carla Hall

Copy Editors: Brian Walls, Teresa Artman, Kevin Kent

Indexer: Angie Bess Martin, RN

Proofreader: Billy Fields

Dedication

Dedicated to the late Dr. Karen Ehrat and Julie Macdonald, former past presidents of the American Organization of Nurse Executives, both exemplary nurse leaders and mentors.

Also . . .

. . . to my younger brother, Todd Emerson Rollins, with considerable appreciation and love, for teaching me my first lesson in sustaining leadership—listening with purpose—and inspired me to . . . "Go confidently in the direction of your dreams. Live the life you have imagined." (Henry David Thoreau)

. . . to the future nurse leaders who will move the profession to great heights and credibility by embracing the philosophy of consistent mentoring and continuing to leave his or her imprint on the nursing profession. . . . "The significance of a man is not in what he attains but rather in what he longs to attain." (Kahlil Gibran)

. . . to colleagues who have consistently demonstrated a lifelong dedication to excellence in nursing leadership and mentoring, it is a significant and humbling honor to mention Roxane Spitzer, JoEllen Koerner, Rita Carty, Venice Ferguson, Rhonda Anderson, Maryann Fralic, Luther Christman, Claire Fagin, Linda Juall Carpenito-Moyet, Debra Townsend, Marie Manthey, Jayne Felgen, Brian Millar, Tim Porter-O'Grady, and Loretta Ford, to name but a few who have positively touched my life. In addition, to the former nursing faculty at Good Samaritan Hospital School of Nursing (now Linfield-Good Samaritan School of Nursing, Portland, Oregon), specifically, Carol Lawson, Pat Hough, Shirley Tighe, Evelyn Smith, Pam Harris (dean emerita), and the late Dean Lloydena Grimes. . . . "Go to the people. Learn from them. Live with them. Start with what they know. Build with what they have. But with the best of leaders, when the work is done, the task accomplished, the people will say, 'We have done this ourselves.'" (Lao Tzu)

. . . to my father, Dr. Troy Rollins, who always said when we do something and do it right the first time we are giving our best, and the times I failed short of this, he was there to support me. . . . "Let me tell you the secret that has led me to my goal. My strength lies solely in my tenacity." (Louis Pasteur)

. . . lastly, to my beautiful and heart-filled mother, Mary Emerson Rollins, who continually provides me the inspiration, unyielding support, and unconditional love for everything I attempt, especially in the profession of nursing. She has forever and consistently been the *wind beneath my wings*—energy, commitment, and life-long goals. . . . "A skillful man reads his dreams for self-knowledge, yet not the details but the quality." (Ralph Waldo Emerson)

Acknowledgements

I want to thank my daughter, Aimee, and my son, Chris, who never let me stop thinking that anything is possible with hard work, dedication, focus, and persistence—even though there were many trips to the university library that they moaned about! This book is the result of their continuous love, confidence, and support. I will forever be blessed they are a part of my life path and lessons.

A special and heartfelt *thank you* goes to all the nursing leaders, current and aspiring, who shared their story and commitment to leadership mentoring, as well as their dedication to our nursing profession through their work for this book. Without their hard work—as well as the support of the phenomenal Cindy Saver, acquisition editor, and Carla Hall, development editor, from the Honor Society of Nursing, Sigma Theta Tau International—this book would not have become a reality.

And to all the 197 plus authors from all over the world who took the time to join this monumental journey in sharing their commitment of mentoring and supporting nursing's future generations of nurse leaders, I thank you. You are the stars that bring nursing to the forefront and truly make a difference to the profession and to the community.

"If you don't achieve success on the first, second, or third attempt, it doesn't mean you have failed. It simply means you must try again from a different angle."

—Linda Aiken, PhD, FAAN, FRCN, RN

SOULPRINTS

"Mentors are souls that dance in and out of our lives, and with each passing, leave a SOULPRINT."

Debra Townsend, RN
CEO, President, Concepts of
  Care, Inc.

The National Center for
  Compassionate Care
Washington, D.C., USA

Each Christmas Eve, I pause to create a story of someone who has extended a surprising act of kindness to me within the year. My story this year is dedicated to Nancy Rollins Gantz; a cherished colleague who has been out of touch but always near at heart.

Many years ago, I was on the American Association of Critical-Care Nurses national stage delivering the most personally memorable keynote of my career. For some wonderful reason, I discovered her in a sea of 6,000 faces. We were two critical-care leaders, each from different areas of service and living worlds apart. That instantaneous moment brought me to this invitation—to contribute to the fabric of this text. It is our mutual hope that sharing mentoring wisdom will take our beloved profession to greater heights. At the very least, our stories may touch you in a way that propels you to care deeply for another within our nursing profession.

Caring for the people that care for the people has become my life's work. I serve a profession that is currently in crisis. The prediction of our shrinking workforce is staggering, and we are all scurrying to try to change that forecast. I have dedicated the greater part of my 40-year career toward nursing retention. Truth be told, we lost focus years ago on protecting our greatest resource—the treasures currently dedicated to nursing. I unite with all the other voices within this text to share an emphatic message: You are never alone. You must have the courage to reach out to us or to someone else. Most of us have not lost the art of compassion. At our very core lies a compassionate heart. That said, we become numbed by the overwhelming demands facing our profession and our world.

This is a text to remind you of our presence. Perhaps within one of these essays you will find hope and the courage to reach out to another in need of wisdom. Quite simply, this is the art of mentoring. Pause to reach out to someone and tell them of their value. Take moments out of your day to practice this engagement. It is a gift to you and to others. Discover someone and leave an imprint on their heart, as Nancy has done for us with this book. I join fellow authors within this text to thank her for the invitation to contribute our unique SOULPRINTS.

Table of Contents

Foreword

The issues related to creating a healthier world are truly within the domain of the nursing profession to address. This book, with its 101+ essays, will help readers prepare for that next step and further demonstrate how nurses around the world make a difference every day. These essays, representing 34 countries and six continents, are told from the perspective of the leader and mentee. They cover nearly every subject area nurse leaders and managers may encounter—from critical thinking to empowerment, influence to negotiation, patient safety to succession planning, theory of practice to writing for publication, and everything in between. The authors share their journeys and lessons learned. With its unique presentation of a mentor/mentee team writing each chapter, this book showcases the power of mentoring in developing new leaders, which is particularly relevant as our profession continues to face projections of unprecedented global nurse shortages in the face of aging populations and emerging health threats.

I encourage you to use your leadership abilities to enable emerging leaders to develop the confidence and skills they need to lead others. This book will provide you with information and examples to guide you in this process. The potential for us, collectively, to make a difference for nursing's global future is real. The key is for each of us, through reading these stories, to accept the challenge and create our own story.

I truly believe that my own leadership journey owes much to my mentors. What I have accomplished in leadership positions can be credited to mentors who took the time to move me into that next opportunity, even when I did not recognize my own potential. My mentors had trust and confidence in my abilities, and they supported me in taking risks. So, too, did all the mentors here.

This book uniquely approaches leadership and mentoring from a global perspective. There is no doubt that these mentees are part of our next generation of leaders who, in turn, will mentor others to influence global health.

—Patricia E. Thompson, RN, EdD, FAAN
Chief Executive Officer
The Honor Society of Nursing, Sigma Theta Tau International

Introduction

"Never lose an opportunity of urging a practical beginning, however small, for it is wonderful how often in such matters the mustard-seed germinates and roots itself."

—Florence Nightingale

During the 19th century and the Crimean War, Florence Nightingale set the foundation for the professional practice of nursing and scientific outcomes. Her profound insight remains applicable and relevant in the 21st century practice of nursing. Because the health care environment creates daily challenges for nurses practicing in all arenas, Nightingale's historic advice and wisdom become more applicable than ever before. Nightingale demonstrated through her practice that "nurses must be leaders who learn and help others to learn" (Joint Commission, 1999). Through her work, we come to understand that developing others in the field of nursing is an obligation that should be accomplished through methodical, strategic goals and objectives, and through mutually willing individuals. Each and every generation of nurses can relate to this belief.

In an environment where health care takes on a matrix appearance, experienced nurses must embrace the philosophy and consistently practice the art of mentoring, coaching, and moving aspiring nurse leaders from novice to expert. Throughout my 30-year career, I have taken this philosophy personally. If the nursing profession is to successfully survive and unquestionably thrive, we—young as well as seasoned leaders—must become mentors at every opportunity. Nurses are the only individuals or groups that can address this significant and critical action.

Any success I have achieved during my career has resulted directly from inspiring, energized, and truly committed nurse leaders. These leaders—some known professionally in nursing and others unknown—motivated my desire to continually educate myself throughout my career, as well as make significant, important contributions to move the nursing profession forward.

They were the epitome of nursing excellence in practice, research, theory, and vision, and they inspired me to be the best in nursing—never compromising patient care or services and teaching me to embrace and practice the nursing philosophy that promotes distinction, consistency, and quality. These individuals identified the importance of mentoring—creating partnerships where someone with experience and expertise shares skills and knowledge with those who are inexperienced in cultivating and promoting growth.

Mentoring: An Overview

In the late 1970s, I met a nurse's aide with the heart, compassion, and intelligence to apply critical thinking and problem-solving skills when the situation warranted. She had nine children, no husband, and financial burdens that constantly occupied her mind. Our paths crossed when I was a young director of nurses, and I was blessed to see her in action at her patients' bedsides, providing quality, compassionate care.

Our friendship developed and blossomed. I could see she had the ability and desire to further her education and become a registered nurse, and even beyond. She had such a desire and drive in her soul that she would not let up until she could make a difference in the nursing profession and in the quality of patient care. It was my honor to become her mentor, and she went on to fulfill her career goals—including a master's degree in nursing, which was not even on her mind when we began our mentoring relationship.

This opened the door for me not only to become a mentor for others, but also to become a mentee of experienced nurse leaders to learn, grow, and be the very best I could be in the nursing profession and make global contributions to the quality of health care.

Goals of This Book

The goals of this book are to

- Illustrate the process and rewards of mentoring for the organization, mentee, and mentor.

- Offer salient, tangible, subject-based lessons for new and experienced leaders alike.

- Demonstrate that mentee-mentor competencies are more readily gained through personal example, channeled practice, or experience than through pure education and training.

Numerous companies all over the world have established formal and informal processes to support new employees or potential leaders through mentoring programs. These companies realize the enormous benefit to both the organization and the individual employee. Benefits include staff satisfaction and retention, education support, heightened customer and patient satisfaction, organizational development, and sensitivity to cultural change and workplace adaptation.

The process of taking experienced individuals and pairing them with the younger generation for professional development has demonstrated successful results for business practice. The business world learned long ago that people are continually learning practices from others, whether good or bad. The nursing profession must adopt these proven programs and apply them in individual organizations for nursing to continue to prosper, survive, and then thrive in the coming years of changing populations and changing health care. Mentoring programs must be a priority for all leadership and clinical staff.

Organization of the Book

The book is organized in alphabetical order by subject matter. Each chapter title begins with the main subject of that chapter's essay. For example, "Academic and Service Partnership" is the first chapter of the book. You will find this title on the first page (chapter opener page) and in the upper-right corner of every right-hand page after the chapter opener.

You may notice that some chapter titles have parenthetical material. This is descriptive text (or language components such as the articles *a, an,* and *the*) that helps clarify the content of the essay, but is not the most critical component of the chapter's subject matter. For example, "(What's Your) Philosophy Own It, Live It." In this case, philosophy is the subject of the essay, but the question "What's Your Philosophy?" clarifies that the essay will help the reader explore his or her personal/professional philosophy. With this approach, the first nonparenthetical word is the most descriptive of the subject, and the chapter essays are alphabetically ordered in that way.

In addition to the usual subject index, we have included both an author index and a country index. These indexes make it easy for the reader to browse by contributing author, including both mentor and mentee, or by country of contributor. References are at the end of the book, beginning on page 633.

The Magnetism of Each Chapter

The creation of this book has been my dream since 1970, when I took my first "101: Fundamentals of Nursing" class. The 101+ chapters (there are two bonus chapters!) in this book cover a broad range of topics, from the perspectives of academic-service partnerships, time management, unity as a profession, multisystem structures, work-life balance, and cultural diversity, all coupling the mentor and mentee in a rich growth relationship. A total of 197 nurse leaders from six continents and 34 countries—including Botswana, Malta, Portugal, Romania, Republic of Moldova, South Africa, Spain, United Kingdom, and United States—share their mentor and mentee experiences.

At the close of each chapter, readers are asked to reflect upon their personal experience and complete self-reflective questions as to where they are in the particular process addressed in the chapter. Overall, the book directs global questions, such as

- How should you select your mentee?

- How should you select your mentor?

- Where will you achieve the richest growth experience that will enhance your career and your personal goals?

- What are the issues in specific countries that can benefit from mentoring?

- What are some of the "success stories" in the nursing profession and the mentoring partnership?

Summary

Energy. Synergy. Early in my career, I learned that both components are essential to mentoring. Leadership gurus such as Max Dupree, Rosabeth Moss Kanter, and Peter Drucker wrote about the importance of mentoring, coaching, and developing support for new employees or aspiring managers. Becoming an effective, well-respected, and knowledgeable leader does not come solely through reading books or attending professional conferences and meetings. Rather, good leadership is a combination of these resources coupled with supportive interactions, collaboration, communication, and learning with colleagues—including nurses and members of other health care disciplines.

Make an impact. Leave footprints in the nursing profession through mentoring. To quote Dr. Loretta Ford (cofounder of the first pediatric nurse practitioner program some 40 years ago), "Be in a hurry; there is not a moment to waste!"

—Nancy Rollins Gantz, MSN, RN, PhD, MBA, NE-BC
President and Senior Consultant
CAPPS International
Sydney, Australia
Mesa, Arizona, USA

References

Joint Commission on the Accreditation of Healthcare Organizations. (1999). *Florence Nightingale: Measuring Hospital Care Outcomes*. Oakbrook Terrace, IL: Joint Commission.

Additional Resources

Ensher, E. A., & Murphy, S. E. (2005). *Power mentoring: How successful mentors and protégés get the most out of their relationships*. San Francisco: Jossey-Bass.

Zachary, L. J. (2005). *Creating a mentoring culture: The organization's guide*. San Francisco: Jossey-Bass.

A Note From the Editors

Please note that the editors have retained the authors' regional spelling differences within the English language. An example is retaining the Australian spelling of "specialisation" that is spelled "specialization" in American English. With the exception of jargon or very localized word choices, we left the author voices intact as much as possible. This was done to respect our global differences.

1

Academic and Service Partnership:
A Stronger Voice

"Clinical and education leaders should come together more to strategize over our future—as nurse caregivers, scientists, and leaders of health care. As a team, we have a stronger voice."

—Kathleen Sanford

Mentors

Frances Vlasses, RN, PhD, NEA-BC
Associate Professor and Research Consultant
Loyola University Chicago
Chicago, Illinois, USA

and

Carolyn Hope Smeltzer, RN, EdD, FAAN, FACHE
Vice President and Partner
PricewaterhouseCoopers
Chicago, Illinois, USA

Mentee

Ashley Currier, RN, BSN
Manager, Inpatient Surgical, Northwestern Memorial Hospital
Chicago, Illinois, USA

In a health care world of increasing complexity, nursing is revisiting academic and service partnerships; the working relationship between service and academia in sharing resources, knowledge, skills set, and decision making. The coming together of resources, an integral part of partnerships, provides not only the opportunity to deliver safer and more effective care, but also holds potential for removing isolated decision making and bringing increased value to the clinical world of nursing. Patients, communities, and the health care profession all benefit from such partnerships.

One challenge, as we dust off the concepts of partnership, is that nursing, patients, and health care are navigating through uncharted waters. The most recent constraints in health care, such as financial challenges, variation in care, and public awareness of quality and safety outcomes concerns, require an environment that seeks transformational and collaborative leaders at the front line.

The Mission

The joining of academia and service provides for a broader vision in the academic world and an enhanced energy in the practice arena. Together, they create the necessary environment to promote the innovation needed to achieve optimal nursing education and care delivery. Despite the heightened intricacies characteristic of health care, an academic and service partnership enhances the resources available, sustains creativity, and leads to innovative solution finding and planning.

For example collaboration can enhance evidence-based nursing practice initiatives. Coupling nurse researchers with those providing daily patient care spotlights the challenges nurses face and leads both parties down a path that pairs a need with the correct solution and implementation. A partnership of this caliber can enhance patient care, provide nurses the expectations and deliverables for performance, and fine-tune the skills necessary to provide optimal patient care in a population of increasing acuity.

The Building Blocks

Although the mission of an academic and service partnership needs to be carefully mapped, the building blocks for success remain consistent for any flourishing union. These include

- Trust.
- Clear communication.
- Careful delineation of needs and expectations.
- Mutual goals and platforms.
- Commitment. This factor is key to a sustainable partnership. A commitment over time is needed, not just for short-term wins.

Nursing has a multitude of opportunities to affect the profession positively. However, development of these partnerships requires careful attention and detail. To achieve a positive impact, careful planning and commitment to maintenance must include:

- **A needs assessment:** Recognizing the external and internal factors that affect patients and our profession helps to identify future paths more accurately and brings areas of opportunity to the forefront.

- **Highlighting strengths, weaknesses, and challenges:** Each partner brings pluses and minuses to the table. Evaluating these can provide a clear division of responsibilities.

- **Identification of the mission and goals of each entity:** In a collaborative partnership, a mutual awareness of each party's mission and goals maintains congruency with set expectations, encourages forward thinking and strategic positioning, and creates new opportunities.

For partnerships to flourish, we must also attend to organizational structure and workload. Existing salary and promotion structures do not support innovative roles and responsibilities that allow for sharing with an equal commitment to both arenas. Leadership must take on the challenge of creating new contractual arrangements that allow faculty and clinicians to be productive while honoring the nuances of each role.

The Potential

With the building blocks for success in place, partnerships in nursing can positively affect the profession on various levels. Consider the possibilities of partnerships with board members, community members, professional association executives, an organization or a leader in a field outside the health care industry, and even global partners. Each of these represents relationships, talent pools, learning, and resources that can positively affect patients and our profession.

Partnership can lead an organization or an individual into a bevy of opportunities for personal and professional enhancement. The power and excitement that comes from collaborating grows as individuals move through their career. A successfully developed partnership not only affects performance, but also motivates further development.

Nursing is at the crossroads of interdependence between the academic and service worlds. Through the collaboration of academia and service, nursing may excel in a diverse and ever-changing environment. With the potential to enhance a multitude of nursing aspects, having partners at the table is imperative.

The Reality

Despite the strengths of an academic/service partnership, they are not easily realized. The authors participated in a think tank with nurse executives from Catholic Health Initiatives (CHI), one of the largest Catholic health care systems in the United States with facilities ranging from community to teaching hospitals in rural as well as metropolitan areas. When asked their opinions about partnerships they spoke with enthusiasm and interest, identifying several benefits of service and academia working together including:

- Partnerships were needed to create a fertile environment for evidence-based practice and research.

- Partnerships could provide opportunities for innovation and creativity.

- The education of nurses could flourish under the watchful eye of the partnership. Additionally, sharing expertise, exposing students to health care realities, enhancing recruitment of practitioners and faculty, and strengthening clinical role models are all benefits of academic/service partnerships. The CHI nurse executive group proposed that knowledge from the practice arena feeds curriculum change, improves competency, and enhances job satisfaction and professional development for nursing leadership (CHI, 2008).

Reflections from Ashley Currier, Mentee

Time, resources, and agendas are often detours on the path of partnerships. However, I've learned that detours can and should be a minor hiccup. Through juggling various demands, I have formed some of my most effective and most creative partnerships.

Fran Vlasses and I began working together on the Nursing Research Council at Northwestern Memorial Hospital after Fran joined as a faculty research consultant from Loyola University Niehoff School of Nursing. There is something magical about hearing your thoughts and passions echoed by another person. Fran often provides the well-articulated sentence that I wish I had said. Her nursing expertise has enhanced my excitement and newness to the field. Fran meets every challenge with an open mind, collaborates effectively with her resources, and champions action towards an innovative solution. As a representative from the academic world, I view Fran and her work at Loyola University as something that enriches my mind.

Successful partnerships, to me, are those you can mold and shape over time and bring along wherever your path may take you.

Reflections from Fran Vlasses, Mentor

Ashley has a natural talent for research and leadership. I have had the wonderful opportunity to encourage her. In this relationship, my job has been to capture and direct her energy. I have guided her and a team of nurses through a research project on medication administration, which came out of her commitment to excellence in patient care. The results have been shared and procedural changes are being designed based on these findings. Working with Ashley as a mentee provides an exemplar of the benefits of the academic/service partnership that we have with Northwestern Memorial Hospital. This partnership has provided an arena within which we could combine my skills in research with Ashley's drive to solve a clinical problem. Through this partnership professional development has taken place and, most important, patients will benefit.

Self-Reflective Questions

1. How do you make the formation of partnerships a personal goal? (What actions do you live out to support it as a personal goal?)

2. In what ways are you clear about your own gaps or the gaps you represent, for example, is there a need for professional development in evidence-based practice that can be addressed by a faculty member? How so? Do you develop the philosophy "We need each other's insights to balance each other's blind spots" (Cronenwett, 2004)?

3. Do you find partners whose talents meet your needs or just fill the gaps?

4. In what way do your partnerships support diversity?

5. In what way do you choose partners who share your vision, values, and culture?

6. How do you display teamwork? Do you adopt a "we're in this together" approach characterized by a daring vision and authentic and well-spoken candor?

7. How do you share the success and the failures of agreed upon projects?

8. Do you think broadly about partnerships? Not limited to education/service, do you develop at least one partner who is not in health care? Do you move beyond getting the work done to offering support for initiatives that are not shared?

Self-Reflective Questions *(continued)*

9. What are the nonimmediate/nontangible rewards, recognition, or resources for partnerships?

10. What forms of power and influence can a partnership provide?

The authors wish to acknowledge the nurse executives from the Catholic Health Initiative Summit 2008 for sharing their thoughts and reflections on partnerships.

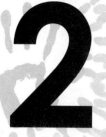

2 (An) Aging Nursing Workforce: A Time for Action

"The great thing about getting older is that you don't lose all the ages you have got."

—Anonymous

Mentor
Gloria Thupayagale-
  Tshweneagae, MSN, RN
Lecturer, University of
  Botswana School of Nursing
Botswana, Africa

Mentee
Tebogo Rapaeye, BNS, RN
Assistant Nursing Officer,
  Tertiary Hospital System
Botswana, Africa

In our youth, we often overlook the fact that we will age. When I took over a leadership position from a senior colleague 10 years ago, I remember hearing him say, "You will also get to where I am." He meant that one day I would also age and have to make room for someone younger. However, realities have changed in my country. Many people in the workforce today are over 45 and will reach retirement in 20 years. When I replaced my colleague, there were many other qualified candidates competing for the position. Today, this is not the case as more nurses are needed to care for clients with HIV and AIDS, and younger nurses are opting to work elsewhere because of the work-related stress associated with HIV and AIDS, as well as other social ills associated with nurses' working conditions in Botswana. In most African countries, younger nurses with two years or less of experience leave their prospective countries to go and work elsewhere (Thupayagale-Tshweneagae, 2007). This movement leaves only older nurses with the required education and experience to work with clients and younger nurses with less than two years experience. These inexperienced nurses need to work with the older nurses who can guide them to attain the necessary experience in nursing.

The Aging Workforce

The world's transition from the industrial age to the information age brought challenges that require reforms. The nature of work has changed from brawn to knowledge, calling for changes in our work policies (Klein, 2007). Those who are knowledgeable, experienced, and skillful are the key players in implementing the mandates of their organizations and institutions.

In many countries (Botswana, South Africa, and Malawi, to name a few), policy and tradition cause people in the workforce to retire in their mid- to late-sixties, irrespective of their skill base, professional status, and work performance despite the fact that the workforce is aging in most countries.

The nursing workforce is also aging. In a study on nursing shortages by Caron (2004) in the United Kingdom, most nurses in the study were between age 41 and 50, with a significant number of them age 51 to 60. The average age of nurses in the United States is over 46 years of age and 41% of the nursing population is 50 or older (United States Department of Health and Human Services, 2007).

At the same time, life expectancy in developing countries is approaching 80 years, according to the Annie E. Casey Foundation report of 2005. The report further states that the number of persons with disabilities also is dwindling because health care technologies have reduced disabilities normally experienced in old age. Given these trends, an implication can be drawn that any active nurse, regardless of age, should be kept in service.

A Worldwide Pandemic

The impact of HIV and AIDS on young people age 19–25 and persons age 25–34 has had a felt effect in nursing, especially in the sub-Saharan region (Tlou, 2005). Motlaleng (2005) studied 40 students who graduated from a nursing post-basic programme in Botswana. The findings showed, on average, a member of the cohort died of HIV and AIDS illness every year. Before the study ended, six members of the cohort died, meaning this nursing workforce was depleted 15 percent in 5 years. This leaves even fewer people to replace aging nurses.

Education Requirements

In Botswana, according to the Nursing and Midwifery Council of Botswana Register (2005), the majority of nurses in managerial positions in practice and education are over age 50. The register also shows no nurses under age 40 with a master's degree, and no nurses under age 45 with a doctoral degree (the majority being over age 50). Educating nurses in most developing countries is dependant on government funding; as a result it takes a minimum of 12 years to earn a master's degree and 16 years for a doctoral degree. For a lecturer to teach in an African university (Botswana, Muhambili, Nairobi, South Africa), they need a minimum of a master's degree. To progress through the ranks of academia, a doctoral degree is encouraged.

However, because of inadequate funding and the length of time required to train a nurse to this level, there are very few nurse educators; therefore, the number of trained nurses is dwindling. This explains why nurses in education and senior administration are age 50 and above. Moreover, the pattern in Botswana is similar to most developing countries, such as Zambia, Malawi, and South Africa (Dovlo, 2001).

The Value of Older Adults in the Workforce

Many employers would like to retain their aging workforce beyond the retirement age. These employers see keeping the aging workforce as cost-effective because it requires no new training. The skills, knowledge, and experiences of the aging workforce also serve in mentoring the younger workforce. In addition, older adults can learn new technical skills from the younger workers.

Reflections from Tebogo Rapaeye, Mentee

These scenarios show that nurse educators, researchers, and senior administrators are aging. Most of the aging nursing workforce are women. Women in the nursing profession at this age are still active and have more than the basic qualifications and necessary experiences the nursing field requires. On average, such persons have a life expectation of an additional 10–20 years after the retirement age. Thus, forced retirement in their 60s is wasteful of their professional experience.

Knowledgeable nurses should remain in service to mentor younger nurses new to the profession. For example, I have been part of the research studies done by the mentor and have assisted in writing for publication. In the clinical setting, I have worked closely with some senior and older nurses and have been able to gain experience from them. To date, I can work independently in some areas such as the general wards and still need to be mentored in other areas such as critical care nursing.

Let us not keep the older nurses for their age; let us instead keep them for their contribution and expertise. Why are we keeping policies that do not work? Imagine if your group (mentor's cohort, age 50–55) retires at 65. Who will continue the work you are doing? The retirement age should be extended for nurses.

Community of All Ages

The aging population is a reality for all sectors. Organizations must prescribe a plan that will enable older adults to remain in service. The authors contend that at age 65, the vast experience and knowledge accumulated is still needed. Rather than remove people from the workplace because of their age, deploy them in less physically demanding positions with flexible hours. Use the aging population as mentors and consultants in their fields of specialty.

Every organization needs to develop retention strategies that use the aging workforce so the valuable experience they have is not lost. Quality nursing can be sustained if the needs of the aging nursing workforce are met without compromising the needs of the younger nursing workforce. We need to consider nursing as a community of all ages.

Self-Reflective Questions

1. How do you view aging? As an opportunity to gain experiences and wisdom? Or as a handicap? Describe why you believe one way or the other.

2. Do you think you can contribute to the nursing profession beyond the age of 65? If so, in what capacities? If not, why not?

3. Does your organization have a policy, formal or informal, about retaining nurses nearing or at retirement age?

4. What are the ways an aging nurse retention policy may help your department or organization?

5. In what ways does the culture of your organization support or undermine the work of older nurses?

6. Do you think older nurses can be good mentors for younger nurses? If so, what can you do within your organization to encourage or faciltate mentoring?

Self-Reflective Questions *(continued)*

7. In what ways do you or can you show you value aging nurses within your organization?

8. Do you think symbiotic relationships can exist between the aging nursing workforce and the younger nursing workforce? How so?

9. How has your career been positively impacted by the work or role modeling of older nurses?

10. When you envision yourself at the end of your career, what legacy do you hope to leave behind?

(The) Art of Nursing: 3
Aesthetic Knowing

"Nursing is an art; and if it is to be made an art, it requires as exclusive a devotion, as hard a preparation, as any painter's or sculptor's work; for what is the having to do with dead canvas or cold marble, compared with having to do with the living spirit—the temple of God's spirit? It is one of the Fine Arts; I had almost said, the finest of the Fine Arts."

—Florence Nightingale

Mentor

Barbara M. Dossey, PhD, RN,
  AHN-BC, FAAN
International Co-Director
  and Board Member of the
  Nightingale Initiative for
  Global Health
Washington, DC, and
Ottawa, Ontario, Canada
Director, Holistic Nursing
  Consultants
Santa Fe, New Mexico, USA

Mentee

Anna Dermenchyan, RN, BSN,
  PHN
Clinical Nurse, Cardiothoracic
  ICU, Ronald Reagan UCLA
  Medical Center
Los Angeles, California, USA

Florence Nightingale's eloquent quote that starts off this chapter fully captures the art of nursing. *Aesthetic knowing,* the art of nursing, is a pattern of knowing that includes the integral and holistic expression of all the other recognized patterns of knowing—empirical, ethical, personal, not knowing, and socio-political (Dossey, et.al., 2005; Dossey 2010). Aesthetic knowing includes knowledge, skills, experience, and instinct. Within aesthetic knowing, we value the inherent dignity of individuals—including ourselves—and how we engage as a facilitator of healing. We recognize that we are part of the healing environment of patients and others. As we explore our individual and collective experiences, we more clearly understand the art of nursing. Take a moment to reflect on the poem, "The Art of Nursing."

Developing Aesthetic Awareness

What can we do each day before our daily encounters with patients, families, colleagues, and health care team members to call forth our aesthetic awareness and to access our inner strengths and resources? One suggestion lies in Anna's (mentee) journal entry, written September 2008 just weeks into her first professional nursing position:

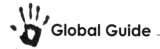

Global Guide

The Art of Nursing

When a nurse
Encounters another
Something happens
What occurs
Is never a neutral event

A pulse taken
Words exchanged
A touch
A healing moment
Two persons
Are never
The same

Used with permission. ©1984 by Barbara M. Dossey and Cathie E. Guzzetta.

A 12-hour shift starting at 7 a.m. waits for me at the Cardiothoracic ICU, my new home after nursing school. Before I left the house, I did my loving-kindness meditation, which helps me focus and think positively for the rest of the day. "May I be free from fear and harm, both internal and external. May I be truly happy and deeply peaceful. May there be ease in every aspect of my life. May I love my life completely just as it is."

When I practice loving-kindness toward myself, I am better equipped to remember the art of nursing, to face the challenging day ahead, and to show loving-kindness to my colleagues, patients, and their families.

It also helps to understand the key elements and qualities of aesthetic knowing:

- **Presence:** *Presence* is a way of approaching a person that respects and honors the person's essence; it is relating in a way that reflects a quality of "being with" and "in collaboration with."

- **Deep listening:** *Deep listening* is being present and focused with intention to understand what another person is expressing or not expressing.

- **Bearing witness:** *Bearing witness* is being present to things as they are; it is the state where skills are enhanced by reflection and mindfulness (the practice of giving attention to what is happening in the present moment to our thoughts, feelings, emotions, and/or sensations). For example, when a nurse encounters a mother who is crying over the acute state of her very ill baby, the nurse who has done all that is needed with giving medications and completing necessary protocols is willing to sit with the mother, not talking or doing any procedures, just sitting or standing in silence. Even if no words are spoken, a therapeutic encounter will occur as the nurse comes together with this mother in the moment to be present to her suffering.

- **Finding inner harmony and balance:** Through our mindfulness, we are more able to achieve states of *equanimity*, the stability of mind that allows us to be present with a good and impartial heart no matter how beneficial or difficult the situation.

- **Intention:** We use our *intention*—the conscious awareness of being in the present moment with self or another person—to help facilitate the healing process. It is the deliberate act of using the will that is often experienced as the act of love.

- **Intuition:** We recognize our *intuition*, the perceived knowing of events—past or future—insight, or uncanny understanding of a personal situation without a conscious use of logical, analytical processes, which may also be informed by our senses, to receive information. Intuition is that experience of sudden insight into a feeling, a solution, or a problem where time, events, and tangible or intangible elements fit together in a unified experience, such as understanding more about pain and suffering, or other experiences of life, health, illness, and death.

Take a moment to read another journal entry as Anna shares another aspect of aesthetic knowing as she reflects on and values the dignity of her patient.

Mr. Galt, my 67-year-old patient admitted to the unit after his open heart surgery, is unstable. . . . When I was doing my post-op orders, I was reminded of sitting in class for three weeks trying to learn about the critical care patient and how a body manages homeostasis. . . . I know Mr. Galt is fragile and that I need to treat him with respect and dignity. Call him by name and explain all the procedures, irrespective of him being on a ventilator or whether he understands. Doing so makes my patient feel like a person and not an organism.

When I take care of a patient, I am part of their personal experience. What I do can either help them feel better and recover to a higher state of health or contribute to the negative part of their sickness. When we have deep and profound respect for the human being, we go beyond the probable and make others see what is possible only through us. This is the heart of the art of nursing.

Daily Exploration

Developing the process of aesthetic knowing requires our own unique exploration each day. In closing, Anna shares a few joyous moments and the novelty and anticipation of future events that invigorates her before she returns from her lunch break to the critical care unit.

I'm reflecting on all the new learning that has taken place. I know more than what I knew at the beginning of the shift, which gives me the encouragement to stay focused. These gardens are filled with green plants, and narrow pathways where I can walk for stretched minutes, and a small stream filled with turtles. I'm watching squirrels do their little dances as they chase each other. This place brings a smile to my face and to the faces of all the people who walk past me.

This peace and beauty gets me thinking of all the exciting events that are coming up on my calendar. I celebrate having a balance of work and fun. Tomorrow, I'm biking for an hour. Next week, I'm attending a lecture on artificial hydration and nutrition in end-stage disease, an ethics lecture given by the director of UCLA's Healthcare Ethics. At the end of next week, I'm going to the World Festival of Sacred Music with my former coworkers. Okay, back to the hospital with a new determination to succeed.

Self-Reflective Questions

1. What does Florence Nightingale's quote on the art of nursing mean to you?

2. How do you live out your values in your own "art of nursing"?

3. How can you integrate presence where you are available with the wholeness of your being?

4. How can you recognize your inner sense of joy?

5. How can you cultivate your intuitive processes?

6. How can you cultivate peace of mind as you move through your busy day?

7. How can you be more of a healing presence for others?

Self-Reflective Questions *(continued)*

8. How can you nurture your ability to be mindful and live consciously?

9. Do you trust intuition in patient encounters and in your personal life? If not, how can you reconnect with your own intuition?

10. Do you recognize your intention where you have a conscious alignment with your creative essence and divine purpose?

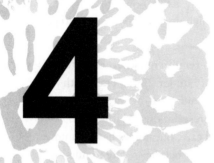

4

Autonomy in Nursing

"Never take a back seat . . . never take 'no' for an answer."

—Vernice Ferguson

Mentor
Sandy Summers, RN, MSN, MPH
Founder and Executive
  Director, The Truth About
  Nursing
Baltimore, Maryland, USA

Mentee
Richard M. Kimball, Jr., RN, MSN,
  MPH
Outpatient Amyotrophic Lateral
  Sclerosis Clinic
Johns Hopkins Hospital
Baltimore, Maryland, USA

The media largely portrays nurses as subservient to physicians who give them "orders." Yet nursing is a distinct, self-regulating, autonomous profession deserving of significant resources to prepare nurses and deliver quality care. Career seekers who have the qualities skilled nursing requires—including intellect, courage, passion, interpersonal ability, and a strong work ethic—value autonomy greatly. When nursing is perceived as a tiny, junior subset of medicine, instead of an autonomous profession, decision makers may not understand why it needs its own resources for clinical practice, education, and research. Nursing suffers, and by extension, so does patient care.

Nursing governs itself through nurse-controlled boards that administer the rigorous examinations nurses must pass to gain their licenses to practice. Nurses in the workplace are hired, fired, and managed by senior nurses, not physicians. They work in a chain of command that reaches to a chief of nursing. Even nurses who work in physician-owned outpatient offices operate autonomously. They are still bound by the laws and ethics that govern nursing, which do not depend on who pays them for their work.

Nursing has its own codes of ethics, which require nurses to educate and advocate for patients (International Council of Nurses, 2005; The Truth About Nursing, 2009). Nurses have decisional authority over whether to participate in procedures or carry out physician prescriptions (Mathes, 2005). Of course, nursing care overlaps with medical care, but nurses have a unique knowledge base and a holistic practice model that belongs solely to nursing (Thornton, 2009). This holistic model gives nurses independent obligations to their patients that do not depend on physicians or other colleagues. Nurses are educated by nursing scholars and use textbooks written by these scholars.

Nurse practice acts hold nurses legally accountable to provide care that nurses deem necessary (Summers, 2006). Many nurse practice acts, such as those in the United States, define the profession in broad terms that do not depend on physicians (California Board of Registered Nursing, 1997). These laws make clear that nursing manages itself, defining nursing practice to include a wide range of important prevention and care functions (General Laws of Massachusetts, n.d.; Texas Legislature, n.d.). The statutes note that *one* aspect of nursing is to administer certain treatments prescribed by advanced practitioners, but that does not create a subordinate relationship. Even in administering these treatments, nurses have a professional and legal obligation to assess the care prescribed, and if necessary, to work for better options. Moreover, nurses are not relieved of nursing malpractice liability or their ethical obligations simply because they are administering treatment prescribed by an advanced practitioner.

Some U.S. courts also recognize that nursing is a distinct scientific profession with its own standards and scope of care. For example, the Illinois Supreme Court recently concluded that a physician was not qualified to testify as to a nursing standard of care because he was not a nurse (Sullivan v Edward Hospital, 2004). The court explained that nursing is an "independent profession with a unique body of knowledge and not simply a subcategory of medicine" (Murphy, 2004). The American Association of Nurse Attorneys argues that only nurses—not physicians—should be permitted to provide expert testimony as to the nursing standard of care in malpractice actions (American Association of Nurse Attorneys, 2004).

The misperception that nurses report to physicians may be common because of the historic gender-related power imbalance between the two health professions. Physicians have an unequalled combination of economic power and social status. They have more years of formal education than most (though not all) nurses (Pankratz & Pankratz, 1974). But this does not mean that nurses are subordinate to physicians or have no independent duties to patients. Nursing autonomy does not cease to exist simply because nurses face practical barriers. Additionally, many physicians wrongly see themselves as being in charge of patient care. Some physicians act abusively toward nurses, which drives nurses from the workforce (Rosenstein, 2002). Some nurses are intimidated by physicians. And of course, allowing the perception that physicians are ultimately responsible for care lets nurses escape blame for errors. This combination of factors leaves many nurses reluctant to challenge physicians or to assert themselves in general (Buresh & Gordon, 2006). But nurses—and their patients—pay for that choice in the long run with a weakened profession that cannot deliver the quality or quantity of care patients need (Mathes, 2005).

Nurses must change this situation. To achieve safe and effective patient care, nurses must routinely practice autonomy—and physicians and hospital administrators must embrace the idea. To advocate for patients, nurses must be able to negotiate in a meaningful way with advanced practitioners, and if necessary, work to prevent actions nurses believe may harm patients. This advocacy is not easy given the continuing imbalance in power; nonetheless, nurses have a duty to protect their patients. So nurses should act and dress like health professionals, use nurse-empowering language such as "prescriptions" instead of "orders," and act as health experts in the media or at community forums. We are working at The Truth About Nursing to change how the world sees nursing (www.TruthAboutNursing.org).

More than ever, career seekers—and the public—must learn that nursing is a distinct, self-regulating profession with its own scope of practice and knowledge base, as well as its own clinical leaders and scholars. Nursing autonomy has been the key to saving countless lives, though relatively few people know our autonomy exists. We must mentor our colleagues to change how the public sees nursing for the profession to gain the strength it needs to meet the global health challenges ahead.

Comments from Richard Kimball, Mentee

Working with Sandy Summers in nursing advocacy pursuits over the years has strongly influenced my perception of the nurse's role in our health care system. I believe that the concept of nursing autonomy she has helped me understand is best for patients and nurses. I use this concept to shape my practice and patient interactions, as well as my relations with medical personnel. In my practice at the outpatient amyotrophic lateral sclerosis (ALS) clinic at Johns Hopkins, my nurse colleagues and I run the show. Nurses coordinate the multidisciplinary team, which also includes physicians and physical, occupational, speech, and respiratory therapists. The ALS clinic also conducts clinical drug trials and quality-of-life studies—coincidentally, with the aim of increasing autonomy for our patients. We assess new and long-term patients and work with them to make a plan of care. Their needs include physical assistance, home care, transportation, education about the disease process, and how to achieve the best quality of life.

Although we work in collaboration with physicians, they do not control our practice or interventions. When we agree on physicians' treatment plans, my nurse colleagues and I help patients carry through with them. When we disagree with physicians' treatment plans, we contact them to discuss our concerns and negotiate for a better plan.

My nursing practice is autonomous, and that is essential for the health of patients. When two professions approach health problems from different perspectives and must come to an agreement about a patient's care plan, patients get better health care. We must work to empower nurses across the spectrum of clinical practice to embrace this autonomy. Residencies of one year or longer with strong mentors would help empower mentee nurses, encourage them to embrace their autonomy and advocate forcefully with physicians who may have prescribed unsafe care, and reshape the health care system that often works against good care for patients. Our patients need strong nurses who can protect them and help them gain better care in the often daunting modern health system.

Self-Reflective Questions

1. When physicians write prescriptions or care plans that you do not believe are in your patients' interest, do you negotiate for a better plan of care?

2. Do you view your role more as carrying out the plans of physicians, or as working with physicians as a peer to provide the best care for patients, even if that sometimes leads to physician resistance?

3. When you and a physician cannot agree on a plan of care, do you do what the physician wants, or do you seek input and support from the relevant literature, your nurse colleagues, the patient, and/or the ethics committee to find the best solution?

Self-Reflective Questions *(continued)*

4. When patients have health care questions about which you have knowledge, do you say "I'll go get the doctor to answer that," or do you answer the questions yourself, using your knowledge and your own authority as a professional whose role it is to educate the patient?

5. When a nursing care error occurs, do you allow blame to shift to the physician, or do you take responsibility for the error and explore ways to improve nursing care delivery to prevent further occurrences?

6. If a patient deteriorates in the middle of the night and needs an intervention from a physician who has been abusive or contemptuous of nurses' views in the past, do you contact the physician right away, or wait until morning for fear of receiving more abuse?

7. Is it subversive or contrary to good team practice to call for an ethics consult if you disagree with a physician on a care plan?

8. If a physician denies or ignores the need for palliative care at the end of a dying patient's life, do you approach the patient and her family about it on your own, or do you stay silent, deferring to the physician?

9. If you are in a patient resuscitation situation in which you are concerned that a cardiac tamponade or tension pneumothorax be ruled out before stopping the code, do you advocate for this intervention, or do you stay silent, believing it is not your place to advocate in this situation?

10. The chief orthopedic surgeon at your hospital arrives late one night to perform an emergency operation, but he appears to be drunk, and he is imperious and intimidating. Do you let the surgeon operate, or call security or other colleagues to ensure that he does not operate while impaired?

Business Acumen and Impeccable Ethics

5

"There are three things that physicians want for their patients and that patients want for themselves. We all want security, or put another way, universal access. We want freedom of choice; that's the American way. And we want to control our costs. The problem is this: it is impossible to do all three simultaneously and to do all three well."

—Catherine D. DeAngelis

Mentor
Pamela J. Maraldo, PhD, RN
Managing Partner,
  PJM Associates
Former Chief Executive Officer
  of the National League for
  Nursing
New York, New York, USA

* The author dedicates this chapter to her mentee, Rene D'aiuta Feuerbach, who was unable to participate due to unforeseen circumstances.

"He who has the gold makes the rules" is a cynical twist on the Golden Rule, but one often proven true throughout business and industry. Business acumen, the ability to make profitable business decisions, has been the stock in trade of "whoever has the gold." By and large, that has not been nurses.

Business acumen can have a positive or negative effect on ethics, since it puts decision-making power in the hands of those who have it. To understand the relationship between ethics and business acumen, we need to take a step back.

A Look Back

By the 1990s, most hospitals in the United States were for-profit, and even not-for-profits began behaving like for-profits by cutting programs that were not profitable, such as women's health. When I was a lobbyist for nursing in the 1970s and 1980s, Washington, D.C., was the center of health care; we used to say *as goes Medicare so goes health care.* By the 1990s, Wall Street became the new center of health care activity.

Health care moved from small cottage businesses in local communities to large corporate businesses, from a pattern of individual practice to mega networks and group practices in hospitals and medical enterprises. This size and complexity of these systems puts inordinate stress on our efforts to recognize the importance of healing and patient-centered values and do what it takes to make sure these values prevail in day-to-day practice. Ethical underpinnings, or the actions that ought to accompany business acumen, too often have been tossed aside like an old shoe. Often caught in the midst of ethical crossfire, nurses have had to abide by decisions that they considered unethical if they wanted to keep their jobs.

Nursing shortages similarly have had a negative impact on the quality of patient care (Clark, Leddy, Drain, & Kaldenberg, 2003). Nurse leaders have known this for a long time, yet chronic shortages persist. For instance, many in health care have frowned upon using staffing agencies to deal with nurse shortages, arguing that they are a costly Band-Aid. Funds could be better spent to increase nursing salaries and benefits, therefore drawing more nurses to the field, but hospitals continue to use agencies in spite of nurses' protests.

Instead of eschewing the existence of such agencies, why not start them ourselves? Nursing leaders could control a profitable enterprise that could have a say regarding nursing salaries and standards of care. Without control over "the gold" (resources), nurses are often in the difficult ethical position of having to abide by someone else's decisions. Denying patients health care because they don't have the means to pay for it is another example. I have spent much of my professional life urging nurses to move toward leadership positions and health care businesses as a strategy to give nurses more economic advantage and decision-making power. I have always advised my mentees to get into the position of decision maker instead of having to live with someone else's unethical decisions.

The ethical expectations held by nurses and the public regarding the medical profession and the health care system are very high. At times, we haven't seen the big picture, yet we recognize that the changes in business and the economy have had a profound effect on the ethics of health care around the world.

The New Perspective

Now major change is on the horizon. The health care system is an enormous economic enterprise. Nevertheless, because of nurses' proximity to patients, we see more. We see an enterprise that assumes an intimate position in our lives. We don't think of medical or nursing care simply as something to be sold anymore than we would think about love as something to be sold, or justice as something to be bought. Health care is indeed a business, but from a nursing perspective, it has to be more than that, and it has a profoundly ethical character that can be given a rich interpretation.

In this era of greed-motivated scandals in countries all over the globe, the public is becoming acutely sensitive to ethical motivations of business activity. Changing rapidly in response to events that capture public imagination, whether computer services fraud in India, Internet fraud in Japan, or the Bernard Madoff Ponzi scheme in the United States, fundamental ethical motivations and values are leaping into the limelight. The link between business ethics and profitability, shareholder value, and success in the marketplace are becoming more and more evident. Business ethics and social responsibility are on the way to becoming the new mantras for success in any business, including health care.

The business and ethical implications of the current environment for nursing leaders are profound. As surveys continue to demonstrate the public's high trust of nurses, nursing has great leverage in restoring trust and confidence in the health care system. Nursing also has wonderful business opportunities around the world.

Brave New World of the Healing Organization

Former U.S. President Dwight D. Eisenhower's famous statement about peace between nations, "We'll never have peace in the world until we have it in the hearts of men" can also apply to business acumen guided by ethical practice in health care. Ethical considerations in health care may be laboring under old paradigms of rule-setting, keeping obligations, and a sense of duty. As one nursing leader said, "A nurse may perform actions out of a sense of duty or moral obligation, and would be an ethical nurse, yet it may be false to say that she cared about the patient. The value of human care and caring involves a higher sense of spirit of self" (Barnum, 1996).

Fraud and corruption seem to be immune to rules and even governmental intervention. Additionally, changing economic incentives alone won't bring about ethical practices. Ethical or moral ideas—moral at the level of individual behavior—fueled by a strong commitment to change are needed. The moral idea functions as a compass, directing people toward some activities and purposes and away from others. As societies support right ways of delivering health care and protecting human rights, the timing is right for nurses to take this opportunity to foster better, more effective ways of interacting with and supporting patients.

Palliative end-of-life care in hospitals stands out as an idea that was taken up and promoted by health care leaders. The hospice care concept illustrates how moral ideas, in conjunction with the concepts of "moral practice" and the relationships among people engaged in this practice, can stimulate program ideas (Gilmore & Hirschhorn, 2006).

Nurse leaders will likely find more receptivity than ever before in promoting the "healing organization" as a powerful ethical idea for the 21st century (Institute of Medicine, 2006). A call for care to be organized around the patient, including using the "natural capital of natural healing," can be seen as a logical, as well as a good moral starting point involving people in decisions about their care and calling for clinicians to work seamlessly together, listening with their hearts as well as their heads (Berwick, 2004).

Healing, the natural way in which all imbalances are rectified so that the symptoms of the stress or illness can be eliminated, has as much to do with spiritual matters as ethical ones. Enlightened nurses understand that the difference between a focus on treatment and healing is reflected in the intentions and the values of the eco-system in which care is given. Yet, it is far easier to order insulin for diabetes control than to help people lose weight by healing the repression and anger associated with their weight. It is much easier to order medications for hypertension than to address the underlying stressors that create it.

Giving the right mediations for diabetes and hypertension are ethical things to do, but we could do better and work toward the changes in behaviors that will heal. New paradigms based on ethical and spiritual ideas that come from the heart and the head—not from the same old rulebook—are needed. Abiding by a sense of duty might be highly ethical, but it is not enough to heal patients.

Sometimes patients' own natural abilities to heal are overwhelmed by pressures and stressors to their systems, so they need the help of medicine and surgery. Drugs and surgery help greatly in the short term, but healing happens separately. This is why it is critical for nurses to create a healing environment so that patients can help themselves back to health.

The Institute of Medicine has stressed that the basic unit of health care should not be visits or encounters, but healing relationships that allow patients to obtain the trustworthy information and emotional support they need. Because emotional support and trust are established not only by continuous attention to day-to-day patient needs, but also by the vigilant anticipation of patient needs, the recruitment and retention of a capable, enlightened, and cooperative nursing and medical staff should form the basic healing nexus of patient-centered environment.

Because health care environments are malleable to the patterns of thought and caring intentions of the people who work there, fostering a healing vision and values must prevail over technical command and control management. In the context of a healing vision, nurse leaders could initiate a host of new businesses that could be of great benefit to people's health and well-being. Innovative approaches to chronic illness, long-term care, global Web-based businesses that bring vital nursing knowledge and skills to the public, and complementary therapy centers are just a few ideas where the business acumen of nurses could bring solutions.

Healing the whole person has traditionally been seen as part of a coordinated program of treatment. However, the scientific approach has tended to separate the treatment of the symptoms from the root causes of the disease. Nursing leaders are capable of bridging this gap and creating business enterprises with healing fields of enormous strength. Additionally, visions that emphasize healing can give rise to new complementary approaches found to be effective supplements to traditional medical approaches.

Societies around the world are ripe for new business initiatives that create new healing alternatives to the current approaches to care. Societies are also craving ethical leadership in health care, in for-profit as well as not-for-profit sectors. Fast technological change, overcapacity in hospital markets, nursing shortages, reduced margins, and changing demographics call for not just problem solving, but new visions and new ways of doing things. Let the change begin with us.

Self-Reflective Questions

1. When you go to work every day, do you feel like you have to put aside ethical considerations regarding patient care that are important to you to get ahead and succeed in your job?

2. Do you believe that you have the power and authority to make decisions that you think are important to give the best care you can to patients? If so, what decisions have you made? If not, what can you do about it?

3. What is your organization's impact on the larger community in which it resides and the international community around the world? Is the impact positive, negative, or more complicated?

4. Have you ever had a situation at work where you knew the right action to take but believed you could not take it because you might lose your job or be reprimanded?

5. Are you involved in voluntary causes or activities outside of work—a professional or community organization, church, or synagogue—where you are involved in activities that you wish you could bring to work? If so, what are they?

6. Do you believe that your work contributes to the promotion of ethical values in your society and to people in other societies around the world? If so, what are the connections between your local community and the larger society?

7. Do you see yourself as a global nursing leader with responsibility for people and events beyond your community? What about beyond your country? If so, what are some examples? If not, how could you see yourself relating to people beyond your immediate circles?

8. What do you consider the greatest ethical challenges facing health care?

9. Do you see any business opportunities in health care that can uniquely use your skills and provide a valuable service? Do you see that they could be profitable as well as ethical? Explain.

10. Do you believe that you engage in healing encounters with your staff as well as your patients? Why or why not?

C-Suite Savvy

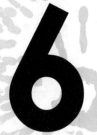

6

"Leadership is action, not position."

—Donald H. McGannon

Mentor
Victoria L. Rich, PhD, RN, FAAN
Chief Nurse Executive
University of Pennsylvania
  Medical Center
Philadelphia, Pennsylvania, USA

Mentee
Sandra Jost, MSN, RN
Associate Chief Nursing Officer
Hospital of the University of
  Pennsylvania
Philadelphia, Pennsylvania, USA

"C-Suite" is the senior executive leadership team of a health care organization. Traditionally, the C-Suite members are the chief executive officer (CEO), the chief financial officer (CFO), chief operating officer (COO), chief medical officer (CMO), chief human resource officer (CHRO), chief information officer (CIO), and the chief nursing officer/executive (CNO/CNE).

Each of the C-Suite members represent a unique, accountable perspective derived from a variety of health care stakeholders. The CEO, COO, and CFO points of view and advocacy focus on the governance of regulations, finance, and community needs. The CIO must provide leadership and direction in the management of data and information. The CHRO must ensure a respective; safe work environment. The CMO provides medical leadership and governance. The CNO/CNE voice is that of the patient and family. The CNO/CNE integrates, synthesizes, leads, and translates bi-directionally these multiple perspectives into nursing practice and patient outcomes.

The didactic knowledge and competencies needed to be a CNO/CNE are clearly articulated by the American Organization of Nurse Executives (AONE). In addition to those competencies, the savviness needed for a CNO/CNE to become an equal member of the C-Suite who can persuade and influence patient care outcomes must come from personal and professional mentorship and coaching. C-Suite nurse executives must mentor the next generation of C-Suite CNO/CNEs not only to hold, but also to enhance our leadership voice and to create a health care culture centered on patients and families.

Personality Hardiness

My doctoral work focused on the personal and professional characteristics of a transformational nurse leader. My research led me to the concept of personality hardiness and the "hardy executive" (Maddi & Kobasa, 1984). Personality hardiness is proven to be an effective moderating variable between stress and health (Kobasa, 1979). Maddi and Kobasa (1987) state that a hardy personality is reasonably stable over a lifetime, although it is amenable to alterations under specific extraordinary events. Hardy executives have a high commitment to work and life, a greater sense of control, and openness to change and challenges (Rich & Rich, 1987).

The three Cs of personality hardiness contain the knowledge, savvy, and wisdom the CNO/CNE mentor should model to the mentee seeking entry into the C-Suite:

- **Commitment:** The ability to feel actively involved with others and a belief in truth, decency, and the value of work/life balance. This dimension represents a fundamental sense of self worth, purpose, and accountability, which protects against weakness during adversity.

- **Control:** The absence of feeling powerless; possessing an internal focus that one is responsible for and/or able to influence occurrences in one's life both personally and professionally. Being resourceful rather than helpless is key to this measure.

- **Challenge:** The belief that change is not a threat to personal security but an opportunity for personal growth and development (Judkins, Massey & Huff, 2006). Challenge represents that failure and crisis offer benefit and opportunity. Challenge also infers the confidence to express beliefs with passion and conviction.

Equipping the Mentee

A mentee must also develop and keep within his or her personal toolbox self-efficacy, self-esteem, self-reflection, life-long learning, and emotional intelligence. My doctoral dissertation taught me three major lessons that I convey to my mentee in a variety of circumstances.

Lesson #1

Build a coalition of social support; this includes peers, family, and friends. It is key to have someone who you trust and are willing to be open with for honest feedback.

Lesson #2

This involves engaging in active problem solving and knowing that avoidance behavior must be honestly realized and overcome.

Lesson #3

Always self-reflect on one's own behavior and understand that each human being is behaving from his or her own world view, wants, and needs.

C-Suite Savviness: Reflections from an Associate Chief Nursing Officer Mentee

One of the many personal and professional benefits of being a mentee of a seasoned CNO is that I am consistently encouraged to be reflective. I find intriguing that often lessons I perceive as salient or paramount upon immediate reflection are not the ones that seem most important over time.

Such was the case in 2006 when our organization, the Hospital of the University of Pennsylvania (HUP), a 704 bed quaternary care facility, was on the journey to Magnet recognition. Magnet Program Recognition is granted by the American Nurses' Credentialing Center (ANCC), an affiliate of the American Nurses Association, to hospitals that satisfy a set of criteria designed to measure the strength and quality of their nursing. A Magnet recognized hospital is described as one that delivers excellent patient outcomes, where nurses have a high level of job satisfaction, and where there is a low staff nurse turnover rate. Magnet is also indicative of nursing involvement in data collection, research, and decision making in patient care delivery.

At that time, I thought I was being mentored about how to lead a team toward a very prestigious award—and indeed I was. However, years later, I see that I also learned a far more important lesson in C-Suite savviness—how to be a "hardy" chief nursing officer through the three Cs of commitment, control, and challenge.

Our Magnet pursuit had started approximately 5 years prior when Victoria Rich, my mentor and our CNO, arrived at our academic medical center following her role as COO at a community hospital. HUP always had a proud autonomous nursing tradition. However, at that time, HUP was in the midst of challenging financial times. Nursing had a 30% vacancy rate and beds were closed as a result of the understaffing in nursing. Despite the challenges, Victoria assessed the patient care culture and declared that HUP should achieve Magnet recognition. She saw potential, talent, and that special something that ran deeper in the nursing department than the seemingly insurmountable problems that would have made a less hardy and committed CNO shy away. Victoria represented vision and hope. She was inspiring and people believed.

In 2006, after years of hard work had rebuilt the infrastructure, clinical nurse specialists had returned to the units, evidence-based practice was flourishing, and quality data brought to the clinicians allowed informed, meaningful decision making. Every one of the 14 Forces of Magnetism was in place. It was, therefore, disconcerting when, as the deadline to submit the Magnet Recognition Program application loomed, Victoria believed something was not right. The clinical nurses and the nursing leadership team seemed ambivalent. The excitement that should have been there was absent. Some felt we were ready, but others did not. Further, we were having trouble pulling together the narratives for the application.

Victoria intuited that something was missing. She was interpreting what was being said but also what was not being said. She resisted the temptation to look at and listen to evidence confirming only the good. Instead, she was authentic and sought evidence that might disconfirm readiness to achieve status as a Magnet Recognized Program. Victoria discovered that the team was having trouble identifying with the Magnet label. The hospital had previously won esteemed awards, and the nursing department seemed to be approaching this as a "To-Do" or an award to be won rather than an approach to care.

Victoria was worried. So worried that despite the intense pressure to meet the submission deadline, she paused. Despite all eyes being on her and nursing to achieve this prestigious recognition that would help the hospital regain rankings on exclusive, sought-after lists, she was committed to Magnet Program Recognition being more than an award. She believed that Magnet status needed to be about patients and delivering world-class care.

For the first time I was exposed to C-Suite savviness that was rooted in the three Cs and that revolved around what was best for the patients and the staff—not what was necessarily best for the CNO. I must admit that I felt trepidation when, after intense deliberation and thought-provoking debate, we made the decision to postpone our Magnet Recognition Program application.

Although we made the decision as a team, the CNO had to have the courageous conversation with the C-Suite members.

To deliver the message that we were "just not there" was difficult. It was made even more complicated by the fact that on paper we *were* there. The clinical and quality outcomes were in place. But, Victoria trusted the advice she received from her lifelong mentors and, perhaps more important, from her intuition and conviction. She knew that if achieving Magnet Program Recognition did not have deep meaning to the clinical nurses, achieving the status would not be good enough. As a result, Victoria convinced the C-Suite to wait despite the tremendous pressure to go forward. Victoria was able to successfully frame this dialogue with the C-Suite around nursing's ability to realize the commitment to achieve Magnet recognition despite obstacles, while maintaining personal control of one's feelings of empowerment versus powerlessness in the face of real challenges. I now realize that I witnessed commitment, control, and a renewed, meaningful challenge that day. I witnessed real C-Suite savvy. We dropped back and regrouped. Under Victoria's leadership, the team took back and controlled the vision of what recognition as a Magnet Program meant to HUP nursing by developing our professional practice model — HUP Nursing Excellence in Professional Practice (HUP NEPP). HUP nursing defined the components that comprise world-class patient care:

- **Authentic Leadership**, as demonstrated by:

    - Communication skills that are not constricted by "either/or" thinking but instead advance solutions that incorporate "both/and" principles.

    - Results oriented behavior that role models collaboration.

    - Self-efficacy in tone and style that guides nursing through change.

    - Strategic and visionary acumen.

    - Effective management of diverse health belief systems that created a gracious space culture.

- **Shared Governance** provides the clinical nurses a voice in decision making.

- **Integrated Primary Nursing,** a balanced blend of classic Primary Nursing care delivery model with Relationship-Based Care delivery model. All care delivered by a professional RN is based on five tenets:

- **P:** Patient and Family focused.
- **E:** Evidence-Based.
- **A:** Accountable.
- **C:** Coordinated.
- **C:** Continuous.

- **Evidence-based Practice,** a systematic approach to problem solving for health care providers that integrates the best evidence from scientific investigations into practice.

- **Partnership** as characterized by trust, mutual respect, consistent and visible support, and open and honest communication.

- **Skilled Communication,** two way dialogue in which people decide together, characterized by active listening and consideration of the other point-of-view.

These components had been built during the five year journey to status as a Magnet Recognized Program, but for the nurses, the dots had not been connected to the Magnet process. The CNO challenged the division to return to our commitment to nursing excellence. We worked hard to help the bedside clinical nurses connect the care they were already delivering to the Forces of Magnetism. They began to see that Magnet status did not simply represent a title, but instead was the excellence in the care they had worked so diligently to develop over the previous years. We messaged tirelessly about the meaning of our professional practice model. We branded the HUP NEPP—lapel pins, posters, clip art, headers, screen savers, posters, essay contests, stationery, and a host of creative ideas flowed organically and proudly from the clinical nurses and leadership team. In short, we saw the culture tip from apathy to authenticity and engagement. In June of 2007, HUP was proud to be designated as a Magnet Recognized organization.

Self-Reflective Questions

1. Who is your defined, dedicated mentor?

2. In what ways are you tenacious and relentless?

3. In what ways do you schedule time to nourish your mind, body, and spirit away from work?

4. How are you able to remain steadfast in your beliefs and values and still compromise?

5. In what ways have you successfully asked for help?

6. How easy is it for you to admit you are wrong and apologize?

7. Do you know when to be silent and when to speak?

8. Are you comfortable with difficult (courageous) conversations?

9. Do you know how to persuade and influence?

10. Are you "bringing the patient in the room" with you?

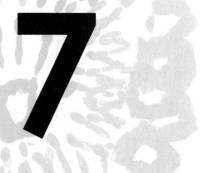

7

Capacities:
Expanding and
Liberating

"Liberation of other people's capacities depends on the liberation of our own capacities that, in each new situation, takes place with theirs, searching for complementarities and adjusting differences."

—Collière

Mentor	*Mentee*
Marta Lima Basto, PhD, MSN, RN, EANS	Maria dos Anjos Pereira Lopes, PhD, MSN, RN, EANS
Member of the Scientific Committee	Lecturer, Escola Superior de Enfermagem
Coordinator of the Advanced Education Program, Doctoral Programme in Nursing University of Lisbon	Researcher and Member, Coordinating Committee, Nursing Research and Development Unit
Researcher, Nursing Research and Development	Escola Superior de Enfermagem
Escola Superior de Enfermagem Lisbon, Portugal	Member, Scientific Committee, Doctoral Programme in Nursing, University of Lisbon Lisbon, Portugal

The following chapter reports a purposeful conversation between Marta Lima-Basto (M) and Maria dos Anjos Pereira Lopes (MA) as a response to the invitation to participate in this book.

M: Let's talk about leadership, taking as an example the situations we have experienced together, where you identified some characteristics worth mentioning.

MA: You display a leadership profile I admire. First of all, you are not power bound, so you stimulate those who are around you to develop their own autonomy. You are a regional and national resource in the nursing area, influencing and developing those around you. The feature I most appreciate is your entrepreneurial attitude, how you are not afraid of making mistakes and how you see risk as a challenge. Being persistent, tolerant, and humble are characteristics you have refined through the years.

I have selected three types of situations to discuss here: your role as a tutor, as a public speaker, and as researcher and scholar. All are qualities essential in uniting our profession.

When I started teaching at the medical–surgical nursing specialization programme (1987), it was one of the post-basic specialization programmes for nurses. At the time, you were teaching nursing models and theories, and you were considered an authority on a subject many did not value, one that was seen to be too "theoretical." Naturally, we asked you to teach the first hours on the subject, and my colleague and I, the least experienced teachers, applied some of the models to practice: caring for adults and older people. That was already hard enough, but one day, during our second experience, you told us in a very straightforward style, "This is the last time I am doing it; you are old enough to take the responsibility from now on." It came like a shock. We're in trouble, we thought! But I see this incident as an example of your way of doing things.

M: Have you done it with colleagues?

MA: I am just starting. When I meet motivated, "alive" colleagues, I grab them. I stay with them, counselling until they don't need me. I really enjoy working with others.

M: I agree that this is the way I behave most of the time. I am sensitive to enthusiastic or curious colleagues, and I remember them when I come in touch with some information that might be useful. I have been surprised by how grateful they are when I pass information along, because I think this is part of my job as a tutor. I am doing them no favour. It's a risk to pay more attention to those who show interest and less to others, and this tendency is something all tutors have to pay attention to.

I do enjoy helping people open new horizons, question the obvious, and maintain a good argument (MA smiles, and we remember occasions when I overdid it). It is true I am direct in expressing my opinion when the time comes. I do prefer consensus, but when necessary I have made tough decisions. Professional unity is very important for the group to enter new stages of development. Making the right decisions can unite us.

MA: That is the opposite of manipulation. You use your power to influence others instead of applying your formal/hierarchical power. You are not afraid of giving your opinion; you don't play the cat and mouse game. I recall the time when you, as president of the school's scientific council, took us on a long journey to uncover the common values of the teaching staff and led us through the discussion of "sub-areas" of the discipline of nursing that would guide the decisions about organizational departments and areas of study for new programmes.

M: On several occasions I have had the chance of participating in new experiments and taking risks. I recall the time we (including the students) decided to evaluate the students qualitatively during the programme. (A postgraduate programme to prepare nurse teachers and supervisors started in 1967, and one of the changes made was to the model of student evaluations.) A strong reaction followed when the former students were confronted with colleagues who were evaluated in the classic way—on a scale from 0 to 20. In retrospect, we could have avoided negative results by informing those who decided about promotions about the change in evaluations. If I did it again, I would take care to inform more clearly. We become wiser with age.

The first time I organized an "experiment" I had only a few months practice as a nurse. I was working at the Cancer Institute in 1962 and on a quiet Sunday morning was in charge of the unit. I suggested to the group of nurses on duty to try the primary nurse work method, which at the end of the shift was positively evaluated. When I came back on Tuesday, the head nurse was furious because I had overruled her. The patient distribution system was never tried again. The only positive outcome was to use the incident in class, years later, as an example of what should not be done.

Another example is the stand I have often taken that it should be the most experienced tutors to teach the most difficult parts of the programme—the practicum. Most colleagues do not agree.

MA: The mainstream opinion about the role of the more experienced tutors remains the same. I recall another "experiment" we made together in 1999 as part of the course "Nursing: History and Epistemology," a first-year course of the undergraduate programme. The students contacted families in different organizations and followed them during the year to develop several transversal competencies. It did not work well, and we know why. It would be worthwhile to try something of the same kind, not repeating but innovating, making sure to have positive results.

M: Let's hear your thoughts on speaking in public.

MA: You seem to always have something to say in public as a reaction to a presentation. With your interventions you enlarge the possible perspectives on the subject, opening up for new ways of looking into a subject, without criticizing the speaker. This leads others to get away from routine or "déja vue" positions. It is as if a little star above your head is saying proudly, "I am a nurse and I like to be one."

M: It hasn't always been like that. It is not easy to talk in public, whether I am presenting a paper that I have prepared at home or participating from the floor. But I agree that lately it has become easier, because the spectrum of my knowledge is larger and I have had the chance of discussing many professional issues. Regarding the "little star," some colleagues say about me that I have a mission in life, and they mean it in a critical way. I don't feel at all I have a mission to fulfill, but it is true that I like to influence people and in doing so bring our profession together.

MA: The "mission" others perceive in you comes from recognizing that you give a good image of the profession. By the way, I have been asked by colleagues to check if you are willing to be a candidate in the next election for presidency of the Order of Nurses, our National Nurses Association, which regulates the profession and has some delegations from the government. Membership is compulsory in order to practice, and as a consequence, the organization has around 50.000 members, all nurses. It would follow nicely on the series of roles you have had. It seems these roles have been planned ahead; they are a natural sequence.

M: Not at all. None of the professional roles I have played have been planned. Circumstances have been favourable, and I have grabbed the chances and taken some risks. When I became a nurse, I wanted to work in the community and that has happened only for a short while, but each time a possibility like a research study comes along that is the path that I choose. I never intended to become a teacher, but the opportunity of having a fellowship to study in the United States (1976) made me accept the challenge. When I retired as a tutor, I was available to start the nursing research and development unit, a natural development because I had been a researcher in another unit. About 3 years later the opportunity arose to participate in the planning of the doctoral programme in nursing at the University of Lisbon.

MA: You make change happen; this is what I appreciate about you. It seems the pathways are linear, that one thing follows the other. The projects exist, and you don't need to be told to join them. You are ready to take some risks. Young people are not trained to take risks, and they are not developing the entrepreneurial capacities that might give them chances of becoming leaders in the profession.

M: Maybe not as much as we would like them to. To unite nursing globally as a profession we do need to increase the number of leaders. I don't mean just hierarchical leaders, but nurses who can take the necessary risks to develop their own leadership capacities within the context of their work, whether they are part of a team of nurses in a hospital, the community, a professional association, or an international workgroup. Nurses all have the chance of developing their capacities at all these levels.

MA: That's true, We need stimulating projects to develop our competencies.

Self-Reflective Questions

1. What have you learned from your own mistakes?

2. In what ways do you turn difficulties into challenges?

3. When you try to influence others, how do you check if they are using their own autonomy?

4. How can you make a point of sharing information, knowledge, and wisdom?

5. When was the last time you took a risk? Was it worthwhile? Why?

6. Do others consider you persistent (not stubborn)? In what ways?

7. In what ways do you feel powerful enough to be humble?

8. How do you exercise your capacity to question/state your views in public?

9. How are you becoming more tolerant?

10. How do you make a point of stating your views clearly while respecting others?

(The Role of) Caring in Leadership Development

8

"Too often we underestimate the power of a touch, a smile, a kind word, a listening ear, an honest compliment, or the smallest act of caring, all of which have the potential to turn a life around."

—Leo F. Buscaglia

Mentor

Carole Kenner, DNS,
  RNC-NIC, FAAN
Dean and Professor University
  of Oklahoma College of
  Nursing
President, Council of International
  Neonatal Nurses
Oklahoma City, Oklahoma, USA

Mentee

Marina Boykova, MSc, RN
Doctoral Student, University of
  Oklahoma College of Nursing
Oklahoma City, Oklahoma, USA
Formerly Neonatal Nurse
  Educator, Children's Hospital #1
St. Petersburg, Russia

Caring is the heart of nursing. This essential feature of the profession of nursing is evident in our everyday practices with our patients, as well as in our everyday lives as health professionals. Caring is a critical issue in leadership if we want to develop our profession and future leaders. Caring includes:

- A feeling of compassion for others.

- Exhibiting concern and empathy.

- Displaying warmth or affection.

- Being concerned with the protection of others.

- Being solicitous.

Leadership, on the other hand, includes:

- Influencing a group of people to move toward its goals.

- The capacity and ability to affect human behavior so as to accomplish a mission.

- A passion, persistence, and imagination to get results.

- Motivating and committing people to action and making them responsible for their performance.

- A first or principal performer of a group.

- A person followed by others.

- Guidance.

- Direction.

How then, is caring and leadership in nursing related? Very simply, both require the fulfillment of people's potential.

My Journey as a Mentee

For me, caring is helping. Leadership is helping, coupled with growth—helping to move forward to achieve one's potential, to set goals and reach them, to withstand difficulties and overcome barriers. Therefore, is caring not an overarching goal of nursing? Leadership through caring occurs in two phases.

1. Learning and experiencing caring from your leaders.

2. Demonstrating caring in your leadership.

I have been lucky to meet incredible nurse leaders. Two people changed my life. They were Carolyn Lund, neonatal clinical nurse specialist from Children's Hospital in Oakland, California, USA, whom I met in the beginning of my career in the early 1990s, and Carole Kenner, dean of the University of Oklahoma College of Nursing, Oklahoma, USA, whom I met in 2005. Both of them were nurses from a country other than my own—I am Russian. Despite our cultural differences, even speaking different languages, we are very similar people. We share the same feelings about nursing, about nursing's role, and our beloved specialty—neonatal nursing. I was amazed at how knowledgeable they were and how much passion they had for nursing. More amazing was to see their love and caring for all people.

What was important for me to feel cared for? Simple things. It was important to receive emotional support, to feel and know that someone, like my mentors, experienced and shared my feelings. These nurses asked how I was doing in my endeavors to change the world where I lived, how many hours I slept, and how my workday went. Simple words of reassurance, loving care mixed with professional questions, and a shared passion. These gave me energy when I felt exhausted or in pain, when I experienced trouble at work, or when I struggled with indifference. For me, these feelings were similar to feeling your mother's love and care.

Feeling connected with the people whom I considered great leaders was also important. Like any relationship, this required work. We e-mailed each other almost daily, and I always received a timely reply, which was so important when I had a problem or was in a bad mood. These actions were evidence of caring about *me* as a person and a professional.

Finally, I valued my mentors' incredible willingness to share their knowledge and experience. Although I was an inexperienced nurse without specialized education, there were no harsh words, judgments, or laughing at me for not knowing something. There was only guidance, motivation, and empowerment—true leadership. They would offer advice, things like "Read this book, it will help you," "Look at this information and let me know what you think," "Try this, and we will see what happens." For me, to receive such reassurance, advice, support, love, and care was significant.

By experiencing such caring in leadership, you begin to believe in yourself. This is what happened to me. I started feeling I could make decisions and take responsibility. My networks were expanding, and I wanted to use the knowledge I received to overcome problems and barriers. I wanted to change the world, and I wanted people to follow me. An in-service education program was established in my unit where I taught new and visiting nurses from other cities of Russia while I remained in practice. I taught them in the way I was taught by my mentors—giving not only knowledge but also sharing my passion for our profession and empowering them to believe in themselves. The number of nurses who wanted to come and see our unit increased; program materials have been adopted by many nurseries all over Russia. The first All-Russian Neonatal Nursing Conference was held in my hospital in 2006, and we had more than 130 neonatal nurses from more than 35 Russian cities and neonatal experts from Sweden, the United Kingdom, and the United States. The idea of this conference came from nurses at my unit, and there was a great enthusiasm for solving organizational issues while preparing this conference. The next step is to establish a neonatal nurses association in Russia—the idea born during that conference. Of course, my mentor, Carole Kenner, was present at this very important event for Russian nurses.

Some argue leadership qualities are innate; others believe leadership qualities are made. I believe leadership can be developed, but you must have a mentor-leader who cares about you. By simply caring, leaders can help us to grow. As we say in Russia, only then can you move the mountains! Moreover, caring—an essential element in leadership—can develop nurse leaders. I am a doctoral student at the University of Oklahoma College of Nursing, and I do believe I can move mountains!

Comments from Carole Kenner, Mentor

Marina's journey illustrates common themes: connection through caring that transcends the professional relationship, and a need to have someone who believes in you so you can believe in yourself. Leadership is a two-way street. People learn from each other. It is bidirectional, mentor to mentee, and vice versa (Hesselbein & Cohen, 1999). You can and do gain strength from the mentee when the going gets tough. You also see someone who can continue your work or legacy. Marina also describes her desire to change the world. She is already accomplishing that. Her aspirations and passion have changed my world and reaffirmed that one person can make a difference. Leadership through caring can change the world one person at a time.

Self-Reflective Questions

1. What do you enjoy about working closely with another person? What do you think others enjoy about working closely with you?

2. Should nurses have to earn their way by years of experience or can they be coached by seasoned nurses early in their careers in order to move forward at their own pace?

3. How can you be a better listener? Cite specific ways to enhance your listening skills.

4. Whose agenda or goals should come first, the mentee's or the mentor's? Why?

5. What are five things you value about your mentor or mentee?

6. What physical (e.g., eye contact) or task (e.g., returning calls quickly) actions can you take to demonstrate caring and respect? Try to list at least five.

Self-Reflective Questions *(continued)*

7. Is the mentee honest and consistent in her willingness to learn from the mentor and to share feelings, experiences, and responsibilities in order to reach a goal together?

8. In what ways can caring promote confidence and positive self-esteem? What are the caring and leadership values of improved confidence and positive self-esteem?

9. What are the benefits of both the mentor and mentee holding caring as a value?

10. In what ways does caring about another person strengthen your ability to foster growth in others?

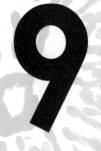

9

Celebrating:
Recognition, Reward, and the Power of Life-Mentors

"Celebrate what you want to see more of."

—Thomas J. Peters

Mentor	*Mentee*
Debra Townsend, RN	Michael Bratton, RN, MA
CEO, President	President, Healthcare
Concepts of Care, Inc. and	Connection
The National Center for	Vice President and Chief
Compassionate Care	Nursing Officer
Washington, D.C., USA	Middle Tennessee Medical
	Center
	Murfreesboro, Tennessee, USA

I (Debra) know a secret about every one of you who have dedicated your lives to this cherished profession. I have watched you care far too often from between the bedrails. As a stroke and cancer victor, I've experienced your art and embraced the comfort of holistic care. Those moments convinced me of my need to honor and celebrate nursing at every given opportunity.

My life's work is designed to help others develop their gifts, reminding nurses of their vital contributions to care. Valuing the work of nursing is critical. Far too often, nurses do not pause to experience the ordinary miracles woven within daily practice. Watch the magic unfold in any given unit, and you will see the following:

- Patients led with compassion and competence through the maze of care.

- Loved ones who are caught in a world of unknown fears being comforted and consoled.

- The gentle art of presence, providing rest for the weary and peace for the fearful.

Celebrating Kindness

One of my cherished memories as a staff nurse involved just a few kind words from a physician. There is a distinctive reason that our National Center for Compassionate Care is dedicated to caregiver advocacy. Somewhere along the health care spectrum, we have become too business-oriented and less people-oriented. "Caring for the people that care for the people" is the mantra within our team. It must become the mantra of every organization. We are suffering as a profession, our stars are falling, our leaders are exhausted, and our new kids on the block are being eaten alive. Someone must stop the madness. Have we forgotten the joy of offering heartfelt praise to a deserving colleague? Have we lost the art of civility? I suggest that we are all accountable for recognizing and rewarding excellence in care. At the very least, it will do something for your soul and help retain the treasures so desperately needed at the bedside.

Celebrating Relationships with Life-Mentors

When we dare to reach out and touch others with meaningful words and compassionate gestures, we become a healthier workplace with more intense spirit and connectedness. True synergy begins to form within individual relationships, teams, and organizations. A cultural transformation can begin with focus on meaningful affirmation and valuing one another.

Speaking and presenting has given me an opportunity to interview thousands of colleagues, enjoying dialog with respected leaders within health care. Many of us have become life-mentors, willing to share wisdom in our global mission to retain nursing professionals. It is my pleasure to introduce you to Michael Bratton, a beloved chief nurse executive who returned to the bedside to study nurse retention. After dedicating more than 20 years to our profession and serving in nearly every leadership role, Michael's mission was to listen to the voices on the front lines of care. In doing so, he captured not only my attention but also my trust. Through years of collaborative work on nurse retention, Michael has become a treasured advisor on interweaving recognition, reward, and praise into the workplace. I invite you to listen to his wisdom.

Celebrating Meaningful Recognition, Reward, and Praise: Reflections from Michael Bratton

As a nurse, sometimes you just need to take care of patients. Between 1979 and 2005, I experienced nursing as a bedside nurse, nurse manager, and nursing director, as well as a chief nursing executive. I had practiced in medical/surgical, critical care, sub-acute care, home care, and rehabilitation. Many years had passed since I provided direct patient care. I needed to get back to the basics, experiencing first-hand what nurses do every day. It was time to experience how a staff nurse feels while navigating the complexity of a hospital.

Don't misunderstand: I enjoy leadership, its challenges, and contributions. The most important contribution that a good leader offers is serving others who are closer to direct patient care. A leader does this through removing barriers, obstacles, and complexity. Leaders also help design patient care delivery systems and processes. Most important, leaders foster an environment that empowers others.

Fortunately, I still remembered what "sick" looks like. That had not changed. However, many other aspects of nursing care had changed—new medications and therapies, new technology, revisions in care delivery processes. My quest was to understand—to re-experience hospital nursing though the eyes of the bedside RN. I took a refresher course and moved to a job within a critical care unit.

This three-year experience as a bedside caregiver rekindled my respect for those who do it every day. Nurses still make a difference. They touch patients' lives in ways that few people will ever experience. Nursing remains the science and art of caring for our human brothers and sisters as they respond to life's health challenges.

I was privileged to work with a group of nursing leaders who embarked on strengthening our culture. Our aim was to foster patient-centered care as well as creating a healthy work environment. Two things became a vital part of our culture. First, we made appreciation a part of every leadership meeting. We did this by distributing blank "thank you" notes at the beginning of each meeting. During the meeting, each nursing leader wrote at least two notes to staff nurses, expressing appreciation for their contributions during the previous week. As a result, thousands of notes were written over the course of a few years.

Second, we established quarterly forums where we met for a few hours to tell stories about our nurses. These stories were profound, highlighting the differences that nurses were making in the lives of patients. Leaders invited a staff nurse to the meeting and then told a story about the nurse—a story reflecting patient-centered care and teamwork.

We measured our nurses' satisfaction ratings as we implemented these two methods. Nurses' ratings of recognition by their immediate supervisor moved from 26% to 47% who strongly agreed, with overall favorable ratings moving from 63% to 78%. (Comparatively, the benchmark hospital's average rating in the survey was 70%.) At the same time, our retention, vacancy, and turnover measurements also improved.

During the first year in my journey back to the bedside, our hospital had its annual Nurses' Week event. As you may know, getting the top speakers for Nurses' Week requires advanced preparation. We were fortunate to secure Debra Townsend to help us celebrate. Debra's presentation at our hospital was the beginning of our life-mentoring relationship.

Debra was an expert speaker and platform presenter. Despite being an experienced leader, I was a novice presenter. However, I wanted to learn to tell our hospital's story so that others might learn from our experience. Personally, I wanted to re-invigorate bedside nurses about the importance of their work. At the same time, it was important to encourage nursing leaders to "stay the course" in valuing their own influence.

I have been privileged and blessed to learn from Debra the art of public speaking and presentation. She has generously invited me to co-present on various topics, including retention, leadership, and storytelling. As a result, our hospital's story about valuing recognition, appreciation, and praise has been presented at several national nursing conferences. Together, our work has affected thousands of caregivers and leaders. Thousands more deserve to be recognized and rewarded, and we encourage you to continue this vital mission.

Nurses make a critical difference in the lives of everyone they touch. Important work deserves to be rewarded and recognized. Take time to value what nurses do every day. There is no better way to retain the treasures within our profession.

Celebrating Life!

I (Debra) remain a joyous victor of many storms that tried diligently to extinguish my light. My faith taught me to rise above those challenges and to rediscover the gift of health. As a patient, I learned about the power generated from gentle words and thoughtful actions. As a leader, I learned how meaningful recognition and reward invigorates and values colleagues. Thank you to all who graced my path within 40 years of practice. Today, and every day, let us pause to celebrate our beloved profession, and the impact that kindness can have on every living soul.

Self-Reflective Questions

1. How do you pause to view nursing through the eyes of a patient?

2. How can you find value in meaningful words and compassionate gestures?

3. Have you considered written notes of appreciation to colleagues for exemplary patient-centered care or teamwork?

4. If you received positive feedback from a patient that should be shared with others, how did you share it?

5. As a leader, what forums or meetings do you participate in where others can be encouraged to recognize a nurse?

6. How do you balance negative feedback with positive?

7. Are there patient care skills that you can participate in, even if you don't regularly practice at the bedside?

8. How can you publicly recognize professional colleagues who further enhance the value of affirmation?

9. As a mentor, how do you seek opportunities on a consistent basis to encourage mentees?

10. Who are your life-mentors who would value a note of appreciation?

Change Management Skills: Setting the Context for Transformation

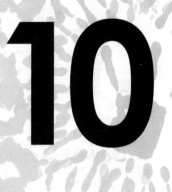

10

"Thirsty, we dream of an oasis, while we rest next to a stream."

–Rumi

Mentor

Tim Porter-O'Grady, DM, EdD, APRN, FAAN
Senior Partner, Tim Porter-O'Grady Associates, Inc.
Atlanta, Georgia, USA
Associate Professor, Leadership Scholar
College of Nursing and Healthcare Innovation
Arizona State University
Phoenix, Arizona, USA

Mentee

Sara Basinger, RN, BSN
Graduate Student, Masters in Healthcare Innovation
College of Nursing and Healthcare Innovation
Arizona State University
Phoenix, Arizona, USA

Sally had an "A-ha!" learning moment. She had been a unit manager on a medical/surgical unit for 5 years and felt that she had seen most everything there was to see of human frailties and foibles. The passions and pains of people, whether patient or provider, all fell within the auspices of her role, and so far, she had handled it all well.

Lately though, she noticed that a lot of what nurses had learned about practice and had traditionally focused on was under fire. For example, time for care was slipping away, and the pace of clinical technology was quickly changing everything. The focus on outcomes and value was now becoming a part of the regulations for practice, patients were staying for shorter periods, and the hospital environment was becoming more difficult to navigate. Sally saw that the staff was finding themselves increasingly burdened with change with little options to know what to do. They all looked to her for the answers to make it better for everyone. What her staff didn't know was that Sally didn't have the answers, and was feeling the pinch and pain as much as anyone else on the unit.

Lately, Sally had been thinking that the changes the staff was experiencing were much deeper and more significant than she had originally thought. This "new age" was ushering in a new reality for practice and calling for a different mental model for patient care. The foundations that everyone expressed in their past practices simply didn't seem sustainable. Everyone would now have to understand the emerging reality and incorporate it into what he or she decided and, ultimately, what he or she did. Sally was beginning to have heretical thoughts that the nursing staff might have to surrender their attachment to old beliefs and practices that may no longer reflect the state of the art and science, replacing them with more relevant and contemporary notions of the role of the nurse and the content of practice.

Much of what the staff complained about was never going to disappear. Many of the emerging realities affecting what nurses did were the very by-products of the clinical and technological innovations that were transforming medical practice and patient experience. Intervention required less invasiveness and time. Patients left earlier and better, and did most of their healing at home. Electronic media, hardware, and processes were increasing mobility and were portability-driven. Documentation, records, and evidence-based systems were now requiring that practice changes occur almost instantly, replacing the old policy and procedure mechanisms for defining practices. And all this was happening now!

Sally saw that her nursing staff would have to come to terms with this shifting reality and transform their practice if they were to continue to thrive and contribute. She couldn't do it for them. They would all need to come to terms with the conflict between attachment to traditional practices and contemporary demands. Staff would have to confront this attachment and begin to leave some treasured practices behind. But how would she engage the staff to begin this challenging and revolutionary work?

The Mentor's Perspective
Sally's Steps for Helping the Change Transition

Three major steps to making this change would be necessary to initiate and sustain this process. First, safe space would need to be created for staff to mourn and grieve the loss of what they had come to know, be, and do. Staff needed a voice for their pain and loss, and Sally needed to give the change a language so that staff named their experiences and allowed their frustrations to be fully expressed. The losses also needed to be left behind, and the door to yesterday's practice needed to be closed and locked so that the staff could turn away to look ahead to what, as nurses, they were to become if they were to thrive.

Secondly, Sally knew that staff needed a deeper understanding regarding what was happening in health care that was radically changing practices and patient experiences. For one instance, Sally would need to have the staff discuss how to change "policy-driven" practice to "evidence-based practice." Staff had to name these many dramatic changes and make them relevant to their own lives. Technology now had to be seen as an extension of the human experience, and not external to it. Technology, now intimate to practice, was a fundamental part of everything that would be nursing practice. Standards, practices, protocols, documentation, patient teaching, and clinical function would forevermore have a technological component to it that would need to be embraced and internalized in all nursing practice. And, all of this would have to be seen as a component of excellent nursing care.

Finally, Sally knew that the staff would have to translate all this emerging reality into practice and application. Staff would need to anticipate, and even predict, what all this meant in regard to their nursing work and what changes needed to be accommodated and how. Staff would have to do this translational work with enthusiasm and commitment, knowing that it ultimately would create a better experience for the patient and provide better tools for both nurses and patients to improve the quality and effectiveness of their experience (Malloch & Porter-O'Grady, 2007).

Sally knew that time was of the essence and that the work of changing perspectives, attitudes, insights, and practices would not be easy. It never was. Nursing was changing dramatically—not getting worse, just becoming different. For her, it was time to change the dialog. Bottom line, it was time to engage the staff more fully. Now was as good a time as ever to get the process going for everyone. Change wasn't going away.

The Mentee's Perspective
Sally's Change Mission: Making Change Work

Sally sat at her desk at eight o'clock in the evening, again. Her husband was calling and inquiring why she was late, again. There was one more project to complete for the chief nursing officer before she was able to go home—the dreaded action plan for quality improvement related to patient falls. As Sally started to put the action plan together, she thought how this action plan would be different from last month, and the month before: There was no difference. The scores were almost identical from month to month, and Sally was at a loss for how she could fix the problem.

As Sally continued to work, one of her clinical nurse leaders, Dave, walked into her office. He asked, "Is there anything we can do to help you so you can go home? You are here every night until at least eight o'clock, and you need to spend more time with your family." Seeing this as a breakthrough moment for her and a chance to put into action what her mentor had challenged her to do—namely, to transfer ownership and engage the staff—Sally replied, "Yes. Can you help me figure out why we are not meeting our quality improvement benchmark for patient falls, and help us all get a handle on it?"

"I have some ideas," Dave suggested. "I'm going to get Nancy and Joan to work with me on this. So go home!"

Dave and his nurse colleagues sat down and identified some areas of focus. They researched the best evidence and best practices from professional organizations' data. Then, they identified what was actually happening at the bedside to cause the majority of falls and compared that to evidenced-based practice. The staff made decisions that closed the gap between practice and evidenced-based practice. The nurses also formed ways to disseminate standards and engage the unit nursing staff, including them in tracking compliance.

Several mornings later, Sally came to work and was surprised by all the effort the staff had already put forth in solving the quality improvement issues in the department. Sally sat and thought, "Why am I surprised? Only the staff can make a difference in patient care. Anyone sitting behind the desk cannot make a difference in quality patient care; directives are management derived and staff chooses to follow or not follow them."

This was a transformational moment for Sally. Dave was at the forefront of building quality improvement teams for the department. After only a few short months, everyone was seeing the difference that the teams were making to the department. Patient falls had almost disappeared—and not surprisingly, patient and employee satisfaction scores were now climbing.

Sally's story serves as a lesson to me. My mentor provides the context, insight, and support for my leadership of change. I have learned what Sally needs to know, through good mentoring and leadership application, that staff drives everything toward real sustainable success. I am a fellow learner in this collective journey confronting the challenge of transforming nursing practice—the chief learner, in fact. I pull together information and resources about the challenges and changes confronting us and make it all known to the staff, gathering the tools and supports necessary to drive our clinical performance and our professional success (Porter-O'Grady & Malloch, 2009). For me now, that's real leadership—oh, yes, and for Sally—who is really Sara—too!

Self-Reflective Questions

1. How can you become a learner in the transformational journey?

2. How can you acknowledge challenges to your own beliefs?

3. How much do you read outside your specialty/field?

4. What tools do you use to assess your core nursing values?

5. What are the changes that most dramatically affect your practice?

6. What challenges currently most threaten your current leader practices?

7. What is the one leader behavior you must now change?

8. Who is a mentor who can help guide your own transformation as a leader?

9. What is your career plan to address your personal leader journey?

10. How willing are you to change?

11

Changing the Future One Mentorship at a Time

"In every art, beginners must start with models of those who have practiced the same art before them. And it is not only a matter of looking...it is a matter of being drawn into the individual work of art, of realizing that it has been made by a real human being, and trying to discover the secret of its creation."

—Ruth Whitman

Mentor
Sabah Abu-Zinadah, BSN, MSN, PhD
Chairperson, Nursing Scientific Board
Saudi Commission for Health Specialties
Riyadh, Saudi Arabia

Mentee
Amal Al Barnawi, BSN, MSN
Medical/Oncology Nursing Program Director
King Faisal Specialist Hospital and Research Centre
Riyadh, Saudi Arabia

After I finished my doctoral degree and returned to Saudi Arabia in 1999, I noticed that even though the nursing profession in Saudi Arabia at that time was 19 years old, we were and still are suffering from poor professional image that affects our recruitment and retention plan for Saudi nurses. Perhaps changes did not occur because all the efforts and actions were implemented outside the full control of nurses and nursing profession, that is, media campaigns, physician-nurse relationship, salary and compensation packages, national nursing development strategies, and so on. If we focus now on plans where nurses take action toward change, we will have an opportunity to improve the image of nursing. Currently, no mentoring programs accurately address the proper training of students for the job market in Saudi Arabia. This reality potentially impacts public confidence, overall support of the nursing profession, and nursing's image.

We also face other issues. Individual pride stands in the face of the mentorship program. Asking for help is against the cultural norm in the Arab world; it is seen as a reflection of weakness. So to be a mentor in Saudi Arabia, you must initiate it voluntarily, as a leader and as a fulfillment of your responsibility toward your profession and community. The relationship between the mentor and mentee can exist, unspoken, without title, at an unconscious level. You know that your mentees respect you, regard you as a veteran, seek your advice, and consider you as role model with such comments as "I am like you" or "People think that I am like you." Your mentees can share their secrets at the professional and social levels, allowing you to help them plan their careers.

Wise People Teach Others

Informal mentors played a significant part in my development, they shared their wisdom, knowledge, and experience with me. Now, it's my turn to become an informal mentor to others, because there are no formal mentorship programs in Saudi Arabia. I benefit from mentoring as well, getting the pure satisfaction of teaching as I facilitate a mentee in learning, self-discovery, and personal growth.

A mentoring partnership is long term and evolves into a mutually beneficial collaboration where mentors learn from the feedback, insights, and self-reflection of mentee. By mentoring one generation of nursing professionals, our knowledge travels into the future; in turn those mentees convey their knowledge to succeeding generations. Without mentoring, even the most talented novice can suffer from a lack of direction or focus that ultimately hinders his or her ability to develop as a professional. Lack of mentoring can cause job dissatisfaction and the loss of high-quality students or qualified employees and impacts nursing's professional image.

As mentor, I adapted Strasen's Self-Image Model (Strasen, 1992) as a framework in establishing my partnership with mentees. This model explains that the person's thoughts and beliefs determine that person's self-image. Self-image determines actions, performance, and achievements. Each nurse's actions and achievements, in turn, affect the collective image of professional nursing. The image of professional nursing then supports or alters the individual nurse's self-image.

Because the majority of the efforts to improve the image of nursing have been aimed at improving the image of the nursing profession, little change has occurred, because achieving such a goal for such a large group of people is difficult. In contrast, my focus is on changing the thoughts and beliefs of mentees. That in turn will determine their self-image, and subsequently their actions and performance will change. I believe if enough nurses can enhance their self-image, the image and achievement of the entire profession will improve. But attainment of this goal is not easy.

Carl Rogers (1961) describes self-image as a composition of thoughts and beliefs people hold about themselves. Personal experiences, heredity, environment, gender, socialization, and reference groups influence our thoughts and beliefs about who we are. Our thoughts and beliefs are a product of gender socialization, past experience, triumphs, failures, and other people's reactions to and perceptions of us. As a result of these influences, we develop an image of ourselves that we believe is true. Consequently, we act in accordance with our self-image because we cannot consistently act differently from what we believe to be true.

Employees with positive self-images tend to have an internal locus of control, so they believe they can make an impact on the organization. In contrast, employees with poor self-images have an external locus of control, and they perceive that they are controlled by the organization. So, changing nurses' perceptions of their power base and influence is one of my major goals in the mentorship agenda. If the person has a positive self-image, the brain directs that person to accomplish significant goals. On the other hand, if the person has a poor self-image, the brain directs that person's body to actualize failure behavior.

Two major principles determine the impact of self-image:

- First, we always act like the person we believe ourselves to be. If we believe that we are not in control of our nursing practice or feel that we do not have any input into the functioning of our department, we behave in a way that is consistent with those beliefs. No matter how much control or authority we are actually given, we do not see it and cannot take advantage of it because we do not believe we have that power. Therefore, by helping mentees to change their thoughts, experiences, environment, and reference groups, I can help them to change their self-image from negative to positive.

- The second principle is this: If you can think it, you can attain it. This means the only factors standing between you and your dreams are hard work, a willingness to take risk, and perseverance. That is why I make it clear to mentees that the total responsibility for their success rests on their shoulders.

A majority of nurses have been women, and women have been socialized to be more dependent on other people, to focus on external sources of power rather than on themselves, and to avoid risk. I encourage mentees to be more willing to take risks and do whatever it takes to be in control of themselves by having a vision and living their vision 24 hours a day. Nurses have been socialized to have the self-image of giving, caring, and dedicated helpers who need to follow directions, be respectful, and never make mistakes. I help mentees to change their self-images to be that of more independent, thinking professionals. The actions of many nurses show that they have compromised self-images and comparatively low levels of self-esteem compared to other professionals. So, I try to help mentees to internalize the self-image of a professional and assume total responsibility of their lives.

Mentorship takes a lot of patience and energy. However, I believe that if I mentor one person, then I have changed someone, and that person can mentor 10 or more people. Then the 10 can each mentor 10 more, and so on. You cannot wait until everybody is ready; you have to make them want to come along. You have to go forward, and as you are moving, others will join.

The Mentee's Journey

I have worked with Dr. Abu-Zinadah for the last 10 years. My informal mentoring relationship with her means I can talk to a true professional and get the information I need to make me feel more comfortable in the professional world. It definitely reassured me that I made the right choice to enter nursing, I am happy with the decision, and I am successful in what I am doing. I could talk to her about plans for my postgraduate study, and she helped enable me to finish my master's degree, which was beneficial for my career. I found it encouraging to know about the other things in the field I could do, which allowed me the sort of freedom and creative initiative I value.

Through this informal mentoring I also learned about a real leader out in the world who had a hard time and still learned what she needed to be successful. Her experience helped make me feel that some people in the world are genuinely interested in supporting me in my endeavors. I receive continuous assurance that I am doing the right things to succeed in my position, and I am given the opportunities and support to develop professionally as a nurse leader.

Dr. Abu-Zinadah is a role model, confident and committed to self-development and the development of others, and she is supportive and respectable. Through the journey of mentoring, I became more effective in my role, have self-confidence, and have developed the knowledge and skills to be successful in complex health care environments. I like having a mentor who was pursuing a job and education that I would like to model.

Rewards of Mentoring

Peter Drucker said that "knowledge is always embodied in a person; carried by a person; created, augmented, or improved by a person; applied by a person; taught and passed on by a person; used or misused by a person" (2001).

Being a mentor, for me, is a lifelong relationship. Mentoring is very rewarding. To invest in someone's success by sharing my insights and experiences is an honor. I'm committing to take interest in someone's life, not just helping that person to prepare for a career. I enjoy providing concrete suggestions my mentees can use right away and offering ideas and encouragement around longer term career planning and establishing a trust that they can come to me with the challenges they face as young adults. I always want them to know they are important to me first as people, and then we can deal with getting ready for the workplace. As with most things in life, the success of a mentoring relationship is a result of both parties approaching the experience with passion, commitment, and honesty, and also remembering to have fun along the journey. My only regret is that we can't offer a mentor to every graduate.

Self-Reflective Questions

1. What is your organization's attitude regarding devoting time to mentoring?

2. What level of confidence do you have regarding talking about the benefit of mentoring to your senior managers?

3. In what areas of your work would mentoring be beneficial?

4. What are your colleagues' attitudes to mentoring?

5. When have you listened to people's concerns about self-development?

6. In what ways can you juggle activities at work to open up more time for mentoring sessions?

7. How can you communicate the benefit of mentoring to your subordinates?

8. In what ways can you invite suggestions about current working practice?

9. How can you display that you trust your staff and invite initiative?

10. In what ways can you shake things up at work?

Coaching as an Essential Skill: the Impact of Presence

12

"The future depends on what we do in the present."

—Mahatma Gandhi

Mentor
Catherine Robinson-Walker,
  MBA, MCC
President, The Leadership Studio
Oakland, California, USA

Mentee
Christina Marczak, MSN, RN
Registered Nurse, Hospital of
  the University of Pennsylvania
Philadelphia, Pennsylvania, USA

Christina (Tina) Marczak, a mentee who is a young nurse leader from Philadelphia, Pennsylvania, USA, shares her memories of learning from an individual who served as a significant role model in her professional life. Catherine Robinson-Walker, a formally trained and experienced leadership coach, provides perspective on Tina's recollections. Tina's formative encounters and Catherine's observations offer us insights into the powerful effect that coaching and mentoring behaviors can have when nurse leaders are in the early stages of their careers.

Tina: As I have grown and developed as a professional, the most memorable coaching and mentoring experiences are ones in which my mentors did not realize they were serving in that role. As a new-to-practice nurse, I constantly observed what the more experienced nurse was doing or saying. I watched, I listened, and eventually, I began to practice. These observations became the foundation for my own professional growth and development.

Catherine: The first insight Tina provides is that many of us are coaches and role models, whether we realize it or not. People constantly watch those of us in leadership. Our habits, what we pay attention to, and how we treat people are just a few of the qualities new nurses and nurse leaders keenly observe when they interact with us.

Tina: I began my nursing career at an inner city Philadelphia hospital in 1993. As a graduate nurse working the off shift on a high acuity medical-surgical floor, I was responsible for the care of numerous post-operative patients. I met many challenges along the way: patient issues, clinical concerns, and overwhelming shifts. Luckily, I was fortunate to have a nurse co-ordinator to turn to for support and guidance. The availability of the nurse coordinator was similar to a security blanket in that her presence offered the support of an experienced clinician who possessed the confidence and the clinical expertise I lacked.

Catherine: In her second insight Tina reveals how a new nurse can feel in situations of high stress and concern. When we serve in mentor and coaching roles, our very presence can provide a sense of safety for people like Tina who are new and somewhat overwhelmed.

Tina: I met Nancy while working an evening shift on my unit that began as any other. However, while busily trying to care for my patients, I heard the voice of another nurse yell, "Mr. Smith, Mr. Smith, are you OK? I need help in Room 2...someone call a CODE." This was my first code experience.

When I ran to the room, I saw that many experienced nurses were already there. I continued to the nurses' station to direct the code team to the correct room. Standing there, I was met by Nancy who greeted me and then quickly went to the patient's room. I stood at the station feeling a little lost and not quite knowing what to do. I am not sure whether a new nurse is ever prepared for this experience, but seeing cardiopulmonary resuscitation (CPR) performed on a 35-year-old man who came in for an elective hernia repair certainly was not what I was expecting. While standing in a daze, I heard a kind voice ask whether I was alright. When I turned around, I saw Nancy's concerned, yet gentle face. She had returned and was genuinely concerned about me, a new, impressionable, and terrified graduate nurse.

Catherine: Tina tells us something important about Nancy and the action she took when the patient coded. Assured that the patient was being treated by others, Nancy came back to see how Tina was faring. Nancy expressed genuine concern for Tina during a demanding event that Tina had not experienced previously.

Many years later, Tina recalls Nancy's kindness and genuine concern. Notice that Nancy did not tell Tina to get over it, or that this is "business as usual" on the shift. Nancy created a powerful learning opportunity for Tina because she focused on Tina's feelings and experience rather than her own comfort with these situations.

Tina: That was my first interaction with Nancy, who would serve as my mentor for years to come. To me, a mentor is someone who role models behaviors you wish to emulate. Nancy is just that person for me. Year after year, Nancy modeled the nurse I wanted to be—honest and caring, determined yet gentle, and ever so knowledgeable. Without ever saying a word, she taught me about the nurse I wanted to be.

Catherine: Here, Tina describes the qualities Nancy embodies and that Tina admires. As a coach and mentor, our presence and our behaviors say much more about us than do our words. Based on Nancy's actions, Tina sees Nancy as honest and caring, determined yet gentle, and ever so knowledgeable. In Tina's eyes, Nancy's behavior consistently reinforced Tina's initial impressions of who Nancy was as a nurse leader. Nancy's presence, her actions, and the trust that they engendered created the basis for the mentoring relationship that became so significant for Tina.

Tina: Nancy has a way of getting you to find the right decision. While she guides you to the correct answer, she always makes you feel successful. On many occasions, I relied on Nancy's expertise to guide me in making the best possible decisions for my patients. Conversations with Nancy would provide the clarity and the information I needed in order to come to the appropriate solution. Nancy would rarely provide the answer, but would instead ask questions. Her choice of questions led me to offer more information which would, in turn, lead me to the answer. I am certain she could have resolved most issues more quickly, but instead, Nancy chose to take each situation as an opportunity to teach.

Catherine: Tina shows that Nancy was focused on Tina's growth as a professional nurse. Her behavior suggests that Nancy was not focused exclusively on herself. Instead of just handling the task alone and perhaps more efficiently, Nancy opted to provide Tina with gentle guidance and thoughtful questions. Nancy's approach supported Tina so Tina could learn, build confidence and eventually develop her own successful approaches and solutions.

Tina: One of the most important messages I received from Nancy is to commit to always doing the right thing for patients and their families. She put aside everything else and gracefully redirected the focus onto what was right for the patient.

As a result of my relationship with Nancy, I demonstrate that same commitment to patient care. Regardless of the situation, maintaining a focus on the delivery of quality patient care has made my decision making much easier. I have been practicing for 15 years, and Nancy has recently retired. Although I no longer have direct contact with her, I strive each day to emulate her example.

Catherine: As a result of Nancy's actions and qualities, Tina has developed a profound sense of her own professional values. These values guide Tina 15 years later, even though Nancy and Tina no longer see each other. Nancy's impression on Tina remains palpable, and Tina's story provides a wonderful tribute to Nancy's coaching and role modeling. Nancy's qualities continue to inspire Tina to maintain her focus on high quality patient care.

Self-Reflective Questions

1. Whether leaders know it or not, they serve as role models and mentors on a 24/7 basis. What are the effects of nurses watching their leaders all the time?

2. How does regularly offering support and guidance benefit individuals who receive such messages?

3. What role does your presence play, particularly on younger nurses feeling stressed or concerned?

4. How much time do you spend finding out how younger nurses are faring after a difficult situation is satisfactorily addressed?

5. How do you show nurses you work with that you are concerned about their well-being and growth?

6. How does regularly practicing kindness affect the nurses with whom you interact?

7. How do you manage your emotions in challenging times so you can focus on the experience that younger nurses are having?

8. What behaviors regularly indicate your sense of character and integrity?

9. How does appropriate and clear feedback allow nurses to learn and gain confidence in their abilities?

10. How do you regularly convey a strong sense of values, such as a commitment to excellence in patient care?

Collaboration and Developing Partnerships

13

"The mentor's mind is like a mirror—impartially reflecting back the truth of the person and the situation. Through this precise and nonjudgmental mirroring, the mentor invites others to engage truthfully in their life, to accept and express their greatness."

—Eric Klein and Nancy Dickenson-Hazard

Mentor
Deloras Jones, MS, RN
Executive Director
California Institute for Nursing
   and Health Care
Berkeley, California, USA

Mentee
Liana Orsolini-Hain, PhD, RN
Nursing Instructor, City College
   of San Francisco
San Francisco, California, USA

The California Institute for Nursing and Health Care (CINHC) is leading the statewide effort to implement a master plan for the California nursing workforce with the goal of ensuring a sufficient supply of nurses to care for Californians (CINHC, 2009). More than 30 organizations in the state have given their endorsement to CINHC to lead this effort. CINHC, a 501(c)(3) public benefit organization, serves as a neutral, nonpartisan entity to develop and implement solutions to the challenges that impede efforts to secure a qualified nursing workforce. CINHC is the only organization in California focused exclusively upon building the nursing workforce and optimizing nursing's contribution to the health of Californians; thus, CINHC has become recognized as California's "nursing workforce center"—one of 29 in the country. Collaboration and developing partnerships is fundamental to the work of CINHC and is also key to its success.

An Effective Organizational Structure

Although a small board of directors is responsible for CINHC policy and fiscal oversight, the steering committee helps shape the on-going work of CINHC, including development of its programs. The Steering Committee represents key stakeholders and endorsing organizations, providing the forum for California nursing leadership organizations, state agencies, and other stakeholders to work together to create nursing workforce solutions. The committee provides a bridge between workforce efforts of the profession, health care industry, the public sector of state agencies, and educational institutions.

Steering committee members commit to act in the best interests of nursing in California rather than those of their own organizations. Information, issues, needs, challenges, and resources are part of the mix in any discussion. Together, the members—in whole or in various committees and task forces—work to develop solutions that benefit all, which means each of CINHC's programs, solutions, and recommendations already have been vetted and accepted by a diverse and representative group by the time they are in final form.

Model for Change

CINHC program leaders use the CINHC model for change to guide the programs they lead, thus ensuring collaboration and partnering (Jones, Patterson, & Jackson, 2009). This model includes convening diverse stakeholders critical to success, facilitating discovery and decision making among the stakeholders, and catalyzing change. CINHC has developed an iterative process through which it leads stakeholder organizations to formulate and agree upon solutions to specific challenges, processes for change, and implementation of the changes. The process includes the following steps to reaching a common approach to any specific issue:

1. Identify and convene diverse stakeholders, including champions of an issue, content experts, and individuals or representatives of groups essential for reaching successful outcomes and broad-based buy-in.

2. Reach agreement on the issue to be addressed.

3. Identify barriers to reaching desired outcome.

4. Determine how to overcome barriers.

5. Make recommendations/strategies that result in action plans to overcome barriers to produce desired outcomes.

6. Build consensus through convergent thinking, thus obtaining broad-based commitment for implementation while designing solutions.

In the past 6 years, CINHC has refined the preceding process and used it to achieve the following general goals for all its major projects:

- **Create an environment that facilitates convergent thinking** and the buy-in that allows change to happen through the development of a common approach or single "voice" for an issue. This includes providing a safe and neutral setting in which controversial topics can be grappled with and worked through to a common approach.

- **Serve as a catalyst for action** through convening and facilitating the process for action through collaboration, thus allowing change to occur. Frequently, CINHC provides the vision for change that draws the stakeholders together.

- **Reach a common approach.** Reaching a common approach can be time consuming, but once achieved, the commitment for implementation is well under way, thus expediting the change process or reaching towards desired outcomes. The process for addressing an issue is part of the process for implementing the action steps.

- **Recognize regional difference and provide for planning and solutions that address local needs.** These are vital in a state as large and diverse as California. Although a single voice is needed for statewide initiatives, solutions often require a more regional focus to be implemented effectively in different communities. Respecting regional difference is necessary for engaging local leaders and stakeholders, as well as for obtaining grants that have distinct geographic boundaries.

The Effects of the Model for Change

This model for change and its resulting collaborative efforts have made a difference in addressing California's nursing workforce issues. The following examples illustrate the effectiveness of this approach.

First, Goal 1 of the Master Plan, *Building Educational Capacity in California Schools of Nursing*, was completed in March of 2005 and has served as a reference document for policy makers at the state capital, the Governor's office, foundations, and regional planners (CINHC, 2009). In 4 years, enrollment in the state's nursing programs has increased 54 percent, and more than $160 million in public funds supporting the increase of educational capacity can be mapped to this plan.

Goal 1 was developed by CINHC convening key stakeholders, which included representatives of all the types of nursing programs in the state, professional associations, employers of nurses, chancellors' offices of the state educational institutions, regulators, and policy makers. The major barriers to increasing capacity were articulated, and solutions were identified to overcome them. Goal 1 reflected the commitments that the chancellors' offices could make as well as those that the Governor's office felt could shape the administration's approach. When Goal 1 was ready to be implemented, it had buy-in from the major stakeholders and served as a framework for a common approach to building education capacity in the state's schools of nursing.

A second example of the effectiveness of CINHC Model of Change is the development of a white paper on education redesign (CINHC, 2009). The need to redesign nursing education is driven by factors, such as the growing gaps between how nurses are educated and the evolving need of the health care delivery system, and the need for a nursing workforce educated at a higher level. This latter driving force needed to be addressed within the context that 70 percent of the state's new nurses were educated at community colleges, but only 26 percent continued to obtain a higher degree in nursing. One hundred thought leaders were brought together by CINHC over the course of a year to grapple with this need to redesign nursing education in the state. Two of the major outcomes were

- The consensus that education and service must agree to the expected competencies of new graduates. This is needed to facilitate the redesign of curriculum in schools of nursing and to define service's responsibility for nursing education, which may best be accomplished through formal residencies of new nurses.

- The development of collaborative models of nursing education through partnerships between associate degree community college nursing programs, baccalaureate degree granting institutions, and health service organizations. These collaborative models would have the elements of dual admission, shared faculty, and integrated curriculum, and would be arranged in such a way that associate degree students can complete the baccalaureate degree in nursing in one year after completing their associate degree requirements.

Responses to request for proposals (RFPs) calling for demonstration of the collaborative model of nursing education have resulted in 13 responses representing 50 schools of nursing in California. Inherent in the RFP is the agreement for participating schools to partner with hospitals that are part of the collaborative to reach agreement on competencies of the new graduates. This building of agreement of competencies will be integrated into an overall statewide effort.

Mentee's Story

When I first met Deloras Jones, the executive director of CINHC, she was presenting the Master Plan for nursing for California to a large group of deans and directors of nursing. She described the six focus areas of the Master Plan: educational systems and capacity, recruitment, nursing practice, workforce diversity, working environments, and workforce data collection. At the time, I did not know what to make of her, and I was not convinced California needed a master plan.

Two years later, I found myself in her office introducing myself as a doctoral student in nursing who was interested in workforce development issues and who was researching the influences of associate degree–prepared nurses who did not return to school for a higher degree in nursing. I'll never forget how she came around to sit with me in the front of her large desk, eliminating any physical barriers between us. She conveyed such confidence that I had a great deal to offer CINHC in the work of the white paper project on nursing education redesign for California and that together thought leaders could make a real difference in improving nursing education in many areas.

Her confidence in me increased my confidence in myself so that I eventually consented to co-chair the committee on collaborative nursing education models. Seeing Deloras in action on the work of this white paper was amazing. She demonstrated an uncanny ability to bring together stakeholders who traditionally came from opposite sides of many issues. It was simply surreal to sit at the same table with directors and deans from associate degree and baccalaureate nursing programs, private as well as public nursing programs, nursing officers from service health care organizations, National League for Nursing and American Association of Colleges of Nursing executives, government officials, and the American Nurses Association of California.

She set the whole project in motion to facilitate consensus-building about what the issues were and helped move us into a doable action plan. Then she procured millions of dollars of funding for implementation of collaborative education models so that associate degree nursing students could seamlessly continue with their education for a baccalaureate or master's degree in nursing. Seeing Deloras in action taught me what effective leadership is and that it can result in significant change for the good of the nursing profession and for the good of the patient. Today I am grateful for CINHC, its Master Plan, and the white paper on education redesign. I currently serve on the steering committee as chair of the California League for Nursing.

Self-Reflective Questions

1. Which issue in your nursing practice or in health care are you the most passionate about?

2. Which stakeholders would you want to have come to the table to achieve broad-based buy-in for your issue?

3. Who are other champions for this issue, including content experts, individuals, and/or groups essential for reaching successful outcomes?

4. How would you have to frame this issue to facilitate reaching agreement among all constituents?

5. How would you bring everyone together to facilitate a process for collaboration?

6. What are all the barriers that could potentially block you from reaching your desired outcome?

7. Which strategies do you and your stakeholders propose to employ to overcome these barriers?

8. What are the possible unintended consequences of your solutions, and how can you prevent these from happening?

9. What are possible funding sources to help support your strategies to overcome barriers?

10. How will you approach those stakeholders who did not participate in this process?

Communication: Verbal and Nonverbal

14

"The most important practical lesson that can be given to nurses is to teach them what to observe."

—Florence Nightingale

Mentor
Carmen Rumeu Casares, MSc, RN
Director of Nursing
Clínica Universidad de Navarra
Pamplona, Spain

Mentee
Leticia San Martín-Rodríguez, PhD, MSc, RN
Nurse Manager, Nursing Development Career
Clínica Universidad de Navarra
Pamplona, Spain

Over half a century ago, Antoine de Saint-Exupéry, the great French writer and pilot, wrote, "If you want to build a ship, don't drum up people to collect wood and don't assign them tasks and work, but rather teach them to long for the endless immensity of the sea." This quote, together with Florence Nightingale's, conveys the importance of setting effective leadership examples when motivating a team to achieve success.

One of the main differences between a manager and a leader is that the manager works on something that already exists, whereas the leader creates the work. To carry out any project the leader should be able to communicate the mission and values of the organization to the staff through oral communication and through modeling the desired behavior.

The leader has a vision of what he or she wants to achieve and can communicate that vision to others in a way that makes people want to be a part of it.

Communicating the Mission

In the 1980s, a leader began to be seen as "someone who defines organizational reality through the articulation of a vision which is a reflection of how he defines an organization's mission and the values which will support it" (Bryman, 1996). According to Cardona and Rey (2008), an organization's mission is the contribution and values that define the identity of the organization. Therefore, the mission includes the contributions the organization, department, team, and professional make up that give meaning to the mission.

The main challenge of the nurse leader is to communicate to his or her teammates the mission, the values that sustain it, and each teammate's contribution to the mission. Achieving this goal develops a strong sense of motivation within the team. Colleagues are not only motivated by extrinsic goals (what they receive as a result of their job) and intrinsic goals (how much they enjoy performing their job), but also by a more inspiring, transcendent reason (Pérez-López, 1991). A transcendental leader is strongly engaged with the staff and generates the same commitment on his or her colleagues (Cardona and Rey, 2008). This leader type is close to nursing leader type, since for the sake of the patient, nurses tend to be altruistic and self denied.

Most nursing departments have a document that reflects the mission and values of that department within the hospital. It is also routine practice to remember the overall mission and values of the hospital. Ideally, however, the mission and values should be reflected in the clinical practice and recognized by patients, their families, and even visitors. Having this goal in mind helps nurses to make changes, become better professionals, and work according to those values. But "how and when do people change? People change something when an issue affects them deeply both personally and professionally" (McKee, Boyatzis & Johnston, 2008).

Role of Values

To communicate the mission, the leader must strongly uphold the values and develop them on a regular basis in his or her daily work (Cardona & Rey, 2008). Verbal communication is quite important, but even more essential is that leaders exemplify their values through their actions. This point underlines the importance of nonverbal communication—the "speech" given by the actions. Mehrabian (1968) emphasizes that the words in a message have only a 7% effect on the recipient, whereas the nonverbal communication accounts for half the response of the person who receives the message (Manning & Curtis, 1988; Mehrabian, 1968). When communicating the mission and values, a coherent consistency between what the leader says and what his or her daily work and actions suggest is necessary.

Two key values within the nursing profession are: attitude of service and respect for each person. *Attitude of service* is described in the literature as a key feature of transcendental leadership (Cardona, 2000) and servant leadership (Russell & Stone, 2002). Upenieks (2002) noted that today's nurse leaders should "lead to serve." Nurse leaders should serve staff nurses by taking care of them as they would care for a patient, and giving them the needed tools to carry out their mission. The leader also communicates the importance of serving others and humbleness. As a result, staff nurses witness this service, understand it as an essential part of the mission and values, and return to incorporate it into their area from headquarters to the patient's bedside. Nursing leaders must be able to understand employee values, beliefs, and motivations and how current nursing leadership roles can be creatively redesigned to engage those staff members (Chambers Clark, 2008).

The second value, *respect for each person*, appreciates the human qualities of each professional. According to Duluc (2000), this attitude fosters a respectful environment, which enables the open, honest communication needed to develop a trusting environment. Ferguson-Paré (1998) suggests that there is a relationship between the nursing holistic visions of the patient and the vision a leader should have about the nursing profession. Therefore, leaders should understand that nurses have a life outside their professional community; a life of personal and familial interests, needs, hopes, and dreams (Ferguson-Paré, 1998). This value also reflects to staff nurses the importance of work-life balance and reinforces consistency between "what is said" and "what is done."

Reflections From the Mentor and Mentee

By reviewing the mission and values of our hospital with all the nurse managers, we are learning to refresh the culture that runs our organization. Part of our strength is that we both have much to learn from colleagues who have many years' experience in our institution. I (Carmen) have worked 17 years in this hospital; 14 of those years in management. Leticia (mentee) has been involved in management for three years since completing her PhD. Her dissertation relates to the managerial field.

As a mentor, I encourage Leticia to learn as much as possible from her new role and to develop her communication skills to exemplify the mission and the values of the hospital. When making decisions, she is realizing the importance of taking our mission and values into account. By getting to know the mission and values deeper, she exhibits the high commitment that managers need to communicate—verbally and nonverbally—to their staff.

As a mentee, I (Leticia) observe that my mentor is working strongly to achieve a further commitment from middle managers to keep a transcendental reason for their jobs, meaning to work on thinking about their staff satisfaction and self-recognition of a well-done job. Our nurse leader sets a clear example of effective leadership for our nurses by being available to all staff members and showing that she is at their service whenever needed. She treats each one as uniquely individual yet part of a larger team. I realize how positive and strong the culture of our hospital is. Our nursing leadership tries to follow the lives, families, and sometimes personal issues of the 1,100 people who are part of our staff. Although it is almost impossible, they try to be close to everyone, especially when the need arises.

Self-Reflective Questions

1. What is the mission of your institution?

2. How does effective communication help you make a difference?

3. How can you communicate the values of your unit and organization with patients and families?

4. How do you attempt to get to know each person who is under your responsibility?

5. How do you handle when a staff member is experiencing a personal difficulty?

6. How can you be available to everyone at your organization?

7. Should a manager be visible to staff, patients, and families?

8. Do you have a plan on how to communicate information to nurses?

9. How do you maintain being approachable and reachable by others?

10. Do you encourage others when talking to them?

Community in Context With Leadership Development

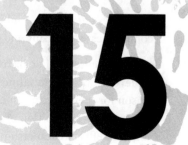

15

"And so is the world put back by the death of everyone who has to sacrifice the development of his or her peculiar gifts (which were meant, not for selfish gratification, but for the improvement of that world) to conventionality."

—Florence Nightingale

Mentor
JoEllen Koerner, RN, PhD, FAAN
Senior Consultant, Dynamis
  Healthcare Advisors
Sioux Falls, South Dakota, USA

Mentee
Sarah Lamkin, RN, MSN
Nurse and Certified Poison Information Specialist in Cincinnati
  Children's Hospital Medical
  Center
Cincinnati, Ohio, USA

In our interconnected universe, everything is experienced within the dance of relationship. Through connection and community we define who we are and how the world works. As our social consciousness deepens, the definition of community expands to include those who have gone before us as well as those who will follow. We increasingly realize that what we do today has an impact globally and also affects future generations.

Each encounter occurs within the context of an environment. Context both forms and informs the experience. For example, we draw from different aspects of ourselves when we are with our children than when we are with co-workers. Each of us interprets life based on our past experiences as well as our hopes for the future. Therefore, no two individuals within a group have the same experience because of differing perceptions and expectations. To align these multiple viewpoints into a synergistic focus requires a co-creative process between an inspiring leader and an authentic community.

Inspiration and Authenticity

An inspiring leader is one who offers clarity by addressing both the issue at hand and the environment in which it is nested. A compelling vision is created that shows expansive new ways to address old problems. Information and resources are provided in a way that enlightens everyone involved; each becomes more in the exchange.

An authentic community engages in the process. Community members feel passionate about the issue and bring both commitment and energy to the work. Thoughtful but candid exchange allows multiple perspectives to be shared. Adoption of the best solution, even if it is not the preferred option for an individual, fosters the greater good rather than a "win" for a few.

Respect and Co-Creation

Two themes that dominate my (JoEllen) global nursing experience with groups and communities include respect and co-creation. Some nurses coming to the United States from the Philippines were experiencing competency challenges in their new working environment. I was invited to assist a community of nurses in their home country to explore the issue at hand. A core team of both U.S. and Philippine nursing leaders was established to investigate this issue as well as its solution. A series of interviews with practicing nurses and new nurse graduates was balanced with a similar dialogue between nursing educators and service leaders in the region. This was accompanied by knowledge and competency assessment of nurses seeking employment as well as nursing students about to graduate.

As we sifted through the data findings, punctuated by rich stories and exemplars, we discovered that although all RNs had a BSN degree, their initial work experience varied considerably based on the health care setting in which they were employed. Some had exposure to hospitals equal in sophistication to large medical centers in the United States. Others found the context of their work environment to be significantly less resourced. In each case, the practice pattern of the nurses was reflective of their clinical settings.

To correct this uneven playing field, a professional development center was established. It offered opportunities for individual nurses to complete an in-depth assessment of current skills and knowledge and a rich array of educational tools. Development opportunities designed to deepen assessment and intervention skills, offered through interactive Web resources based on national standards, strengthened core nursing capacity. Initial on-boarding orientation programs for some U.S. hospitals were also offered through a Web portal of the hiring hospital. Each of these learning endeavors helped strengthen the competency of the nurse, easing some of the culture shock experienced when the nurse moved to another country (Curato, Jiongco, & Koerner, 2008).

Reflections from Sarah Lamkin, Mentee

I think some of my favorite conversations with JoEllen have centered on respecting the wisdom of each person based on who they are, where they live, and the importance of authentic presence (the offering of self in the healing process). She has helped me realize that nurses have the opportunity to discover a different component of health care as they are increasingly thrust into the global community through travel opportunities and access to the World Wide Web. I have started to realize how integral preventative care is to wider socio-cultural issues, such as malaria and women's health issues. Collaborating with communities often requires an open mind and a willingness to forego many western frameworks, such as delegation of nursing and other patient care activities in order to truly develop a connection with communities and address the needs of the relationship between environment, nursing, person, and health.

As a profession, nursing is committed to assisting communities and contributing to their health by providing information on health education and management. It is an ongoing intellectual challenge because nurses must take into consideration geography, demography, economics, politics, religious beliefs, and cultural patterns of interaction. Every nurse must understand the importance of supporting community participation in the process when working with a community to solve problems.

Partnerships and Sustainability

Two themes dominate my nursing experiences with communities: partnership and sustainability. Partnerships, with active participation by community members, increase understanding of how nurses can best meet the needs of the entire community. Creating sustainability, or implementing long-term solutions to problems, is crucial to guaranteeing lasting success.

In nursing school, I participated in a one-day food and clothing drive that provided food and clothing to people in need. The conversations I had with the people who came to the drive changed my worldview. I learned that most of the people I was interacting with were unhappy with their economic status, and to my astonishment had made no plans or attempts to better themselves through education or hard work. Those who received the handouts and give-aways seemed to have less motivation to work. This partnership was unsuccessful because we did not provide a long-term solution to their suffering or promote a sustainable means to improve their health.

In contrast, after I graduated nursing school, I became involved with the not-for-profit Village Life Outreach Project. This organization fights poverty in rural Tanzania, East Africa, by empowering villagers to address the issues that most affect them, such as lack of clean water, substandard health care delivery, and poor nutrition. Instead of simply providing hand-outs, Village Life Outreach works with communities to enact long-lasting, sustainable improvement measures. Avoiding a top-down approach develops a sense of dignity in the community as well as self-reliance.

Importance of Interrelationships

Nurses practice in traditional and non-traditional health care settings and communities worldwide. For the nursing profession, the way forward is to consider the interrelationship between the community and the environment with passion and enthusiasm. Nurses need to be inspiring leaders, creating multi-disciplinary research and education collaborations that foster the greater good for all within communities.

Self-Reflective Questions

1. What is changing or needs to change? Why?

2. What opposing factors are causing resistance to the change?

3. How are the beliefs, values, and capacities of the involved parties affecting the process?

4. How much of people's actions are due to the environment and cultural norms in which this change is embedded?

5. What physical, fiscal, and human resources are needed to facilitate the change?

6. How will you implement the change without negatively affecting the culture?

Self-Reflective Questions *(continued)*

7. Describe the role of a leader and the role of a community group in true partnership.

8. Will this change include such a partnership? Why or why not?

9. Are the changes sustainable? Should they be?

10. How will you define and measure success?

16

Competency Evaluation and Leadership

"Effective nursing leadership is important in all nursing roles, whether the nurse practices in the field of education developing future leaders, as a researcher who mentors new researchers, as an administrator who provides support and guidance to staff, as a practitioner who provides exemplary care and shares professional knowledge, or as one who provides direction and support to practice through policy development."

—A. Squires

Mentor
Margarita Peya, RN, MMANS, MHCR
Professeur
School of Nursing, University of Barcelona
Barcelona, Spain

Mentee
Maria Eulàlia Juvé, RN, MMSN, MNLM, QRD
Catalan Institute of Health
Barcelona, Spain

The aim of this chapter is to explain the theoretical framework of the COM-A project. The project defined nursing competence and established evaluation parameters as a part of nursing leadership and strategic plan for the Catalan Institute of Health of Catalonia, Spain; the project included use of competency evaluation as part of "pay for performance" (Juvé et al., 2007a).

Seven hundred nurses from the eight public hospitals participated in the project, which was led by Mrs. Maria Eulàlia Juvé and mentored by an academic group from different university nursing faculties of Catalonia.

The titles of most of the sections of this chapter describes the mentor's challenging question for the mentee in the hopes of discovering the main theoretical and conceptual topics to guide the first steps of the project development.

Two in One: Defining the Concept

Competency comprises the sum of knowledge, skills, and attitudes, allowing complex decision making processes to determine the proper performance/execution in each case and situation (Benner, 1984; McConell, 2001). Competency implies a dynamic process through which a professional uses knowledge, skills, attitudes, and "wisdom" related to his or her profession in order to develop it effectively in any situation within his or her area of practice.

In their review, McMullan et al. (2003) also noted that the terms "competence," "competency," "performance," and "capability" were frequently used inconsistently and interchangeably. These authors suggested that *competences* are job related as well as descriptive of action, behavior, or outcome of performance. Comparatively, *competencies* are person oriented, referring to underlying characteristics and qualities that are indicative of effective or superior performance in a job.

In this project, we use the term "competence" in this same sense: namely, to define the job-related standards of practice. We use the concept of *competency* to encompass individual-related attributes, qualities, and traits, indicating effective and differentiated performance or "the added value" that one brings to the practice (Ordre des infermières de Quebec, 1985; Sociedad Española de Enfermería Oncológica, 1997; Teixidor et al., 2003).

Competency or Expertise?

The Human Skills Acquisition Model (HSAM) of Professors Stuart and Hubert Dreyfus, (Benner, 1984) was developed in the 1970s within the artificial intelligence program at the University of California in Berkeley. This model describes the evolution process to competency/expertise first through theoretical knowledge application, and then lived experiences accumulation analysis and discrimination. It posits that in the acquisition and development of a skill, one passes through five levels of proficiency

- Novice.

- Advanced beginner.

- Competent.

- Proficient.

- Expert.

Thus, in this sense, competency and expertise are synonymous concepts.

The main premises of the HSAM are

- Acquisition of competency is a dynamic process.

- Getting to a level of expertise depends upon individual traits and the context.

- Not everybody will achieve the highest levels (proficient/expert).

- The highest levels of competency can be reached only through reflective and continuous practice.

- Competency distribution in a professional population usually draws a normal curvature of Gaus' Bell.

Identifying Individual Traits That Define Competency

The competency stage depends upon individual determinants and also upon the context. Personal traits constructing competency are known as *competency dimensions* and comprise allied knowledge, skills, and attitudes articulated in five areas (Choudhry et al., 2005):

- Cognitive and learning dimension.

- Technical dimension.

- Integration dimension.

- Relational dimension.

- Moral and affective dimension.

Cognitive and learning dimension includes basic knowledge, the capacity to learn from lived experiences, the ability to generate questions and hypothesis, curiosity, attention capacity, self-acquisition of new knowledge, analysis capacity and abstract problem-resolution skills, observation, and self-criticism of one's thinking processes.

The *technical dimension* embodies manual abilities and skills for technical procedures execution as well as mental skills for organization, and time and resources management.

Integration dimension refers to critical reasoning strategies; knowledge application in real situations; relational incorporation of human, scientific, and clinical judgement elements; and uncertainty management.

Relational dimension explains the capacity to share knowledge, abilities, or attitudes (teaching skills); team-working capacity; communication skills; and conflict management.

Moral and affective dimension includes issues related to emotional intelligence, skills to care for and look after the others, sensibility and respect, and stress tolerance.

Expertise: Culture or Genetics?

Traditionally, competency has been associated with an intensive education on a knowledge area or discipline. However, expertise is closer to tacit knowledge than explicit recognition patterns that construct neural networks, explaining intuition as a result of complex learning processes and the integration and contrast of experiences. The interpretation of experiences builds a conceptual network, easing problem-solving processes in ambiguous, stressful, emergency, or uncertain situations. That is why decision making in expert or proficient professionals overpasses or omits, in many cases, the norm. Expert performance is guided by neural network functioning.

Neural networking can explain not only recognition patterns but "learning from errors" skills. The relationship between competency and context is well described in the scientific literature cited at the beginning of this text

What Is Competency Assessment?

Competency assessment is the process used to evaluate the level or interval of expertise of a professional in a concrete context. Traditionally, competency assessment has been achieved by separately measuring knowledge, skills, and attitudes, in the middle or lower level of Miller's Pyramid (Juvé et al., 2007a).

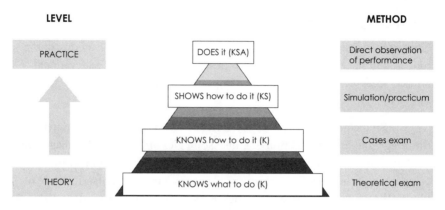

K=Knowledge; KS=Knowledge and skills; KSA=Knowledge, skills and attitudes

Figure 1   Miller's Pyramid

Competency assessment is based upon two main components: the evaluation tool and the evaluation method.

The characteristics of the assessment evaluation tool have to adjust authenticity (inclusion of relevant concepts of the construct of interest), validity (including face validity and sensibility), and reliability (reproducibility) (Juvé et al., 2007b).

In their clinical practice and management, health care professionals combine a wide range of cognitive, psychomotor, and affective skills to achieve a cohesive focus on patient care. So, competency should not be assessed from the context in which decision making has to be made. This means that competency must be evaluated directly, from performance in the context of clinical practice.

No method is completely objective, yet any competency evaluation process implicates two main sources of potential bias: the evaluator's subjectivity and socialization between the evaluator and the evaluated individual.

Described formulas to minimize the impact of these two effects in the final result of the assessment (Juvé et al., 2007a, 2008; Winskill, 2000) are:

- The use of valid and reliable tools.

- Establishing a threshold of competency.

- The use of direct performance evaluation methods.

- Assessment triangulation.

Conclusions to Start Up the Project

Competency assessment not only depends upon reliability and validity of the tool used in the evaluation but also its proper use as well as the educational impact, acceptability level, economic impact, and transparency of the process as a whole.

Assessing competency is not only a matter of measure, but it is related to the design and implementation of global strategies of leadership, management, education and learning, application, and marketing. Thus, as an essential component of the "pay for performance" program in the Catalan Institute of Health (Juvé et al., 2007a), competency assessment should be guided by the following principles, tending to minimize the subjective effects of evaluation:

- Assessment has to be done comprehensively—directly integrating knowledge, skills, and attitudes—as well as observing clinical practice.

- Competency assessment is located at the top of the Miller's Pyramid (Juvé et al., 2007a).

- The assessment tool has to cover nurses' clinical competences and the indicators of competency/expertise.

- The assessment tool has to be valid and reliable.

To neutralize subjectivity and socialization, a multimodal assessment method is recommended, including self-evaluation and in critical cases, external evaluation.

Project Status

The project has been developed from this starting point and has been implemented since 2008 as a part of the "pay for performance" system in the hospitals of Catalan Institute of Health. Approximately 700 nurses have already been evaluated with the COM-VA expertise assessment system since then.

Self-Reflective Questions

1. How do you compare competency and leadership?

2. How do competence and competency differ?

3. From your leadership style, how would you use competency assessment and for what purposes?

4. Using the principles of the Human Skills Acquisition Model and Benner's works, how would you describe the different levels of expertise?

5. How do competency dimensions relate to each other?

6. How does the model described in this chapter explain the use of intuition?

7. How do you define a competent leader?

8. What are the features needed for a competency evaluation tool?

9. What are the formulas to minimize the impact of the two bias effects?

10. What competencies do you think you have as a leader?

Confidence

17

"What could we accomplish if we approached every day with confidence and an attitude of 'I can do whatever it takes'?"

—Karren Kowalski

Mentor
Diana T.F. Lee, PhD, RN
Chair and Professor of Nursing
Director of the Nethersole
  School of Nursing and Assist-
  ant Dean of the Faculty of
  Medicine
Chinese University of Hong
  Kong
Visiting Professor
University of London, United
  Kingdom
Advisory Professor of Fudan
  University and Guangzhou
  Medical College in China
Hong Kong SAR, China

Mentee
Carmen W.H. Chan, RN, BSN,
  Mphi, PhD
The Nethersole School of
  Nursing
Chinese University of Hong
  Kong
Sha Tin, Hong Kong SAR, China

Confidence is often regarded as a building block for success—an energy that strengthens one's mind to expect positive outcomes. Fearlessness or careless-ness that makes one bold is not confidence (Murthy, 2008). In an exploratory study on determinants of success among nurse managers, nurse managers ranked self-confidence as one of the most important competencies related to success of management (Dubnichi & Sloan, 1991). Self-confidence is a belief in one's capability to accomplish a task, demonstrated by a willingness to ex-ercise independent judgment (Dubnichi & Sloan, 1991). This belief leads to an expectation of a positive outcome of self-performance. A confident leader conveys to the team that the leader can confront and successfully deal with adversity and hardship. In other words, confidence conveys feasibility and workability in a workplace.

Becoming confident is a learning process. Many behaviors originate in childhood. Most children hear negatives about their behaviors or personalities far more often than they hear positives. As we grow older, negativism carries over into our working lives, making it harder to enjoy our job and feel confident. However, behaviorists now know that, with enough praise, even a difficult child can quickly turn into a well-behaved one. Vestal (2005) advocates that the most lasting form of confidence is not self-generated but nurtured by others. Therefore, the best way to nurture confidence is to replace negativism with a culture of praise and affirmation. Creating an environment that includes positive reassurance from colleagues and supervisors encourages people to do their best and instills in them a belief that they can succeed. Confident leaders almost always inspire confidence in others.

Nurse leaders serve in a fast-paced environment with an endless list of problems to solve and multiple crises to handle (Vestal, 2005). For a leader assuming a new role or expanded responsibilities, feeling overwhelmed and powerless is especially common. Jeffers (1987) states the core fear of all humans is the perceived incapability of handling what life can bring. This negative self-talk contributes to fear, which can limit and paralyze a leader.

A leader can increase self-confidence by facing fears and substituting negative thinking with a positive approach (Kowalski et al., 2003). For example, plan to resolve fear and replace it with action. For example, take a course or share your feelings with a mentor. Positive statements, such as, "I'm great at my job," "I'm noticed and appreciated at work," and "I love what I do" are powerful in changing attitudes and behavior. By thinking and believing you will succeed, fulfilling the prophecy becomes more likely. Being confident means expecting a positive outcome and improving your ability to make that outcome happen.

Lessons Learned by Carmen Chan, Mentee

The bachelor of nursing programme at The Chinese University of Hong Kong carries the largest number of students and credit units of study in Hong Kong. During my first year of appointment as the programme's coordinator, I had to revise the curriculum structure and content drastically. A new team of workers and a new curriculum challenged my ability and character, and created a high degree of anxiety. This state did not just happen *to* me; it happened *in* me. I examined whether I was a worker or a leader, a peacemaker or a revolutionist. Additionally, I reflected on what motivated me, challenged me, and pleased me.

After determining that I was truly passionate about the new curriculum, I went through a painful process of stepping from my comfort zone and proceeding. I needed to share my vision with a trusted mentor to help guide me through the process. Diana was that person for me. Her affirmation that I follow my heart and do the necessary work boosted my confidence. In her capacity as the director of the Nethersole School of Nursing, she reiterated the need to revise the curriculum. She played critic so that I could rehearse defending my position. The more affirmation I received, the more confident I became. The experience became an opportunity to learn and grow rather than a battle to win or lose. I realized I had to be open to new possibilities and alternatives, and that a perfect curriculum liked by everyone simply did not exist. Additionally, I realized that I had to play multiple roles—sometimes advocate, sometimes peacemaker.

It took me quite some time to reflect on what happened *in* me. This experience became an important milestone of liking my ideas, my actions, my motives, and my values. Although I still aim for self-improvement, my self-confidence brings me closer to achieving my goals. I believe confidence is built on a foundation of values, integrity, and worthiness independent of others' approval. These qualities are inherent in a person's spirituality.

Self-Reflective Questions

1. Do you take charge of your actions?

2. Do you act assertively, speak calmly, and listen properly?

3. Are you able to give genuine praise and accept constructive criticism?

4. Do you evaluate yourself realistically?

5. Do you appreciate your achievement?

6. When an opportunity comes up, do you say, "Why not?" rather than "Why?"

7. Are you flexible towards people, circumstances, and all things new?

8. Are you truly willing to learn from your mistakes?

9. Do you feel you can influence situations and outcomes?

10. Do you practice positive self-talk, such as, "I am great at my job"?

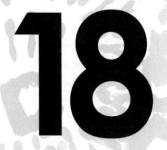

18

Conflict Resolution and Improving Cooperation

"Conflict is inevitable… and can be constructive or destructive."

—Ruth M. Tappen

Mentor

Naomi Mmapelo Seboni, PhD, RN, RM
Head, School of Nursing, Faculty of Health Sciences, University of Botswana
Director of World Health Organization's Collaborating Centre for Nursing and Midwifery Development, Africa Region
Gaborone, Botswana

Mentee

Tshepo Rothi Monau, PhD, MS, BSc
Lecturer, Pathophysiology/Physiology, School of Nursing
University of Botswana
Gaborone, Botswana

Conflict refers to a relational position in which there is tension between two parties, and neither is willing to succumb to the power of the other. Usually conflict has painful emotional involvement as two antagonistic impulses clash. Conflict is inevitable and can be constructive or destructive (Tappen, 2001). It can occur at various levels within an individual, a family, a community, and even an entire nation. Much attention and effort can be placed on avoiding conflict, but conflict inevitably arises. Whether it becomes constructive or destructive depends on how it is managed. Note that conflict should not be confused with a healthy, constructive argument or discussion in which two parties hold opposing ideas or opinions.

Causes of Conflict

Conflict can emanate from political, economic, legal, cultural, and technological issues. These include competition, power struggles, cultural differences, different approaches to tasks, invasion of another's space, and lack of respect for the views and feelings of others. Some of the most common causes of conflict in the workplace are dissimilar knowledge, skills, values, and interests; scarce resources; rivalry for rewards; and role ambiguity. Also noteworthy is that working environments are increasingly encroached on by factors that can easily be viewed as threatening to health personnel. For instance, litigation against health facilities and health workers is creating a threatening environment that calls health professionals to "self-defense" and shifting blame. The increasing demand for health care and limited staffing put health workers under tremendous workloads. These factors increase the propensity of nurses and other workers to interpret situations in ways that might yield conflict. Additionally, nurses are educated and socialized to work assertively and to handle differences of opinions with assertiveness, yet there is a very fine line between assertive behavior and bullying (Kelly, 2006).

Effects of Conflict

Conflict can have both positive and negative effects. Looking at conflict as an opportunity for positive change and/or deeper knowledge can alter the way people interact and deal with challenges and injustices. If approached with an open mind, conflict can push individuals beyond their comfort zones to find creative and innovative ways to promote cooperation. It may also open the door to other ideas than group mentality and thus prevent conformity. Expressing difference of opinion, also called disagreement (Saltman et al, 2006), does not always have to cause harm to interpersonal relations.

Conflict wastes resources, especially time and money. The psychological well-being of those involved can be compromised. Conflict also creates rivalry and mistrust. Therefore, resolving even the smallest conflict is essential. Unresolved conflict may create an unpleasant work environment or escalate a simple discord between work colleagues into avoidance, verbal assaults, resentment, and an inability to work together as a team (Teambuilding Inc., 2007).

Conflict Resolution

Conflict resolution is the process of settling the differences between conflicting parties and re-establishing or improving the relationship. This betterment is achieved through clearing misconceptions, admitting and apologizing for wrongs, reaching an agreement, and/or accepting differences. The resultant relationship allows the two parties to work together and bring out each other's best (win-win situation). Van de Vliert (1998) observes that effective conflict resolution minimizes frustration and provides opportunity for mutual understanding, cooperation, and increased productivity.

The extent and nature of the conflict determines the approach to its resolution. The avoidance approach, commonly used by both nurse managers and nurses, leaves issues unresolved and prolongs tension. This approach practically ignores the conflict, hoping that the conflict, with all its inherent problems, will be "accidentally" resolved. Approaches to conflict resolution need to be specific, culture sensitive, and informed by objective information (Kelly, 2006).

Proactive Conflict Resolution

Specifically for nursing personnel, research has shown that conflict resolution style predicts level of staff morale, burnout, and job satisfaction (Montoro-Rodrigues & Small, 2006; Williamson & Schultz, 1993). The same studies and others have also shown that failing to resolve conflict increases emotional exhaustion and the feeling of job depersonalization.

Nurses who are proactive in resolving conflict in their workplace recognize four stages of conflict management:

1. Information gathering.
2. Developing a relevant and positive plan.
3. Developing a framework for the process.
4. Developing activities toward settling matters between conflicting parties.

Information gathering allows both parties to be present to convey their view of the situation. In a warm, friendly, and supportive environment, the conflicting parties must be interviewed to identify the source, nature, and perceived cause of the conflict (Anderson, 2005).

A relevant and positive plan adopts a team approach that emphasizes common ground. Those in conflict should show some degree of empathy (Anderson, 2005) and establish confidence that the parties' feelings will not be trivialized. Recognition of prevailing power dynamics should be demonstrated and cultural mannerisms of communication must be understood (Winter & Cherrier, 2008). The mediator must not seem to trivialize the issue or feelings. The culture in which conflict resolution takes place must also be taken into account in order to be aware of details such as body language.

To guide the process of conflict resolution, adopting an appropriate perspective embraces fairness. The nurse must identify differences, demonstrate a clear understanding of the problem, and speak specifically and clearly to its contributing factors. Unclear messages and other undoings, such as taking sides, can harden attitudes.

Nurses must also develop activities that constitute the steps to be followed in the process of resolving a conflict, which must include evaluation of the procedure followed and its outcome to ensure mutual satisfaction of both parties. Factors that shape listening and reassurance must be outlined. These would include choosing the setting, presence of both parties at the hearing, etc, for transparency and reassurance. Additionally, managers must help develop possible solutions from the parties involved and then evaluate the effectiveness of the resolution based on the satisfaction of those parties (Teambuilding Inc., 2007). Negotiation techniques should be adopted to avoid unnecessary obliging, which may be construed as favoritism of one party at the expense of the other. In obliging, the mediator deliberately elevates the other party to make him or her feel better about the situation (Schilling, n.d.). Obliging is more appropriate in situations where conflict is between a nurse manager and his or her subordinate and they themselves attempt to resolve it.

Improving Cooperation

Cooperation is purposefully working together toward the same goal. Conflict deters cooperation in the workplace and, therefore, should not be ignored. To practice constructive conflict management, all parties involved need to adhere to values of cooperation, such as effective communication, colleagueship, collaboration, fairness, and respect for others (Siu et al, 2008; Kantek & Kavla, 2007). Leaders of every health facility, together with their team, must develop a conflict management process that should be understood by all, empowering them to mediate conflict in a timely manner. This conflict management approach reduces the frequency and intensity of unresolved conflict and improves cooperation.

Lessons Learned by Tshepo Monau, Mentee

I have worked with nursing lecturers my entire career. I remember a situation that involved one female nurse lecturer and a male nursing student. The student was brilliant but arrogant. The student consulted with me after being failed on a test question he believed he had answered correctly. The student gave me the test paper and his responses, and sure enough the student was right. Without telling the student my analysis of the situation, I requested him to leave me with the papers for a discussion with his lecturer. I requested the company of another lecturer, who was friends with the lecturer involved, to sit in at the discussion between me and our colleague. Since I did not want to aggravate the arrogance of the student, we initially talked in his absence. The lecturer admitted the mistake, blaming it on the arrogance of the student that creates a negative attitude in her. She promised to correct the grade for the student. Her friend and I advised her to admit her mistake to the student and to acknowledge his abilities. I did not hear any news of strained relations between the two again. This process prevented a new conflict and resolved an existing one.

Self-Reflective Questions

1. How do you recognize conflict when it occurs?

2. Do you usually resolve conflict in a timely manner or try to avoid it?

3. What do nurses need to learn about conflict?

4. Who should be empowered to resolve conflicts among colleagues?

5. What would you describe as your preferred approaches to conflict resolution?

6. What are the effects of ignoring conflict in the workplace?

7. How is improving cooperation important?

8. What is the connection, if any, between conflict resolution and improving cooperation?

9. Why should health facilities have a conflict resolution process?

10. How would you contribute to a conflict resolution team?

Creativity in Nursing

19

"I have an almost complete disregard of precedent, and a faith in the possibility of something better. . . . . I defy the tyranny of precedent. I go for anything new that might improve the past."

—Clara Barton

Mentors

Carolyn Hope Smeltzer, RN,
  EdD, FAAN, FACHE
Vice President and Partner
PricewaterhouseCoopers
Chicago, Illinois, USA

and

Frances Vlasses, RN, PhD,
  NEA-BC
Associate Professor and
  Research Consultant
Loyola University Chicago
Chicago, Illinois, USA

Mentee

Shabnam Noordin, RN, MSN
Registered Nurse and Clinical
  Information Analyst
Advocate Lutheran General
  Hospital
Park Ridge, Illinois, USA

Does creativity have a place in nursing? Creativity is often associated with art and poetry, but we believe the definition is much broader and often goes unrecognized. We believe creativity is an innovative way to find solutions to problems or group of ideas that are not the norm or highly recognized in many disciplines. It is a silent art that has existed in nursing since the birth of the profession. Florence Nightingale improved poor public health conditions with new ways of thinking. She initiated innovative methods in hospital organization, nursing education, and nursing practice with limited resources, providing a template for creativity that has become a strong asset in nursing practice throughout our history.

Creativity still occurs daily in the interactions between nurses and their patients. Hospitals are inundated with technology, standardization, and tools for nurses to provide the best possible care to their patients, and this overshadows the basic acts of nursing care that define our profession. Despite availability of such resources, nurses continue to find creative ways, "workarounds," to provide nursing care. They find creative ways to bring the very essence back to the bedside.

The following examples show nurses, staff, and leaders who found ingenious ways to provide care to their patients. For these nurses, there is nothing extraordinary about what they do for their patients or their work environment; their creative and unconventional ways to provide what is best for their patients is what makes them truly extraordinary. Each story illustrates a tip that you can use to encourage creativity.

Give time, freedom, resources, and opportunity to try new ideas, rather than follow "what is."

Try New Ideas

When Carol's request to purchase bulk underwear for her patients was denied, she was shocked. The hospital administrator told Carol it would be too difficult for the accounting department to create a new account for the underwear. How was it possible that her patients, who suffered from mental illness, could not have underwear? Carol worked hard to collect donations for clean clothes for her patients but always fell short on collecting clean underwear. Having clean clothes improved self-esteem of her mentally ill patients and motivated them to maintain their personal hygiene. Carol wouldn't take "No" for an answer. Soon she came up with an unconventional solution to her problem. She began ordering bulk underwear and charged the expense to the office supply account, itemizing the purchase as paper clips (Smeltzer & Vlasses, 2003).

Reward creativity, not just with monetary gifts but with praise and recognition.

Reward Creativity

Janice was inspired to make pillows after an elderly patient asked her for a pillow so she could clip her call button to something. Eventually, Janice was making about 150 pillows each week and paid for them from her budget. She did not mind the expense because the pillows were her way of providing added comfort to her patients, and the look her patients gave her when they received the pillow was priceless. Janice has sent shipments of her pillows to military hospitals as far away as Iraq and Afghanistan. Her efforts are recognized through the letters she has received from patients and family members who are grateful for a caring touch. These pillows are a source of comfort, joy, and hope. For Janice, making pillows for her patients was a way to release stress after a long day of work (Smeltzer & Vlasses, 2003).

> Make creativity visible, not silent. Put into place systems and procedures that value and emphasize creativity as a priority.

Make Creativity Visible

Nurses at a long-term care facility started a program, Angels Passing By, inspired by a dying resident who lived in their facility for many years. They wanted to help the patient and her devoted husband through the dying process. The nurses placed a journal at her bedside and placed an angel on the cover of the journal and outside her door. The symbols represented how the staff saw nurses as angels of mercy who were always visible. Nurses placed many comfort care items at the patient's bedside and were prepared to put all the comfort measures they had learned in nursing school to practice. Staff members who cared for her wrote their name and date in the journal with a message or a prayer. This was the staff's way of letting her and her husband know that someone was always watching her. After her death, the staff realized the magnitude of their initiative and continued the program. Now each dying resident of the facility receives a pre-made angel cart that includes a journal, comfort items, and angel logo (Smeltzer & Vlasses, 2003).

Creative Nursing

As frontline leaders, nurses know what works best and what doesn't work for their patients. They use their expertise and innovative thinking to find solutions to problems that are unconventional or unheard of. Nurses identify their role as provider and share many moments of their patients' lives through nursing interventions. These moments of interactions, sensitivity, kindness, and generosity shared by nurses and their patients become an unforgettable part of our memory and the patients' history. It is this exchange of experiences that is marked by attributes of a creative act. They can only be reflected upon and not shared again. Creative nurses are nurses who have the capacity to ask new questions, seek new answers, create new standards, and see what others see, but in a different way. Creativity exists in all of us, and it requires time, energy, support, discipline, and recognition to flourish.

Challenging Times

In baccalaureate programs, nursing students learn critical thinking skills and practical aspects of nursing. When nurses enter graduate education, they must learn to challenge ideas and adapt creative thinking skills; they learn to question the status quo.

When nurses transition from school to the bedside or from the bedside to a leadership position, challenges to their questioning and creativity arise. The new leaders are at risk of losing their creativity as they become more visible and they lead by example. Nurse leaders often work in environments bound by the rules and regulations of bureaucratic leadership that often obstruct creative solutions to problems. They are submerged in the day-to-day duties of finance, staffing, and quality improvement. They must devote time and energy to problems of productivity and crisis avoidance. Nurse leaders place great emphasis on the pragmatic and the objective.

To overcome these challenges, nurse leaders need to become creative. Creative nurse leaders use their knowledge and expertise to find innovative solutions to health care problems, challenge existing solutions, provide intellectual challenge, assess and refine their own creative skills, and reward and recognize nurses who use creative skills at the bedside or in management (Amabile & Khaire, 2008).

A key attribute of creative nurse leaders is their ability to listen for boredom. When nurses are "bored," they lose motivation to excel in their work environment. Creative nurse leaders are perceptive and tune into the nurses' boredom by intellectually stimulating them. They listen to and value nurses' ideas, giving them freedom to experiment and pursue their passions.

However, being creative is not always easy. You will likely experience resistance from those invested in the "traditional" way of doing things. Finding a place and time to be creative may be perceived as wasting time by some. Anticipate resistance, identify the sources, and develop strategies for overcoming objections before any change takes place. For example, provide frequent opportunity for conversation, discuss (and role model) how to take a creative approach to problem solving, and understand that change requires you to consistently support staff as they take small steps forward.

Creating the Creative Work Environment

Creative nurse leaders use their authority to create environments where nursing creativity can foster.

Nursing creativity flourishes in environments where nurses and nurse leaders share similar values, trusting relationships are abundant, risk taking and exchange of ideas is encouraged, and nurses have autonomy to work freely and independently. Environments that foster innovation are characterized by nurse leaders who embrace the certainty of failure, where creative ideas are rewarded, and expert nursing practice is recognized and supported. Nurse leaders can role model a creative lifestyle and make every effort to provide nurses opportunity to try new ideas, make mistakes, and begin anew (Amabile & Khaire, 2008).

Energy from Creativity

Creativity brings energy, excitement, and solutions to patient care and work environments. Staff and management can examine practices with a different perspective to improve productivity and staff satisfaction.

Creative thoughts and actions often take time and reflection, yet offer new and different solutions for problems. Assess your nursing or leadership practice, and your creative abilities in your work environment, by using the self-reflection questions at the end of this chapter. Think about times you have been creative. What results were achieved? What feelings did you have? More importantly, try to recreate the feeling, passion, and reason you had when you were creative.

So, to answer the question at the beginning of this chapter: Yes, creativity has a place—an important place—in nursing, and leaders can establish an environment where creativity is valued.

Mentee Reflections

In the process of collaborating on this chapter with the mentors, I learned what creativity means in the nursing profession and how nurses apply it in their daily practice. During this journey I reflected on my personal experiences as a bedside nurse and how I questioned the status quo and applied creative thinking to implement unconventional practice solutions. As I transitioned into a professional role, my method of thinking was often challenged because it did not always conform to the conventional standards of the professional environment. However, when placed in an environment where creativity was fostered through support from leaders and mentors, I was encouraged to tap into my creativity to find the most effective solutions. I was also able to understand the importance of having mentors who can encourage and guide mentees in creatively collaborating and developing solutions that may not follow the path of least resistance.

Self-Reflective Questions

1. Are you prepared for resistance to creative initiatives?

2. Does your organization allow time, freedom, resources, and opportunity to try new ideas rather than follow the status quo?

3. Do you embrace the inevitability of failure?

4. Can you be an appreciative audience for staff and leadership?

5. Do you promote dialogue as a way of exploring new ideas?

6. Are you listening for boredom?

7. How can you make creativity visible, not silent?

8. How do you reward creativity?

9. Do you motivate employees through intellectual and social engagement, such as regularly scheduled opportunities for conversation?

10. What are the rules and practices of your organization that fail to stimulate creativity?

Credibility

20

"Watch your thoughts, they become words. Watch your words, they become actions. Watch your actions, they become habits. Watch your habits, they become character. Watch your character, it becomes your destiny."

–Author unknown

Mentor

Siu Yin Lee, RN, MHS
Director of Nursing, National
  University Hospital (member of
  the National University Health
  System)
Associate Professor, Alice Lee
  Centre for Nursing Studies
National University of Singapore
Singapore

Mentee

Catherine Siow Lan Koh, RN,
  MSN
Assistant Director of Nursing
  National University Hospital
  (member of the National
  University Health System),
National University of Singapore
Singapore

The health care profession is one that places great value and emphasis on credibility. As an industry with ethical practices at its core, one would undoubtedly and very commonly find credibility, or its synonymous terms—integrity and honesty, weaved into the corporate statements or core values of many health care organizations. Being highly conscious of the significance of credibility in the industry we work in, I wish to relate its importance to you as a leader. Because two decades of cross-cultural comparisons indicate honesty as the top characteristic of admired leaders (Carroll, 2005), it is tremendously important that health care leaders share aspects of credibility with aspiring nurse leaders.

Credibility in Leadership

Deducing that credibility is a key ingredient of successful leadership is not difficult. General Dwight D. Eisenhower, 34th president of the United States of America, said, "To be a leader, a man must have followers.

And to have followers, a man must have their confidence." A leader is surely set for failure if his or her peers and colleagues fail to place their trust in his or her words and actions. Perhaps a cliché, but one of my guiding principles in work and life is to practice what you preach. Squaring your words with your behaviors exemplifies trustworthiness and integrity—the attributes required of a leader to succeed.

Petrick and Quinn (2000) defined integrity as consistency between word and deed, in line with a consistent set of principles, especially in the context of a temptation or challenge to the contrary. At the most fundamental level, leaders must speak of things they truly believe in, viewpoints that align with their value systems. Credible leaders cannot hope for acceptance until they speak truthfully to themselves and to others. One of the building blocks of a credible reputation is integrating speech and behavior consistently with beliefs. To act with consistency, leaders must know who they are and what they stand for, and then act within those values (Carroll, 2005). Extending this into our day-to-day actions and words, the quality of being credible is best demonstrated in a leader's willingness and courage to stand behind their words when situations threaten to compromise their core principles.

Credibility in Your Staff

Besides building credibility in your leadership, instilling this characteristic in your staff is equally important to foster an honest and open environment within the institution, which ultimately contributes to the building of a credible organizational reputation. Behavioral hallmarks, such as honesty, ethical standards, and maintained moral principles, define workforce integrity (Strubblefield, 2005). One of the early lessons in nursing education urges ethical practice, a fundamental and integral trait of the health care profession. One of the Nurse Executive (leader) Competencies recommended by the American Organization of Nurse Executives (AONE) is the ability to build trusting, collaborative relationships with different parties involved in the patient care as they champion patient care, quality, and nursing professionalism (Chase, 1994, AONE, 2005). Nurses are entrusted with the responsibility of ensuring, to the best of their ability, a quality of life, care, and well-being befitting a patient's condition. Such a responsibility requires nurses to always be ready to play the role of the patient's advocate, and be able to communicate honestly and openly with fellow health care workers in determining the most ideal care plan for the patient. Additionally, open communication with patients throughout their care has a dramatic effect on a patient feeling in control and a part of the health care team.

Integrity in practice can also be seen in the way health care organizations deal with mistakes. Misrepresentations or mistakes by any caregiver can potentially result in fatal consequences. Does your institution emphasize the need to disclose errors? When faced with such errors, how should leaders react? An open discussion of the error, within the guidelines of state and federal law, has shown positive settlement outcomes between health care organizations and patients. That is, an organization that deals with mistakes in a transparent manner builds credibility. Increasingly, the preferred environment is one that preempts such problems from manifesting and is free of fear of reprisal (Hader, 2005), which will only be made possible by an open and honest culture upheld by an informed team of professional health care workers.

Reflections from Mentee

I am a firm believer that the behaviors and decisions of leaders must be consistent with their values and be demonstrated. A leader with conflicting and wavering behaviors will never reach his followers with his words or intentions. Kouzes (2003) aptly articulates this point: "Leadership is personal… It's about you… If people don't believe in you, they won't believe in what you say. And if it's about you, then it's about your beliefs, your values, and your principles."

Before asking others for a certain behavior, it is critical that one first sets an example and role models the behavior consistently. A leader has to adopt the habit of setting his or her example in all circumstances so that the followers are able to "assure themselves that the person is worthy of their trust" (Kouzes, 2003). Staffs are highly cognizant of what their leaders value. If a leader exalts patient-centered care but does not support or provide an environment that facilitates such care, staff may soon see "empty promises" and conclude that the leader is at best, not really serious or, at worst, an outright hypocrite (Kouzes, 2002). Staff members need to see for themselves what the leader stands for, have similar beliefs, and appreciate the leader's values. Only then will there be willing followers.

Finally, credibility should not only matter to leaders and to staff. Credibility should be present and evident in the health care organization and its processes on account of the patients receiving the care. Because patients place their utmost trust in a health care facility, its leaders, and its staff during vulnerable and weakened moments, we might reflect on and be constantly mindful of the importance of credibility in our daily lives.

Self-Reflective Questions

1. How do you reflect on decisions you have made?

2. How do your behaviors exemplify your decisions, actions, and words?

3. When do you feel most comfortable with the decisions you have made?

4. What methods do you use to justify and rationalize your decisions?

5. How do you react to policies and practices that contradict your principles?

6. If you changed your decision on an issue, how would you communicate this with those affected?

7. How do you create opportunities for building relationships or trust between you and your staff?

8. What level of importance do you place on integrity and credibility with your staff?

9. Describe the environment of a non-punitive culture that encourages reporting of mistakes and oversights?

10. What requirements are needed for your staff to function independently with a clear understanding of what you advocate and what the department/organization stands for?

Critical Thinking 21

"Great mentors tirelessly demand complete and honest analyses and accept only sound inferences and explanations, guiding insights about the world's most challenging problems. Building these critical thinking skills and dispositions is the mentor's finest gift."

—Noreen Facione

Mentor
Agnes Tiwari, PhD, RN, MSc, DN, RNT, RCNT, MCMI
Department of Nursing Studies
The University of Hong Kong
Pokfulam, Hong Kong

Mentee
Peter Lai, MNurs, BN, RN, ET
Adult ICU
Queen Mary Hospital
Pokfulam, Hong Kong

Critical thinking, a fundamental goal of higher education, is essential to expert clinical decision-making and competent professional practice. Although research shows that critical thinking can be learned and nurtured (Facione & Facione, 1997; Tiwari et al., 2006), it can also be stifled if educational or workplace environments are not conducive to its development. In this chapter, educational experiences designed by the mentor to help the mentee enhance his critical thinking are described to illustrate how the mentee's critical thinking skills have expanded.

Critical Thinking in Chinese Culture

The disposition to courageously and fair-mindedly question and seek the best possible answers is the very essence of critical thinking (Facione et al., 2009). Compared to his Western counterpart, the mentee in this chapter is likely to have different critical thinking skills and a different disposition toward critical thinking because of differing cultural, educational, and workplace contexts. Specifically, the emphasis of the Chinese culture on social harmony (Gabrenya & Hwang, 1996) may cause him to believe that asking questions and challenging assumptions is not desirable for preserving harmonious relationships. Also, coming from an examination-oriented and teacher-dominated educational system (Salili et al., 2001), the mentee may not be prepared to seek the best possible answers in a courageous and fair-minded manner.

To help the mentee become more proficient in critical thinking, a constructivist pedagogical approach, in which he actively pursues and understands the critical thinking skills of analysis, interpretation, inference, explanation, evaluation, meta-cognition, self-monitoring, and self-correction (American Philosophical Association, 1990), was used. Additionally, as an advanced practice nurse (APN) in an adult intensive care unit in Hong Kong, internationalization of his critical thinking was achieved through his diligent and persistent efforts to engage the skills in his professional practice. Two experiences that enhanced the mentee's critical thinking are highlighted. They are the use of dialectical discussion and the translation of research to practice.

Dialectical Discussion

Dialectical discussion is the use of discussion as a learning strategy (Brookfield & Preskill, 1999) in which dialectical thinking is conducted to test the strengths and weaknesses of opposing points of view (Paul & Elder, 2002). Dialectical discussion promotes the mentee's critical thinking by:

- Encouraging him to achieve a more critically informed understanding of the subject under discussion

- Enhancing his self-awareness and capacity for self-critique

- Fostering an appreciation of the diversity of expressed points of view

- Acting as a catalyst for questioning and changing rote practice

Guidelines, stated as critical thinking questions based on problems, help the mentee and his fellow discussants to question, explain, analyze, reflect on, evaluate, and theorize about the specified issues. The extent to which the mentee and his group engage in dialectical discussion is evaluated through peer review using the Holistic Critical Thinking Scoring Rubric (HCTSR) (Facione & Facione, 1994). Peer review offers the mentee a learning opportunity to rate and provide factual and objective feedback to his peers. Through the practice of dialectical discussion and peer feedback, the mentee becomes more skillful and confident in asking questions, expressing his views, conducting analyses, drawing inferences, providing justifications for his decisions, and evaluating his judgments.

Examining Policy Dialectically

Through his participation in dialectical discussions, the mentee began to question the policy on visiting hours in his workplace that restricts visiting to two hours per day. Reflecting on the fundamentals of Chinese beliefs and values, he became increasingly aware of the implications of the restricted visiting policy for the family. Specifically, when family members are prevented from staying by the bedside of the patient, they are unable to fulfill their familial duties expected of them in the Confucius tradition. Furthermore, the patient dying unattended by his or her children is a serious violation of filial piety and likely to be a permanent regret for the children.

Although the mentee understood the need for a restricted visiting policy in his intensive care unit, he was open to the possibility of a more cultural-friendly alternative. In searching for an acceptable alternative, he listened to his colleagues' suggestions. In response to those who opposed relaxing the visiting hours, he tried to see the argument from their perspectives and examined the reasons and contexts for their objections. Even when he had sound evidence to counter his colleagues' arguments, he ensured that the counter-argument was presented in a harmonious and respectful manner without making the opposition lose face. Through a series of reflective, deliberate, and analytical discussions, he patiently worked with his colleagues to find possible alternatives to the existing visiting policy. Although he, as a charge nurse, had the authority to relax the policy on special occasions, he made sure that a top-down approach was not used when making the change.

During the process, the mentee learned the importance of combining critical thinking with flexibility and cultural sensitivity. At the time of writing this chapter, the mentee has successfully introduced an alternative to the existing visiting policy based on clinical judgment conducted on a case-by-case basis. Although the more flexible option in visiting has yet to be evaluated, the following serves to illustrate how it has made a difference.

An elderly woman was admitted to the unit in a critical state. Her elderly husband, a retired lawyer, was very agitated on finding out that he would not be able to stay by his wife who was very frightened by the unfamiliar environment. This was further aggravated by the fact that their children were abroad at the time and would not be able to come home immediately. The mentee carefully considered the circumstances before making the decision to institute flexible visiting hours for the husband and daily telephone briefings for the overseas family members. The results were a more relaxed patient, a much calmer husband, and less anxious children.

Translating Research to Practice

Learning how to translate research to practice through the process of translational research has also helped the mentee to enhance his critical thinking. Translational research involves scientific investigation of methods, interventions, and variables that influence adoption of evidence-based practices by individuals and organizations to improve decision making in health care (Titler, 2004). It promotes the mentee's critical thinking by encouraging him to:

- Take an increasingly independent and self-directed role to formulate a clinical issue into searchable and answerable questions.

- Find the relevant evidence for the questions identified.

- Critically appraise the evidence.

- Select appropriate models and/or strategies for translating research evidence to clinical practice.

- Assess the implementation potential of the proposed evidence-based practice.

- Develop the evidence-based practice guidelines.

- Develop plans to implement the proposed practice and evaluate the outcomes.

- Generate and justify the basis for deciding whether to adopt or modify the proposal.

Unexpectedly, the mentee found that such skills were not only useful for translating research to practice but also for planning new educational programs when he was charged with the responsibility of planning and implementing an intensive care nursing program for nurses from China. He first developed a program team of experienced intensive care health professionals. Leading the team, he held focus group sessions with stakeholders to appraise and justify the need for the program, assess implementation potential, formulate implementation plans, and negotiate for resources. Even though the program was initially a controversial one for many of his colleagues, he was able to gain their understanding, trust, and cooperation by using the above skills. As a result, existing communication channels were enhanced and a better balance between service and trainees' needs was achieved through regular reviews. Thus, by applying the concepts of continuous monitoring and periodic evaluation borrowed from translational research, the mentee has successfully instituted a new and challenging program. During the process, he has also become more competent in the use of a reflective, deliberate, and analytical approach to decision making when articulating his suggestions and justifications to the stakeholders.

Culture and Critical Thinking

Although culture has an impact on the expression of thinking and judgment, educational mentorship can enhance the growth of critical thinking, resulting in improved clinical judgment for the benefits of the patients, their families, and the profession.

Self-Reflective Questions

1. Do you think about what the issue is before making a decision?

2. Do you have the desire to ask difficult and insightful questions?

3. Do you diligently seek relevant information when solving a problem?

4. Do you take a step back and ask yourself what you may have missed in your thinking process?

5. Do you monitor your own thinking for possible errors?

6. Do you follow reasons and evidence wherever they may lead in order to find the truth?

7. Do you reconsider or suspend judgment when you realize that perhaps the evidence that you are using is not accurate?

8. Are you honest enough to face your own personal biases?

9. Do you use an orderly approach when dealing with complex matters?

10. Would colleagues consider you a role model for asking questions and seeking the best possible answers?

22

Cultural Diversity: Integration, Spirit, and Education

"We need to use our minds, hearts, and imagination to generate images of the future, use our voice, hands, and feet to create our destiny."

—Martha Rogers

Mentor

Professor G. Rumay Alexander, EdD, RN
Director, Office of Multicultural Affairs
University of North Carolina at Chapel Hill
Chapel Hill, North Carolina, USA

Mentee

Angie Ramsey, RN, CPN
Associate Clinical Professor and Director, Office of Multicultural Affairs
University of North Carolina at Chapel Hill
Chapel Hill, North Carolina, USA

Diversity issues come bearing a gift. They require a deeper understanding of the universe and our place in it. Diversity beckons us to find the acceptance, self-awareness, and humility to affirm each other and create a better future for the next generations. The central issues are power-sharing, language, culture, gender, religion, sexuality, physical ability, body size, and so on. Difference—in whatever forms it takes—does not create the challenges we encounter; our judgment produces them. My mentee, Angie Ramsey, brings these lessons front and center as she gives an account of what can happen when teachable moments, whether formal or informal, are grasped and exploited.

The Gift that Keeps on Giving

When I began attending meetings for our nursing shared governance diversity council, I was intimidated by the task before me: co-chair of a council of nurses from different backgrounds with different ideas about diversity and the role of a diversity council. Dr. Alexander attended our meetings as an advisor. By sharing some of her challenges and experiences, and engaging us in dialogue regarding diversity, she quickly helped us create a safe environment and cohesive group with a common goal. More importantly, she affirmed for us the enormity and importance of creating a more culturally relevant environment for not only our colleagues but for those we serve. I remember thinking, "What a gift!"

Recently, I was participating in an exercise on diversity with our council that examined stereotypes and first impressions. This is when I received the second gift. While writing down my responses, I had a moment of self-awareness that took me by surprise. I looked up and made eye contact with Dr. Alexander. I could tell from the way she looked at me that she knew what I was thinking and wasn't going to let me off the hook. In her silence, I could hear her saying, "Ask the question!" So, I did. "What if the first thing we notice about someone is their gender, or their race, or their ethnicity? What does that mean?" The lesson I learned that day was that diversity is a process, a life-long commitment to self-awareness, openness, and letting go.

Whether I'm taking care of my patients, interacting with my co-workers, or orienting a nurse, I now focus more on commonalities than differences and search for ways to be more accepting and inclusive. I am thankful for the mentors of our profession. They give us hope and inspire us, through leadership, to help remove the inequities of our world and to be, as Dr. Alexander would say, "less about health care and more about health caring." That's the gift that keeps on giving.

Courageous Dialogues

We do not spend nearly enough time asking the questions and holding the courageous dialogues that will propel us to a preferred future where oppression does not flourish and differences are accepted without fear. Both of these acts are deceptively simple yet often avoided. We are dependent on language—our choice of words—to help us ask the questions begging to be asked, to convey a lived experience or to consider that multiple realities can and do exist simultaneously. Often, it seems words fall short. Poetry, paintings, music, dance, theatrical performances, or movies can give insight and voice to that which eludes us as comprehensible (Van Manen, 1990). A truth can be manifested through the arrangement of the words but can also be found beyond words. African American, Lorrie Davis-Dick, in her insightful poem "Dance Professor Dance" demonstrates how this can be accomplished. She reminds us that success and achievement are neither race or gender specific goals. They are the desires of all humanity.

Dance Professor Dance

Professor you don't know me but I am sure that you have seen me around.
Who am I? What do I look like? Well that's not important right now.
I am truly amazed by all of your certifications and nursing degrees.
I see you each day as I sit and listen attentively to you speak.
Boldly I begin to think, that may be me someday.
A prolific nurse educator with diverse knowledge, flare, and no-nonsense ways.

Professor you don't know me but I am sure that you have seen me around.
Who am I? What do I look like? Well that's not important right now.
At first, it seemed that you wanted me here but as time passed, it became
     crystal clear.
Today when I approach you, I feel instantly rejected.
I start to think no, this cannot be true of all of you.

Professor you don't know me but I am sure that you have seen me around.
Who am I? What do I look like? Well that's not important right now.
I sit in your class day to day and we have even stood side-by-side.
I make no excuse for my silky caramel complexion, long black wavy hair or
     even my urban style.
The grades I earn speak for themselves and my nursing skills are always
     above the rest.
It's true I know what you see in me is not your vision of the trailblazing
     nurse of the 21st century.

Professor you don't know me but I am sure that you have seen me around.
Who am I? What do I look like? Well that's not important right now.
Please remember that I not only see you as a disseminator of nursing knowledge.
Unfortunately, what you cannot see is that you truly are the mentor and I
     the mentee.
Together we dance invisibly.

Professor you don't know me but I am sure that you have seen me around.
Who am I? What do I look like? Well that's not important right now.
I too represent the future and plan to become the new Nightingale, Peplau, Roy, or
     the prolific Wykle.
Now please do not be ashamed that you overlooked my talent, worth, and skill.
Do not look back at the past.
Look ahead to change your perspective this academic year.

Once again there I will sit in your class listening to you teach.
Professor let's not again begin our mentor-mentee dance invisibly.

—Lorrie Davis-Dick

Value of Diversity

All encounters are cultural encounters that provide, if we are paying attention, opportunities to teach. Significant insights occur about the experience of difference when democratic dialogue, inquiry, and mindful, reflective practices are employed. Without diversity, we limit our intellectual and social development. We limit our visions for the best future possible. We are all instruments of hope. It takes courage to create a caring society, which is the spirit of nursing. Acts characterized by inclusion, justice, and appreciation of diverse individual knowledge can support changing the environment for the ultimate success of all.

Self-Reflective Questions

1. When you make decisions, do you include people of different lived experiences in the discussions?

2. When did you operate on assumption rather than fact?

3. What questions would you like to ask of someone whose culture is different from mine? Why have you been afraid to ask these questions? What conditions are needed for you to ask these questions?

4. Did you ask to be forgiven when it became apparent that you unintentionally hurt someone?

5. When did you demand respect from another but failed to give it?

6. Because multiple realties coexist and thus provide a context for our actions, what can you do to support the creation of a welcoming, inclusive, and trusting environment?

7. If diversity is a priority, what does it take to treat it like other priorities?

8. How can you be more sensitive to the perspectives of others?

9. Think about a conversation you had with someone you did not trust. Why did you not trust them? How congruent was the conversation with what you were thinking?

10. How have you demonstrated your commitment to diversity and inclusion?

23

Customer Focused:
Delivering Care They Want and Need

"Nursing is one of the few things one can do to earn a living that really does offer hope for a meaningful life."

—Leah Curtin

Mentor
Franklin A. Shaffer, EdD, RN, FAAN
Executive Vice President, Cross Country Healthcare
Chief Nursing Officer, Cross Country Staffing
Founder and Chief Learning Officer University Cross Country
Boca Raton, Florida, USA

Mentee
Carol A. Tuttas, MSN, RN, CNA, BC
Clinical Liaison and Interview Services Manager, Cross Country Staffing
Boca Raton, Florida, USA

Patients have developed from passive recipients of information and care into eager online researchers and active participants in care plans. Hospital transparency and increased access to information technology have empowered patients to "shop" online to help them decide which facility offers the best care. The recent addition of the Hospital Consumer Assessment of Healthcare Providers and Systems (HCAHPS) to public reporting re-defined "best care" to include patients' perceptions of the care they have received. Patients have transformed into consumers and customers.

The health care staffing industry contributes to the provision of professional services to patient consumers/customers in a vast array of health care facility settings. The direct consumers/customers of the staffing firm are two-fold: health care facilities and health care professionals. This competitive sales/business environment must be tempered and regulated by a strong nursing presence to ensure compliance and quality to satisfy both sets of consumers, and ultimately, the patient consumer/customers whose needs drive the health care system. Nursing leaders in the health care staffing industry are presented with challenges unique to the business. A nurse with leadership experience in health care facility settings brings highly valuable skill sets and experiences to the table, but must be prepared for a transition to a sales/business environment. Such nurse leaders can transition to the health care staffing industry more effectively and are more likely to be retained, when a relationship with a mentor, seasoned in the industry, is built and sustained.

Setting the Scene

Cross Country Healthcare Inc. is a public-traded, for-profit, human resources management company that owns 10 distinct health care businesses. One division is Cross Country Staffing (CCS), a leading staffing firm providing temporary nurses for 13-week assignments to more than 3,000 medical centers in the United States. Cross Country employed Dr. Franklin Shaffer in February of 1996 as the vice president for education and professional development. He founded Cross Country University (CCU), a non-degree granting, corporate university serving nurses and allied professionals primarily working for Cross Country Healthcare. In 1997, the American Nurses Credentialing Center's Commission on Accreditation—the gold standard for continuing education (CE) for nurses—accredited CCU as a provider of continuing education (CE).

Offering practical programs that focused on jump starting professional skills, CCU helped Cross Country grow dramatically. With that growth, Dr. Shaffer had to ensure that each business entity—and each professional—had the right people with the right skills at the right time. Fortunately, the combined networks of Cross Country attracted several excellent nurses to CCU, including Carol Tuttas. Carol and Dr. Shaffer each discuss the mentorship experience to illustrate the relationship from both perspectives.

One Such Nurse: Mentor's Perspective

Carol Tuttas joined CCS in 2006 as the professional services educator (later to become a clinical liaison and interview services manager) with a high level of competence and solid foundations in clinical and managerial nursing. Our challenge was to transfer the knowledge and experience she gained in the hospital arena into the corporate world, specifically into the staffing segment. Carol's clinical and managerial experience—and her desire to learn and make a difference—served her well in the transition. Her management experience prepared her to deal with staffing, scheduling, and financial management—essentials in the staffing and corporate worlds. Her clinical experience prepared her to function efficiently and effectively when centering on the business of travel nursing.

As her mentor, I collaborated with Carol to put her expertise to effective use in the company. Carol had a natural curiosity and desire to learn about the corporation. Many customers want to eliminate the need to use our services, but cannot; other customers see a helpful solution to seasonal demands. Both perspectives present unique challenges in meeting customers' expectations—especially for someone new to both the industry and the firm.

The next paragraphs describe how the mentor/protégé relationship served to facilitate Carol's adaptation to the sales/business environment while preserving, recognizing, developing, and utilizing the valuable skills she brought to the table.

Effective and frequent communication between us helped Carol address the communication challenges of the business. The staffing firm is set up to communicate "virtually," with fellow employees, health care facilities and health care professionals across the nation, mainly via information technology and telephonic means. Coming from an acute care nursing management background, Carol had been most familiar and comfortable with face-to-face communication with staff, patients, families, and colleagues. Carol's love for writing provided an excellent platform to build on and exposed her to publishing for the purpose of educating and developing internal employees and traveling health care professionals. Through our frequent (often informal but in-depth) discussions about her new role and its potential, Carol learned to provide a presence and voice for our travel nurses by encouraging them to write and publish with her—a very successful initiative.

Navigating Transition: Mentee's Perspective

My successful transition from 10 years of acute care and long-term care nursing management to corporate RN educator and clinical liaison in the health care staffing industry was facilitated through mentorship.

Beginning in 2006, Franklin Shaffer (chief nursing officer and chief learning officer for CCS) helped me navigate through and adapt to this new and very different environment. Dr. Shaffer developed a methodical and comprehensive on-boarding (orientation) schedule designed to familiarize me with the many facets of the business. Perhaps one of the biggest adjustments for me was the broadening mindset adjustment from acute care nurse manager to corporate nurse. The health care staffing industry is a sales-driven business with some unique (sales/business) goals and indicators in addition to those I was accustomed to in direct patient care nursing management settings.

That being said, the core product of the health care staffing industry is still clinical in nature. Dr. Shaffer acclimated me to the means by which the quality of the contract staff supplied by the company is measured, recorded, monitored, and maintained in a virtual setting for thousands of CCS health care professional employees across the nation. This process and the daily decisions made as a result of it influences the satisfaction of health care facility clients perhaps more than any other aspect of the service the firm provides. In frequent discussions and interactions with Dr. Shaffer, we assessed and evaluated as a team what my learning needs were, what resources I needed to gain the necessary insight, policy knowledge, and technical skills to succeed in this aspect of the business, and what progress I had made. Now, in the role of the clinical liaison, I enjoy daily opportunities to interact directly with the health care professionals of CCS, to listen to their feedback, provide coaching, guidance and counseling, and to evaluate placement suitability to name just a few of the corporate responsibilities in the scope of my role.

Hospital cultures vary greatly, and contract staff must learn to be flexible and adaptable in order to succeed. In my role as a clinical liaison in the corporate headquarters, I apply my nursing management and clinical background to address concerns of the nurses in the field, offer coaching and guidance pertaining to the adaptation skills unique and so critical to travelers. I often refer travelers to CCU for CE products to enhance their knowledge base. Dr. Shaffer facilitated the application of my existing nursing management skills and background to build and maintain favorable "distance relationships" with CCS customers (contract staff and nursing management contacts at health care facilities across the nation). The mentoring process (the career developing relationship I continue to enjoy with Dr. Shaffer, to provide guidance, information-sharing, and support) has broadened my awareness of the diversity of customer needs, organizational cultures, and expectations across the country relative to the health care staffing industry. Much attention is directed to the evaluation of nurses' profiles and the necessary skills specific to traveling professional nurses in order to facilitate correct placement decisions, and success for both set of clients as well as the firm.

The successful transition from acute care hospital nursing management to the unique role of a corporate nurse can be attributed to the continued attention and interest of my committed mentor. The mentorship experience helps me adapt to the goals, strategies, processes, and relationship-building techniques within an environment where a multifaceted, nationwide customer base is not only served from a distance, but is characterized by the need to meet progressively intensifying customer service expectations.

Hospitals and health care providers require impeccable service and expect health care professionals from a staffing firm to meet the customer service demands of their specific patient and health care team populations. The corporate nurse leader in the health care staffing industry contributes significantly to both the quality and safety of care delivered at the bedside in addition to the satisfaction of both health care facilities and health care professionals, and to the company's bottom line. Mentorship, as I have experienced it, has undoubtedly and notably contributed to my development as a corporate nurse leader in the unique world of health care staffing.

Self-Reflective Questions

1. How might this mentee's experience have differed in the absence of a committed, experienced nurse leader as a mentor?

2. What characteristics of a mentee transitioning into a new role or career field contribute most favorably to the outcome of the mentorship?

3. How might the development of a nurse leader differ in the corporate setting of health care staffing, as opposed to direct care settings?

4. Why is nursing leadership development essential at the corporate level of the health care staffing industry?

5. How do corporate nurse leaders in the health care staffing industry influence the delivery of quality health care at the bedside?

6. What might be the effect if corporate nurse leader mentors were absent from the health care staffing industry?

7. Which corporate leadership roles at health care staffing firms should be performed by RNs? Why?

8. What is the minimum preparation (formal education and nursing experience) that should be required to qualify for nurse leadership positions in corporate health care staffing firms?

9. What characteristics should a nurse seek when selecting a nurse-leader mentor in a corporate setting?

10. How and when does the mentee become established and distinguished as an individual nurse leader through mentorship in the corporate setting?

Data Collection: Care Model Validation

24

"So what makes more sense? Increasing the number of nurses on a shift, or doubling the amount of time nurses spend in direct patient care? Both scenarios may result in nurses spending more time in direct patient care, but reducing inefficiencies and redesigning processes of care is not only less costly, but will also improve nursing morale and satisfaction."

—Pat Rutherford

Mentor

David W. Byres, RN, BA, BScN, MSN
Vice President, Clinical Programs
Chief of Professional Practice & Nursing
Providence Health Care
Adjunct Professor, University of British Columbia School of Nursing
Vancouver, British Columbia, Canada

Mentee

Darlene MacKinnon, RN, BScN, MHA
Director, Clinical and Non-Clinical Programs
Providence Legacy Projects
Providence Health Care
Vancouver, British Columbia, Canada

Maximizing the efficiency and effectiveness of the health care team is essential in the delivery of safe, quality care. It is also integral to the functioning of the hospital and is dependent on a care delivery model that has the appropriate number and types of health care professionals who are able to work effectively and efficiently within the organization (Hendrich, Chow, Skierczynski & Zhenqiang, 2008).

Reports of increased workloads by staff combined with growing workforce shortages across most of the health care disciplines has been the impetus for many health care organizations to explore different care delivery approaches in an attempt to get the *right* model.

Care Model Redesign

For Providence Health Care (PHC), the right model would allow for safe, quality care by a team of dedicated health care professionals (HCPs) who feel valued and respected. PHC leaders realized that this model might differ across acute care and specialty areas. Thus, they began their journey toward care model redesign by implementing collaborative practice between RNs and LPNs in the acute medical and surgical units. The process across all sites began in 2008 and is expected to conclude in early 2010. The identified goals of collaborative practice were to:

- Optimize scope of practice for RNs and LPNs.

- Utilize a patient acuity scoring system.

- Redesign patient assignment and care processes on units.

Data Collection

To identify the *right* care delivery model, PHC leaders believed they needed to understand how their HCPs were working. To do this, they embarked on an observational study aimed at gaining an understanding of the components of the clinical work related to direct care activities, caregiver movement, and communication between HCPs. The goal of the communication and movement analysis was to estimate the extent to which care unit layout hampers communications (between HCPs) by categorizing and quantifying communication patterns among caregivers on the inpatient study units. Subsequent data collection was directed at the type and categories of care that were occurring. Data was also generated on the population served on the unit.

Direct observational studies were completed on four inpatient units. The study units were a 25-bed surgical unit, a 25-bed medical, clinical teaching unit, a 57-bed medicine unit, and a 37-bed geriatric medicine/rehabilitation/family practice unit. Data was collected by using handheld PDAs, that allowed the observers to track location and activities of the HCPs. All activities were time-stamped. The observational study included HCPs: RNs, LPNs, unit clerks (UCs), social workers (SWs), occupational therapists (OTs), physiotherapists (PTs), and physicians.

To analyze the data in a constructive manner, PHC leaders identified seven initial questions:

1. How do caregivers spend their time?

2. Where do caregivers spend their time?

3. How do caregivers communicate?

4. Where do caregivers communicate?

5. Who talks to whom?

6. How do caregivers document?

7. Where do caregivers document?

Transforming Care

The next step for PHC was using the findings of the observational studies as the preliminary data for the transformational work of nursing practice care changes. PHC leadership adopted Rutherford, Lee, & Grelner's (2004) Transforming Care at the Bedside (TCAB) model as their framework for care model redesign. Launched in 2003 with the Institute for Healthcare Improvement and the Robert Wood Johnson Foundation, TCAB:

- Engages direct care staff and leaders at all levels of the organization in quality improvement.

- Uses high leverage changes that result in achieving one or more design targets in pilot areas that are then spread through the medical-surgical units of the organization. Uses an All-Teach-All-Learn model for participants.

PHC is now applying the TCAB principles to the 37-bed geriatric medicine/rehabilitation/family practice unit, which was part of the observational study. The staff on the unit are using the data to identify areas for improvement, and—with the guidance of leaders in professional practice, quality improvement, and change initiative—are trialing small tests of change within the Plan-Do-Study-Act quality improvement framework. To monitor changes and identify areas for improvement, the nursing staff on this unit is collecting data monthly. PTs, OTs, and SWs will soon begin participating in the data collection.

Professional practice and nursing leaders at PHC are discovering the type of clinical work that occurs and whether the provider doing the work is actually necessary based on the observational data, research literature, and the needs of the patient population. For example, are there non-nursing tasks completed by nurses that could be completed by another health care provider to increase the time nurses spend in direct care?

Design and Implementation

When the study was being designed by Darlene MacKinnon and Stantec Architecture, David Byres, vice president and chief of professional practice and nursing, stressed the importance of statistician involvement to ensure that the amount of data collected (observations) corresponded to a representative sample. This was important to ensure valid and reliable results and to maintain a high level of confidence in the data, which proved invaluable as PHC leaders presented the results to internal and external stakeholders.

The initial desire by strategic development and renewal at PHC for the observational studies was to understand how unit configuration affects HCP movement, travel time, and communication. The data gathered was used in two ways: to inform future design decisions and to identify potential opportunities and recommendations for improvement to existing unit environments. Simultaneously, David also identified the need for PHC to examine its care delivery models and recognized the opportunity to collect some detailed baseline data regarding caregiver activities. Expanding the goals of the study at the onset allowed PHC leaders to answer the questions related to designing the ideal inpatient unit and how HCPs used their time.

The HCPs on the inpatient study units were very supportive of the observational studies. Nurses especially welcomed the observers to record and report their work. Having clinical staff involved in all aspects of the design and implementation of the study was critical to gain buy-in from the staff. Additionally, a foundation of trust is instrumental in changing existing work and practice cultures. The study was implemented in a respectful, transparent manner and the research consultants followed through on promises concerning observational schedules and presenting data to the staff—essential when using the data for care model redesign. Data from our last measurement period indicates we have increased the time nurses spend with patients by 20 percent.

Lessons Learned

As a mentee working with David, the lessons have been many. David's approach is very open and honest. Individuals at all levels of the organization feel his respect and respect him for his "get things done" attitude and his ability to create a comfortable, caring atmosphere. He asks for advice and consults with nurses, allied health professionals, health care leaders, researchers, architects, and hospital administrators. David expects this approach from all participants he works with and exemplifies it in his interactions with the patients and families we serve.

As I move forward working with other groups, being open, honest, and clear ensures that leaders and frontline staff feel confident, comfortable, and trusting. Ensuring a sound methodology allows solid data integrity for answers to all the stakeholder questions. With a statistician involved through the entire study, the product is reliable. Additionally, collaborating respectfully and transparently with clinical staff members involved in the research is critical in gaining buy-in and support for the study and the potential changes to their work and practice cultures. Using this approach helps me find a model for care delivery redesign that reduces inefficiencies and process costs yet improves nursing morale and satisfaction.

Self-Reflective Questions

1. Does your organization have staffing issues specific to frontline HCPs?

2. Has your organization identified a need to examine their care delivery model(s)?

3. Do your leaders have a good understanding of how care is delivered across the different health care disciplines?

4. Does your organization know how much time HCPs spend in direct patient care?

5. Does your organization know the effect documentation time has on direct patient care?

6. How does the layout of your unit affect walking time and patient care?

7. How do HCPs communicate? Is technology that enables efficient communication between the health care team used?

8. Does your organization promote quality improvement at all levels?

9. How do you engage your staff during change?

10. Does your organization have a formal approach for supporting staff during change?

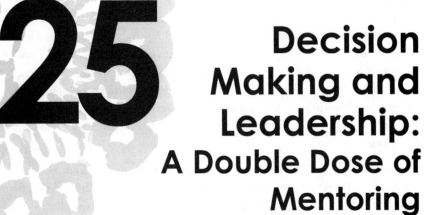

25 Decision Making and Leadership: A Double Dose of Mentoring

"You have to sleep on important decisions for at least one night. Decisions must grow and become mature."

—Maria Mischo-Kelling
(15 years experience as a leader, CNO)

"I try to look ahead and estimate the consequences. After I have made a decision, I stop thinking about it. I do not trouble myself with long drawn-out doubting."

—Karin Maechler
(3 years experience as a leader, head nurse)

Mentors
Renate Tewes, PhD
Professor for Nursing Science
  and Nursing Administration,
  Protestant University of
  Applied Science
Dresden, Germany

and

Barbara Gebert
Principal of the School of
  Nursing in Berlin
Berlin, Germany

Mentees

Maria Mischo-Kelling
Hospital CNO
Bozen, Italy

and

Karin Maechler
Student in Nursing Science &
  Nursing Administration,
  Protestant University of
  Applied Sciences
Dresden, Germany

Decision making can be seen as the heart of leadership. But what is needed to make a good decision? And how does personality affect decision making? What rules are to be followed? Dijksterhuis (2007) studied decision making in management by comparing three groups of managers. The first group decided spontaneously by gut feeling, and the second group thought about the issue repeatedly before deciding. The third group researched the issue, slept on it for three nights while working on other tasks during the daytime, and then decided according to gut feeling. The result was that the third group made the best decisions.

According to Dijksterhuis and Nordgren (2006), our conscious mind's ability to understand information is limited. Thus, collecting information first and then sleeping on it gives us time to sort data "by night" to produce a good decision. Although this method is good for making decisions about complex matters, decisions about simple issues are best tackled by conscious thought. Therefore, scientifically based rules can aid good decision making.

In their Theory of Unconscious Thought, Dijksterhuis and Nordgren (2006) explain the relationship between the quality and the complexity of a decision. For conscious thought (CT), quality varies as a function of complexity; for unconscious thought (UT), it does not.

Methods of Decision Making

Taylor (2005) researched the process of decision making in ICU nursing. The results can be generalized and are transferable into management and leadership. The four methods of decision making are

1. Decision analysis
2. Hypothetical-deductive method
3. Pattern recognition
4. Intuition

Each are discussed next, with thoughts from Maria and Karin.

Decision Analysis

Decision analysis is often used in management. It is a rational way of systematic data interpretation and offers a set of different instruments. Decision analysis often starts with measuring and modeling uncertainty and includes a cost-effectiveness analysis. Other instruments can be decision trees, clinical pathways, objective risk analysis, program evaluation, or flowcharts.

For example, a nurse director of a university hospital wanted to determine if implementing primary nursing would help to reduce turnover of his nursing staff by modeling group decision-making. First, the group listed all reasons for staff turnover, then all the reasons for staff to stay. Then the group listed the advantages and disadvantages of primary nursing. When they found out that nurses have more room for decision making and range of possibilities (autonomy) with primary nursing, they knew implementing it would be the perfect answer. The most important element in primary nursing is "the clear, individualized allocation of responsibility for decision-making about patient care" (Manthey, 1980: 32). Compared to team nursing, the autonomy of nurses grows in primary nursing. Autonomy is strongly correlated to job satisfaction in nursing (Blegen, 1993; Mrayyan, 2003; Kramer & Schmalenberg, 2003).

Hypothetical-Deductive Method

With this method, data is collected and a hypothesis is built. Then, more data is collected and the hypothesis is changed until a decision is made.

For example, a nurse team member is late again. The team leader comes to the hypothesis that this nurse is unreliable and also irresponsible toward the other team members. The head nurse collects more data about the lack of punctuality and talks to the nurse. The decision is made that the next time this nurse misses shift report the head nurse will report this to the nurse manager (Tewes, 2008).

Pattern Recognition

Pattern recognition is defined as grasping the whole situation at once—not just an aspect of it. This process of awareness can be analytical or intuitive.

For example, a nurse director becomes aware that the board of management has more meetings than usual without inviting her and, thus, she gets less information about the meeting results. Because she already experienced such a situation, she recognizes the pattern from past experiences—her company plans to sell the hospital or will merge with other partners.

Intuition

Intuition, a process of unconscious decision making, does not follow linear thinking. Intuition is often quick, easy, and you can validate it. The knowledge base of intuition results from experience and pattern recognition (Easen & Wilcocksen, 1996). Dijksterhus' research (2007) shows how effectively unconscious minds can work for leaders.

For example, the CEO of a new hospital who has to decide what company she wants to contract with for orthopaedic equipment asks the two companies in town for offers. Although one is the most cost-effective, she decides by intuition to choose the other one. It turned out that her decision was good because the chosen partner offered such good service that her patients were very pleased.

Decision Making as a Process

The process of decision making includes temporal stages or phases (Carroll & Johnson, 1990; Bandman & Bandman, 1988). Before the goal is reached, the decision maker moves through the process to compare and analyze related information. The process of decision making is purposeful and goal directed (Grohar-Murray & DiCroce, 1997).

Grohar-Murray and DiCroce (1997) described six stages for decision making in leadership and management in nursing, which are outlined in Table 1.

Factors that influence the decision-making process are knowledge, experience, stress, role models, and values. Grohar-Murray and DiCroce (1997) also described decision making in nursing as "teamwork that calls for both cooperation and coordination. It is not sufficient to agree on a common goal, but each participant must also understand the plan. Coordination of group efforts provides stability in the face of differing opinions about the issue."

While I've known Maria Mischo-Kelling for 13 years, Karin Maechler became my student only 4 years ago. Maria is the CEO of a large health care company in Italy, and Karin the head nurse of a medical department. When it comes to questions about decision making in their leadership positions, I am functioning as a coach. What I practice mostly in coaching is asking questions; this helps my mentees to find their answers themselves.

Putting Decision Making to Practical Use: Maria

My favorite method of decision making is to make a draft and give it to my leaders so that we can discuss the issue on a deeper level and are well prepared for a decision. The advantage of this discussion is to have different perspectives so that all can be engaged in finding a consensus.

Table 1   **Process of decision making.**

1. Identify participants	2. Gather pertinent facts	3. Generate alternative decisions
Determine qualified decision makers. Base selection on: • Nature of issues • Experience • Knowledge • Interest • Personal traits that foster group efforts	Employ fact-finding techniques. Survey others. Remember that each fact is a premise and that decisions are a combination of multiple premises.	Use techniques that cultivate creativity. Don't judge ideas and aim for quantity of options. Entertain what seems ridiculous. Look for variations in ideas.

4. Predict outcomes	5. Select best alternative	6. Plan for managing consequence
Recognize desired and undesired outcome of each alternative. Concentrate on quality. Form list determining undesirable outcomes that cannot be managed. Condense list accordingly.	Weigh the undesirable outcomes against the value of desirable outcomes of remaining alternatives. Select the best alternative.	Secure support of the whole group. Communicate to all who are affected by the decision. • Be honest about the pros and cons. • Show how the pros outweigh the cons. • Suggest ways to handle undesirable outcomes. • Offer to assist where possible.

Decision Making as Goal Setting: Karin

I always have goals for a year. One year, my aim was to achieve better cooperation between my team members. Before, everyone just worked on their own. Now my team members help each other. As a result of the good team atmosphere we have established these last few years, University of Dresden independent research has shown us to be the number one ward with less strain and less absenteeism.

Factoring Fairness into Decision Making: Karin

In her article, "Why do good people do bad things?" Leah Curtin (1996) tries to find a reason for unethical behavior in management. Organizational culture and moral intelligence influence leadership decisions. "The business environment seems to cultivate a condition of moral schizophrenia" (Nash, 1990). An organizational culture based on "hire and fire" is focused more on economic aspects than on employees' needs and carries a higher potential for unethical behavior (Tewes, 2008: 110). The moral intelligence of the leader is a factor of success in many companies (Lennik & Kiel, 2005).

Here are three different and helpful methods for leaders to improve their ethical decision making:

1. Establishing moral intelligence.

2. Reflecting their own behavior: for example, by coaching, leadership training, or counseling.

3. Establishing good communication with all levels of employees of the organization.

Magnet hospitals know how important leaders' reflection and good communication are (Laschinger et al., 2001).

Learning Experiences from the Mentees

Karin Maechler: I was curious about the research of Dijksterhuis, especially when I saw his findings and compared it with my experiences. As a rational person, I mostly try to distance myself from emotions and find my solutions by thinking over them. When reflecting on the research results from Dijksterhuis, I became aware that unconsciousness could play an important role in professional decision making in management. It is exiting news, that my intuitive part is still waiting to be discovered.

Maria Mischo-Kelling: I realized that I do a lot of unconscious decision making, and I will explain my strategies more clearly to my team in the future. I want to do more conscious decision making and take my time for reflection.

Self-Reflective Questions

1. Think about an example of a decision-making process you followed as a leader that satisfied you.

    What was the challenge?

    What influenced the process (helped or hindered)?

    What did you learn?

2. Think about a decision-making process that did not satisfy you.

    What was the challenge?

    What influenced the process (helped or hindered)?

    What did you learn?

3. What type of decision making do you prefer?

4. What are your favorite instruments in decision making?

5. To expand your skill set, what other instruments would you like to try in the future?

6. How could you develop your abilities of professional decision making?

7. If you should give advice in professional decision making for the next generation of leaders, what would this be?

Delegation Skills 26

"I have found in life that one must be visible in fighting for what one is passionate about, and hope the rest will follow."

—Claire Fagin

Mentor

María Mercedes Duran de
  Villalobos, RN, MSC
Nurse, Universidad Nacional de
  Colombia
Full Professor and Professor
  Emeritus, Universidad
  Nacional de Colombia
Bogata, Colombia

Mentee

Lorena Chaparro Díaz, RN, BSN
Nurse, Universidad Nacional de
  Colombia
DNSc Candidate, Universidad
  Nacional de Colombia
Bogata, Colombia

Transformational leadership motivates people to transform those under their supervision into independent professionals who can think critically and make assertive decisions. This type of leadership inspires followers in the search to satisfy increasingly complex needs. It also encourages stimulating relationships that contribute to the growth and development of leaders and followers, casting the leader as more of an ethical agent than a controller of action (Burns, 1978 quoted by Valiga & Grossman, 2007). In short, the leader is portrayed as a mentor who obliges others to develop leadership skills and abilities in a way that encourages their potential and affords consciously created opportunities for development.

Delegation is an important tool for transformational leadership. The National Council of State Boards of Nursing (1995) defines delegation as "The transfer of authority to a competent person to perform selected nursing tasks in a particular situation. The delegating nurse retains responsibility for the delegation." In this chapter, however, we deal with the need to address the root need for delegation. The leader cannot do everything, the leader does not know everything, the environment, with its bureaucratic foundation forces the leader to delegate, and changing paradigms creates the need for transformation.

Defining a Leader

Certain features and elements must exist if a leader is to feel comfortable. These features and elements usually are developed consciously because it is crucial to be sensitive, to be able to transmit, without words, the profound meaning involved, besides being alert to the overall benefits and striving for improvement, quality care and assistance, and quality monitoring that is well timed. Cohen (2004) proposes it is also important to decide what to delegate and to whom, how often, and why.

Delegation by Potential

The ability to delegate begins with the need to be fully conscious of the other person's potential (Feltner et al., 2008). This is crucial if responsibility is to be assigned in a way that is consistent with how that person performs best. A good leader must understand that he or she does not need to be responsible for a solution, but must constantly look for new ways to grow personally and professionally to mitigate any conflicts that might arise, such as competition with the other person (mentee) or anyone else under the leader's supervision. Another aspect of delegation is to create propitious environments for the performance of new duties and to provide constant feedback. When this philosophy is applied, the tendency is for others, including mentees, to replicate the model, either consciously or unconsciously.

The Benefits of Delegation

The ability to delegate saves time by permitting a number of processes to be undertaken at once. The result can be an opportune and effective contribution to the organization. It also allows skills to be developed simultaneously among various members of the team. This helps to create a solid group of persons to whom responsibility can be delegated. The leader must not focus on a single member of the team. The lessons of what has been accomplished and the problems encountered in each undertaking must be shared.

Several 19th century theories of leadership share the idea that leadership is related directly to personality. However, current understanding is that leadership skills and the ability to delegate at every level of professional practice need to be strengthened to constantly have the opportunity to make appropriate decisions quickly. Some nurses (Sullivan et al., 2003) claim that perfecting leadership skills—and, hence, the ability to delegate—can be done through feedback provided to a novice by an expert nurse in an environment that allows for trial and error and also constant communication with feedback.

Delegation in Nursing

Nursing practice, as a scenario for developing these skills, has been outlined within the managerial aspects of how human talent is handled in nursing services and is framed by a leadership-skill model that facilitates decisions on delegating responsibility (Sherman et al., 2007). In this model, the attributes of care are interrelated, and propitious environments are created, along with one-to-one relationships. There is time to learn and grow, to evaluate and appreciate, to encourage space or an opportunity to know one another and to share experiences, to consider the options for change if required, and to rely on other people.

Institutional policies that facilitate leadership also allow delegation skills to be developed. Delegation is not an alternative course when there is an overload (Cohen, 2001); rather, it must be regarded as a policy of the organization. The ability or capacity to delegate varies according to the nature of the environment (care, teaching, or research), the degree of possible risk to others, the capabilities of those concerned, the frequency of contact with similar situations, and the extent to which other persons are involved (colleagues-patient-family) (Fisher, 1999). In a policy sense, delegation also contributes to one generation taking over for another: for example, an expert nurse leaves his or her legacy to a novice, who surely will be the one to maintain a school of thought. Delegation is something done consciously.

Delegation in nursing has become a necessary skill, given the wide variety of roles in the professional environment. The nursing professional acts as director, teacher, communicator, technical adviser, facilitator, and source of support and supervisor, in addition to performing many other functions that emerge from progress in science and technology. This necessitates different levels of training, which must be consistent with the person's plans, characteristics, and skills for the job.

In terms of actually delegating responsibility to the mentee, some of the aforementioned elements are present. The academic environment that a university offers—particularly research and academic projects, such as care for chronic patients and caregivers—has been a motivating scenario. The mentee's personal experience includes professors who take on the task of mentoring a nurse with basic leadership skills, such as responsibility, devotion, dedication, and efficient and opportune performance of an assigned task. Postgraduate training is, perhaps, the best tool to empower those skills, inasmuch as the complexity of acquiring this knowledge is progressive yet practical when it comes to assigning a specific task that also becomes more complex in duty and responsibility, but always with the mentoring of a tutor who neither judges nor gives a grade, but provides orientation and the tools to regularly perform the task well (Cohen, 2001).

The mentor must consider the alternative possibilities of being satisfied delegating to the mentee or having poor judgment of his or her abilities, expecting outcomes impossible to reach because of poor assessment in the first place. In the process of delegation, experience shows that a mentee who initially has potential and goodwill can turn out to be superficial, with no commitment to the task. At any time, the mentor must be clear in his or her own goals and learn to perceive distractions that can result in a less-than-optimal outcome.

Personal relations and effective communication play an important role in successful delegation. To properly convey what is to be delegated, the leader must show empathy toward the person to whom a task is being given. This is complemented with synchronization in cognitive, affective, and intuitive dimensions (Barter, 2002). The ability to delegate also becomes the cornerstone of a leader and is acquired when he is able to identify needs and the viability of resources, communicate clearly, and use motivational techniques to effectively authorize someone to perform a particular task (Barter, 2002).

How Delegation Has Benefited Me (Mentee)

My experience as a mentee, as a leader-to-be, has been through the implementation of caregivers for chronic patients program. Its Spanish name is *Cuidando a cuidadores*, which translates to Taking Care of Caregivers. This program runs along with the research line of Care for Chronic Patients and Their Families (Barrera et al., 2006).

I began my participation with the group as an undergraduate student, helping as an instructor in several curricular and noncurricular activities, but mainly working as a research assistant. Later, my participation as a research collaborator in a master's program and during the last four years as a doctoral student have given me more and more responsibilities, and the growth opportunities have increased as well. These challenges have increased in complexity but have given me the skills and competency to guide students, patients, and caregivers.

The opportunity to place myself in different situations in nursing practice, always with my mentors close to me, has improved my ability to help others—patients, students interested in research, and faculty who trust my commitment and dedication. I only hope to be able to pass this philosophy to many students, nurses, and caregivers.

Self-Reflective Questions

1. What is your motivation for being a leader?

2. To be a transforming leader, do you need to acknowledge and understand the needs of your practicum arena? If so, how can you do that?

3. How can you understand the potentialities, strengths, and limitations of the people you choose to work with?

4. What sort of strategies do you use to select your team members and to encourage them to recognize, develop, and use their abilities and skills?

5. How do you delegate functions among your team members?

6. What should be your reaction or attitude about the success or failure of one of the members of your team?

7. How are personal and professional values important for both the mentor and the mentee?

8. How does your attitude as a mentor motivate the mentee to receive guidance and gain knowledge?

9. How can you gain insight into others so you can be a better leader?

10. As a mentor or mentee, are you prepared to receive feedback from others in an attentive and effective way?

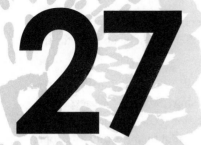

27

Diversity

"We are only on the threshold of nursing. In the future, which I shall not see, for I am old, may a better way be opened! May the methods by which every infant, every human being, will have the best chance of health—the methods by which every sick person will have the best chance of recovery, be learned and practiced!"

—Florence Nightingale

Mentor
Jeanette Ives Erickson, RN, MS, FAAN
Senior Vice President for Patient Care
Chief Nurse, Massachusetts General Hospital
Boston, Massachusetts, USA

Mentee
Deborah Washington, RN, MS
Director of Diversity
Massachusetts General Hospital
Boston, Massachusetts, USA

According to the Sullivan Commission's 2004 report, African Americans, Latino Americans, and Native Americans make up 25% of the U.S. population but only 9% of the nation's nurses. Increasing diversity in the health care workforce has been identified as a key factor in reducing health care disparities. The Institute of Medicine's report (2004), *In the Nation's Compelling Interest: Ensuring Diversity in the Health Care Workforce*, called national attention to this issue. Advancing an organization's diversity agenda requires commitment and teamwork. This chapter focuses on the mentoring relationship as it relates to this important work.

The word "mentor" has deep historical roots. Today, mentoring requires new attributes because individuals of background and ethnicity that is diverse—like me (Deborah), an African American—are part of the equation. A different social ideology now opens doors through which I can step. The time-honored concept of one person benefiting from the experience, wisdom, and professional acumen of another should be updated for the diverse workforce of which I am a member.

Historically, mentoring, whether intentionally or unintentionally, has fostered the status quo. It rarely involved relationships of dissimilar backgrounds or worldviews. Mentoring put a career on track for success. Mentees gained access to educational preparation that placed them in the proximity of people of influence. Talent garnered attention for up-and-comers. For the marginalized, though, education was frequently a financial challenge, and talent wasn't enough to overcome all the other considerations. The first cracks in the "glass ceiling" that traditionally hindered individual progress were impacted by a greater social unrest that led to legal action. Such steps focused attention on the rights of individuals who wanted to "win" at work without social discrimination blocking their path. I am heir to those actions and social movements. Issues of social justice have influenced health care in many ways, and the emergence of a diverse, professional workforce is but one illustration.

The Benefits of a Diverse Workforce

The implications of mentoring on a diverse workforce are yet to be fully recognized. The more examples we have of inter-ethnic mentoring, the more comprehensible the unexplored becomes. Individuals from marginalized groups seldom have a strong presence in the organizational culture. Lack of a critical mass and uncertainty about inclusion are difficult barriers to overcome for individuals who do not conform to the status quo. The introduction of social differences to an organizational culture in the forms of ethnicity, sexual orientation, and country of origin create an expanded new workforce. The means by which workplace inclusion is accomplished depends upon leadership. My mentoring relationship is a case in point.

An Effective Mentor Sees No Barriers

An effective mentor is a trusted teacher who passes on skills and knowledge and also teaches good judgment without dominating the relationship nor requiring the mentee to work in his or her shadow. My mentor exhibited these critically important qualities. My role as director of diversity is the first of its kind in the organization in which I work. There was no roadmap; I was a novice leader in an organizational structure that included clinical directors, associate chief nurses, and administrative leaders. The role was daunting for someone who had thought of herself as "just a staff nurse."

My mentor neither tried to move me from my personal or cultural context nor let any aspect of my identity get in the way of teaching me organizational savvy and helping me build a social network. An environment conducive for development was structured to include self-awareness programs and leadership courses. I was given every opportunity to demonstrate what my role contributed to the team. I was never made to feel that my position was a sidebar to the overall work of the leadership team.

I viewed my mentor's language as her instrument of connection. The language she chose guided me along the way to attain my goals and dreams. When she wanted to encourage me to do or think about something, she said, "It would be important to . . ." or "I think this would be good for you." As the recipient of her feedback, I have never felt manipulated or uncomfortable. Her feedback is always supportive and strengthening.

From the Mentor: The Goals Supersede Boundaries

I (Jeanette) have been fortunate to be surrounded by strong and giving mentors throughout my life. During my career, I had mentors whose passion and lessons shaped me as a person and informed my clinical and leadership practice. As someone who has benefited greatly from mentorship, I feel that it is not only a privilege but also a duty to mentor others.

My mentee and I became partners looking to change our organization and profession. Our conversations were of great importance. We shared a common goal and had common values. Together, we wanted to build a multicultural workforce that mirrored our diverse patient population. We knew that we wanted to address health disparities and could advance both agendas by addressing what was important for every person.

My mentee has become a trailblazer. When she assumed the role of director of diversity nearly 15 years ago, "diversity" was an unfamiliar concept at our institution. Through her inspiring vision and steadfast commitment, diversity today is an integral part of our culture—prominently reinforced in the hospital's recently revised mission statement. She has led initiatives to promote diversity within the workforce, translate cultural competence into practice, and engage the Massachusetts General Hospital (MGH) community in frank conversations. She taught us that to avoid becoming victims, individuals need training, education, coping strategies, and positive role models. Along the way, she cautioned us about not letting our diversity efforts become "window-dressing."

Despite all that I have tried to pass along to my mentee, she in turn has taught me great lessons. I recall her saying, "When a Caucasian person goes into a hospital knowing she will receive the highest quality care, and a minority individual goes into the same hospital worried she will receive less than adequate care, something is wrong with the health care system." I felt compelled to act.

Just as Patricia Benner (1984) applies the Dreyfus brothers' (1980) "skill-acquisition theory" to describe clinical nurses' advancement from novice to expert, I find this is an invaluable framework with which to view my mentee's advancement. I have seen her transition from a highly competent staff nurse to a director. Over time, through lessons, listening, and inquiry, she has emerged as a great teacher, coach, and change agent.

Her contributions are far-reaching, innovative, heartfelt, enduring, and visible throughout our hospital and beyond our walls. She has embedded diversity into our cultural DNA, and components of her work are replicated nationwide. Here are some of the tangible ways in which she has excelled:

- **Promotes culturally competent care:** Facilitation of an 8-hour, interactive culturally competent care curriculum program offered monthly to staff and leadership.

- **Creates opportunities to celebrate diversity:** Launching the African American Pinning Ceremony, which recognizes the contributions of African American employees in fostering a positive and open organizational culture. This is a powerful tradition of community sharing and healing.

- **Establishes pipeline programs:** Programs supporting people from diverse backgrounds to pursue and/or advance a career in health care. One such program is the Hausman Student Nurse Fellowship, in which fellows have the opportunity to work with a minority mentor, while developing essential skill sets needed to thrive in the workplace.

- **Initiates innovation programs:** Foreign-born nurses supporting foreign-educated nurses with mentorships to facilitate the achievement of career goals. For example, studying for licensure, transition into the workforce, and identifying the best work environment for their individual goals and aspirations.

- **Fosters community outreach:** Led a team that created a wallet-sized "Basic Medical Card" for distribution at a New Bostonian event to help new immigrants navigate language and other barriers to accessing health care. The U.S. State Department commended the team on this work and now distributes the card to newly arrived immigrants nationwide.

Nothing, however, is more gratifying than knowing my mentee as a person, friend, and colleague. She offers a wonderful balance of admirable traits—she is driven and determined, humble and light-hearted, serious with a rich and ready humor, and scholarly but a true listener. She is an eager student of life.

Self-Reflective Questions

1. In what way does your team reflect the guidance of your leadership regarding inclusion?

2. What organizational conventions have been changed because of nursing commitment to diversity?

3. How does attention to diversity inspire others to make uncommon connections with a potential mentee?

4. What perceptible evidence indicates that inter-ethnic dyads are unsurprising in your organization?

5. Why is mentoring a multicultural, multilingual, multiethnic workforce vital to the future of nursing?

6. What competencies are necessary for a mentor preparing a leader to function in a U.S. health care system with a proliferating global perspective?

7. Why is a focus on diversity in mentoring relationships well timed for attention to such issues as health disparities, competence in care, health reform, and the nursing shortage?

8. What are the narrative themes in diversity-based mentoring relationships that inform the novice-to-expert paradigm?

9. What microcultural rules of your organization are made more apparent by a diversity-based mentor/mentee plan for career success?

10. What is the proportional representation of diversity of people whom you have helped as a nurse leader and led others to do the same?

Empowerment

28

"You can buy a man's time, you can buy a man's physical presence at a certain place, you can even buy a measured number of skilled muscular motions per hour or day. But you cannot buy enthusiasm, you cannot buy initiative, you cannot buy loyalty, and you cannot buy the devotion of hearts, minds, and souls. You have to earn these things."

—Clarence Francis

Mentor
Gilda Pelusi, PhD, MS, RN
Tutor and Teaching Professor at
  School of Nursing
Università Politecnica delle
  Marche
Italy

Mentee
Dania Comparcini, RN
Clinical Nurse
Hospital Ospedali Riuniti
  Umberto I Ancona
Italy

According to Kuokkanen et al. (2007), empowerment means encouraging and allowing individuals to take responsibility for improving how they do their jobs and contribute to an organization's goals. Empowerment refers to increasing the strength of individuals and often encourages those who have been empowered to develop confidence in their capabilities. Empowerment also means leading individuals to become more autonomous in decision making (Kanter, 1993). Empowerment can also induce organizational and personal changes (Huber, 2000).

The Mentor's Perspective

My personal belief of leadership coincides with Conger and Kanungo (1988) and Kantor (1993).

Conger and Kanugo say an innovative and non-authoritarian leader is able to stimulate employees to improve their quality. The role of the leader is to give support, guidance, and encouragement during challenging moments.

Kanter highlights how people's behavior is closely related to the workplace. Situations where people can develop and increase their own power increase the likelihood of achieving organizational results.

Conger and Kanungo

Conger & Kanungo (1988) associate the concept of empowerment to self-efficacy. The leader's role is to create an environment in which collaborators develop a strong sense of efficacy to reduce their sense of powerlessness. Conger and Kanungo present four behaviors of a leader:

1. **Increases work meaning:** The leader improves collaborators' productivity through motivational reinforcement.

2. **Strengthens decisional involvement:** The leader enhances group discussion; making decisions this way is collective and is not imposed in an authoritarian manner.

3. **Facilitates goals:** The leader is in charge to provide resources to help collaborators reach goals.

4. **Reduces bureaucracy by supplying autonomy:** The leader stimulates autonomy in the organizational work process, with appropriate and incisive choices. The organizational process becomes modern and adapts to changes.

Rosabeth Moss Kanter's Theory

Rosabeth Moss Kanter is considered an expert in management theories and empowerment. Kanter theorizes that one's empowerment can be positively affected by organizational structure (Kanter, 1993). Power in this context, considered the ability to reach goals, is related to structural environmental conditions. Kanter speaks about formal and informal power sources. Formal power is legitimized by the organization, whereas informal power results from personal relations with collaborators. The necessary organizational characteristics to develop empowerment are the following:

- Leaders and collaborators offer support for a common goal and provide feedback.
- Resources for the goal's achievement are accessible.
- The possibility of professional and personal growth exists.

Leadership Behaviors That Foster Empowerment

Empowerment means enabling to act or giving ability to. Comparatively, power—being able to control others—consists in the ability to influence other people's behavior to produce determined effects. Power can take several forms (French & Raven 1968):

1. **Legitimate:** A hierarchical position inside the organization; strictly linked to the concept of authority.

2. **Reward:** Giving something in exchange for service or merit (whether good or improper).

3. **Coercive:** Issuing punishment for those who don't respect one's orders and procedures.

4. **Experience:** Knowledge of a particular ability or the mastery to solve a problem.

5. **Referent:** Using charisma and a strong ability of persuasion to influence and lead others.

Additionally, three environments that relate to power and leadership are

1. **Power over:** Control and dominion of subordinates; the instrument to maintain an order or essential value.

2. **Power with:** Collaboration and partnership; parties interpret and elaborate together. In this type of power, communication has a vital role. The purpose of the leader is to help his or her employees to make better choices and to interpret events and process conflicts.

3. **Power of:** The ability to create, to elaborate projects, and to achieve goals. The leader must have crucial personal attitudes that can guide and direct employees.

In leadership theories, more importance is given to *influence*, or the ability of a leader to affect the behaviors of the collaborators and to achieve organizational goals. Therefore, empowerment means to confer responsibility and liberty to act in a mature vision of the power, in which it evolves from an idea of having "power over" to sharing "power with." In this way, people can have control of their professional life and on the important decisions with which they are concerned.

Empowerment and Type of Leadership

The concept of leadership concerns the capacity to encourage the collaborators' self-confidence. In the literature, there emerges the concept of adaptive leadership, which allows the leader to adopt the best behavior in regard to the experience of collaborators and also the environment in which they work. This behavior improves and fosters the goal's achievements and the organization. It is, therefore, very important to understand the complexity of work conditions. In a highly professional work environment, such as nursing, it is paramount to adopt a leader who can encourage decision making, creativity, and freedom of communication (Welford 2002). Transformational leadership is considered the most adequate and coherent to the empowerment approach. Its main characteristics are the creation of a common vision, positive relationships, development of confidence, and self confidence. Bass (1985) describes four main characteristics:

1. **Charisma:** The leader can present a clear vision of the goals to be reached by obtaining confidence and respect from collaborators.

2. **Inspiration:** Through this process, the leader increases the confidence with and among collaborators, thus positively influencing their performances and enthusiasm.

3. **Intellectual stimulation:** The leader increases the focus on problems and gives a positive perspective.

4. **Individualized consideration:** The leader supports and encourages development of the team and of the individual.

The exchanges of know-how, knowledge, and experiences are tools with which to improve the quality of work as another important element of the transformational leadership.

How My Leader Empowered Me (Mentee)

Gilda has been the kind of leader who exemplifies the meaning of empowerment. She empowered me upon graduation to help me realize my thesis project (an experimental thesis regarding the psychiatric area). She has furnished me all the information I need when trying to make the most autonomous decisions possible. Above all, she understood my desire to deepen nursing research. Subsequently, she has continued to validate my potential, involving me in other projects. This has increased my self-awareness in relationship to workplace competencies. She empowered me not only by giving me the possibility to grow professionally, but she also taught me to improve the ability of analysis related to alternative choices—and at the same time, she has made me stronger and more active inside the university context.

The Relationship between Empowerment and Motivation

Several surveys have focused upon the relationship between empowerment and job satisfaction (Anderson, E.F.F., 2000). Recent studies show that managers who feel validated by an organization don't become frustrated and unsatisfied with their roles. In particular, Laschinger et al. (2001) present the relationship between structural empowerment, psychological empowerment, job strain, and satisfaction.

Structural empowerment refers to the necessary organizational character-istics that promote an empowerment approach, offer access to information and resources, and also support opportunities for professional development and growth. Psychological empowerment is defined as the attitude that the individ-uals should have to profit from the empowerment approach—a sort of logical result of the structural empowerment.

Recent studies (Lucas, et al., 2008; Manojlovich, et al. 2002; & Allison, & Laschinger, 2005) show that managers with access to strategic information about the hospital and their organizational unit have a high psychological em-powerment. This result shows the relationship between structural and psycho-logical empowerment and the capacity of the latter to increase satisfaction and to reduce job strain.

Can Empowerment Improve Nurses' Motivation?

Especially in health care systems, human resource characteristics represent the main element to ensure service quality. The health care system should, there-fore, focus its goals upon nurses' motivation. Some surveys show how job dis-satisfaction negatively influences productivity. To facilitate motivational growth, creating a work environment where individuals can develop and improve their performance while getting support to reach organizational goals is very impor-tant (Lancaster, 1985). Nurses can be motivated, giving them the possibility to grow considering their own needs and promoting their own responsibility while reducing resistance to change (Breisch, 1999) to implement organizational in-struments. My personal experience as a chief nurse taught me that implement-ing innovative organizational instruments can be done only through the in-volvement of the nurses in an environment in which everyone has the occasion to take part in its design and feel the design is part of their creation.

Mentee Comments

My experience has taught me that it is very important to have a team leader who can validate an individual's abilities and who can transmit his own knowledge to share the attainment of common objectives.

A Fundamental Process

Empowerment is a fundamental process in nursing that allows the development of human potential while increasing motivation and job satisfaction. To render everyone empowered, leaders need to be in a position to love their collaborators and to feel satisfaction in seeing them grow and develop their own potential. Giving staff responsibilities and opportunities while showing confidence in their abilities results in increased job satisfaction, commitment, and effectiveness.

Self-Reflective Questions

1. How do you share the information that concerns the organization with your collaborators, with the purpose of improving both the sense of individual responsibility and performance levels?

2. During a process of change, if your collaborators become frustrated and discouraged, how are you able to listen, and at the same time, share information?

3. How can you become better able to listen and to consider new ideas coming from your collaborators?

4. What needs to change so that you believe you have enough information to be able to influence the organization?

5. What are the goals you want to reach with your team?

6. How can you better give responsibility to your collaborators, encourage them, and validate them to promote moving from a hierarchical culture to one of empowerment?

7. How could you improve the distribution of leadership among the members of your team?

8. How do you guide your team and encourage decisional group actions?

9. How do your collaborators actively use the information given to them?

10. How can you better succeed in strengthening internal motivations to change?

Energy Crisis: Energize Your Work and Life

29

"Your first and foremost job as a leader is to raise your own energy level, and then help orchestrate the energies of those around you."

—Peter Drucker

Mentor
Laurie Shiparski, RN, BSN, MS
President, Edgework
  Institute, Inc.
Grand Rapids, Michigan, USA

Mentee
Jennifer Bishop, RN, BSN
St. Vincent's East
Birmingham, Alabama, USA

Health care is facing an energy crisis. Health care leaders and care providers are experiencing an energy drain in many settings instead of an energizing work environment. This translates to less-effective care to energy-deprived patients. Where is the energy? Where are the passion and purpose? The caring and presence? The joy and satisfaction in serving? Why are we all so tired? Is there anything we can do about it? This is a call to all health care leaders to take this energy crisis seriously and consider what we can do to address it.

Thinking about Human Energy

Jon Gordon has committed his life's work to helping us with energy management: "We are energy beings more than human beings. Einstein's $E = MC^2$ tells us that anything that is matter is composed of energy, and since we are matter, we are energy. So if we want to improve and transform our lives, we must transform our energy" (Gordon,

2006, p. 7). In physics, energy makes things happen—so do we, as energetic beings. We are powerful and have the ability to change our own energy levels as well as to affect the energy of others. It is time that we gave some intentional thought to managing our human energy because it is the key to delivering effective health care.

What We Can Do to Manage Our Energy

On a personal level, each of us can identify those behaviors that energize us. Our resilience to deal with challenges and our ability to serve others will be greater if we do the following:

- Get enough rest.

- Eat a healthy diet.

- Get appropriate exercise.

- Do things that we love to do (hobbies, nature, family, interests).

- Have a positive outlook.

- Connect with others who energize us; create a "court of support."

- Take time for ourselves each day (make breathing space).

- Learn to work with change and manage our stress related to it.

Many of us know these behaviors and want to incorporate them into our lives, but somehow we succumb to our workloads and end up with little healthy energy left. In this burned-out state, our negative energies take over, and we transfer that energy into the work place. We bring negative energy home, too, which affects our personal relationships. How can we transform our negative, heavy energy into healthy energy?

The first step is to recognize we are in this de-energizing state and make a choice to change. Then, even the smallest behavior changes can begin to move us forward. Sustaining the change is difficult on our own but can be supported by asking friends for help and by signing up for coaching sessions with a life coach. More help may be available if the organization has supportive programs or employee assistance programs.

One recommendation is to create a "court of support" that includes friends or family who can provide specific support to you (Daily, 2008). Think of a person who can support you in the following areas:

- **Thinker:** Who will stimulate me to think of the perceptions, judgments, patterns, and options I have related to life situations?

- **Challenger:** Who gets me to see the real truth—the risk—and helps me take action?

- **Supporter:** Who will love me unconditionally and be compassionate, helping me to feel what is happening to me?

- **Sage:** Who will help me see the big picture, see the purpose in what is happening, and bless me in my efforts? This is a mentor: a wise one you admire and trust.

This "court of support" can offer a balance of energy needed when working with life challenges and dilemmas. Another great strategy comes from the Four Gateway Coaching Model (Daily 2007).

Identifying Draining and Energizing Behaviors

A valuable exercise to do with yourself or a work team is to identify energizing and draining behaviors. Take a sheet of paper and make two columns. In the first column, write down all the behaviors that energize you. In the second column, write down all the behaviors that drain your energy (see Table 1 for examples). If you are having trouble identifying them in your own life, you can think of a person who is energizing. What are his or her behaviors? And think of a person who drains your energy: What are his or her behaviors? Now look at all the behaviors listed: You might notice that you have the capacity to have both kinds of behavior—and that some are so conditioned that you might not even realize when you slip into them.

Table 1   Examples of energizing and draining behaviors.

Energizing Behaviors	Draining Behaviors
Encouraging and accepting	Complaining
Forgiving	Critical and judging
Open communication	Talks about others negatively
Good listener	Takes all the credit
People/relationships are first	Self-serving
Caring	Cranky
Calm	Overexcited, dramatic
Creative in offering new ideas	Abandon situations; withdraw
Problem solver	Victim stance (poor me)
Appreciative and grateful to others	Demanding

The key is to try to stay in the energizing column and notice when you slip into the draining column. Make a conscious choice to get yourself out of the draining behavior. When you feel yourself slipping, take a step back and look at the situation. What is the situation that is causing the draining behavior? Can the task be broken into sections, making it easier to complete? Is there something that you can delegate to lighten the workload? Some people take on too much, and it causes them to exhibit draining behaviors.

Enhancing Communication/Relationship Skills

Our energizing and draining behaviors have a lot to do with relationships. Therefore, if we make a conscious effort to be more effective in communicating and connecting with others, we will minimize the loss of energy. It can feel overwhelming at times, and we might wonder where to begin on this topic. Five key principles of dialog that we can focus on to energize ourselves and others are listed in Table 2. They are adapted from the book *Can the Human Being Thrive in the Workplace: Dialogue as a Strategy of Hope* (Wesorick, 1997).

Table 2   Principles of Dialogue

Principle	Definition	Behavior we can manifest
Intention	The willingness to create a safe place to learn collectively, share thinking, listen to the thinking of another, be surprised, and honor the presence of each other's body, mind, and spirit.	Think and hold the intent. Invite others.
Listening	The willingness to learn to listen to self and others with the body, mind, spirit without judgment and competition.	Listen with the ears of your heart. Listen to what comes up in you and others, the collective, and between the lines.
Advocacy	The willingness to share personal thinking and how you came to think that with the intention of exposing not defending it.	Speak from your heart. Suspend your judgments. Share your thoughts and feelings to reveal a perspective. Be courageous—speak your truth.

Table 2   Principles of Dialogue *(continued)*

Principle	Definition	Behavior we can manifest
Inquiry	The willingness to ask questions and dig deeper to uncover insights and new learning.	Ask genuine questions of curiosity. Reveal why you are asking.
Silence	The willingness to experience and learn by reflecting and discovering the lessons from personal awareness, words unspoken, and the quiet of the soul.	Be present to each person and situation. Take silent time for yourself each day. Slow down conversation. Pause and reflect when someone says something heartfelt and wise.

On an individual level, these principles and practical behaviors can help us use our energy in the best ways with our loved ones and in the work setting. Often when trying to master these behaviors, we make some progress and then experience a setback. This is because we are changing how we relate, and others will have to respond differently. There has to be a restabilizing period during which we create new norms. We are also most at risk for this when we are tired, stressed, or overworked, because when our resilience is down, we fall back into known patterns that are not always healthy.

Natural Cycles of Change

A critical factor in energy management is how we manage change. Change is a part of life. No matter whether it is change that we make or that is forced upon us, we have a choice of how we respond. There are beliefs, as illustrated in Table 3, that could help us act and lead with positive energy.

Table 3   Beliefs on change that are energizing

Beliefs	Explanation
Expect change and seek the learning.	Know that we learn something from every life experience and change; it is how we progress in our journey.

Table 3   Beliefs on change that are energizing

Beliefs	Explanation
Believe that everything happens for a reason that may not be revealed to you.	Example: You didn't get a job because your perfect job is being offered to you in the next interview. When one door closes, another opens.
Identify your best practices to manage change.	Think of a time when you managed it well. What got you through it successfully? What did you learn to do?
Work with the natural cycles, not against them.	Are there changes that are taking too much energy and feel like they have to be forced? Maybe they are not meant to force. Example: Trying to save someone's life at any cost when they are meant to die.
Know there are ongoing polarities and dynamics to manage.	Some things are not problems to fix, and fixing will take a limitless amount of energy to no avail. Stop trying to fix them and learn to manage them.
Realize your resources.	You don't have to do it alone. Remember that there are people to help. Be grateful for all the help and things you have at your disposal.
Forgive yourself and others.	If a change doesn't go well, don't be so hard on yourself and others. Take the learning as a gold nugget and move on.

Concerning working with ongoing dynamics, there has been great work done by Barry Johnson, PhD, who describes ways to understand polarities and manage them over time. The polarity to explore here is stability verses change. Which one do we need? The answer is both: They seem like opposites but are interrelated, and we need both to balance our lives.

Johnson developed a way to look at these polarities in a map format. There is an upside and downside to each side of the polarity; and, if we only focus on one, we actually experience the downside of both. This helps us manage energy by teaching us that these dynamics are predictable and that we can manage them by realizing that tension and resistance are necessary.

There is wisdom in resistance because it signals us to act to balance out the situation. For example, a person might have a busy month and begin to notice a longing for some quiet, stable, at-home time. Or, a person has had the same job for a long time and is feeling stagnant. These are signals to seek solitude in the home or new experiences in the job. The polarity map in Table 4 shows the upside and downside of this dynamic.

Table 4   Managing the change-stability dynamic (Johnson, 1996)

Goal: Effective Energy Management	
+ Upside of Change	**+ Upside of Stability**
New energy	**Continuity**
New perspectives	Loyalty
New challenges: skills, knowledge, experiences	"Felt" job security Avoiding foolish risks
Willing to take risks	Know how to work with each other
— Downside of Change	**— Downside of Stability**
Chaos	**Stagnation**
Reduced loyalty	Unwilling to take risks
"Felt" job insecurity	Feeling stuck
Take foolish risks	No forward movement
Constant readjustment to working relationships and work ways	No new perspectives or new challenges
No time to evaluate effective ness of changes	

The goal is to keep ourselves in the upper two quadrants as much as possible, although we will slightly dip into the two lower quadrants long enough to feel the downside and then course-correct.

Call to Health Care Leaders

This call to health care leaders is to be an energizing leader. We should take care of ourselves by engaging in healthy behaviors that enable us to give more to those we lead. As a result, we will have the energy to focus on creating energizing cultures for health care providers and patients. This includes living from our passion and purpose, engaging all levels in decision making, promoting healthy relationships and communication, working with the natural cycles of change, showing gratitude to colleagues and staff, and being a beacon of hope for those around us.

Lessons Learned by Mentee

As a new nurse, maintaining the energy in my life has become a priority. I have learned that it is easy to be caught in chaos when so many new tasks and challenges happen so quickly for a novice nurse. During my first few months of work, I was completely overwhelmed because I had so many new things to learn and so many new responsibilities to carry out. I am very conscientious and wanted to do my best to serve patients and be a good co-worker. Keeping up my energy suddenly became one of my top priorities. I had to identify the stressors at work and find ways to deal with them in a positive way. There were times when I felt like I could not make it through the day. There were moments when I cried to my mentors because I thought I could never make it in the world of fast-paced emergency nursing.

However, they taught me important tools that I have to use every day. That is why I think this topic and the work that Laurie is doing is so important to keeping people in the health care workforce. Now, I take time out of my busy schedule for exercising, reading inspirational articles, and surrounding myself with people that support me. My mentors have taught me that the energy I possess affects the people around me, both positively and negatively. They have taught me that what I put into my job is what I get out of it. Having a positive energy when I am at work not only makes the day better for me, but it also makes it better for my patients.

Self-Reflective Questions

1. As a leader, what do you believe about energy management?

2. What are your energizing and draining behaviors?

3. Who makes up your "court of support" to help you be an energizing leader?

4. What programs, or supports, have you put into place to support those you lead?

5. What are you doing to constantly improve your communication and relationships?

6. What are your best practices to manage change in your life?

7. Are you forcing things to happen or working with the natural cycles of change?

8. What are the points of tension in your life, and is there a polarity to manage instead of a problem to solve?

9. How can you express gratitude for your life and to those around you?

10. In what ways are you a role model for being an energizing leader?

(The) Environment Plays a Role in Health Care

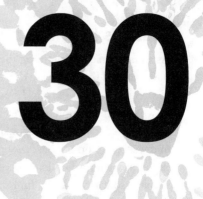

30

"There is only one humanity."

—Arthur Miller

Mentor
Frances Kam Yuet Wong, RN, PhD
Professor, School of Nursing
The Hong Kong Polytechnic University
Hong Kong SAR, China

Mentee
Shaoling Wang, RN, BSN
Doctorate student, School of Nursing
The Hong Kong Polytechnic University
Hong Kong SAR, China

In the spring of 1983, Arthur Miller was in Beijing, China, assisting the Chinese Theatre Association with the production of his famous play, *Death of a Salesman*. The task was a challenge for Miller because China is a socialist country and the concept of a salesman was little understood when the country's market economy was in its infant stage. Miller documented his first encounter with the cast in his book *Salesman in Beijing* (1984) as follows:

The way to make this play most American is to make it most Chinese. The alternative is what? You will try to imitate films you have seen, correct? They [the actors and actresses] nod and laugh. But those films are already imitations, so you will be imitating an imitation. Or maybe you will try to observe how I behave and imitate me. But this play cannot work at all—it can easily be a disaster—if it is approached in a spirit of cultural mimicry. I can tell you now that one of my main motives in coming here is to try to show that there is only one humanity.

Arthur Miller's experience to produce his play *Death of a Salesman* in China intrigues me when I relate the experience of mentoring Shaoling Wang, my doctorate student. The theme of sharing "one humanity" resonates in me.

Shaoling was born in mainland China and trained as a nurse in the 1970s. She spent two years in the late 1980s studying in Hong Kong full-time. Other than the period studying in Hong Kong, Shaoling's learning and working experiences are mainly based in Guangzhou, China.

I was born and raised in Hong Kong when it was under the colonial rule of the United Kingdom. I received my baccalaureate nursing education in the 1970s in the United States. I also spent a year studying in the United Kingdom. Most of my working experience is in the United States and Hong Kong.

Basically, Shaoling and I came from two different worlds before we met. However, we shared a similar aspiration. We both wanted to work in an area that helps clients attain optimal health, particularly when returning home after hospital discharge. To be specific, we were both interested in the design and evaluation of service models that strengthen transitional care in support of the clients to stay well in the community. (To help the readers appreciate the health care systems of the two places where Shaoling and I are coming from, please refer to the *note* at the end of this article.)

Mainland China and Hong Kong share similar issues in health care systems. The hospitals in both places are overcrowded. One of the key goals in health care is to empower clients, particularly for those with chronic diseases, to self-management so that they rely less on hospital care. The incentive to contain cost by maintaining the clients in the community and reducing the use of hospitals is shared by the central government of China and the regional government of Hong Kong. Shaoling and I have common goals but different interpretations of the goals because of the different health care systems that we have been living in.

In the United States, the pioneer works on providing support for post-discharged clients by Brooten et al. (2002) and Naylor et al. (1999) have successfully demonstrated the value of transitional care using research evidence. The aims of transitional care are to provide coordinated services with continuity and to prevent unnecessary hospital readmissions. The reduction of readmission is a means to save cost in Hong Kong, just as it is in other places. The reduction of readmission is less of a concern because each episode of patient hospitalization generates revenue. The provision of care after hospital discharge is not governed by the national health care pricing regulations, and the hospital cannot charge patients for post-discharge services. In other words, the provision of transitional care after hospital discharge consumes resources rather than creates monetary gain. The incentive to develop transitional care in the system of mainland China is therefore not strong.

So, I tried to introduce the concept of transitional care by using an analogy of "post-sales service," and Shaoling appreciated this concept immediately. The idea of post-sales service is common in the current commercial market in mainland China. Though transitional care as a kind of post-sales service does not generate immediate revenue in the hospital, in the long run it brings about a phenomenon called "social effect." The phenomenon of social effect refers to the increased reputation that results because of the quality service provided by the hospitals. This social effect can turn into economic effect when more patients are willing to use these hospitals that provide post-discharge follow-up care. Also in the very busy hospitals, when patients are discharged home early with follow-up, beds can then be made available for the admission of more patients that need them. Our ultimate goals are for the well-being of the clients so that they can access the appropriate level of care for optimal health.

This explanation of the value of transitional care to Shaoling and the nurses in mainland China is similar to an episode when Arthur Miller was trying to explain the relationship of Willy Loman with his second son, Happy, to the cast. The actor who played Happy, after some discussion, was enlightened and said, "One thing about the play that is very Chinese is the way Willy tries to make his son successful. The Chinese father always wants his sons to be 'dragons.'" This is what Arthur Miller means when he refers to sharing one humanity. Similarly in health care, all governments who love their people would aim at providing essential comprehensive coverage to protect the health of its citizens. This is also the goal of the central government of China. One of the chief goals in health care is to enable people access to appropriate level of care at the right time to promote improved health outcomes (Andersen and Davidson, 2001).

Human beings can be masters of all creatures because of our ability to pass on our accumulated culture from one generation to another. We nurture our younger ones through love and passion for humanity, the one humanity that we share. How can we do it? Confucius is the great ancient educator in China, and he once said in *The Analects* (n.d.), "Those who are quiet treasure knowledge, those who are eager to learn are not tired, and those who are educative do not feel weary." We nurture the next generation by being students ourselves at all times as we assume the role of being a mentor to others. We can become more effective mentors by learning from Confucius who reminds us to keep learning ourselves as we pass on what we know to others. The relationship between the mentor and mentee is developmental and dynamic in this challenging health care environment. The world is now flat, and we are now living in a global village. As the world becomes more homogenous, we begin to share similar life issues and solutions. We have to think globally and at the same time act locally.

Comments from Shaoling Wang (Mentee)

In July 2006, I started my post-graduate study under the supervision of Professor Frances Wong. As a novice, I knew little about how to conduct research with sound methodology to produce strong evidence. My supervisor shared with me her knowledge without reservation and facilitated me to learn actively. She was always there for me when I needed her. We experienced the ups and downs of conducting a clinical research together, and I have gradually learned how to face the challenges in the particular context of the Chinese health care environment and overcome barriers encountered in the research process.

One of the larger goals Professor Wong and I share is to strengthen transitional care in mainland China. I chose the development and evaluation of a transitional care model for Chronic Obstructive Pulmonary Disease (COPD) patients as the topic of my doctorate study. The management of COPD in mainland China usually focuses on the acute phase of care using hospital services. The concept of transitional care supporting patients as they resume normal life at home after hospital discharge is relatively weak. The experience in Hong Kong and overseas is that transitional care can help promote the well-being of patients in the community so that they rely less on hospital services. Usually a nurse helps lead the transitional care service and is supported by a multidisciplinary team. The development of such a transitional care program in mainland China is not easy because some roles are non-existent. For example, physiotherapists play an important role in pulmonary rehabilitation, but this category of care provider is just now emerging in China. Another key element of success of the program is to empower the nurse to lead the team and prepare him or her for the mastery of transitional care. To design an effective program that is locally applicable, we solicited advice from 20 experts in respiratory care with background in nursing, medicine, physiotherapy, occupational therapy, and dietetics in mainland China and Hong Kong. We also provided a structured training program for the nurses from both the hospital and community settings in support of the study. As the study progressed, the study nurses and I witnessed the value of transitional care to the patients whom we serve. It was most rewarding to watch the improvement of the patients in the intervention group. Patients' knowledge of, skills in dealing with, and self-efficacy in COPD disease management were enhanced.

Throughout these 2 1/2 years, apart from knowledge and technique on conducting research, I learned a lot from my supervisor. Her serious attitude in scholarly work, commitment to the nursing profession, and passion for mentoring the younger generation are great lessons for me, both as a nurse and as a person!

Note

China is a communist country and her health care system has been evolving since the establishment of the new government in 1949. Between 1950 and 1980, China established a health care system that provided health care to almost everyone (Blumenthal and Hsiao, 2005). In the early 1980s, China reduced the central government's share of health care services, which went from 32% in 1978 to 15% in 1999 (Gao et al., 2001). This reduction in government support encouraged the generation of revenue via privatizing health care facilities (Blumenthal and Hsiao, 2005). The payment of fees-for-service resulted in the overprovision of services and over-use of drugs and high-technology tests (The World Bank, 1997; Blumenthal and Hsiao, 2005). Patients could choose the level of provider they could afford, so overlapping functions and frag-mented service delivery responsibilities existed at different levels of care (Liu et al., 2002). At the turn of the 21st century, the Chinese government identified a need for the country to build a more effective health service system for her people.

In Hong Kong, the government always had a stated policy that no citizen should be deprived of adequate health care. The Hong Kong Government subsidized heavily all the services, adapting the British social health care system during the colonial rule (Fung, Tse, and Yeoh, 1999). The public hospital system is overloaded, shouldering most of the secondary health care services for the people in Hong Kong. A lack of coordination and cohesion exists between primary and inpatient care, acute and community medicine, and the private and public sectors in Hong Kong (The Harvard Team, 1999). The Hong Kong government is now planning for major health care review. The key mission is to reconstruct a sustainable health care system by reducing the need for hospital care by strengthening ambulatory and community care (Hong Kong Government, 2008).

Self-Reflective Questions

1. In what ways do you consider nursing as an important profession that contributes to people's health and well-being?

2. How do you take responsibility for caring for clients both in the hospital and in the community?

3. In what ways should a professional nurse be a direct care provider as well as a designer for effective service models?

4. How important do you think transitional care to support patients who return home after hospital discharge is?

5. What differences and similarities do you see in health care issues among countries?

6. In what ways is cost-effective care important?

7. How is the reduction of hospital readmission beneficial to clients?

8. How can a mentor learn continuously?

9. How can a mentor-mentee relationship advocate mutual growth?

10. In what ways can you think globally and act locally?

Evolving Leadership

31

"In the past a leader was a boss. Today's leaders must be partners with their people."

—Ken Blanchard

Mentor

Mally Ehrenfeld, RN, PhD
Head Associate Professor,
  Department of Nursing
Stanley Steyer School of Health
  Professions
Tel Aviv University
Tel Aviv, Israel

Mentee

Merav Ben Nathan, RN, PhD
Senior Teacher
Pat Mattews Academic School
  of Nursing, Hillel-Yaffe Medical
  Center; Department of Nurs-
  ing, Stanley Steyer School of
  Health Professions
 Tel Aviv University
Tel Aviv, Israel

On May 8, 2008, Israel celebrated its 60th Independence Day. Its first Prime Minister, David Ben-Gurion, declared the new state 60 years earlier after receiving worldwide recognition at the United Nations summit. This Zionist leader had captured the hearts of the people of Israel, as well as those of Jewish communities around the world. As the first to claim and to receive acknowledgment, the Zionist leaders, especially Ben-Gurion, received the faith and support of their nation. The leadership of the pioneer generation exemplified glory and pride but was also based on ideals and support. Ben-Gurion's model of leadership characterized the pioneer generation in many fields, including nursing. Several leaders in nursing, such as Professor Rebecca Bergman and Mrs. Steiner-Freud, led the battle for academization of the profession in Israel. This approach differs considerably from contemporary leadership.

21st Century Leadership

Today's leaders need to find new ways of motivating and encouraging their followers. The fine art of leadership aims at recruiting and inspiring. Leadership today involves carrying out daily commitments and responsibilities while maintaining achievements.

Critical Attributes of a Leader

These forward-moving, step-by-step efforts require vision, creativity, and occasionally the courage to take risks. Unlike previous generations in which leaders were imbued with heroic meaning, today's leadership is more transparent and is not easily forgiven by the public.

Effective leadership is associated with better and more ethical performance (Chiokfoong-Loke, 2001). Leaders must emphasize and exemplify positive values when discussing the importance of their goals in order to motivate team members (Upenieks, 2003). One way of doing so is to encourage the reporting of mistakes to learn how to manage them, prevent their reoccurrence, and recognize the factors that caused them (King, 2001). To quote a well-known Hebrew proverb: "Making a mistake once is human, repeating it is a fool's choice."

True leadership has other attributes, such as persistence and creativity, but it ultimately encourages others to progress. This requires patience and time, emphasizing the message of teamwork. The team's atmosphere and sense of togetherness might help compensate for the lost heroics of the early days of the State. Good relationships, encouragement, initiatives, special skills, and talents provide positive contributions to the nursing team, thereby increasing their motivation and minimizing burnout (Scott-Cawiezell et al., 2004; Medland, Howard-Ruben, & Whitaker, 2004).

In today's nursing world, leaders must listen to the team and enable them to participate in the whole process. Encouraging new skills among workers can be prompted by developing new ways of thinking, using reflective skills in their work, empowering them to grow and take more responsibilities, and nurturing them to become leaders. The work of today's generation of leaders is an ongoing dynamic process. Modern leaders must keep inspiring their workers to maintain enthusiasm in their work and emphasize tolerance and integration.

The case of academization of nursing in Israel demonstrates the need for flexibility in order to adjust to changing realities. This process can no longer be achieved through revolutions, but rather gradual and steady development.

Initially, nursing was perceived as a profession that required skills that could be obtained in the clinical field. Massive efforts to maintain a high rate of knowledge accelerated the process of nursing academization. The state of nursing today is the product of many long, intensive efforts to motivate people to fulfill the ambition. These efforts made the vision reality.

The Leader as a Moral Compass

Today's leader serves as a significant role model and guide for the group, recognizing that the whole is larger then the sum of its parts and that the leader is only one of those parts. Such an attitude characterizes the Jewish way of thinking, namely that humbleness and modesty are values to cultivate. It further enables the leader to rely on his subordinates to provide new and improved ideas.

In recent years, we are witnessing more complex styles of management and leadership than in the past. Reches and Tabak (1995) stated that the role of the leader in light of the development during the last century has raised new ethical dilemmas. Their research focused on leadership in the field of health professions, and mainly on legal dilemmas. The rising number of malpractice lawsuits in the field of health care has led to the development of new protocols in the workplace. Leaders are required to give group members a sense of responsibility while fulfilling the aim of helping patients and protecting their health. Risk management units in many hospitals are a direct result of the cases presented by Tabak, Reches, and Wagner (1995). Such changes have led to a policy transformation in health institutions and governmental regulatory processes that is still evolving in understanding and application (Street, Robertson, & Geiger, 1997).

Leaders are also required to make decisions in situations where dual loyalty exists. Such decisions in health care might occur when a new ward is opened at a hospital and a lack of human resources exists. The leader's job in this case is to identify ethical and moral dilemmas. This ability is critical for decision making. As a result, an ethical culture can be developed at the workplace.

The Role of Ownership in Creating a Vision

Providing a forum for discussions and idea sharing among team members is essential for the team to feel as though they are part of the decision-making process. Furthermore, it motivates and gives them a sense of ownership and responsibility. These methods allow leaders and the team to discuss their targets and ensure that they accomplish their vision. A vision is essential to the nature of leadership. Whether nurses are involved in one-to-one care or advocating at a national level, they need to ascribe to a vision of what they want to accomplish. It is only by holding such a vision, that clarity of purpose and execution of function will be achieved (Graham, 2003).

Evidence-Based Practice Leadership

Evidence-based practice is a fundamental framework for contemporary leadership. Examining recent research and clinical knowledge provides a fact-based framework for the leader, promotes the quality of work, and influences the team's satisfaction (Laura & Joanne, 2006; Cullen & Titler, 2004; Caramanica et al., 2002). Such leadership serves as a model for team members to seek and learn new knowledge.

The Role of Technology

Technology is also a changing factor for contemporary leadership. The development of technology and its increasing affordability has made information highly accessible (Heller, Oros, & Durney-Crowely, 2005). This accessibility has further improved work processes to become more transparent (Perednia & Allen, 1995). The access to information enables a wider range of new clinical knowledge and a faster way of learning, which leads to better health care. Therefore, this component must be part of the tools used by all contemporary leaders.

One should look toward the future in preparation for potential leadership challenges. Further developments in technology, forces of globalization, and processes of politicization of health care, might soon become more prominent to leaders in the nursing field. This outlook sheds light on leadership as a product of its time and era.

New Ways of Thinking

In the years since the 20th century, the goals, learnings, and technologies achieved have altered and expanded the role of the nurse leader. Positive, collegial relationships and supportive environments are still essential components of leadership and teamwork. However, the 21st century requires developing new ways of thinking about teamwork and the individuals who contribute to the process. Leaders must strengthen, satisfy, and motivate collaborators, further investing and involving them in achieving their goals within an organization's vision. Leadership in nursing, an evolving, rapidly changing act of influencing, is being influenced by an ever-changing society.

Reflections from Merav Ben Nathan, Mentee

As a student and a rather young nurse, I was blessed to learn from individuals in the nursing field whom I respected and considered role models. They influenced and shaped me personally and professionally. By developing my talents and abilities with the guidance and support of my mentor, it was easy for me to follow their example.

Early in the course of my career, my mentor encouraged me to develop my computer and Internet skills, which are now essential in our field because of the rapid changes and developments in technology. Because these technologies have made a dramatic impact on health services and the nursing field, I am fortunate that I was advised to improve my skills with these applications and that I continued to develop them throughout my professional life.

Similarly, the implementation of evidence-based practice and the development of effective learning by attending clinical conferences have molded my professional attitude and influenced my practical application of the role. This type of experience has enhanced my ability to speak to a large audience and to present issues professionally supported by evidence-based nursing. Additionally, this exposure to problem solving and critical thinking, initiated by my nurse leaders, allowed me to effectively prioritize my tasks, manage conflicts, and cope with teaching-related issues.

Although various attributes of a leader in this field have been discussed, the reality is that it takes a mixture of these independent ingredients in just the right doses to be successful. Each situation encountered in managing a team requires a different mixture every time an obstacle arises.

Self-Reflective Questions

1. Do you manage to carry out daily commitments and responsibilities while maintaining achievements?

2. Do your creative efforts require vision and the courage to take risks?

3. In your work, do you find that you emphasize the importance and positive values of your goals?

4. Is your leadership associated with better and more ethical performance?

5. Do you encourage workers to report mistakes in order to improve risk management, prevent reoccurrence, and recognize possible causes?

Self-Reflective Questions

6. Do you contribute to the nursing team through the development of good relationships, encouragement, initiatives, special skills, and talents?

7. In your work, do you give attention to the small details as well as the general aspects?

8. Do you keep up with recent research and clinical knowledge?

9. Do you encourage new skills among workers through development of new ways of thinking, use of reflective skills, empowerment to grow, and their assuming more responsibilities?

10. Do you inspire your workers to maintain enthusiasm in their work and emphasize tolerance and integration?

Excellent Care

32

"Some people have greatness thrust upon them. Very few have excellence thrust upon them . . . they achieve it. They do not achieve it unwittingly by 'doing what comes naturally,' and they do not stumble into it in the course of amusing themselves. All excellence demands discipline and tenacity of purpose."

—John Gardner

Mentor
Sabah Abu-Zinadah, BSN, MSN, PhD
Chairperson, Nursing Scientific Board
Saudi Commission for Health Specialties
Riyadh, Saudi Arabia

Mentee
Nada Massode, BSN
Infection Control Coordinator
Security Forces Hospital Program
Riyadh, Saudi Arabia

The nursing profession is a young profession in Saudi Arabia. The first baccalaureate of science in nursing (BSN) degree program started in 1976. I (Nada) am in the third group to graduate from this program, and the majority of Saudi nurses are at a diploma level.

It became our mission as pioneers to prove that the BSN graduate brings something different that we like to call "an excellent care." The message involves practicing quality every day, in many ways, while infinitely improving both practice and care. One day, though, I realized that I had unconsciously done things based on certain principles, yet I kept wondering why I had conflict with others. I sat down and started to reflect, why?

What Excellence Means to Me: Mentee

The answer is that not everyone is willing to pay the price. Achievement has a price tag. For example, how much are you willing to "pay" with hard work, patience, and sacrifice to survive to become a person of excellence? The answer is important because the cost is great. Then I had to face a major decision: Am I willing to sacrifice the standards that I built over the years? Am I willing to compromise my value system—the base of who I am? Is that worthwhile?

Excellence means achieving quality standards. Most people could not tell the difference in quality by the naked eye. Quality is about how we live, love, care, work, and value things around us. Quality is not a substance; rather, it is a choice of style, it is a choice of standards, and it is an identity. Quality is about pride, and quality is a commitment. Quality is started by people at all levels: One influences the other. We cannot own quality and keep it to ourselves; it has to be shared to enjoy it. That is why we continuously strive to achieve and establish quality to create quality culture, and we continuously influence others to do the same by example and not only "walking the walk" but by "talking the talk." The best mentors are apt to be among those executives who have a strong passion to excellence in their characters.

Seeds of Greatness

Denis Waitley (1988) reveals 10 basic principles of success. Because these 10 principles are seldom practiced, I (mentor) used those principles as the main framework for this chapter. They are a good guideline if you want to be successful. They also promote effective mentoring. Having practiced these principles even before I read about it, I am a believer. It is quite challenging to put these principles in practice when the majority behaves differently.

Successful people believe in themselves and hold on to their dreams and visions because they have a strong feeling of self-worth, greater than the feeling of rejection or acceptance of their ideas by others. Every completion for them means a new beginning. The sense of ability to be innovator provides great courage to move forward. Successful people feel love inside themselves before they can give it to another. Self-esteem, then, is the start of the road to success.

Successful people are blessed by having a good mental picture of self through interaction with healthy role models and positive family support, which is continuously nourished and cultivated through positive interaction with surrounding environment. It is the ingredient for happiness and success. Successful people do have an "I can" attitude; when things do not go smoothly at first, they develop persistence to help them to keep trying by getting more information or trying something a different way until they get it right. Visual-ization and affirmation of success is the key to healthy development. Remember you are your most important critic.

Successful people understand the true reward in life depends upon the quali-ty of the contribution that they make for their profession and community. Being a self-reliant adult means holding higher professional standards, being a distinct individual within the group, investing more effort, and taking risks. Successful people realize that they are responsible for what happens in their own life. They tackle the hardest and the most challenging things first and understand that their fulfillment will come after achieving the job at hand. Before they ask for a pay increase, successful people tell their employers what they can offer for the organization.

Successful people are characterized by being knowledgeable. Most people believe that graduation day is the end of study. Most people are better prepared and motivated in their hobbies than they are in their lifework. Knowledge is power. It controls access to opportunity and advancement. Knowledge is the leading edge of tomorrow. Wisdom is the combination of honesty and knowl-edge applied through experience. Successful people consistently think, do, and say what they believe to be true. Every time individuals engage in dishonest activities of any kind, the results come back to haunt them. Successful people honestly consider the well-being of others before they look after themselves.

Successful people, who realize that many individuals fail to achieve their goals in life because they never really set them in the first place, master goal-setting strategies. They have clearly defined purposes. Things do not just hap-pen in their lives; they make life happen for them. They know the difference between achieving planned goals and falling into chaos. Successful people are good communicators. Effective communication depends upon the ability to recognize others' needs and help them to fill those needs.

Successful people know that the good old days are here and now. Every generation sees its position as the one that is living under the most pressing and difficult circumstances in history. By complaining about the unkind world, they will never have to solve their problems, but playing the scapegoat game will not be the solution. To develop adaptability to the stresses of life, you need to view those stresses as normal. Successful people develop strength of character.

Successful people do things that the majority of the population is not will-ing to do, and do so with perseverance, which means hanging in there when the odds stack up against them, knowing that they are right. Perseverance shows how someone succeeds in the face of incredible odds. Successful people know that perseverance makes a difference.

Successful people have the ability to see life from within; their attitude and responses are developed because of seeing the world more clearly. When we see clearly, we value ourselves more, and our self-esteem grows stronger. When we see clearly, we can imagine and understand our responsibility for self-development. When we see clearly, we develop our wisdom, know our purpose, and have faith. When we see clearly, we have the ability to reach others, the ability to adapt to change, and to persevere when we are overwhelmed.

My Dream

I heard about Dr. Abu-Zinadah in 1996 when I was a student at King Saud University, studying nursing. She was known as a strong Saudi leader in nursing with a vision to promote the nursing profession in Saudi Arabia.

Since that time, I hoped to work under her command. One day, in 2004, my dream came true. She supported my nomination as a member for the Saudi nursing board—the one she chairs—representing my hospital. Even though I wasn't qualified to be a member (because I did not have a master's degree), she supported me. She faced all kinds of resistance from the Saudi Commission for Health Specialty and my hospital, but she believed in me, and I won the membership.

I have learned many things from the fantastic working relationship and various experiences she provided for me. Her leadership helped me to reflect upon my previous experiences and future goals: how to be successful, how to achieve excellence, and how to hold high professional standards. The interaction with her helped me to understand others and myself. She demonstrates for me effective communication, interpersonal, and decision-making skills, as well as a willingness to be flexible. Additionally, her firsthand knowledge was helpful in giving me a deeper understanding of the profession, and helped me address some of my special interests and concerns. I truly appreciated this wonderful working experience.

I cannot fully express my respect and admiration for Dr. Abu-Zinadah as an individual as well as a professional; her support, thoughtfulness, and understanding of others are truly inspirational and demonstrate characteristics that I wish to possess as a leader and an educator.

Finally, I can't forget her messages:

- Don't give up on your goals.
- Believe in yourself. You can do it!
- Remember that achieving one excellent goal is better than reaching many insignificant goals.

She always ignites the ambition, the drive, and the desire of how to take full advantage of all the opportunities that have been presented to me. I learn to give my best for all projects I have at hand, to be honest, to treat people with respect, to observe a strong work ethic, to know my strengths and improve my weaknesses, and to plan my personal growth and development. She taught me that I have to do whatever it takes to keep my knowledge up-to-date and pursue my postgraduate study. I am planning on finishing my postgraduate study and coming back to be part of the nursing development team in Saudi Arabia. During this journey, Dr. Abu-Zinadah has proven that where there is a will, there is a way.

Passion for Excellence

Tom Peters said, "Success is not a destination, it is a journey" (Peters & Waterman, 2004). The true passion for excellence is the ability to look people in the eye and watch things happen.

Self-Reflective Questions

1. How can you accept yourself just as you are?

2. How can you see yourself as a real winner in life?

3. Do you give more than you are expected to give? If so, how? If not, why?

4. How can you be more honest with yourself and others?

5. What professional goals do you have that can be shared by someone who can reinforce your purpose?

6. What are ways in which you look for the good in others with an open mind?

7. Would others view you as an optimist? If not, why?

8. How can you better adapt easily to change?

9. Do you hang in there when you believe you are right?

10. How do you convert stumbling blocks into stepping stones?

33 Facility Design and New Construction

"The opportunity to take shell space and not replicate the present and familiar, but instead integrate environmental design, technology, and a new care delivery model is imperative."

—Ann L. Hendrich

Mentor
Carol A. Watson, PhD, RN, CENP
Professor, University of Iowa
  College of Nursing
Iowa City, Iowa, USA

Mentee
Beth Houlahan, MSN, RN
Senior Vice President,
  Nursing and Patient Care
  Services
Mercy Medical Center
Cedar Rapids, Iowa, USA

Nurse executives have an unprecedented opportunity to create new, transformative space for patients and nurses. The recent surge in hospital construction gives nurse executives a unique role in the design of new facilities to create healthful and healing environments. But, it's a role with which many nurse executives have limited experience. To avoid merely replicating current design configurations, new knowledge and skills are needed.

The Evidence for a Different Design

Mercy Medical Center in Cedar Rapids, Iowa, completed a major renovation of its inpatient departments, moving from a mix of private/semi-private patient rooms to private patient rooms entirely. But, the project was more than just creating private rooms. Evidence-based facility design, embedded technology, redesigned work processes, and participation by all stakeholders were integral to the design process.

Extensive renovation or new construction is costly, but evidence exists that supports an impressive return on investment. Private rooms require fewer patient transfers. Every patient transfer costs $500–$1,000 and is reported to increase the length of stay for patients by one-half to one day (Hamilton, 2000). We did our own evaluation of intra-department transfers and found that we averaged five intra-departmental transfers per day in each inpatient department. After renovation, we reduced intra-departmental transfers by 70%.

Quieter, less stressful environments translate into less pain, decreased need for narcotics, and more rest for patients (The Advisory Board, 2003). Of Mercy patients responding to a 2007 Hospital Consumer Assessment of Healthcare Providers and Systems (HCAHPS) survey, 64% reported the area around their rooms was always quiet at night, and 69% reported their pain was always well controlled. This compared to 57% and 67% of patients from all hospitals on HCAHPS quietness and pain control items.

Private patient rooms are safer for patients. Fewer health care acquired infections occur with private rooms (Bilchik, 2002), and private patient rooms result in fewer medication errors (Hendrich, Fay, & Sorrels, 2004). When patients share the same space, transmission of infections and misidentification of patients is more likely to occur than when patients are provided care in private rooms.

The design principles to create a safe, healing environment for patients are more than just moving a bed out of a semi-private room. Evidence-based facility design is not about just designing a physical environment but also designing a delivery model and philosophy of care (Lowers, 1999). If the focus is predominately on the physical design, the care delivery model will remain as the status quo.

Much of the research on facility design focuses primarily on the design of patient rooms. However, the design of support space, such as the size of the medication preparation areas and decentralization of equipment and supplies, is equally important in improving patient outcomes. Additionally, nursing staff benefit from innovative facility design. A true healing environment doesn't meet the stated objectives unless it exists for everyone in the facility (Watson, 2005). Nurses need space to rest and recover from physically and emotionally exhausting work, so sound design principles need to be incorporated in break rooms as well as clinical and support space.

Basic Design Principles

The involvement of the nurse executive is critical to expanding the focus from facility design to creating healthier environments that support new models for care delivery. The steps that we followed in redesigning the patient space at Mercy serves as a good reference point for nurse executives undertaking a redesign effort.

The first step is to put together an interdisciplinary work group, including the nurse executive, frontline managers, and clinical staff, to lead the design planning and oversight of implementation. The next step is to conduct a review of the literature to make sure that all members of the workgroup are current about basic design principles. Many resources now exist that provide sound evidence about the most effective development strategies to create safer and healthier environments for patients and staff (Ulrich, Quan, Zimring, Joseph, & Choudhary, 2004; Marberry, 2006; & Reid, Compton, Grossman, & Fanjiang, 2005).

Benchmark tours to new or renovated facilities that have taken an innovative approach to redesign are critical. We challenged our architects to find the best examples of innovative flow and design in health care facilities across the country. From the benchmark tours, the work group developed a list of our top 10 priorities to guide the design process.

When the initial design work was completed, a mock up of the proposed space was built, and all staff who would work in the new space was encouraged to explore the space and provide feedback to the workgroup by using a structured survey. Patient, family, and physician feedback was also solicited. That input was used by the work group members with the architects to finalize the design. The same basic design was adhered to within each floor to create a standard blueprint. The only variation allowed was in office space.

Some of the design basics included creating space to accommodate family members who stay around the clock, decentralizing patient care supplies and equipment both inside and outside of the rooms, increasing patient control over the environment (including remote control for window blinds and thermostat within patient's reach), and incorporating ergonomic principles to minimize bending and stooping for staff.

Embedded Technology

In addition to radically redesigning the environment, embedding technology and principles of a wireless environment was critical. A survey in 2001 of more than 300 companies with more than 100 employees, which included health care, explored the relationship between a wireless environment and productivity of employees (NOP World-Technology, 2001). The survey found that employees working in wireless environments increased productivity by 22%. The impact of a wireless environment on productivity in health care was even greater.

Mercy's wireless environment began with the installation of a voice over IP system, placing voice information and data on the same network. After research and discussion by our staff, the wireless computer on wheels was adopted as the basic device for electronic documentation, although we have a mixed hardware environment (that is, hand-helds for assistive staff, tablets for physicians, and fixed computers or thin clients for centralized work areas).

A voice-activated communications system is a core part of the network. The system is a fully functional phone that interfaces with the nurse call system and sends patient calls directly to the care nurse. It also interfaces with the monitors in critical care, so alarms are sent through the communications system and not broadcast throughout the unit. Development is underway that would enter basic numeric information from the communications system directly onto the electronic chart, allowing for voice-activated, hands-free electronic documentation.

All acute care patient rooms are set up for digital video cameras. In the acute care departments, cameras are used primarily for surveillance of patients at high risk for falling, seizures, and other safety concerns. In critical care, video cameras are installed in each room, and physicians can access video images of patients through PDAs or smart phones. We have just begun to tap the potential that digital video offers to enhance quality and safety.

Another important use of a wireless environment is telemetry monitoring. All acute medical-surgical patients can be monitored wirelessly. All patients on telemetry are monitored within their own department but also in the cardiology department. In that department, monitor techs watch all the monitors 24 hours a day, every day. When arrhythmias or other cardiac abnormalities are noted, the monitor techs confer with the charge nurse of the cardiology department, if needed, and then with the primary nurse of the monitored patient through the wireless communications system. The care nurse is advised on what further steps should be taken and what should be discussed with the attending physician.

Redesign of Work Processes

Building different physical space and embedding technology in the design doesn't guarantee that staff will work more efficiently. Efficiency also requires focus on redesigning the work processes. This is the toughest part of any design effort. As part of our work, we incorporated Lean principles and participated in the Institute for Healthcare Improvement's Innovation Communities—taking action to transform care at the bedside, improving perinatal care, and operational and clinical improvements in the emergency department—to help with redesign of work processes. Redesign of work processes requires a structured performance improvement methodology and a look outside health care to other industries that have approached transformational redesign of work processes.

Integration of Technology and Design

The integration of technology and facility design to create healthier, more positive environments for patients and nurses is an exciting opportunity for nurse executives. But, it means that nurse executives must be aware of the available evidence and incorporate this information into decision making about changes in work environments. Nurse executives must continue to evaluate the impact of facility and technology design on patient and nurse outcomes and communicate the evidence of their investigation to transform not only the physical environment but also the models of care delivery.

Mercy has continued to use this framework—private rooms, wireless technology, work redesign—for any subsequent design of all new spaces or programs, including the emergency department and behavioral health. The result is truly transformational environments for our patients and staff.

Self-Reflective Questions

1. How did you set a clear vision for the facility design project?

2. In what ways did you use the American Organization of Nurse Executive's Guiding Principles for Creating the Hospital of the Future?

3. Did you appoint an interdisciplinary steering committee to work with the architects and interior designers on the facility design project?

4. In what ways did you include the voice of patients and families in the design of the facility?

Self-Reflective Questions *(continued)*

5. Did you review the most current evidence-based design resources?

6. Did you take benchmark tours to evaluate implementation of design best practices?

7. Did you establish goals for the design project?

8. Did you establish measures of success for the facility design project and collect pre- and post-build data?

9. Did you have a mock-up of the proposed space built and have all users of the space evaluate the space?

10. Did you include embedded technology in the facility design?

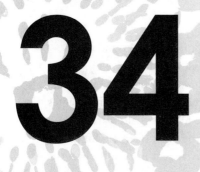

34 Financial Management in the Hospital: The Nurse's Role

"Get to the table and be a player, or someone who does not understand nursing will do that for you."

—Loretta Ford

Mentor
KT Waxman, DNP, MBA, RN, CNL
President and CEO, Waxman &
  Associates, LLC
San Ramon, California, USA

Mentee
Nicole Schaefer, MSN, BSN, RN
Co-Patient Care Manager and
  PACU staff nurse
Palo Alto, California, USA

Mentor perspective: Without question, the role of the nurse and nurse manager is different in today's health care environment than it was 25 years ago. In the past, we took care of patients, wore white uniforms, comforted families, and gave little thought to the business side of health care. Today, every nurse, whether he or she is a manager or a staff nurse, needs to understand that hospitals are businesses. For businesses to be successful, they must make a profit. Many hospitals in the United States are not-for-profit. Such organizations generally use earnings to construct new buildings, provide raises for staff, or buy new equipment. For-profit hospitals follow suit, but only *after* they have paid their shareholders (Waxman, 2008). This concept might be difficult for some to accept, but it is an important piece of information for all health care workers to realize and understand.

Cost of Health Care

Many factors affect the cost of health care today. Both nationally and at the state level, the number of people who are uninsured or underinsured is on the rise. More than 47 million people went without health insurance in 2006, including 8.7 million children, according to data released by the United States Census Bureau in 2007. The United States has the highest health care costs per person in the world, at over $6,000 per capita, per year (Centers for Medicare and Medicaid Services, 2008). In addition, the current nursing shortage is not specific to the United States. We have a global nursing shortage, and that shortage affects the business of the hospital.

The cost of technology plays a large part in the cost of health care. Available technology has exploded in the past 20 years, and the more technology that is available, the more the need exists for specialists to run that technology. Hospitals, competing for the best doctors to come on staff to attract more patients, purchase these expensive technologies. I remember years ago that each time the hospital performed a procedure, it was paid by the various health insurers. Today, however, with managed care and diagnosis-related groups (DRGs), procedures performed are not reimbursed separately; the hospital often receives a flat rate reimbursement, thus increasing costs of health care. Hospitals need to have the most current technology to attract patients and physicians, but with that comes greater expenses for training and managing the technology. Lastly, with increased litigation in the industry, physicians are more apt to order pricey, high-tech tests to ensure that they have covered all bases to avoid a lawsuit. They essentially order tests for the benefit of the medical record, not for the patient. Though these tests might be good for some of our patients, this practice is often not as good for the hospital's "bottom line," because insurance companies seldom pay for them.

The number of new medications developed in the pharmaceutical industry has skyrocketed over the past 20 years, thus increasing the cost of health care and the competitiveness of the pharmaceutical industry. As these drugs are available and utilized by physicians, the costs of patient care rise. When we see two companies begin to sell the generic version of a high-priced drug, the average cost drops significantly. The cost to develop, test, and approve new medications is high and can take years. When the medication is finally available to the public, the manufacturers must charge enough to cover these costs and pay their stockholders, who expect to see a return on their investment (National Coalition on Health Care, n.d.).

Nurses and Cost Management

As nurse managers or staff nurses, we are responsible for helping manage costs with the hospital. Even though we have little to do with payor mix, cost of technology, physician practice patterns, or insurance coverage, nurses can control costs. By being sensitive to the number of supplies we bring into a patient room, the amount of line used, staffing, discharge times, and overall patient management, we can make an impact on the hospital's bottom line. Nurses should always keep the big picture in mind. Each patient-care unit is its own business, and the nurse manager or director works as the chief operating officer of that unit. Knowing the payor mix makeup or how your hospital is reimbursed helps you understand why length of stay is so important and how using fewer resources equates to increased profit for the hospital.

Finance and Budgeting

I was not taught finance in nursing school; I learned finance on the floor as an RN. Working in the for-profit sector, I became knowledgeable about writing and managing budgets and controlling costs in the departments I managed. Now, I help new nurses and nurse managers understand the business side of nursing. In nursing school, we are taught a vocabulary specific to the profession. To the untrained ear, this nursing language can seem confusing. Such is the same with finance and accounting professionals—they use their own terminology to communicate within the field. My advice to new nurse managers and staff nurses in leadership roles is to learn the language of finance to make your job easier and help you gain the respect of finance personnel.

Mentee Perspective

I had been practicing nursing for 10 years when I was promoted to the role of nurse manager, and the responsibility was overwhelming. I had not learned about finance or budgeting in school, although I had always been intrigued by numbers. I attended a few conferences and heard KT Waxman speak about finance and budgeting. That's when the light bulb in my brain turned on. Her style was comfortable, her words easy to follow, and a year later, I attended yet another workshop where she remembered me! I was deep into the nurse manager role at that time and told her that her workshop had helped me in that position. She actually made finance and budgeting seem fun.

After a few years, I decided to go back to school and get my master's degree in nursing. My final semester ended with a project that required a preceptor. Because we both lived in the same area, I turned to KT, who took me on as her mentee. I found that I was able to apply to the practice what she had taught me years before, and I was much more confident in my role as a student. I understood the big picture of health care, and I believe that nurses at all levels need to understand the business side of health care. Managers always seem to be asking us to do more with fewer resources, and until I understood why, I was disgruntled. While it still is not easy, at least now I understand the business side of health care.

Self-Reflective Questions

1. What responsibilities do you have for your budget?

2. How much do you understand about the language of finance?

3. What key financial acronyms can you define?

4. How often do you meet with the finance team?

5. In what ways are you equipped to explain monthly budget variances?

6. What is the payor mix at your hospital? On your unit?

7. How do you convert hours to full-time employees (FTEs) and FTEs to hours?

8. How is your unit productivity measured?

9. How well can you interpret an income statement or balance sheet?

10. How do you keep your staff informed about, and involved in, the budget process?

35

(The) First 100 Days:
Accelerating the Learning Curve for the New Nurse Leader

"Sit down before fact as a little child, be prepared to give up every conceived notion, follow humbly wherever and whatever abysses nature leads, or you will learn nothing."

—Thomas Huxley

Mentor

Chua Gek Phin, MN, BN, Grad.
  Dip (Onc), RN
WHO Fellow in Ambulatory
  Nursing
Director of Nursing
National Cancer Centre
Singapore

Mentee

Eunice Nah Swee Lin,
  MSc, HRM, BHSN
Senior Staff Nurse
SingHealth Polyclinics
Singapore

In Singapore, after a nurse becomes a nurse leader, he or she is considered to have attained the pinnacle of his or her nursing career. However, we are no longer like emperors ascending the throne, as of old. Times have changed. Generational culture has changed, and there are things to learn about becoming a more effective nurse leader. It is in the first 100 days of assuming the role of nurse leader that crucially sets the branding and pace for the rest of the leadership term.

As the director of nursing at the National Cancer Centre (the first of its kind in Singapore), I faced an uphill task of setting up shop, with no predecessors to consult and a lot of resentment from my former bosses who felt I had betrayed them for glory. Rumors erupted that I was robbing my former institution of its talent pool. In fact, its staff had taken a pay cut upon resigning so that they could work at the new center. In spite of how people began to view and ostracize me, I had to muster courage with a clear conscience and walk with my head held high. My only hope for redemption would be to remain humble and grow a center of excellence.

This chapter is a conviction from our hearts to prepare future leaders with straight talk gleaned from personal experience and not mere theory alone. The first 100 days could be the loneliest in your career, and you need to equip yourself with the patience, maturity, and strength to go on. Make plenty of friends because you'll need them for emotional and tangible support. Most of all, you have to work hard and believe in possibilities. The day you choose to step forward to create a new future, you cannot look back.

Determine What Is On Your Plate

Mentor

- Take the proactive stance. Ask questions; as a leader as you cannot say, "I didn't know."

- Ask your boss what is expected of you before you start.

- Ask peers in other institutions how they view their roles and what is their list of top five recommended "To-Do's" for their position.

- If you have predecessors, ask them for advice.

- Seek feedback proactively.

Mentee

The best way to understand your new role is to discuss goals and expectations with your supervisor and seek advice on how you can excel in your first year of "office." Without seeing eye-to-eye on what is expected, you may be disappointed at your next appraisal that your expectations may have differed.

Find time to seek feedback each quarter to ensure that you are on track. Adopt a partnership approach with colleagues and peers. Accountability and transparency through clear communication is paramount to understanding the role of a nursing leader.

Developing Personal Vision, Mission, and Core Values

Mentor

Leadership without a planned and communicated vision of the future lacks depth and heart. It is essential to consider how you want to lead your people and where you want to take them, and then communicate it well. There's nothing more demoralizing than a leader who can't clearly articulate why we're doing what we're doing (Kouzes & Posner, 2003).

Mentee

Interestingly, people appreciate being in touch with their leader—to know what you believe in, how you envision the future, to be informed of new developments, and what they need to do to excel. When they do not know, they can become uncertain and demoralized. Develop your personal leadership vision, mission, and core values, and celebrate your new leadership with your team. Plan the way, share the plans, and build the legacy together.

Apply the Pareto (80/20) Principle

Mentor

- Do only what is necessary.

- Do not take on more than you can handle so that you can complete what you begin. Know how much you have to accomplish in the next 6 months.

- Plan your days with time to spare. If there are fires to fight at work, it will allow you a time buffer.

- Delegate and empower.

- Hire diligent, teachable staff whom you can delegate important yet less-urgent matters to help get things done.

Mentee

Vilfredo Pareto, Italian economist, spoke about the effect of diminishing marginal benefit, which is known as the Pareto, or 80/20, Principle. It is a principle often employed in management efficiency.

For example, in a list of 10 items in a To-Do list, decide what the top (two or three) most important items are that require your attention and that cannot be delegated. To gain best results, focus on the 20 percent that is most important to accomplish that no one else can help you with. The first 100 days can be a whirlwind of learning and doing, so being organized is critical.

Build Your Team

Mentor

- Know your staff members' skills and employ their strengths.

- Understand your staff at a more personal level to build camaraderie.

- Hire the best and choose people you want to work with when you hire them.

- Do things together with your team to let them know you are with them and for them.

- Build trust.

Mentee

Don't hire for the sake of credentials alone. Hire those with whom you can talk easily with and enjoy being around. Hire for shared values and complementing strengths that you can maximize to build a high-performing team. Socialize with team members to get to know them better. They need to know that you are a leader who understands their plight. Working as a team to achieve goals requires relationship building. Build strong relationships with your team that will last through tough times.

Find Mentors

Mentor

- Find a mentor who is or was a nurse leader who is willing to share.

- Find mentors who are in the business field for a breath of fresh air and a different perspective.

- Find a mentor who is a family member or friend who is close enough to be your confidante and knows you well enough to tell you the truth.

Mentee

In Singapore, former prime ministers hold an active advisory role as senior minister after their term is over. This gives the new prime minister counsel and experience should he or she require it because the decisions made are of utmost importance. Although a nurse leader's decisions are not as comparably life changing, leadership is a journey that can get lonelier and heavier the longer you are on it. Therefore, it is good to find a few mentors to guide you and to share your heart with. Mentoring is an effective reflective aid with which to assess and improve how we lead and do things, especially when there is no hand-over of portfolio. Read widely, too, because authors can be mentors who we haven't met.

Impact Your World and Leave a Legacy

An ancient Chinese proverb tells us, "A good beginning is half the battle won." The first 100 days of leadership can be intimidating or overwhelming because the learning curve is high for most. Therefore, it is all the more important to be organized and to carefully plan out how we intend to lead the way while learning as much as we can from those who can impart good advice and share knowledge. After you know what you have to do, build your team because you can't do it all on your own. It takes a good team to do great work.

The beginning of any leader's challenge is always an unknown, unwritten adventure, waiting to be authored. With a parent's loving passion, make plans to grow the work and people, sift from the wisdom of those who have been there before, and surround yourself with those who would help you. Beginnings are all about audacious courage: the practice of humility with an unceasing thirst to be in touch, learn, and progress.

Self-Reflective Questions

1. How can you better understand your role from more than one perspective?

2. If you are not spending enough time with your team to build relationships, what can you do to improve?

3. How can you best determine the individual strengths of each staff and maximize their potential?

4. How can you better surround yourself with effective and talented people who can partner with you?

5. What is your vision for tomorrow?

Self-Reflective Questions *(continued)*

6. How can you clearly articulate your thoughts and ideas, based on feedback?

7. How can you help your staff take ownership of their work and projects through helping them understand why they need to do what they are doing versus issuing a directive?

8. How can you prevent yourself from taking on more than you can handle?

9. How can you best maximize your time through effective empowerment and delegation?

10. Who are the mentors who are willing and able to guide you toward greater success?

36 Gifts: Discovering Earth Angels and Rocky Roads

"A Nurse is . . . a kaleidoscope of potential and promise, offering hope for compassionate and competent care."

—Debra Townsend

Mentor
Debra Townsend, RN
CEO, President
Concepts of Care, Inc., and
  The National Center for Compassionate Care™
Washington, D.C., USA

Mentee
Jeff Doucette, MS, RN, CEN,
  FACHE, NEA-BC
Senior Consultant/Partner
  Doucette & Associates
Durham, North Carolina, USA

We, who are called to do this work called nursing quickly realize that we are never alone. Before us, treasured souls have paved our path, making our particular journey less chaotic. We marvel at their sacrifice and cherish the wisdom they leave behind. When we feel lost, it takes just an instant to realize we are surrounded by present-day mentors, earth angels who care enough to make our contribution meaningful and the care we provide safe. They guide our hands, stimulate our minds, and touch our hearts.

I (Debra) have grown more appreciative of the art of mentoring throughout my 40 years in nursing. Perhaps our most important legacy work is to reach out to others, embracing them as nurse-mentors have done for us. What we usually discover is that the gift is ours. No words can describe the joy of knowing that our moments of shared wisdom might have an impact on patients, cherished caregivers, and future leaders.

It was the beginning of a new millennium and a "hospital in paradise" had partnered with The National Center for Compassionate Care. I was invited to serve as their chief spirit and synergy officer, establishing a healthier work culture and focusing on retention. Few have the privilege of "caring for the people that care for the people," the foundation for our Caregiver Advocacy Model. In this role, my primary joy was being present, offering mentoring in the moment and serving nurses on the front lines of care. One of the best gifts of my career was discovering a young leader named Jeff Doucette.

I asked him two simple questions during our first interview. First, "Why do you have a waiting list of 50 nurses who want to work with you?" and "Please describe yourself like a bowl of ice cream. What flavor would you be?"

His first response was "I love my teams, and let them go. It is my job to get them what they need and get out of their way." In 25 years of teaching leaders, I've discovered that few truly understand or practice the art of empowerment. This young leader already knew the secret and how to use it in daily practice.

To the second question, his emphatic answer was: "I'll tell you what I'm not. I'm not vanilla! I'm rocky road—a little nutty, a little fluffy, and there is a surprise in every bite!"

For 10 years I've watched Jeff in a variety of roles, from nursing director to his first chief nursing officer position. His energy, insight, and unwavering commitment to customer and caregiver service are refreshing. He is becoming the epitome of new leadership for health care, and I find myself in constant awe of his servant heart. Our profession needs a million more "surprises" like Jeff. Perhaps our work as mentors is to be more aware of the gifted and to encourage them in every facet of their growth.

After 10 years of cherished friendship, an interesting awareness and question has evolved: Which one of us is the mentor? Perhaps the most wonderful outcome of the mentor-mentee relationship is the realization that we continue to teach one another. Jeff reminds me of the continued gifts that are still mine to discover. I am blessed to watch him, and thousands of other new colleagues each year, as they create their own care story. I encourage you to explore the art of respectful mentoring and embrace the wisdom you receive with a renewed spirit. What you might encounter is an adventurous rocky road or an earth angel to be your guide. I guarantee they will leave a soul print on your heart and contribute their own stories to this cherished profession.

Passing on the Gift

From the time I (Jeff) was a 14-year-old volunteer in a community emergency department, I knew that I wanted to be a nurse. I also knew that the only way to get to my goal was to have great coaches and mentors along the way. Here are some simple steps to get the most out of your mentoring relationships.

You will find your mentors in the most unlikely of places. Always be on the lookout.

The first mentor I remember was Virginia Ball. She was the school nurse where I went to high school. I clearly remember thinking about nursing, but I was unsure of how to pursue my chosen career. Though guidance counselors were helpful, no one was more encouraging and understanding than Mrs. Ball. What was so unusual about this mentoring relationship was that I didn't even know that I needed a mentor, but I found one I kept in contact with for many years to come. Her depth of experiences and knowledge left me in awe. In a most interesting turn of events, Mrs. Ball also worked per diem at the local hospital in my hometown. In my first nursing leadership role as a house supervisor, Mrs. Ball worked for me! It was incredibly rewarding for both of us to collaborate after all the hours of mentoring and coaching she had given me.

Mentoring is a two-way street. Understand the needs of your mentor and clearly articulate yours.

I can't begin to recall the number of times that people ask me, "Will you be my mentor?" I always respond with the same answer: "Tell me what's in it for me." This seemingly flippant response always catches people off guard until I explain that a true mentoring relationship is a "win-win." I have yet to be in a mentoring relationship where I did not learn as much or more from the person I was mentoring. You should give clear thought to what you expect from the mentor and what the mentor can expect from you. I always write out a mentoring agreement with my mentees. This simple document clearly outlines the expectations and accountabilities of both parties in the mentoring relationship.

One mentor is never enough!

Great athletic teams have a head coach and a series of assistant coaches for a good reason. The more minds you have to solve a problem and strategize, the better the outcome. The same is true for the mentoring relationship. No one person can be all knowing. You need to understand the strengths of your mentor and your needs as a mentee. In doing this, you inevitably find that having more than one mentor is a well-rounded approach to improving your leadership. I have a mentor who I engage primarily for my non-hospital professional growth and several I call upon to help me better lead within my organizations. I strongly recommend that you consider your needs and seek mentors that fit the many facets that make you unique.

A good mentoring relationship enhances your strengths and exposes your hidden talents.

Don't expect the mentoring relationship to be an easy road. A good mentor pushes you to your limits and beyond. As I prepared to sit and write this, I found many reasons why I should not or could not complete the task. As usual, I could count on one of my most cherished mentors to push me to get it done! Mentors push you to grow your strengths even while they work to expose your hidden talents. The art of giving and receiving feedback is a critically important core value in the effective mentoring relationship.

Establishing an effective mentoring relationship can help you to develop your career and develop your potential. Choosing the right mentor, establishing a mentoring agreement, and fostering the ongoing relationship benefit both you and the mentor. Be prepared to commit to your mentor. Just as with any other relationship, this relationship is a unique sharing of information and talents that requires extraordinary commitment from both parties. So whether you are vanilla or rocky road, your commitment to fostering mentoring relationships will help you reach heights you might have never imagined!

Self-Reflective Questions

1. What joy do you find in mentoring others, knowing the impact your wisdom might have in guiding future leaders?

2. In what ways can you create moments in your day to offer the gift of presence to mentees?

3. In what ways do you follow mentees over extended periods of time, thereby witnessing their transformation and progress?

4. How do you embrace the exchange of wisdom that occurs between mentor and mentee, regularly expressing appreciation toward one another?

5. In what ways are you consistently seeking mentoring opportunities?

Self-Reflective Questions *(continued)*

6. What do you expect from a mentor and what can a mentee expect from you?

7. How do you orchestrate a mentoring agreement, outlining the expectations and accountabilities of both parties in the mentoring relationship?

8. Do you understand the strengths of your mentor, and in what ways do you seek a variety of advisors to complement your professional growth?

9. How do you value the art of giving and receiving feedback?

10. In what ways does mentoring involve a unique sharing of information and talents, thereby requiring an extraordinary commitment from both parties?

Global Nursing at Its Best

37

"The world has become so small and is a global village, and everyone is free to move around this village with so much ease! How great."

—Esther Seloilwe

Mentor

Esther Salang Seloilwe, PhD, RN, RM
Senior Lecturer
University of Botswana
Gaborone, Botswana

Mentee

Lame Gaolatihe Bakwenabatsile, RN
Nursing Officer
Princess Marina Hospital
Gaborone, Botswana

Global nursing at its best. Globalization is a modern cliché, but certainly not a new phenomenon. It dates back to the era of exploration and colonialization. The partition of Africa, the slave trade and the movement of traders, and traveling around the world all show that globalization has been around for centuries, if not longer, though perhaps now it is more pronounced.

Globalization is defined as a process of transformation of local or regional phenomenon into a global one. Herman Daly (1999) argues that sometimes internationalization and globalization are used interchangeably. It is erasure of national boundaries for economic purposes. It encompasses a broad range of activities, such as production and distribution of material goods but also non-material services, notably financial and information services. Modern globalization has been accelerated by information technology. The microchip, internet, fax, cellular phones, electronic banking, and e-learning are technologies that have drastically and quickly changed the world. In particular, they have created a new type of economy, the knowledge economy. Knowledge is no longer the domain of the few advantaged people and for particular areas; it is for everyone, everywhere, just a click away (Seloilwe, 2004). Modern technology and globalization have profoundly transformed the world.

Factors That Have Influenced Global Nursing

Perle Cowen and Sue Moorhead (2006) argue that nursing as a profession is increasingly confronted by global health issues such as HIV and AIDS, global warming, displacement of persons by wars and disasters, and so on. Although these health issues are mostly negative, globalization also presents opportunities that are positive. The nursing profession cannot ignore these issues. Nursing has to embrace this global integration and exploit it for its benefit and for the improvement of health care across the world and between nations. Some historical developments have occurred that illustrate globalization has long been embraced in nursing.

- International nursing dates back to the era of Florence Nightingale when she took nurses to the battle at Scutari, during the Crimean War, to assist wounded soldiers.

- Isabel Hampton Robb communicated with other nurses across the Atlantic Ocean to form a body of nurses that could advance the development of nursing internationally. Today, the International Council of Nurses (ICN) is one of the most powerful and influential organizations of nurses in the world.

- Since the 1970s, Sigma Theta Tau International (STTI) has been advancing global nursing scholarship in the world. Currently, this organization is becoming even more global, with chapters at large all over the world pursuing the advancement of nursing knowledge and scholarship. The establishment of the African chapter at large, which I have been instrumental in forming, was a breakthrough, showing that nursing indeed should transcend boundaries.

- Modern technology, including e-mail and the internet, has also accelerated these developments. These technologies have made communication easy, quick, and global so that issues can be discussed and resolved within seconds. Nurses across the globe have formed listserves and created forums to discuss issues that concern them. These nurses provide nursing care away from their homelands.

- International nursing has evolved to include a broad range of activities. Nurses are working around the globe at both the individual and organizational levels. While serving as chair of the department of nursing at the University of Botswana, I have had the opportunity to serve as a member of STTI's futures council. The brainstorming of this work and the completion of the vision all occurred through technology— e-mail and teleconferencing.

- The establishment of links between educational institutions is another example of global nursing. For example, in Botswana I have been instrumental in establishing these links, including the University of Botswana (UB) and the University of Pennsylvania, the UB School of Nursing and Jonkoping University in Sweden, and a Faculty of Health Science link. We have many international exchange scholars and students at UB, and students and scholars have gone abroad on exchange programs.

- Forums have also brought nurses together, such as international conferences to promote global nursing. Nurses have also conducted collaborative research projects across nations, promoting the development of knowledge across the globe.

Requirements for Global Nursing

To achieve global nursing, the strengthening of the nursing workforce worldwide is imperative. Strengthening the nursing workforce leads to better access to preventive, curative, and rehabilitative care, which in turn improves the performance of health care systems. It requires determined advocacy, leadership, and a deep and sustained political and financial commitment on the part of individual nations and the international communities. Strategic planning for nursing development is also critical to the realization of global nursing goals. According to the ICN, appropriate planning and management of nursing workforce is fundamental to achieving and maintaining an optimal workforce and well functioning health care system (ICN, 2005).

Whereas each country plans nursing personnel in accordance with its local context, global nursing calls for a comprehensive and global nursing education system that encompasses a wide range of issues aiming at producing a nurse who is more competent to perform at a global level.

Challenges

International Recruitment and Migration of Nurses

International recruitment and migration of nursing personnel have become issues of global concern in the past decade. Nurses have always embraced the opportunity to move across national borders in search of better pay, career advancement, better working conditions, and quality of life (Kingma, 2006; Connell et al., 2007; Tshweneagae, 2005).

The main argument explaining the relatively high levels of nurse migration today is a combination of nursing shortages in the developed world and "push" factors that cause nurses to leave their home countries, such as low wages, poor career opportunities, unsafe practice environment, and political instability (ICN, 2005).

Practice Environment and Organizational Performance

The varying and often poor quality of environments in which nurses practice is recognized as one of the factors contributing to the global challenges of attracting new recruits into nursing and retaining existing ones. Inadequate staffing and heavy work loads; excessive overtime; inflexible schedules; exposure to occupational hazards; violence; abuse; lack of autonomy; poor human resource management practices and leadership; lack of access to necessary supplies, medication, and technology; inefficient incentives; and poor career development opportunities (Kingma, 2006; Connell et al., 2007; Tshweneagae, 2005) are some of the factors that impact the quality of nursing practice environment. Buchan (2006) argues that the challenge for health care systems is to identify and put in place a package of incentives best suited to meet the specific needs of nurses.

Nursing Education

Central to ensuring the production and retention of a competent nursing work force is the need to educate nurses using a curriculum based on the knowledge, skills, and competencies needed to practice. Nursing education varies in many countries with different levels of preparation, and countries educate nurses for various reasons, especially to meet the health care needs in their own countries and for export. To ensure that the nursing curriculum reflects all these needs, all relevant stakeholders—regulators, employers, educators, and clinicians—must be involved in the development process. Nursing education globally is evolving, and some programs are being improved through international collaboration. Nursing knowledge has to adapt to meet cultural and contextual needs (Upvall, 2006).

Nursing Leadership

Addressing the challenges facing the nursing profession requires effective leadership and management abilities at all levels. Leadership development is a critical aspect of positive and sustainable change today and into the future. Nurse leaders and managers need to be prepared to manage rapid change in a globalised and technologically driven world, with limited financial and human resources.

Nurse leaders and managers, both today and tomorrow, need to demonstrate competence in such areas as strategic thinking and planning, staff development and management, performance appraisal systems, organizational culture and development, communication, negotiation, interpersonal relations, problem solving, conflict resolution, customer services, equipment and resource management, quality improvement, safety and disaster networking, politics and policy development, teamwork, and fundraising.

Nurse leaders also need to understand global governance and regulation and how to build alliances and coalitions, use political leverage, and articulate the value of nursing with key players in national, regional, and international, organizations.

Reactions from the Mentee

Globalization is defined as a process of transformation and has been accelerated by, and is now dependent on, information technology that has created a new type of economy—the knowledge-based economy. This knowledge-based economy is especially evident and accessible nowadays because of the internet. As a student studying at the university, I accessed a lot of information through the internet, which facilitated my learning.

International nursing has long existed, but today it is being amplified as the world has become smaller and smaller. Things we used to just read about, we can now see for ourselves. My generation is fortunate to bear witness to this great development.

The formation of the Africa Honor Society for Nursing is also a good example of global nursing at its best. This organization affords us beginning nurses a platform to collaborate with other scholars not only in our region, but also around the world. We can interact with fellow nurses and share ideas on how to improve nursing care delivery, thus implementing evidence-based practice, which is simply the integration of the best possible research with clinical expertise to meet patient needs. Individual clinical expertise requires a level of proficiency of judgment acquired through both formal education and experience. The ICN in collaboration with Blackwell Publishing has a book titled *Advanced Nursing Practice* by Madrean Schober and Fadwa Affara (2006) that elaborates on the role played by the nurses with advanced knowledge and skills required in health care services world wide. The book explores international commonalities and differences in advanced practice nursing (APN) and addresses issues in practice, education, regulation, research, and role/practice development that are central to the distinctive nature of APN. STTI's *Journal of Nursing Scholarship* also affords an opportunity to use knowledge that experts generate to improve patient care. As a clinical nurse, I refer to these works in my every day practice, and what an opportunity it is that I can use such a resource!

Self-Reflective Questions

1. How do you define global nursing?

2. What factors have influenced the development of global nursing?

3. How do you think global nursing can be achieved?

4. What are some nursing organizations that are engaged in promoting global nursing?

5. How is your country encouraging global nursing?

6. How have you been involved personally in the process of global nursing?

7. What are your views on the issue of promoting global nursing?

8. What has been your interaction level with nurses of other countries?

9. Have you ever been involved in an exchange program? In what ways?

10. What suggestions do you have on how globalization in nursing can be promoted or improved?

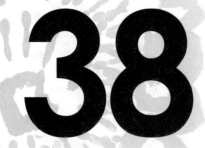

38 (Gaining a) Global Perspective

"Never doubt that a small group of committed citizens can change the world. Indeed, it is the only thing that ever has."

—Margaret Mead

Mentor
Ged F. Williams, MHA, RN
Founding Chair/President,
   World Federation of Critical
   Care Nurses
Executive Director Nursing &
   Midwifery Services
Gold Coast Health Service
   District
Queensland, Australia,

Mentee
Wilson Cañon Montañez
Founding Member, Colombian
   Committee of Critical Care
   Nurses
Nurse Educator and Research
   Assistant, Cardiology Group
Autonomous University
Bucaramanga, Colombia

Most leaders aspire to have a "global perspective." But how do you obtain a global perspective? And how can you inspire others to develop an interest and to make a contribution in the global nursing community? In this chapter, we share the journey, the process, and lessons learned in establishing nursing organisations with an international and global perspective.

A popular Australian vocalist, John Williams, sings a children's song: "From little things, big things grow." These sentiments reflect our experience in developing a global perspective as nursing leaders. (The inspiration for the song was, in fact, the early civil rights protests by black Aboriginal people who started a movement for equal rights and recognition in what was a racially divided society in Australia at the time.)

In August 1997, Ged attended the 7th World Congress on Critical Care in Ottawa, Canada, where he attended a meeting of critical care nursing leaders at a session jointly hosted by the Canadian Association of Critical Care Nurses (CACCN) and the American Association of Critical-Care Nurses (AACN). Approximately 80 nurses attended the meeting where the participants agreed to communicate, collaborate, and cooperate beyond the meeting to form a network of international critical care nurse (CCN) leaders. Inspired by the meeting, Ged (then 33) spoke to senior and experienced Australian CCN leaders and asked how communication, collaboration, and cooperation could be facilitated in a practical sense. The response was not positive: "Ged, these guys meet every four years and say the same thing, but nothing ever happens!" Disappointed, Ged waited for two years hoping that some action might come from the Ottawa meeting. Nothing ever did.

By this time, e-mail was reasonably common in the western world, and Ged began e-mailing the "younger" leaders (people around his age in similar positions in their own countries). A group of about eight from different countries decided to try to establish a list of known CCN leaders throughout the world, to survey these leaders to identify the issues and views on critical care nursing in their respective countries, and to identify the readiness of these nurses and their national associations to support the establishment of an international critical care nursing collaboration or federation.

In two years, led by Ged, the group surveyed 23 leaders from 23 different countries, and found that the support for an international federation of critical care nursing organisations was strong. (Williams et al., 2001).

In October 2001, the World Federation of Critical Care Nurses (WFCCN) was formed at a meeting similar to the one in Ottawa four years prior. This time they met in Sydney, Australia. A global perspective evolved for those who participated in the program. Eight nursing leaders representing eight national nursing organisations established the first council of the WFCCN. A subsequent study was conducted in 2005 that profiled 51 countries (Williams et al., 2007) (see Table 1), and a third study is being undertaken in 2009 to profile 70 countries. WFCCN now has a web site (www.wfccn.org), journal, publications, position statements, international research projects, and conferences with more than 30 formal organisation members.

Table 1   Participating countries in 2005 WFCCN Survey.

Africa	The Americas	Asia/Pacific	Europe
Botswana	Argentina	Australia	Belgium
Ghana	Bolivia	China	Ireland
Malawi	Brazil	Hong Kong	Britain
Namibia	Canada	Japan	Italy
South Africa	Chile	Korea	Croatia
Tanzania	Colombia	Macau	Netherlands
Uganda	Mexico	New Zealand	Cyprus
	Peru	Philippines	Norway
	United States	Singapore	Denmark
	Venezuela	Sri Lanka	Poland
		Taiwan	Estonia
			Saudi Arabia
			Finland
			Slovenia
			France
			Spain
			Germany
			Sweden
			Greece
			Switzerland
			Hungary
			Turkey
			Iceland

On reflection, Ged realized that all this did not start with a single moment of inspiration. Instead, the roots of the organisation's development stemmed back to his experiences as president of the Queensland Branch of the Confederation of Australian Critical Care Nurses (CACCN) in 1994-96, National President of CACCN in 1997, Founding President of the Australian College of Critical Care Nurses (ACCCN) in 1999, and many other life experiences along the way that taught him about the cultures, issues, and needs of CCNs in different yet similar circumstances and contexts to his own.

So, how did Ged develop this passion for a global perspective on nursing? Among other things, he allocated time to travel and to visit hospitals and nurses in other parts of Australia and the world, listening to people's stories, dreams, and aspirations and providing reciprocal encouragement and fellowship, often through interpreters.

Mentee Experiences

Wilson and his colleagues have a similar but different experience in South America. In August 2005, the WFCCN co-hosted the 9th World Congress on Critical Care with the World Federation of Societies of Intensive Care and Critical Care Medicine (WFSICCM) in Buenos Aires, Argentina. This was the same international conference as the one held in Ottawa in 1997 and Sydney in 2001. At the Buenos Aires conference, WFCCN called nursing leaders from Central and South America to participate in a meeting of critical care nursing leaders to explore communication, collaboration, and cooperation opportunities that might lead to the possible formation of a regional Latin-American network of critical care nurses.

In true Latin-American style, the Spanish speaking people expressed overwhelming enthusiasm and passion for the concept. Everyone exchanged e-mail addresses, and in the ensuing two years, these leaders held a series of meetings in Venezuela, Columbia, and Peru to discuss, develop, and draft the constitution and plans for FLECI (Federacion Latino-Americana de Enfermia en Cuidado Intensive—Federation of Latin-American Intensive Care Nurses), which was launched in Lima, Peru, in November 2007.

Wilson has been one of the key participants and supporters in these meetings, leading up to and including the formation meeting of FLECI. (Wilson even designed the FLECI logo.) He quickly learned many things about nursing and nurses in other parts of South and Central America, making many new friends and establishing a broader view of nursing practice and professionalism. In 2008 Wilson organised a five-month education program for himself in Australia where he enrolled in a full-time English language course, visited many hospitals and ICUs, and explored Australian cultures, landscapes, and art.

Wilson is now a member of the newly formed Colombian Association of Critical Care Nurses, he regularly participates in the activities of FLECI, has written and published in English (Cañon, 2007), and plans to present at the 10th World Congress on Critical Care in Florence, Italy, in August 2009—in both Spanish and English. At just 34 years of age Wilson is developing a global perspective early in his nursing career. Wilson is currently a research assistant and teacher at Autonomous University and is studying for a master's degree in epidemiology. In the next 10 years, Wilson will likely have a strong global perspective on nursing, will be multilingual, and will be a key leader in the international nursing arena. Time will tell!

Here are some simple things to remember if you wish to develop a global perspective as a nursing leader:

Grow your skills and competencies in change management and leadership locally.

Lead small changes and incrementally take on bigger, broader challenges.

Overseas travel and networks help to expand your knowledge and understanding of nursing in other cultures and countries.

Be patient. You will find so much to know, learn, and experience. It won't happen overnight but it will happen.

Allow yourself to be humbled by the stories and experiences of others.

Learn to have the serenity to accept the things you cannot change, the courage to change the things you can, the wisdom to know the difference, and the grace to understand the perspective of others.

Self-Reflective Questions

1. How often do you go out of your way to visit new hospitals/wards when travelling?

2. In what ways do you try to understand different cultures, languages, and perspectives from other nurses?

3. What opportunities have you sought to work with small groups of people to pursue worthy humanitarian causes?

4. What mentors do you have who can guide you with national and international linkages?

5. How do you get others involved in your activities, and how do you share the learning?

6. What overseas conferences have you attended and what hospital, health, and social learning did you participate in while visiting overseas?

7. What profiles of nursing from other countries and regions have you read?

8. What steps do you take to inform yourself when a health crisis in a foreign land is reported in the media?

9. What nursing friends in non-English speaking countries do you have? How can you make more?

10. What web sites do you check regularly to increase your global perspective?

Goal Setting

39

"A goal without a plan is just a wish."

—Antoine de Saint-Exupery

Mentor

Ged F. Williams, MHA, RN
Founding Chair/President,
   World Federation of Critical
   Care Nurses
Executive Director, Nursing and
   Midwifery Services
Gold Coast Health
   Service District
Queensland, Australia

Mentee

Katie A. Scarlett, BSN
Recent Graduate,
   Bachelor of Nursing
Charles Darwin University
Northern Territory,
   Australia

Have you ever felt overwhelmed, almost sickened, by the thought of a major long-term goal that you have to accomplish? Whether you are beginning a nursing baccalaureate program and know 3 or 4 years of hard work are ahead of you, or you are starting as a newly appointed chief nursing officer knowing how much change will be required to get your new organisation to meet accreditation standards, nursing is a field of endeavour that places enormous challenges in front of us all on most days.

Of course, we have a choice. We can ignore the challenge and follow a different, less difficult path, or we can seize the opportunity to accept the challenge and hopefully create a better situation, for ourselves, our organisation, or our broader community.

To accept a challenging goal we must first look at the planning and goal setting requirements. It doesn't matter if the goal is personal, professional, organisational, or societal, goal setting and planning processes follow the same simple principles.

Personal Goal Setting: Katie

Ged is my father. As a teenager I was quite confused about who I was, what I wanted to do, and how I would live my life. After I left home, I experimented with different lifestyles, but I found emptiness in some of these choices. Finding a partner and making a commitment to follow a path together formed the start of a personal goal, which is to share my life and experiences with a very good friend with similar personal goals, values, and interests. Along the way, however, I felt a yearning to "be something." I enrolled in a social work degree program for a while, but that did not suit me. Eventually, I worked in our local hospital as a patient care attendant and as a ward clerk. This work enabled me to interact with many patients and to help care for them with many nurses and other health professionals. With the encouragement of theses nurses, my friends, and my family, I set a personal goal to become a registered nurse.

Professional Goal Setting: Katie

Academic study has never come easily to me. But trying to juggle a marriage, a job, and full-time study was even harder. Some personal sacrifices and compromises are necessary when you set an ambitious goal, and being a registered nurse became my goal.

Planning and determination have been key elements to my success to this point. Having a mentor to keep me focused and encouraged is also important. Each semester I write a study plan. It identifies where the key milestones are, for example, assignment due dates, online discussion dates, and examination dates. For each week of the semester, I identify what subjects or chapters I must read and summarize.

With my mentor, I identified dates and times we planned to talk through the work I am doing and clarify concepts and issues, check on progress, and review the plan. Finding a knowledgeable and understanding mentor is an important first step on the journey to achieving an important professional goal. Discussing and planning the journey together and regularly reviewing the plan and actions are necessary to stay focused on the many sub-goals to be achieved along the way.

Organisational Goal Setting: Ged

Setting goals for an organisation such as a hospital or health service uses the same principles of planning and determination that an individual might use. The primary difference is that organisational goal setting has many more participants and stakeholders. When I start in a new organisation in a senior nursing role, I follow a consistent consultation and fact-finding process that starts with a personalised visit and discussion with every manager in my area of responsibility and with every senior director that influences my area of responsibility. Early clarification of goals, expectations, ambitions, and frustrations of these key "opinion leaders" is vital to my early assessment of the culture, climate, and potential that exists in the organisation.

For me to show a human face and to commence positive friendly relationships is critical to getting the mood right for the interventions I may later want to start. I have a simple process for business planning with the nursing service. The seven steps to writing a business plan are summarised in Table 1. I also provide a simple template to each sponsor of each goal or issue to be addressed (see Table 2).

Table 1   Nursing business planning process example.

Step 1 (Week 1)

a) Environmental scan:
- Survey nursing staff—strengths, weakness, opportunities, and threat (SWOT).

b) Nursing leadership and management team:
- Review existing nursing business plans.
- Review existing organisation-wide business plans.
- Review state/province nursing strategic directions plans.
- Review recent nursing/organisation staff/patient satisfaction surveys.

Step 2 (Week 4)

Nursing leadership and management brainstorming session:
- Identify/pre-empt key issues that require immediate attention.
- Agree to allocate key issues to individual "sponsors."
- Agree to template format for documenting each issue and strategy.
  Template headings: Issue/impact, action, who, when, cost, expected result.
  Must also include a "no-cost" option.
- Sponsor is responsible for consulting key stakeholders to inform strategy.

Step 3 (Week 7)

Sponsors write up individual plan and provide to secretary 2 weeks prior to business planning day.

Table 1   Nursing business planning process example.

Step 4 (Week 10)

Business Planning Day (All senior nurses and shared governance committee members):

- Venue—choose a comfortable motel, convention centre.
- Introduction and keynote address(es).
- Outline of existing nursing, district, QH plans.
- Sponsors present issues/strategy, one-by-one, with time for discussion/refinement/endorsement or deletion.
- Morning/afternoon tea, lunch, and conclude with drinks.

Step 5 (Week 11)

Sponsors modify template presentation based upon agreed feedback from business planning day and submit to secretary within 1 week.

Step 6 (Week 12)

Nursing Leaders and Management Regroup (2-hour session):

- Review and modify issues and strategies. Endorse plan within 2 weeks of business planning day.

Step 7

Review issues/strategies and progress periodically via:

- Nursing leadership and management meeting/shared governance committee.
- Formally review and repeat in 12-months time.

Table 2   Nursing services business plan (single page for each issue).

Issue:				
Sponsor:				
Description:				
Tasks/ Actions	Result to be achieved	Who Responsible	By When	Progress Report

A 12-month nursing business plan has about 30 goals or issues, and I expect 75% of the plan to be achieved in the time frame set. Others might be delayed, and some might be discarded as no longer being required or relevant.

Organisational goal setting requires broad consultation and input from many stakeholders. You need time to invest in the consultation and planning process so that most stakeholders can have some ownership and acceptance of the plan.

Societal Goal Setting: Ged

Societal goal setting and change involves many more stakeholders than organizational goal setting and change. This is the realm of the politician; that is, a person who understands the interests and power of other strong opinion leaders, advocacy groups, and the broader community.

As a nurse and leader within the profession, I find it is sometimes necessary to take on a role as a change agent for society. This role can take many forms such as advocating for improved infant health services, establishing a community organisation to coordinate self-help programs for disadvantaged groups, or leading a school parents and citizens committee. In any such role we choose to take on, leadership skills such as goal setting, planning, and influencing are essential.

In my own experience, I have chosen to live and work in the Australian outback for 7 years. As director of nursing at Alice Springs Hospital, I was confronted by the living conditions and challenges faced by many in the community. The indigenous aboriginal people of Australia had, and continue to have, very poor health, education, and social outcomes. According to the Australian Institute of Health and Welfare (2008), childhood illness and death are many times higher in the aboriginal community and life expectancy is 17 years less for an aboriginal person compared to a non-aboriginal person.

Of great concern to me was alcohol and substance abuse resulting in serious violence and injury, particularly that directed at young to middle-aged women and children (Williams et al., 2002). Academic, professional, political, and personal activism were all elements of my response at what was a serious social issue that not only impacted negatively on the health system but almost every other facet of society. My small but important efforts were part of a much larger response by many others to lobby for serious social reform to address this important issue—an issue that is going to take decades or generations to change.

Leadership and Goal Setting

Adair (1983) identified the important distinctions between transactional and transformational leadership. Transactional leadership focuses on achieving a task, taking into account the needs of individuals (self), and the needs of the group (others). Katie's leadership activities and examples are primarily transactional.

Transformational leadership focuses on the relationship of the leader with team members and the inspiration that leads to organisational transformation/change. Ged's leadership activities and examples are primarily transformational.

Transactional and transformational leadership styles are not mutually exclusive. Depending on the scale and scope of the goal to be achieved, either style might be appropriate, although Musker (2004) suggests transformational leadership is the preferred style in caring professions, particularly at the organisational and society level.

Leadership and Planning

In his book, *First Things First*, Stephen Covey (1999) notes that the typical organisation or person spends too much time managing interruptions and crises and much less time planning, wheras a high performing organisation or individual spends much more time on planning.

After an important goal is identified, significant time and energy should be allocated to the planning phase. If planning is done well, then much less time is required initiating, controlling, and supporting the activity, and the goal is ultimately achieved. A useful checklist to the goal setting and planning process is "WRITE IT UP and Publish" (see sidebar); it's important to document and share these learned lessons.

Making Choices

As nurses, we can choose to follow a safe and predictable career path and lifestyle, or we can choose to accept daunting and challenging responsibilities. With either choice, we must set goals for ourselves, our profession, our organisation, or our broader society. Communication and consultation are inevitable and important aspects to the goal setting process. The larger the goal or stakeholder group, the more consultation and communication are required, and the more important a transformational leadership style is. However, no matter how experienced any of us are, we are all well advised to surround ourselves with trusted mentors to help guide us through the challenging and daunting periods so that we are encouraged to pursue the goal and ultimately succeed.

Finally, to achieve our goals, we need clearly documented, well thought-out, and tested plans. We have both found that transparent, documented, and shared planning help us and our colleagues achieve our goals.

Checklist for Goal Setting and Planning– "WRITE IT UP and Publish"

1. **W**rite your goal with a simple explanation as to why it is important and how it will be achieved.

2. **R**esearch the issue to be addressed.

3. **I**dentify interested parties and stakeholders and involve them.

4. **T**est the various ideas and options available to fulfill the goal.

5. **E**ngage others in the planning process to ensure different skills and expertise inform the final approach.

6. **I**nitiate the actions that have been planned and monitor progress against each sub goal.

7. **T**ime is needed to implement your actions; never underestimate the time required to implement change and achieve complex goals.

8. **U**se many evaluation methods to ensure all aspects of your goal are achieved.

9. **P**raise and recognise those who help to achieve the goal.

Self-Reflective Questions

1. In what ways do you record your goal(s)?

2. In what ways do you research the issue? Who, what, when, and how have others done this?

3. What feedback do you seek from others as to the focus and direction of your goals?

4. What mentors do you have that can guide you with your goal setting and planning?

5. How do you get others involved in your goal and plan?

Self-Reflective Questions (continued)

6. How much time do you spend documenting, refining, and testing the plan?

7. How much time have you allocated? And are the timeframes realistic?

8. How do you re-check your plan at stages throughout the process and adjust it?

9. In what ways do you show the focus, determination, and perseverance to reach the goal?

10. What learning lessons, successes, and failures can you share with others?

Grant Applications and Initiations

40

"Writing a sound research grant application is probably the most intellectually challenging of all research tasks. It takes a long time to become a skilled research grant writer, so learn, as I did, from—and with—more experienced researchers with a proven track record of success."

—Alison Tierney

Mentor
Debbie Tolson
Head of Research, School of
  Nursing, Midwifery and
  Community Health
Glasgow Caledonian
  University
Glasgow, Scotland, United
  Kingdom

Mentee
Dr. Joanne Booth
Senior Research Fellow, School
  of Nursing, Midwifery and
  Community Health
Glasgow Caledonian
  University
Glasgow, Scotland, United
  Kingdom

In the broad scheme of things, three types of grants are of interest to nurses: research project and research programme grants, grants for infrastructure and equipment, and grants for everything else, including scholarships and personal study awards. These range from contract awards with clearly defined terms and deliverables (for example, research project awards) to true grants that support a more general aim and allow the recipient more flexibility. Most grant applications involve two strands: the proposal (describes the planned activities) and the application for funding (maps costs and funding request). The lessons we can share on grant writing apply irrespective of the type of grant you seek, so for brevity we concentrate on writing grant applications for research.

In this chapter, we talk as a research professor (mentor) and former nurse consultant (mentee) who both moved to the academy mid career.

Mentor: General Considerations

Applying for grants can be daunting, and you should not underestimate what is involved. Each time you submit a grant application, it tells the funding agency something about the quality of research within the university, about your profession, and about you as a researcher. Therefore, you and your colleagues have a collective responsibility to prepare proposals that are well crafted and display scientific rigour. Proposals prepared in haste rarely achieve the coherence, quality, and realistic costing demanded, and at worst they produce reputational damage and personal distress. On the rare occasion they are funded, they often cost the organisation more to deliver than the grant income received. Dealing with rejection for well-crafted proposals is tough; dealing with rejection for poor quality proposals is humiliating and best avoided.

Writing a grant application is a blend of science, parsimony, and politics. Science includes selecting appropriate methodology and methods to answer research questions. Parsimony is about applying careful attention to detail and editing skills to succinctly communicate ideas with precision and clarity. Politics involves knowing how to convince those at the funding agency that your proposed project satisfies their requirements and offers value for money. You need to convince them that your project should be done now, by your team, in the way you propose. This means you need to understand the internal and external context and the strategic thinking that shapes the perceived merits of your project. Lesson 1 is to know your funder, both who and what they are likely to fund.

Writing Grants

The planning stage is critical to designing a research study, and the discerning nurse researcher must juggle science with legal-ethical and research governance requirements and must think carefully about the practicalities of real-world research and what is possible given the available resource (grant).

The skilled grant writer translates the research proposal and its underlying complexities into an application that is straightforward and clear, convincingly argued, and well edited. Evidence of an applicant's track record in the form of research publications and previous grant completions with appropriate outputs (reports, publications, and conference presentations) speak volumes to the review committee. If you are new to writing grants then team up with more experienced people. Everyone, no matter how experienced in grant writing, can benefit from a critical peer who provides honest and informed feedback. Don't rely on your friends; seek out established scientists, preferably those with experience of making and reviewing grant applications. Be prepared for multiple revisions and challenging feedback and accept that you have to invest a lot of effort and emotion. For your first few applications, or when you raise your ambition in terms of the scale of award sought or prestige of the funding agency, you can gain much from talking to experienced scientific reviewers from nursing and other disciplines. Another way to learn about the pitfalls and essentials of grant writing is through observer status at fund awarding committee meetings.

On a practical note, you need to stay aware of Murphy's Law during grant preparation—if anything can go wrong, it will! A corollary of Murphy's Law is that "everything takes longer than you think," so you might find it helpful to draw up a timetable by working backward from the submission deadline date (Table 1). Remember to tell others to complete their contribution several days ahead of the absolute deadline—longer if possible.

Table 1   A submission backward: time planning.

Key Dates	Actual Date	Key Development Steps
Award announcement		Prepare for success or rejection. Be sensitive to your team's feelings and share news good or bad with due thought to the impact on others.
Review Committee Meeting Date (you might be invited to make a presentation so be available).		
Funder's grant submission deadline.	Start Point!	
Deadlines for obtaining administrative signatories from your own/co-sponsor institution.		Final refinement and proofread.
Your deadline for co-applicant signatures.		Internal peer review of draft proposal.
Your deadline for final draft of proposal and accurate costings.		Clarify the ethical-legal considerations/required permission procedures, and management pathways.
Your deadline for receipt of all documentation required from co-applicants, for example, curriculum vitae, equal opportunity forms.		Estimate budget and adjust plans to fit grant.
Funder's deadline for expression of interest (if required).		Involve stakeholders, users, and collaborating institutions as appropriate.
		Draft proposal.
Funding announcement/ invitational bid or you decide to pursue an open grant call.		Identify a critical peer/supervisor. Assemble your team.

Mentee: Personal Reflections on the Journey from Novice to Lead Applicant

As a senior practitioner, I was accustomed to an autonomous role, leading practice, and being consulted for my knowledge and clinical expertise. Working in research demanded a re-evaluation of my knowledge and skill base. Through reflecting and sensitive mentoring, I realised that a PhD, and the learning gained during its achievement, were merely an effective embarkation point for a research career. I reclassified myself as a novice with respect to grant applications and the leadership of externally funded research, and I realised that I could not develop the necessary new skill set through traditional routes of academic learning. In my view the key to developing the abilities to lead research is the considered identification of a mentor who has knowledge, skills, experience, and strategic vision and is willing to share those with you to facilitate your development.

This relationship is crucial to your success because very little written guidance encompasses the multiple considerations inherent in successful grant application. A plethora of advice exists on research designs and methods, on writing robust scientific proposals, and on getting findings published, but almost nothing exists about negotiating the complex maze of activities that form the grant application process and that ultimately allow you to put your research plans into action. In effect, the current situation revisits the apprenticeship model of learning. In the United Kingdom it is known as "coattailing" an expert researcher. From a mentee's point of view, choosing the right mentor is critical to your ultimate progression and indeed to your career.

As a novice, you need to develop a vision about the direction of your research work and the goals you aim to achieve. A long-term career can be constructed only where a sustained passion drives it forward. Finding your "niche" is fundamental, yet might be particularly challenging. This was the case for me: As a new member of staff, I joined an already established team of researchers on a funded programme of research (Tolson et al., 2008, 2007, 2006) about which I had peripheral understanding through work undertaken in my previous role. Though I could and did indeed want to contribute to this programme to learn about contract research, I had an ever-present need to develop my own research and take a lead in grant writing.

To help me identify my niche area, my professorial mentor reminded me of the need for an area fertile for funding and something that I was truly interested in developing. After I had committed to investigating urinary continence promotion with older people, pursuing several grant opportunities seemed possible. Understanding the risks and benefits of each was key to selecting my first bid. I examined my chances of success and targeted a small international collaborative project award from the British Academy (www.britac.ac.uk/funding/index.cfm). At the time, I did not appreciate the importance of targeting a prestigious organisation, even for a small grant, but I have gained valuable experience and confidence through the international collaboration and have had papers accepted at international conferences and a publication in an international journal (Booth et al., 2009). Since this first grant success, I have gathered in a few larger grants and am building up a programme of work. I still work backward from the grant submission date and have developed a better feel for how long various stages in the application process are likely to take.

Of course your initial development is not the only important component in building your long-term research career. Your mentor can encourage and support your transitions, from novice research team collaborator to taking on leadership roles and ultimately to leading the application and initiation process. A key feature of this for me is learning about horizon scanning and the importance of anticipatory research idea formation. Being "ahead of the game" can be fruitful, and your mentor's advice on where and when to invest time and effort is often invaluable.

Any person involved in the grant application process can attest to the absolute necessity to adopt an objective approach to the business throughout. How to deal with rejection is one of the first and most painful skill sets that must be developed (rejection is not a "lesson to learn"; it is an "experience that must be coped with"). Learning to take the criticism that arises from the review process (some of which you might consider harsh) and using it constructively to improve your application is an essential survival strategy, but one that you must experience to fully comprehend.

Practice, Resilience, and Determination

Great researchers are not automatically great grant writers; it takes practice, resilience, and determination to gather grants. Learn the craft from someone who can help you grow confidence and guide you through moments of success and challenge—a mentor who believes you have what it takes to succeed in this competitive business.

Self-Reflective Questions

1. Are you considering applying for this grant just because you can or is there a compelling strategic organisational/career reason?

2. What are the reasons for applying for this grant and do the reason(s) outweigh the reasons why you should not proceed?

3. What is the funding ceiling and does it offer sufficient resource to cover the full economic cost of the research you wish to undertake?

4. What is the potential gain? Do your chances of success and the potential gain offset the effort involved?

5. In what ways are you the best person to lead this application?

6. What systematic reviews should you know about or undertake before proceeding?

7. Who can you assemble to be a strong team of co-applicants and appropriate critical peers?

8. How likely is it that your co-applicants can deliver what is needed within the time available?

9. If the grant application is successful, will you be able to deliver? In what ways?

10. If rejected how do you plan to take the reviewer feedback on board and recycle the proposal? (If you can't answer this question, pause and reconsider how you answered the first two questions—and be honest!)

Groups and Individuals: Managing Relationships

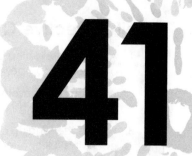

41

"Recognize the talent of others and acknowledge it."

—Gloria Smith

Mentor

Rose O. Sherman, EdD, RN, NEA-BC
Director, Nursing Leadership Institute
Christine E. Lynn College of Nursing
Florida Atlantic University
Boca Raton, Florida, USA

Mentee

Susan MacLeod Dyess, PhD, RN
Project Director, Novice Nurse Leadership Institute
Christine E. Lynn College of Nursing
Florida Atlantic University
Boca Raton, Florida, USA

Casey Stengel, the beloved manager of many major league baseball teams in the United States, once noted that "Finding good players is easy. Getting them to play as a team is another story." Guiding work groups and individuals to get past their day-to-day problems, conflicts, and communication issues and to aim toward a goal of working as a high-performance work group is a significant challenge for today's nursing leaders. High performance work teams or committees in any setting rarely occur naturally. They must be created and managed by nurse leaders who are attentive to the needs of both individuals and the group. Leaders play a key role in helping a team develop the ability to collaborate effectively, build relationships and trust, innovate, and achieve results at a consistently high level.

Managing Relationships and Trust

Consultants who work internationally with both individuals and groups have noted that healthy productive work teams have a common element. They pay close attention to relationship management (Koloroutis, 2004). The most common behaviors that create obstacles to effective group work include blaming others, turf protection, mistrust, and an inability to directly confront issues. In the absence of complete trust, people are more likely to withhold their ideas, observations, and questions. Trust begins with communication. Relationships live within the context of conversations that individuals and groups have, or don't have, with one another. Establishing a culture of respect for the needs of the individual and the group is an important initial step. Recognizing that different generational groups might have a different world view on problems and issues is significant leadership consideration (Sherman, 2006).

Building Individual and Group Commitment

Stephen Covey (2004) wrote in his *Seven Habits of Highly Effective People* that one should begin with the end in mind. This is good advice for leaders to apply when considering the needs of groups and individuals. Alignment to a vision that is clearly defined and agreed upon by all can be a unifying force to create high performance. It provides a frame of reference against which behavior and performance can be measured.

In 2005, nurse leaders from health care agencies and educational settings throughout Palm Beach County, Florida, were challenged by a local foundation to develop a collaborative initiative to address a complex nursing workforce issue. Nurse leaders, many of whom were major market competitors, pledged to work together to develop a program that would create value and sustainable change in the nursing community. The overarching goals discussed by the partners were these: to strengthen the competencies of new nurses along a variety of dimensions, to provide ongoing support to reduce turnover in the first year of practice, and to create a pool of future nurse leaders to serve the community by developing a leadership mindset in the first year of practice. I (Rose) was asked to recommend a nursing leader with the organizational skills and leadership talent to meet the needs of the varied groups and individuals who were part of this partnership. Without reservation, I recommended Susan Dyess. Susan was a passionate young nursing leader with the skill to meet the needs of the leadership in the health care organizations who participated in the project and the enthusiasm to inspire the young novice nurses who would attend the institute. This is her story.

Leadership Exemplar

Thirteen health care organizations in our community were involved in the project called the Novice Nurse Leadership Institute (NNLI). The program is a year in length, offers academic credit and links practice situations with leadership education and activities. Over the past three years, 81 new graduates have participated in three different cohorts. Collaboration in the planning and delivery of the program has been critical. Also, I (Susan), as the project leader, had to understand the needs of the partnership group and the individuals involved in the project.

Providing leadership to the group while not neglecting the individual is consistent with the profession of nursing that allows one to "see the whole while attending to the part" (Newman et al., 2008). Also, consistent with professional nursing practice is intentionally providing meaningful and caring leadership that supports transformational outcomes (Boykin and Schoenhofer, 2001a, 2001b; Newman, 1994, 2008). I sought to live out a leadership style that involved knowing others and being responsive to them using strategies similar to those identified by Ray, Turkel, and Marino (2002) for successful organizational change. The strategies I used (and that I discuss in the sections that follow) included the following:

- Regular meetings to maintain relationships with everyone linked to the project.

- Decision making grounded in consensus.

- Thorough communication in meetings and throughout the project.

- Valuing the input of every individual while fostering a group mindset.

Regular Meetings and Relationships

I found it important to be present and visible as a leader for both the organizational partners associated with the NNLI and with the participants. Visibility was an important aspect of building and sustaining the trust within and among the multiple professional relationships. Representatives from partnering organizations were invited to face-to-face gatherings every three months at a centralized location for the purpose of information sharing and discussion of the project. The program participants met every two weeks at an academic campus where we shared content related to leadership and reflected upon situations from practice. During the various meetings, we shared successes of the project, addressed challenges, and considered areas for improvement and solutions.

The meetings fostered collegial relationships in our community among organizations that viewed themselves as competitors. We established a culture in these meetings based upon authentic respect, trust, and critical inquiry. Additionally, the meetings strengthened the group's cohesive alignment to the overarching goals. Each of us individually and collectively worked to strengthen the competencies of new nurses and assist them to develop a leadership mindset and thus reduced the attrition of our new graduates in their first year of practice.

Decision Making

Although the process was extremely time consuming, we brought all decisions that directly impacted the NNLI to the organizational partnership meetings for consideration and consensus. Our leadership needed to secure the "buy-in" from everyone involved, and seeking consensus invited rich dialogue among the group and enabled the appreciation of various perspectives. Often good ideas improved when more people got involved. A technique we used to facilitate discussions included the following comment, "These are great ideas. Could we expand any of these ideas, and how?" The agreements we reached within decision-making discussions created supportive enthusiasm for the project.

Thorough Communication

After we made decisions, we had to disseminate the information. We maintained a variety of communication efforts to keep both individuals and the group engaged in the project. Electronic communication proved to be the most readily used mode, but personalized meetings, phone calls, and good old fashioned mailings supported the communication efforts as well. Other communication strategies centered on managing the group and individual discussions. We didn't formally establish group ground rules but allowed them to evolve informally. They included the following:

- Listening and paying attention to one another.

- Discussing topics from an agenda one at a time.

- Working through conflict, not avoiding it.

- Allowing everyone an opportunity to express his or her views.

Valuing Input

With the many persons involved, we knew we needed to recognize the wisdom brought to the project by each collaborative member. We shared generous and sincere affirmation when appropriate as a way to strengthen the individual and the bonds among the various project members. Generally, individuals and the group reported personal and professional gains from their experiences associated with the NNLI.

For simplicity, we developed the following **LEADER** acronym that summarizes key strategies used in our partnership for understanding group and individual needs.

> **L**isten to individuals and then consider emerging ideas arising from the group.

> **E**xpect high performance, do not underestimate the old saying "together everyone accomplishes more."

> **A**ppreciate diversity and then capitalize on the uniqueness of the individual to expand the sum total of the group performance.

> **D**irect clearly the general expectation of group performance and then allow for the individual to identify their particular contribution.

> **E**valuate regularly to allow for modification of actions.

> **R**eflect on individual and group occurrences to be mindful of goals and contradiction to goals noted.

Final Thoughts

Providing leadership to the NNLI has allowed me to develop comfort with facilitating a group while still appreciating the needs of individuals. Though it is true that I was given the opportunity to provide leadership to the community project, I was also provided with a group of diversely capable and engaged representatives from the various partnering organizations committed to the success of the project. Dr. Sherman assured me that she would provide me with necessary guidance as I assumed leadership in planning, implementation, and outcome evaluation of the NNLI, and so she did. Dr. Sherman was and is the consummate nurse leader/mentor who encouraged me as I sought excellence as a professional nurse leader. The experience of the NNLI was invaluable and has proven to be an incredible source of professional development for me. The following checklist of questions has worked for the members of our partnership. It might prove helpful to other nurse leaders to understand group and individual needs with a goal of achieving high performance.

Self-Reflective Questions

1. How do you observe and reflect on various aspects of individual and group behaviors?

2. In what ways do you support authentic communication?

3. How can you identify or clarify the ultimate outcome or goal?

4. How can you facilitate critical inquiry to ensure high quality performance?

5. In what ways do you model versatility for advancing the successful attainment of goals?

6. How do you build upon individual and group talent and competency?

7. In what ways do you support decision making based on consensus?

8. How can you resolve or reconcile conflict quickly?

9. In what ways do you consider all aspects and possibilities offered from individuals/the group?

10. How can you recognize and value individual contributions to group efforts?

Growing Through Lifelong Learning

42

"Ultimately, you will find that if life is the real meditation practice, then everything and everybody in your life becomes your teacher, and every moment and occurrence is an opportunity for practice and for seeing beneath the surface appearance of things."

—Jon Kabat-Zinn

Mentor

Debra K. Pendergast, MSN,
  RN NEA-BC
Chair, Division of Nursing
  Services/Associate
  Administrator
Mayo Clinic
Arizona, USA

Mentee

Jessica N. Charles, MSN, RN
Nursing Supervisor, Neurology/
  ENT/Plastics
Mayo Clinic
Arizona, USA

Blazing the trail on the journey of life has often mystified me with the twists, turns, and unprecedented lack of predictability. My (Debra's) human spirit has had to demand time for rest and reflection from the unrelenting mind, which often prefers a frenetic pace.

Human growth and continuous learning is as vital as oxygen in sustaining and nourishing the human potential. I have come to accept that the antidote to premature aging that might manifest as resistance to change is to seek out and commit to mastering the attributes of the perpetual student. Curiosity, tolerance, reflection, and self-compassion for being a beginner are the prerequisites for this mindset.

A student of life knows that with a learner's mindset comes the opportunity and choice to transform data and information into knowledge and wisdom. Wisdom in action is like experiencing a beautiful, fragrant flower, often perceived as living and thriving in the midst of unkempt weeds.

Sharing the Wisdom of Life

Recently in a conversation with nurse leaders, I heard one colleague mention a favorite definition of wisdom. She shared that wisdom is the application of knowledge with compassion. Sharing the journey of continuous learning with my partner (mentee) in this chapter, I have come to experience wisdom as a powerful gift, one that we receive and give with intention. Wisdom, coupled with compassion, is an incredible source of leadership energy, fueling us to propel forward on our interdependent journey as human beings.

Leaders know that lifelong learning is essential to inoculate us against inflexibility and intolerance. Compassion is the glue that holds us together during the difficult times.

To maximize our human growth and learning experiences, we must accept our vulnerability and be able to show it to others. This is a crucial competency for both experienced and novice leaders.

At a recent meditation retreat, I heard a speaker tell us, "Believe nothing, and be open to everything as a possibility." His words sparked controversy among many. My reaction was to pause and think of how many situations in my life are catalogued as clearly black-and-white, and thus easily dismissed. In my early days as a leader, I was steeped in believing that there was always a "right way to do things" and people who did things "right."

As a young leader, I had extensive knowledge but often lacked the wisdom of experience. I was quick to judge and had an ample supply of intolerance for ambiguity. I didn't appreciate the unlimited and glorious "shades of gray."

Early in my career, I sought out clear-cut paths to any problem presented to me. Problem solving and finding solutions were highly regarded attributes. However, these solutions, although technically correct, often lacked wisdom. I am convinced that one of the greatest gifts we can share with our aspiring nurse leaders is to describe our journey of wisdom. This includes nourishing the pursuit of life-long learning through mentoring and sharing the authentic stories of our own leadership travels.

I was introduced to a learning model that reminded me of a personal story. A wise friend told me that we often stall on our life journey because of our reluctance and fear to move into unfamiliar territory. We don't want to be vulnerable or take time to learn new skills, or we lack self-confidence as beginners among accomplished peers. A recent story is my own journey of the last five years. For most of my adult life, I told myself that I didn't have an artistic bone in my body. I loved other people's art, but convinced myself through defeating inner dialog (the silly voice in my head) that I couldn't draw a straight line—and, therefore, had no talent.

Through leadership coaching, I worked on turning the voice of the inner critic into an inner ally and decided to remove my self-imposed learning barriers. This decision has unleashed a pent-up artist within me, resulting in more joy in all levels of my life, including my professional leadership role. The learning model is four stages:

1. Blissful Incompetence

We don't know what we don't know and are oblivious to it. However, other people often know and are very aware of our "blind" spots.

2. Conscious Incompetence

We are painfully aware of what we don't know as we try to master new skills. We experience incredible self-consciousness and discomfort. This stage requires wisdom, courage, and the ability to acknowledge our lack of mastery as we proceed forward. A great example is the doctor or nurse who is embarrassed to try to use the new computer system. Instead, they reject it. In my own example, I take beginning classes on the same art topic repeatedly. I will often ask the same questions to the dismay of the instructors, who often think that I should have grasped the concept in their first class. However, I have made a conscious decision to allow myself the time to be incompetent and compassionate with myself. The pain lessens as the learning increases!

3. Conscious Competence

When we learn something new but are very aware of all the steps because our learning and mastery are not on autopilot yet. For instance, think of the new supervisor initiating performance counseling for an employee using a specific human resources–rules-based format.

4. Unconscious Competence

On autopilot, and so comfortable that we forget those people who are not at this stage yet. An example is a very experienced staff nurse partnered with a new graduate. As leaders, we must be aware of how quickly we can increase the pain of those learners who are still consciously incompetent. That awareness comes from life-long learning and wisdom in action.

Jessica is my writing partner and a newly selected unit supervisor. On her journey of growth and learning, she has focused on self-awareness through seeking out wisdom and knowledge from nurses who have walked the trail before her. She demonstrates courage by showing her vulnerability in order to grow and transform learning into wisdom.

I met Jessica a few years ago on the night shift in our critical care unit. Jessica was the nurse caring for my mother during the last three days of her life. I was inspired by Jessica's outstanding care, her presence as a human being, and her innate wisdom as a caregiver. I was not surprised when she was selected as a unit supervisor several months later.

Breaking Free from My Comfort Zone: Mentee

My first interaction with Debbie was during one of the most vulnerable times a human can experience—the loss of a loved one. Every shift is different as a nurse; the patients and their families are unique and deserving of holistic care. Although I had never met Debbie, I knew that she served as the top nurse leader at the organization where I work. My heart reminded me that Debbie was a loving daughter saying good-bye to her mother. The empathy ran deep.

At this moment in my nursing career, at the bedside, I was working under unconscious competence. My time spent giving care to others was giving back just as much—true reciprocity. The 12-hour shifts never seemed long because of the flow, ease, and comfort.

After meeting Debbie and spending time getting to know her, I learned about the heart and knowledge of nursing administration. She was not just a nurse executive, she was the reflection of the nurse I could become. Her story was one of humbleness and hard work. She was making a difference. I continued to complete master's level courses in nursing leadership and business. Through the process, I discovered how many more lives I could touch through directing and coaching others. I left a critical care staff nurse position to accept a team leader role on a medical surgical unit. When a supervisor position opened several months later, I was up for the challenge. The support that I felt I needed to succeed was within reach.

However, this was new and outside my comfort zone. The first month of working as a supervisor was spent finding out what the expectations were and meeting my people resources throughout the organization. This was a stage of blissful incompetence for me. I was excited to get the chance of learning something new and gaining experiences every day.

A few months later, an almost surreal "imposter" syndrome set in. At this point, I was aware of the accountability and expectations of my new position, yet I felt I wasn't measuring up. I began to find the courage to show my vulnerability and seek guidance, which enabled me to gain new mentors as well as knowledge from many people.

Now I find myself in a state of conscious competence, feeling good about the work I do and the career path I have chosen. My inner voice reminds me that with time, I will return to that unconscious competence that brought comfort and success as an accomplished staff nurse. Reviewing the process tells me that when the time is right and the opportunity arrives, I can take that step back into blissful incompetence and start over. Although the path to wisdom is long, nurse leaders like Debbie make continuous learning possible by sharing their journey.

Self-Reflective Questions

1. How do I embrace the concept of being a life-long learner?

2. How can I become open to seeing and embracing ambiguity?

3. If I am someone whose comfort lies in seeing the world in black-and-white, how can I become open to shades of gray?

4. How can I become open to being vulnerable and showing it with others?

5. As I advance in my leadership journey, how can I cultivate compassion and actively transform knowledge into wisdom?

6. How willing am I to understand the stages of learning?

7. How willing am I to move beyond "painful incompetence" as I move forward as a continuous learner?

8. How do I cultivate the attributes of a life-long learner's curiosity, tolerance, reflection, and self-compassion?

9. How can I become aware of the inner critic and my ability to transform it into an inner ally?

10. How can I share my journey and hard-earned wisdom with others?

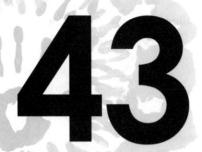

43

Healing

"Healing is a lifelong journey and a process of bringing together aspects of oneself at deeper levels of harmony and inner knowing, leading toward integration. This process includes knowing, doing, and being."

—Barbara Dossey

Mentor

Barbara M. Dossey, PhD, RN, AHN-BC, FAAN
International Co-Director and Board Member of the Nightingale Initiative for Global Health
Washington, DC, and Ottawa, Ontario, Canada
Director, Holistic Nursing Consultants
Santa Fe, New Mexico, USA

Mentee

Jennifer L. Reich, MA, MS, RN, ANP-BC, ACHPN
PhD Nursing Student, University of Arizona College of Nursing
Predoctoral Fellow T-32: Arizona Complementary and Alternative Medicine Research Training Program (ACAMRTP)
Tucson, Arizona USA

We are born with healing capacities that are naturally inherent in all living things. Nurse leaders model healing through self-care and reflection. As noted in the quote above, healing is a process that is with us each day. Sometimes in the fast pace of everyday we forget that we actually know how to take time for a healing moment. An example is to focus with awareness on a slow breath in and a slow breath out several times and then to become aware of the increased space between the breaths when we drop into the relaxation of this healing practice.

No one can take this type of healing away from life. However, when we fail to use this innate capacity, we may hinder our healing process or even forget we have this potential. Although there are many responsibilities in our practice as nurse leaders, as well as in life's continuous challenges, it is this type of healing that allows us to take our full presence into a clinical situation. Reflect on Jennifer Reich's poem "Dignity."

Dignity

To gently wipe the chin
Freeing the saliva that runs down
But cannot be reached-
To wash the hair
Matted and damp with sweat
And brush the teeth that haven't touched real food-
To lotion dry skin
To keep skin dry,
To hold sacred space
For one to cry-
Florence Nightingale
Gandhi
Martin Luther King, Jr.
Mother Teresa
All knew
What was worth living
and dying for
Nurses know this
Live this-
Let us come together
So we never forget
For ourselves
For our patients
For the world
Dignity.

Used with permission. © Jennifer Reich, 2008.

Healing can take place at all levels of human experience, but it most likely does not occur simultaneously on all levels, such as physical, mental, emotional, social, or spiritual. Yet, even with a small shift in a given moment, a person might still perceive that healing has happened. Healing is not predictable. It might occur with the curing of symptoms, but it is not synonymous with curing. Curing might not always happen, but the potential for healing to occur is always present even until one's last breath. Take a moment to read the following, Jennifer's journal entry written in New York City, 2005.

I have become quite close with Mitchell, a 38-year old man with end-stage AIDS. His only family is his sister, Alice, a postal carrier, who finishes her route and comes and visits every day. They don't talk about their parents, who are living but out of the picture. Mitchell is chachectic, weak, but desperately struggles to stay alive. For his sister, he tells me in confidence. Alice is sometimes difficult for our team, demanding, bossy. I feel her fear of being alone. I know it is something we all share as humans, and I weep for her at night when I finally crash in my tiny 18th floor studio apartment. I reflect on eight million human beings in Manhattan, a pea-sized speck of the planet, yet so much isolation, separation, and desperation. Mitchell is dying. He soon is at a point where speaking becomes difficult. There is no hope for a cure now, but healing is possible. I tell our attending physician that I would like to try guided imagery with Alice and Mitchell. She smiles. I love when she smiles; there is so much pain here. During the session, I find myself transported from the cramped inpatient room to a space where suffering is no longer a creation. Alice and I stroke Mitchell's head and he falls asleep. She gives me a hug, as tears run down her cheeks. I tell her I will pray for her, and I mean it. I walk across the street to my apartment and chat with the building supervisor. He likes the cookies I made him. For the moment, I am at peace.

After reading this journal entry, use your reflective lens to identify two key factors in healing—intention and intentionality—that are recognized in integral and holistic nursing (Dossey, 2008; American Holistic Nurses Association and American Nurses Association, 2007) and are Florence Nightingale's legacy (Dossey et al., 2005; Dossey, 2010). *Intention* is a conscious awareness of being in the present moment to help facilitate the healing process. It is the focused mental state using a conscious determination to do a specific thing or to act in a specific manner. It includes being committed to, planning to, or trying to perform an action (Dossey, 2008). *Intentionality* is the quality of an intentionally performed action (Dossey, 2008). So how can we as busy nurses recognize our healing process and integrate intention and intentionality when we are currently faced with health care systems dysfunctions, a global nursing shortage, and many other professional and personal challenges? In each moment we can remember and increase our awareness of maintaining a sense of balance and can address our own suffering or woundedness as shared by Jennifer in the next journal entry written in Tucson, Arizona, in 2008.

No car or plane or train has been successful in distancing me from the old stories that accompany me to every new residence. My feet and legs, strong but worn, have traveled miles upon miles in search of peace, sometimes finding it in the rhythm of the stride, other times in the release of pain. Mostly, though, it is momentary.

"She's a nomad," a mentor mentions casually to another doctoral student sitting down at the table with us as we catch up on the six months since I left Arizona. It's

true, and it doesn't bother me to talk about it. It is my story to this point. I value the rich experiences and deep friendships I have made across many state lines. Still, my soul begs my flesh to drop the baggage and run freely into the flow of life, to allow the suffering to pour out in my sweat, to dance.

I want to create my story now. Not control, create. The old themes just don't fit anymore; just like my jeans from my obsessive days, they are tight and constricting. I cannot keep running away from my heart's desire, it is calling me home, to the only home that is truly infinite. And so I stop, I breathe, I refocus. No need to panic or obsess whether I am good enough, whether I am an imposter. There are no imposters on the stage of life, only roles we play.

I walk in the light of calmness, though the darkness cannot be avoided. I must learn to find calm there too. There is a peace in knowing that I am. Not alone. Intricately connected. Breathing the same air as my sisters and brothers on the East Coast, West Coast, all over the planet. I am thirsty for life and the glass is always waiting; full, to quench my thirst. Today, I pick it up, and drink.

The healing process leads us towards deeper reflection where each nurse can touch the roots of healing and his or her "calling" and can feel a sense of joy. Best wishes in your healing journey.

Self-Reflective Questions

1. How can you acknowledge your own healing and wholeness and the significant connections in your life?

2. Identify your physical, mental, emotional, social, and spiritual potentials in your personal and professional life.

3. How do you nurture your spirit?

4. In what ways do you explore what healing is in your personal and professional life?

5. What are the daily opportunities you have to be consciously aware of your healing potentials?

6. In what ways do you reflect on your vision of healing, caring, and a holistic health care system?

7. How do you reflect on your values, beliefs, and assumptions about healing?

8. In what ways do you consider yourself to be an instrument in the healing process?

9. How would you assess the current quality of your life?

10. How do you create opportunities in which to heal yourself to increase your therapeutic capacities?

44

Image: Self and the Nursing Profession

"Nurses dispense comfort, compassion, and caring without even a prescription."

—Val Saintsbury

Mentor

Elena Stempovscaia, PhD
Chief Nurse, Ministry of Health
  of Republic of Moldova
President of Nursing Association
  of Republic of Moldova
Republic of Moldova

Mentees

Maria Munteanu
Nursing professor, National
  College of Medicine and
  Pharmacy in Chisinau
Republic of Moldova

and

Ludmila Sanduţa
Teacher, Continuing Education
  Centre for Nurses in Chisinau
Republic of Moldova

The nursing profession has an ancient history of at least a thousand years, and in that time it has embraced different shapes. Nursing is one of the noblest professions. Too often, nurses are seen and treated as doctors' helpers rather than as the professionals they are. Promoting and protecting the professional image of nurses is important to maintain the level of respect that nurses deserve. This respect must start with nurses themselves.

Professional Image

The image of nurses in society remains in the shadows, often creating only the impression that we do our jobs well and at a low salary. At the same time, new concepts and theories show us the importance and role of nurses in the health system. Understanding the principles of nursing is an important step to ensuring a positive image with the public.

The nursing profession is based on the idea that everyone deserves all our efforts and care to maintain dignity as a free, responsible, and happy being. It is a noble profession because it addresses life and spirit. We say that nursing is a moral art, because the nurse takes care of human beings and respects life, dignity, and rights. At the same time it is a practical science because it decides, develops, and improves its actions.

Current Concepts and Image

Today, nursing in Republic of Moldova comprises specific actions of prevention, treatment, and recovery to manage the health situation of our patients, with an understanding of past, present, and possible future. Nursing, through care teams, seeks to help patients retain autonomy and regain their joy of life.

In 1989, the Republic of Moldova became independent of the USSR and began the struggle to stand as an independent nation in the world. This struggle encompassed a struggle with our habits and old concepts, with a lack of understanding of the new concepts, and with the inevitable hardships of change.

Understanding new theories of nursing requires solid documentation so we can avoid incorrect interpretations, confusions, and improper application of care models, all of which can negatively impact our professional reputations and the image of our profession.

Training and Transition to Practice

Additionally, understanding new concepts of patient care and applying new procedures properly requires systematic training, the use of correct learning methods, and a constant emphasis on exercise and improvement. Training begun in educational institutions should continue in hospitals and health centres.

The move from theory to practice is sometimes a confusing one. Nursing students enter medical institutions with new ideas and excitement, but in the real-life medical setting they find other practices than those they learned being used and that can lead to confusion and misunderstanding. If the new concept is not developed further, students' enthusiasm from college can gradually turn into discouragement, disillusion, and boredom, which leads either to losing nurses or retaining bored, ineffectual nurses.

When integrating participating students and new concepts of care, we kept the following ideas in mind:

1. All communities or wards should include a newly trained nurse because most of the existing personnel don't realize what must be done to apply new concepts of care to satisfy fundamental needs.

2. Most of the personnel don't show interest for the new concepts because they don't take into account the patient's view. That is why the new nurses seem indiscreet to them or seem to push intimacy.

3. The years of experience non-nursing personnel, such as social workers and medical assistants, should be used to facilitate new nurses' learning.

4. Medical institutions should have enough personnel to spend time on communication with patients

5. To apply and integrate new concepts, doctors need to be acknowledged and included, too.

6. The understanding and application of new practices of nursing depends on the quality of each person on the involvement, skill, and affability of chief nurses and mentors.

In our experience, third-year students managed to incorporate these ideas into an intelligent and sensible way of thinking about health care and learned to adjust and apply them in creative and efficient ways. It is truly satisfying for professor-nurses or mentor-nurses to see graduates understand that application of the new concepts becomes a real, tangible, and beneficial force in the patient's experience. After three years of study, students learn to listen and to exclude distrust and coyness from their professional demeanor, gain confidence in them, and learn to be responsible and proud that they are capable professionals working in a rich and beautiful profession.

To Be a Nurse

For me the present day represents the end of a long road that lasted a whole life. The nursing world is unique in these ways because of the obligation and responsibility we have in working with people's lives. Everything we do is based on that responsibility.

I am honoured to be a nurse and a mentor, one of those people who give their knowledge and their solidarity of spirit to a job that helps to re-establish and keep people's health, honoured to be one of those in a unique position to help create a healthy planet and guide others to do the same.

Maria Munteanu

My name is Maria Munteanu, and I am proud to be one of the mentees of Mrs. Elena Stempovscaia. She is a guiding light in the development of a strong self-image for nurses, which promotes the profession as a whole.

Elena has been the president of the Nursing Association of Republic of Moldova for 15 years. In this association, I feel like I am in a big, united family where love, kindness, professional nobility, and compassion are at the highest level. Elena promotes quality in professional practice, management, leadership, and knowledge, as well as the necessary skills for education and quality practice in nursing. At the same time she promotes the profession and the people who are in this area with the authority and the community that has become a voice of the profession.

Elena is like a spring well with clear water that rises from professionalism, respect and dignity, transparency, collaboration, honesty, loyalty, tolerance, love for people, and medical ethics.

If rivers are measured by their length, width, and depth, then a human's generosity might be said to be determined by his or her thoughts, feelings, and spirit. During the whole period I worked with Elena, I saw her as a strong person with deep feelings and unconditional love, a person who is not afraid to show her tears or laughter. I cherish her because she is a true treasure for the association: kind, intelligent, motivated by justice, strong-willed, tireless, strong, and patient.

Through my relationship with Elena and other mentors, I have come to see that patients need us, and our lives are heroic, stirring, and sublime. Life gives us choices. It shows us the paths we have to choose from—good or bad, life and death. Each moment from life leaves an inscription in the big book of the universe. If we look down deep in our hearts, we find that the nurse was created to give care, to do well, and to reach the divine's heights. In our profession like in no other we must gain people's trust and respect their dignity. Otherwise, how can we ease their pain?

Ludmila Sanduţa

My name is Ludmila Sanduţa. My first step in the health area was my graduation in 1982 from the National College of Pharmacy and Medicine, where I received the specialty of general nurse. Destiny has brought into my path a teacher, an extraordinary guide who energized me not only to love my chosen profession but also to desire to go on, to grow professionally, and pass on the knowledge to others. I am speaking with an immense respect of Mrs. Elena Stempovscaia. She cherishes a special love towards this profession and the nursing history. Thousands of nurses have listened to her precious practical guidance. My decisive step to graduate from the Medicine University in 2005 also was because of Elena.

She has helped me form a self-image that will help me influence nursing now and in the future. As Lucian Blaga, the great Romanian philosopher, poet, and playwright said, "You can get great achievements and victories only by your own participation."

Self-Reflective Questions

1. What do you consider is the current image of nurses in society?

2. In what ways is nursing an autonomous profession?

3. Why is it important that theory and practice in nursing be integrated in equal measure?

4. Who should manage the training of nurses?

5. Why do doctors need to know the new concept of nursing?

6. Why is it important that future nurses show interest for the new concepts?

7. How important is the mentor's role in practice process?

8. How can the mentor form qualified specialists through their own examples and experiences?

9. What can students learn and take about the art of care and communication from their mentors?

10. How can mentors show they are proud of the mentees they have taught and guided through their profession and lives?

Influence and Influencing

45

"Our greatest responsibility is to become a good ancestor."

—Jonas Salk, Microbiologist

Mentor
Jacqueline Filkins
Non-Executive, Cumbria Part-
  nership NHS Foundation Trust
Honorary President,
  European Nurse Directors
  Association (ENDA)
Vice President, European
  Specialist Nurses Organisation
  (ESNO)
West Woodside, Wigton, UK

Mentee
Phil Robertson
Executive Director, Cumbria
  Partnership NHS Foundation
  Trust
North Cumbria, UK

Let me lead you straight into the heart of the matter. This chapter focuses on only one small component of leadership: influence and influencing (or pushing and pulling). To place matters into context, the working relationship between this author and the co-author is briefly outlined.

I am a non-executive director in a national health foundation trust in the United Kingdom (Cumbria Partnership National Health Services [NHS] Foundation Trust) where, integral to board responsibilities, I chair the Clinical Governance Committee. Also as a non-executive director, I work closely with Phil, the director of nursing, who has a particular remit, as executive lead, for Clinical Governance. Phil reflects on our working relationship as follows:

We have a shared value system which is at the heart of our working relationship and influences us. It is built on a personal and professional drive to

*provide the very best care for those who through ill health are vulnerable and in need.
I believe this relationship has developed out of respect for the importance of being nonjudgmental whilst having a clear understanding of the standards one wants to achieve.
Inherent within this relationship is the ability to be challenged and be supported. The
balance of these two dimensions has led to my professional and personal development
which ultimately, I believe, has improved the services we deliver. An example of my
personal development has been the challenge to present a paper at a recent European
conference of health experts.*

To influence patient quality and safety effectively through sound clinical
governance, the board has a critical responsibility. It owns the strategy and ap-
proves the Clinical Governance Committee's terms of reference, and ensures
that it is appropriately resourced.

A wish to influence and effect change without credibility on the part of the
key players remains just that—a wish. The following background information
of the two authors provides some assurances.

Influence and Influencing: Mentor

My career started as a missionary nurse in central Africa and Madagascar.
These postings were my first appointments following nurse training. The
choice of career was influenced by talks heard from missionary nurses (influence) while a child in Switzerland and working as a volunteer in a hospital
after school hours. Being in Africa also gave me the insight that in order to
make things happen (such as obtaining supplies, raising funds, and so on), one
needed to know whom to influence and work with—and how.

My husband and I returned to England, where I worked from staff nurse
to senior clinical nurse, hospital manager to executive director of nursing. My
last appointment was as dean of faculty for health and social sciences. To shape
patient care, involvement in working parties (influencing) and further studies
(influence) led me to a number of national and European honorary appointments relating to education and workforce development and to present-day
involvement in European organizations and the voluntary sector.

Influence and Influencing: Mentee

I entered nurse training directly from school, having been influenced by
undertaking voluntary work with older people. Training took place in a traditional English institution, qualifying as a mental health nurse in 1982. This
was a significant period of my professional socialisation. I was exposed to a

mental health system that was striving to deliver individualized care but was held back by a depersonalized, institutionalized framework without the local vision to radically change models of care. The most important aspect that I was taught throughout the training program was to remember at all times patients are people who deserve respect, dignity, and a care environment that enhances self-worth.

After qualifying as a nurse, I worked primarily in acute psychiatry, taking on a charge nurse's role after one year. I went on to work within the organization I trained in for an additional 20 years, progressively taking on positions of increasing responsibilities. I started to develop the ability to introduce changes that would support service transformation. This continued through a number of senior nursing roles with the remit expanding to include community-based, primary care services, including district nursing, health visiting, and child protection.

Throughout my career, I developed professionally. Having a keen interest in promoting the quality of care, I obtained a master's in total quality management, which has influenced me further regarding the importance of the leadership role and behaviors to deliver effective and sustainable change. I was appointed director of nursing in 2001, and recently have taken on the additional responsibility for integrated governance within the Trust.

Influencing on a Small and a Large Scale: Mentor

The Trust Board in which Phil and I, respectively, have executive and non-executive director responsibilities covers a very large geographical area and includes primary and secondary care for mental health and learning disability services. Effective patient care is dependent upon having the right people with the right skills in the right place, together with the appropriate structures and systems to support delivery of care. Our different backgrounds, experiences, and responsibilities allow us to influence organizational change and to learn from each other. Recently, I was invited to address a conference outside the UK but due to another commitment, I was unable to respond. The organizers responded positively to my suggestion to identify another colleague. Phil was the person I was thinking of and after a moment's hesitation, he responded positively although it was a new and somewhat challenging experience for him. The ripple effect of this is that this has been viewed as a positive learning experience and that other nurses in the organization are being encouraged to share their expertise within a wider audience and to benefit from new learning opportunities.

It is often perceived that influencing policy makers is the role of others. Or that it is difficult. Let me compare the concept of influencing to a marbles game. One could be forgiven to think that it is indeed a complicated game, played with spherical shapes made from semi-precious materials. The reality is that for play to begin, you use balls made from materials that are most readily available where you live (sand transformed into glass). You also need more than one marble and, lastly, the best games (results) are achieved if there are two or more players.

In nursing leadership terms, the marbles are your key players, and the goal is the policy or option proposal or quality goal that you wish to influence and achieve. As with the game of marbles, you need to know your key players and how they interact with each other in order to achieve best results.

Working within Europe and wishing to influence draft health care policies, the stakes are even higher. It is then essential that nurse leaders in each country replicate their own marbles game to achieve desired outcomes.

An example of such an achievement emerged from a meeting of nurse directors who, at a conference, met by chance during a coffee break. Although each of the five directors represented a different country, they identified shared values and challenges. They kept in touch and decided to work together. From this emerged an association (European Nurse Directors Association [ENDA]) that has developed into a recognized policy-shaping organization. I am a co-founder of this organization, and it is hoped that my colleagues do not mind being referred to as key marble players! In this situation it became possible that a body of trusted colleagues (ENDA) became mentors to other organizations who asked for facilitation during periods of change.

Mentee and mentor do not work in isolation. Phil and I are aware that others will be influenced by the way we work. The ripple effect of successful mentoring allows the influenced to become the influencers of the future.

This chapter describes only a small component of the many leadership attributes that are required to be an effective leader. The words "ability to influence" can evoke feelings of negativity and are more likely to be hidden in the more global term of "is able to make change happen." It is our view that to be able to give the best patient care and prepare nurses for the future, present-day nurse leaders need to be able to influence collectively as well as individually.

Self-Reflective Questions

1. How well do you understand each others' roles?

2. What can you do to take sufficient notice of the knowledge base of your mentee/mentor?

3. How do you become skilled at challenging in a nonjudgmental way?

4. Do colleagues seek you out to be their mentor? If not, why?

5. Can you describe the scope of your influence?

6. What are your priorities for influencing?

7. What influences your own values?

8. How are your skills and experiences put to best use?

9. How can you strive to ascertain that your mentoring is based upon mutual respect?

10. How can you promote good mentorship as investment for the future?

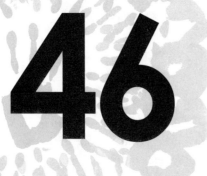

46

Information Technology: The Nature of Health Care Information Systems

"Man and his environment are continuously exchanging matter and energy with each other."

—Martha Rogers

Mentor
Thomas R. Clancy, MBA, PhD, RN
Clinical Professor, School of Nursing
The University of Minnesota
Minneapolis, Minnesota, USA

Mentee
Gregory Clancy, MS, RN
Coordinator for Strategic Projects
Mercy Hospital
Iowa City, Iowa, USA

Over time, all systems become increasingly more complex (Skyttner, 2001). In biological systems, organisms increase their complexity through diversification. For example, natural selection and diversity in a species population result in improved fitness for adaptation and survival. Through such mechanisms as mutation and crossover at the genetic level, this diversity is communicated to future generations.

The metaphor of biological evolution also applies in social organizations such as health care systems. In this context, diversity comprises the range of new ideas, services, and technological innovations the organization generates to adapt in the marketplace. Success depends on how well organizations communicate and execute those ideas through their workforce. To survive and thrive in today's dynamic environment, a health system needs to build an infrastructure that supports a rich social network and enables the rapid implementation of new ideas, services, and technologies.

Organizational Complexity

The paradox faced by health care systems is that as the need for diversification increases, the overall complexity of the organization also increases, often exponentially. In fact, organizational complexity is now considered one of the leading causes of waste and expense in health care systems today (George, 2003). Many tout information systems as the solution. But for those nurse executives who have introduced information technology into the workflow of nursing processes, the difficulties can be formidable. The challenge for today's health care leaders is to plan, design, and implement systems that provide the right information to the right providers at the right time. To do so requires nurse executives to look at improving nursing processes from the perspective of Occam's razor, where the simplest solution is usually the best. I (Thomas) consider such organic systems found in nature (e.g., the human body) to be elegant and to resemble natural processes. The objective of this chapter is to discuss how growth in information is driving increased complexity in health care today and how nurse leaders should reflect on the underlying laws of nature as a guide to improving nursing processes.

Hospitals as we know them today have evolved into sprawling integrated systems with a diverse range of specialties and services. This explosive growth stems from a number of factors. One important reason is the exponential rise of new information being created as a result of the Internet. For example, since the year 2000 more information is now created annually than was created for the previous 300,000 years of human history combined (Clancy and Delaney, 2005). The communication and information sharing capacity of the Internet has fueled new technological advances and increased the diversity of alternative treatments and services available in health systems, which in turn has led to considerable improvements in overall survival rates and quality of life for the population as a whole.

Though the Internet has spurred advances in the diagnosis of disease and treatment of patients, it has also significantly increased the information requirements of nurses in hospitals. A key challenge facing nurse executives today is that growth in information and new knowledge is increasing at an exponential rate, but its adoption in hospitals occurs at a much slower or linear rate (Kurzweil, 2005). In today's environment hospitals are collecting and exporting an ever-increasing amount of date to satisfy the demands of government, insurance, and professional certification agencies. This is a paradox with far more data being generated than the means or tools to evaluate its relevance to patient care and the organization. This has led to an ever-widening gap between the information required by nurses and the information available in the organization. Complicating matters are highly publicized reports, such as the Institute of Medicine's *Crossing the Quality Chasm* (Institute of Medicine, 1996), fueling new requirements regarding the transparency of hospital clinical performance to state and federal agencies. These requirements have resulted in explosive growth in the number of clinical and administrative performance outcomes that must be tracked and reported by hospitals. For example, the typical community hospital now tracks more than 500 indicators, 140 of which are required (Clancy, 2008).

The number of performance indicators in hospitals certainly represents a problem, but choosing which *combination* to monitor at different levels of the organization is an even greater challenge. As the number of indicators monitored increases in a linear fashion, the *combination* of indicators that can be monitored goes up exponentially. For 450 indicators you could report on an amazing 1.73×10^{1000} different combinations at different levels of the hospital! This example represents just one of the enormous problems occurring in hospitals today as a result of increasing health care complexity. Growth in technology and the information generated by it are converging to create an environment so complex that it is becoming unmanageable.

A Natural Systems Approach

As a nurse leader, where do you begin to solve a problem of this magnitude? I have come to the conclusion the answer can be found by observing natural systems. A natural system might be the formation of a neural network in the brain or the evolution of an ecosystem along a coastline. I'm not suggesting you reproduce a natural process, but rather that you study how nature itself deals with increasing complexity. Biological systems are just as prone to complexity as human-made systems. Simply look at how the first single cells evolved into the multicelled organisms of today. However, in contrast to artificially constructed systems, biologic systems have the benefit of time; their evolution has occurred over millions of years. These systems are elegant or, as defined by Webster's, scientifically precise, neat, and simple (Webster, 2009). To illustrate the idea of elegance, I want to compare two similar systems: the branching pattern of the tracheo-bronchial tree in the human lung and the typical computer network in a community hospital.

The tracheo-bronchial tree (TBT) and arterial-vascular system comprise an immensely complex network of arteries, veins, and alveoli that transport oxygen-rich blood throughout the body. Though the oxygen transport system is complex, it is also elegant, just complex enough to maximize its primary function: the transportation of oxygen throughout the body. As you view the branching pattern of the TBT as a whole, you see ever smaller sub-units of the network resemble the same pattern at all scales. Organisms that display self-similar properties such as that shown in the TBT have what is known as a fractal dimension, and it is a measure of how many new self-similar sub-units are revealed at ever higher resolutions (Clancy, 2008). Fractals represent how evolution has culled down an enormous space of solutions to produce an elegant design.

In contrast, human-made systems such as hospital information system networks are a tangled web of computer servers, cables, wireless devices, manual collection processes, and other components that grow far beyond their benefits. Hospital networks do not evolve naturally, but rather are heavily influenced by cost and regulatory pressures. In natural systems when the cost of growth outweighs the benefits, evolutionary pressures generally limit further growth. However, this process doesn't occur in health care because of the centralization of decision making at both the hospital and government level. Because hospitals are mandated to collect and report so many performance metrics, the costs to the organization often outweigh the benefits. When you compare the design of artificially constructed systems to natural systems, natural systems always outperform the artificially constructed ones and at a much lower cost.

Comments from Gregory Clancy (Mentee)

Understanding the process of data collection and flow provides insight and enables you to modify and emulate systems found in nature. You can learn by assessing the types of data being collected and how they are processed. As you track the data transferred from one system to another, several things become apparent. First, the sheer amount of patient care information being collected is astounding. Second, how this data is transferred among databases, individuals, departments, and external agencies creates vulnerabilities. For example, clinical outcomes data is often sent electronically to public web sites through claims data before it is even reviewed internally for its accuracy.

Many organizations have integrated key strategic information into scorecards that merge benchmarks from organizations, such as The Joint Commission, with more recent or concurrent data abstracted from the health care record. Scorecards that electronically send data to target audiences such as

unit managers, bedside caregivers, service line leadership, and upper management are now available. Nurse leaders might find that working with current
data collection processes in the hospital is overwhelming, but using nature
as a model to create elegant collection and reporting processes can provide a
framework to approach an overwhelming situation.

Human Elements Network Design

The number of performance metrics currently being collected in hospitals today is becoming a problem in and of itself. The complexity of how data is collected, stored, and reported within hospitals is, in part, driving the increased
cost of health care today. Unconstrained growth in the number of metrics,
the staff required to collect those metrics, and the technology needed to store
and retrieve data have all led to a state where the costs of maintaining such a
system clearly outweigh the benefits. Although solutions to such problems are
challenging, the answer might be right under our noses. As far-fetched as it
seems, more and more, organizations are turning to system designs that have
evolved through natural processes. Network designs for the optimum transport of essential human elements such as blood and oxygen are a realistic metaphor for many artificially constructed systems such as computer networks.
This fact isn't surprising given that evolution has perfected such systems over
millions of years. However, to achieve the same elegance seen in the simplicity
of nature, you need to wipe the slate clean and evaluate what really makes a
difference in improving care.

Self-Reflective Questions

1. When you are searching for a solution to a complex nursing
   problem, how do you proceed to understand how information
   flows?

2. How do you approach gathering information regarding complex nursing problems and solutions from many different stakeholders and perspectives?

3. Why would you look for repeating patterns when investigating
   the source of a problem?

4. Why prioritize and recommend solutions that solve 80% of the
   problems first?

5. What are the benefits of building consensus with key stakeholders around the number one problem to solve and how does that
   improve clinical outcomes?

Self-Reflective Questions *(continued)*

7. What steps should you take to study the new workflow and its impact on the nursing staff before implementing new information technology?

8. How can you assess whether or not the new workflow, enabled by information technology, is more elegant than the prior workflow?

9. In what ways can you take a new, elegant design and repeat it throughout the information system network?

10. How can the introduction of information technology enable nurses to provide more direct care to patients?

47

Innovating Nursing Education to Transform Future Leadership

"Innovation distinguishes between a leader and a follower."

—Steve Jobs

Mentor

Kathy Malloch, PhD, MBA, RN, FAAN
President, KMA, Inc.
Clinical Professor, Master of Healthcare Innovation Program
College of Nursing & Healthcare Innovation
Arizona State University
Glendale, Arizona, USA

Mentee

Sandra Davidson, RN, MSN, CNE
Director, Master of Healthcare Innovation Program
Clinical Associate Professor
College of Nursing & Healthcare Innovation
Arizona State University
Glendale, Arizona, USA

An important philosophy in my (Kathy's) life has been the belief that there are no accidents, only opportunities presented in many forms and situations. As a student of complexity theory and quantum leadership, I am always looking for ideas, approaches, and colleagues to assist and guide others in being all that they can be as nurses and leaders in the health care world. My recent role as the first director of the Arizona State University College of Nursing & Healthcare Innovation's Master of Healthcare Innovation (MHI) program is an example of a situation that presented itself without my searching for it. To be sure, being director was an exciting and energizing undertaking. The opportunity to create an environment in which innovation was the norm and the expected behavior was also intimidating. I have never been a traditional, tenure-track faculty member. Also, finding colleagues and others to carry this foreboding torch would require significant effort. Innovation in the educational setting requires a unique perspective and a very thick skin because you must continually challenge traditions in the process.

I had no idea where this role would lead—only that innovation in nursing education was needed to develop leaders who could advance health care so that innovation was readily embraced. My experience as a health care leader could be applied to the academic setting. As part of this role, I met with many individuals at the college; one informal meeting proved to be a very important connection to advance the work of the MHI program. My philosophy of leadership—a respectful, proactive, empowering, evidence-driven approach—guided me in developing an important new relationship with Sandra Davidson, a junior faculty member in the college.

Sandra and I met at a small coffee shop in Tempe, Arizona. This meeting between Sandra, a relatively new junior faculty member, and me, the current MHI program director, was destined to be the first of many conversations and ultimately would lead to Sandra being selected as the next MHI program director. As I reflect on this meeting, I find that principles of chaos theory, uncertainty, and vulnerability leadership were present and hard at work. While the goal was to advance innovation, the foundational work was relationship building and developing shared expectations so that innovation could occur.

Sandra's interests and work as a doctoral student studying leadership fueled the discussion to uncover core values, work ethics, and decision-making skills that were strongly aligned with the MHI program needs. Core values of respect for others, presence, making a difference, resilience, and risk taking were quickly evident in our conversations. In addition, Sandra shared a high level of understanding of the role of technology and its use in advancing the work of leadership. One of many innovations incorporated into the MHI program is the use of the mind map tool for communication, documentation of progress in coursework, student assignments, and meeting agendas. (There are many mind mapping tools available. To see samples of mind mapping, visit your library or search the Internet for them.)

I continue to serve as Sandra's coach, colleague, and friend in our work with the innovation students. As busy individuals, we have the potential to be either overwhelmed or fully engaged in the reality of our complex systems. Taking time to meet new colleagues and to explore their interests and goals is important leadership work and necessarily the first step in supporting innovation.

Sandra Davidson: Mentee

Like Kathy, I have always believed that there are no accidents in life. Each interaction, relationship, and encounter has the potential to be transformational. The day I first met Kathy at the coffee shop was a transformational interaction. As we began our conversation, I recall feeling a sense of mutual presence, respect, and openness to the potential. Neither of us knew where our conversation would lead, and as I reflect upon this several years later, I believe our mutual openness to possibility and commitment to be fully engaged in the moment allowed for the emergence of a highly synergistic relationship. Those same patterns of behavior and communication that began at the coffee shop that day are still embodied in our relationship today and are the foundation for both ongoing innovation and our educational approach to leadership and that innovation.

As we have learned, the innovation process is largely conversational. Conversations that result in idea generation and innovation are enabled by quality relationships. The characteristics of relationships that foster innovation are as follows:

- Mutual respect

- Trust that enables risk taking

- Openness to creative emergence

- Ambiguity tolerance

- Shared commitment to the ongoing conversation

These leadership traits of paying attention to the present, focusing on relationships, living in the potential, and suspending judgment have shaped the development of the MHI program and our work of creating innovation leaders. Both Kathy and I have gone on to establish mentoring relationships with students and new faculty in the MHI program. Nothing is more joyful or empowering than "paying forward" and perpetuating the transformational relationships that we ourselves continue to be transformed by. As we engage and invite those around us to contribute to our vision for health care innovation, we build the matrix of conversations and grow the relationships that create the potential for increased novelty and innovation.

Self-Reflective Questions

Here is a 10-step checklist and questions to help you be more innovative.

1. Be flexible: How do you react to changes in your schedule?

2. Be open: In what ways can you enjoy learning about the activities/accomplishments of others?

3. Embrace failures: How often do you share missteps or failures with others?

4. Be creative: What is something "creative" you did in the last 7 days?

5. Abandon your ego: Do you give credit and recognition to the team, not just yourself?

6. Explore differences: Do you work to learn more about individuals who think and act differently than you do?

7. Be resilient: What have you attempted to accomplish more than five times? (Remember WD-40, the lubricant, was named WD-40 because the first 39 formulas failed.)

8. Enjoy: How long did it take you to find humor in your last failure?

9. Explore technology: When was the last time you learned about a device or toy that someone 20 years younger than you uses?

10. Coach: When is the last time you helped someone with their idea or project without giving your advice?

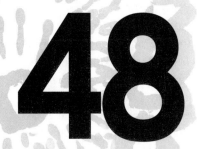

48 Jobless and Searching

"Success is not to be pursued; it is to be attracted by the person you become."

—Jim Rohn

Mentor
Kimberly Richards, RN
President, Kim Richards and
  Associates, Inc. and NurseFit
Littleton, Colorado, USA

Mentee
Jennifer Campbell, BSN, RN
  Staff Nurse, ICU
University of Wisconsin
Madison, Wisconsin, USA

For many reasons, at some point in our careers, we may find ourselves in the difficult pursuit, and endless possibilities, of looking for a new job opportunity. This situation can be a trying yet transformational time to step back, re-assess, and gravitate toward your true calling. Unexpected job loss or the realization that your current job is not a good match can feel like a career-ending event, but if you are resourceful, humble, and believe in your own abilities, you can survive to find an opportunity to contribute your talents in a way that elevates you to a higher purpose and clearer perspective. If you find yourself in this crisis—and it's highly likely that in a nurse's career, he or she will encounter such a situation—you must be careful not to get stuck in a downward spiral. You need a strong, nonjudgmental support system from family and friends, and a mentor's perspective of how failure to find the right niche early in a nurse's career can be a great opportunity. Success is the process of turning *away* from something to turn *toward* something better.

From Kim

As an executive recruiter, potential clients are interviewing me on a daily basis. Each encounter is a new opportunity for me to become more skilled, more emotionally intelligent, and more aware of the impression I make on others. I spend time preparing myself, mentally and emotionally, for my interview journey. I check my attitude at the interview door because any anger, resentment, or negativity might prevent me from receiving an offer of employment. I prepare for each interview by investigating the client's Web site, writing down critical questions, and listing examples of my accomplishments on the side of my notebook. This information helps jumpstart my memory if I get nervous or sidetracked, and I can then clearly answer a client's questions by providing proven solutions and specific experience.

Assess Yourself

Self-assessment can be brutal, but necessary. If I need to update my image, I invest in myself. I have several interview outfits that I always feel great wearing. Do not be fooled into thinking image doesn't make a difference; it does. It is not always the most experienced candidate who lands the job; people hire those whom they connect with, respect, and like being around. Make sure your image is professional without being fussy. If you are unemployed, you might question your ability to afford an update in your wardrobe, but the investment you make in yourself pays off in the form of uplifted self-esteem and an improved attitude, which translates into a healthy self-confidence. No matter what role you are seeking, your appearance speaks volumes.

Act Fast

Knowing your own skills and expertise is essential and can translate into opportunities that present themselves in unlikely places. You need to recognize those opportunities and take quick action before they evaporate. If you hear of something interesting, pursue it—make the call, send an e-mail. Create a sense of urgency without desperation. Cast a wide net. And follow up, follow up, follow up.

Scan the job boards of various professional organizations for opportunities. Most nursing associations have a "career center" you can access. If you can't relocate, consider an interim role that allows you to travel home. Contact employers who are geographically close to you and speak with a hiring authority. Who is the "hiring authority"? Depending on the clinical area and level, it is the person you would report to if you got the job. Though some human resources representatives are extremely helpful and knowledgeable, take it a step further if you really want an opportunity at a particular facility. Find the decision maker and schedule an on-site visit to meet them, even if they do not have a current opportunity vacant. Things can change overnight! Employers often like to hire people in their region because of cultural similarities, familiarity with the environment, and potential savings on relocation costs. Again, follow up, follow up, follow up.

Network with Others

Contact your professional colleagues and let them know you are looking for a new opportunity. Call upon your network. Attend professional conferences and "make the rounds." Make it your "job" to distribute your resume and develop as many contacts as possible. One contact typically leads to another, so stay focused yet open to discussion with potential employers. This is not a time to be shy or embarrassed. Everyone has experienced or will experience a similar situation at some point in his or her career. Sending an e-mail to colleagues can prevent you from being bogged down with answering questions about particulars. The particulars of how you found yourself in this situation aren't important. You need a job, and you are open to all opportunities. This is the time to ask for help, and to make a personal commitment to remember how humbling and difficult the struggle is so that if you are ever in a position of authority, you can provide the same help by extending an opportunity to someone else in need.

Care for Yourself

This is not a time to be "hunkering down" in your house. Get out, exercise often, and participate in whatever brings you joy. Job hunting can be exhausting and stressful and requires diligent mindfulness of the need to refill your reservoirs of energy, resilience, and self-confidence. You must be equipped to sell yourself as a leader, one the potential employer would not want to lose to a competitor. It has been said, "Money doesn't buy you happiness, but being happy has a lot to do with earning money." That adage has proven true in my career. I have never met a truly successful person who is not happy and passionate about their work. I am often asked how to be successful and my answer is always: Find a career/life path that continually re-ignites your passion and touches your soul. For sure, there will be difficult and trying times, but the authentic joy you are able to share with those you meet will naturally attract success. Happiness is infectious, and you will find that people will want to associate, collaborate, and ultimately elevate you to a more global network of success. Opportunities will become abundant when you master a strong personal sense of well being and genuine happiness in your work. Financial reward is sure to follow as you begin to project your personal value, worth and expectation for fair compensation. There have been times in my career when, on paper, I may not have looked like the most "qualified" person for a particular job, yet my ability to convey my love for my passion, my happiness, and my gratitude ultimately won my firm the contract. People tend to want to work with people they like and they aspire to emulate.

From Jen

Starting a new job as a new nurse is a daunting experience, and not necessarily because of patient population, difficult doctors, policies and procedures, or understaffing. In fact, the most challenging aspect of being a new hire is learning, translating, and negotiating the intricate communication of nurse-to-nurse relations.

I recently learned to appreciate the complicated workings of nurse relationships as a new hire and a relatively new nurse at a university Intensive Care Unit (ICU). A large unit, complicated patients, heavy assignments, understaffing, and the many specialist teams meant I could only hope to know my own name by the end of my orientation. New to the area, new to the hospital, new to nursing, I found that my only constant was my preceptor.

Whereas mentors teach mentees clinical skills, assessment techniques, and critical thinking, I have found the more important role of a mentor is to exemplify what it means to practice the "art" of nursing—a common phrase often used but never truly defined. I have attempted a solid definition but have come up short. However, I can identify qualities of nurses who practice an art versus those who just simply practice. Mentors who share this art prepare mentees not only for success on the job, but also for growth within the entire career of nursing.

From observing mentors through preceptorship, I find that the art of nursing is illuminated in communication. Beyond the technical skills and rationale are the abilities to form trusting and positive relationships with other caregivers and team members; to speak freely with tact; to include patients and families in conversation; and to know when to ask for help, when to give it, and when to step back. The art comes in how we act in and react to adversity, to challenging patients, and to heavy assignments. I admire the nurses who practice with ultimate transparency with the patient as the focus, setting aside petty preferences and personality conflicts to provide professional care. Just as we have parameters for vital signs, drug dosing, and interventions, the art of nursing practice is our personal parameter for how we react, communicate, act, and reflect at work. It is truly an art in practice.

After you have celebrated the acceptance of a new job with family and friends, what can you do to prevent being caught "off guard" again? The health care industry provides no guarantees. However, you can make it a practice to stay connected in the future. Continue to attend conferences, serve on committees, and stay abreast of opportunities by keeping in touch with executive recruiters. Learn from the painful experience that it is up to you to manage your career; make a personal commitment to keep yourself at the center of knowledge and opportunity. Begin the next chapter by being proactive, keeping a sensitive ear to the ground, and always looking forward!

Self-Reflective Questions

1. How is the work I perform meaningful work?

2. How can I ensure that my image projects professionalism?

3. What professional associations can I participate in and what benefits does such participation yield?

4. What are the benefits of remaining open to hearing about new opportunities and to having a current resume?

5. In what ways are my job responsibilities in alignment with my talent and passion?

6. In what ways are my actions reflective of my values?

7. How can I provide mentoring for others?

8. How can I consistently challenge myself?

9. How can I keep up with current market trends?

10. In what ways do I take my job for granted?

Leadership Models: Shared Governance as a Path to Professional Involvement

49

"So much of what we do now in health care is team oriented, and I think the opportunity to work together and address issues beyond patient care is very important. There is no real training ground for that outside of nursing organizations."

—Pamela Cipriano

Mentor
Diane J. Mancino, EdD, RN, CAE
Executive Director, National Student Nurses' Association
New York, New York, USA

Mentee
Jenna Sanders
President, National Student Nurses' Association
Senior Nursing Student, University of Saint Francis
Fort Wayne, Indiana, USA

The National Student Nurses' Association (NSNA) is unique. NSNA membership consists of 50,000 undergraduate nursing students enrolled in nursing programs throughout the United States, the District of Columbia, and U.S. territories. An elected board of directors (all nursing students) holds the fiduciary responsibility for the organization. New board members are elected annually, and generally an entire new board is elected. As the executive director of NSNA, I work closely with the president, who is elected by the annual house of delegates to serve in the role for one year. Working in close association with the nursing student leader holding the highest elected position in the United States is a privilege for me.

Since 1952, the NSNA has engaged nursing students in a leadership development practicum rooted in a framework of shared governance. The annual house of delegates immerses nursing students in the art of debate where they learn parliamentary procedure and gain a good working knowledge of *Robert's Rules of Order*. Following election at the convention, the newly elected board of directors participates in a week-long orientation and formal board meeting in New York City. My work with the president begins with a day-long, one-on-one meeting reviewing the role of the president, discussing the president's goals for the year, and exploring strategies to work with the board of directors.

Here, the current president of NSNA and I discuss the value of a historical perspective, shared governance, and the importance of taking a broad view.

The Value of History

Mentor: Because of the transient nature of the NSNA Board of Directors' tenure on the board, the historical context for the organization is conveyed by those with long-term involvement in NSNA—the staff, consultants, and past leaders. My doctoral dissertation and subsequent book, *50 Years of the National Student Nurses' Association* (Mancino, 2002), along with my long-term association with NSNA (I joined the staff in 1981), has earned me the informal title of resident historian. Since my appointment to the executive director role in 1996, I have enjoyed mentoring NSNA presidents during their service on the board and during the course of their nursing career. Sharing the experiences of past presidents with the current president helps the novice leader to understand the complexity of the role of president and how others have faced similar issues.

Mentee: The ability to work with the executive director has proven a blessing on more than one occasion during my term as NSNA president. Since the moment of my election, she has been a wealth of information that has saved me from more than one error in judgment.

Throughout my term, whenever I was faced with an issue involving either one of our constituents or another board member, I approached the executive director—a virtual walking encyclopedia of NSNA history—for historical perspective. For an organization that turns over leadership as frequently as we do, that perspective is vital in preventing us from reinventing the wheel or repeating past mistakes. After all, those who don't know their history are doomed to repeat it. Having such a source of information has enabled me to make informed decisions.

However, the effect is greater than this, because even though I sought the historical information for specific situational needs, I added that information to my broader bank of knowledge. I now have working examples of how to deal with a variety of critical situations in the workplace, in a house of delegates, with a constituent, in an educational setting, and so on. I can honestly say I've learned more in a year from my executive director about working with people than I have in most other situations.

Skills of Shared Governance

Mentor: Shared governance is a democratic decision-making process filled with detailed rules, complex structure, and plenty of politics. Understanding and practicing shared governance is one of the many benefits of NSNA involvement. Several health care delivery organizations now engage staff nurses in shared governance, which offers collective decision-making opportunities and control over nursing practice issues. Nursing students that master the elements of the shared governance model are better prepared to participate on committees and in decision-making councils in the workplace as registered nurses (RNs). Facilitating a board of directors meeting or the house of delegates meeting requires skill, finesse, diplomacy, and courage. Over the course of one year, the NSNA president becomes more comfortable in the role of facilitator. My role as executive director is not to solve problems or direct solutions, but rather to guide the president in the art and skill of facilitating the decision-making process. This might simply mean helping to formulate the right questions to be asked at the right time to stimulate thinking, or it might involve the development of a detailed strategy to overcome conflict and adversity.

Mentee: Before my experience with NSNA, the concept of shared governance was foreign to me. After a few years of involvement, I am a stronger nursing advocate for the lessons that I have learned. As Dr. Mancino mentioned, shared governance is complex and rife with politics. For many, it can take a lifetime to master its intricacies. Three years of NSNA involvement, culminating in an intensive year as president, has been a crash course.

The executive director has worked closely with me throughout my term to prepare me for my role as facilitator of board meetings and the house of delegates and has prepared me for both situations that I knew were coming and those that popped up unexpectedly. I've learned skills necessary to diffuse a tense boardroom situation and strict procedures to maintain a positive atmosphere in a house of delegates with 600 student representatives.

Understanding these rules and regulations and practicing diplomatic skills has certainly helped with my own board and committee meetings, but one particular situation really brought home for me the advantage that NSNA members have over their counterparts. As NSNA president, I attend the meetings, conferences, and conventions of a number of professional nursing associations. During one such event, I was pleased to be joined by a handful of other NSNA members to witness a house of delegates. What we found the most surprising was that for many of the delegates present at this professional meeting, this meeting was their first real exposure to Robert's Rules of Order.

At NSNA meetings, we have specific sessions to help members learn the procedures *Robert's Rules of Order* put forth. As president, I receive a great deal of one-on-one guidance from both the executive director throughout the year and the parliamentarian at our meetings. When things are going smoothly and quietly in a house of delegates, the need to be highly familiar with the intricacies is not as great. However, when the stakes are high and the debate intensifies, knowing the rules can be the difference between winning and losing the issue at hand. At this meeting, we realized for the first time that as students who had participated in NSNA, we knew the rules on a deeper level than many of those in the professional association. As a future nurse advocate with goals of advancing health policy, I know that walking in the door with the knowledge I have gained from my association and my executive director can only increase the odds of me reaching my goals!

A Broader View

Mentor: NSNA leaders are highly sensitive to the image of nursing and how the public perceives the profession. Over the years, many articles on this topic have been published in *Imprint*, NSNA's official publication. Policies and guidelines for standards of ethical behavior, professional conduct at meetings, and appropriate attire have been established and enforced. Although individual freedom of expression and generational and cultural differences are important considerations when developing standards, shared values emerge as the critical component for mentoring students about the image of nursing. As NSNA leaders develop a broader view of the profession and see the bigger picture, they begin to understand the significance of a positive image of nursing students and RNs. Mentoring NSNA leaders to develop professional behaviors that portray a positive image of nursing involves conversations that critically explore the values of nursing and the anticipated and unanticipated consequences of decision-making in this area.

Mentee: As a non-traditional college student, I came into my role with NSNA with a bit of business background and a relatively good understanding of professional image. Though I have had a long running concept of my own professional image, I had never stopped to consider the image of an entire profession before my NSNA involvement.

I find that broadening my outlook has been one of the largest influences NSNA has had on me. Before, I had thought that my behavior and habits were only a reflection of me and what people think of me. I now reflect on how they affect what people think of a multimillion dollar organization. An experience with one student nurse affects the level of respect someone has for the next student nurse encountered and for a generation of future nurse leaders. Further, it could affect whether or not an advertiser, exhibitor, or sponsor takes our organization seriously and makes the determination to invest in NSNA. Additionally, a positive image of nursing students and NSNA makes a big impact on professional nursing organizations. And ultimately it affects whether or not a student decides to become a member.

It is a challenge to get this message across to a multigenerational membership at various stages of life and with varying priorities, but it has always been a priority of NSNA. From the top down, we work to put forth an example of professionalism that serves our members well while they are in NSNA and strives to enhance the profession of nursing as a whole. The more nurses we have out there carrying themselves in a professional manner, the more respect we'll receive, the higher our salaries will rise, the more input we'll have at the decision-making table, and the fewer "naughty nurse" nights we will see at the local bars.

It is a large weight to carry, but not a difficult one when given the education that our organization provides to our members and our executive director provides to the president. We're told over and over again as students that we are the future of nursing. The image that we portray determines what that future will be.

Self-Reflective Questions

1. Think about a situation in nursing that you recently experienced that made you feel uncomfortable. What were the elements of this discomfort? How can you improve the situation should it reoccur?

2. How can a mentor facilitate your participation in professional organizations?

3. How do you portray a professional image of nursing and how can you help other nurses to improve the image of nursing?

4. How can you optimize relationships with your peers to facilitate your professional growth and development?

5. Think about what areas of nursing practice you enjoy the most. What are the career paths available to you to develop your career and educational advancement in these areas?

6. As you prepare for an interview for your first RN position, consider the image that you want to portray. What changes do you need to make in your wardrobe to enhance your professional appearance?

7. Think about your involvement in social networking sites that might not portray the image you want to have professionally. What changes can you make to ensure a professional image?

8. How can your experiences be helpful to a newer nurse or student nurse as a mentee?

9. Is there anyone that you work with that would really help you learn more about your career goal and how to reach these goals?

10. What personal and professional skills do you bring to the nursing profession and how can you best utilize these skills to contribute to the profession's mission?

Leading Interdisciplinary Partnership at the Point of Care

50

"True partnership is not nirvana, utopia, or heaven on earth. It is a new way of looking at the world that provides access to solutions for issues and problems not apparent to most people, and at the same time it also opens the door to new opportunities that we do not know exist."

—Carl Zaiss

Mentor
Bonnie Wesorick, RN, MSN,
  DPNAP, FAAN
Founder and Chairman
CPM Resource Center
Grand Rapids, Michigan, USA

Mentee
Hiliary Siurna, RN, BSN, MSNc
Nursing Practice Leader
Toronto East General
  Hospital
Toronto, Ontario, Canada

Both those who give and receive care know the importance of interdisciplinary partnership. We must stop fragmentation, duplication, repetition, and omission to assure the safety of both those who give and receive care. Leading interdisciplinary partnership is not just another task to be accomplished but part of a greater whole to transform health care. It requires a commitment by everyone to transform practice at the point of care, where the hands of those who give and receive care meet. Carl Zaiss said it well; he noted that when seen for what it is, interdisciplinary partnership opens the door to new opportunities that we do not know exist (Zaiss, 2002).

Why do we not know the opportunities that true interdisciplinary partnership bring to us? The reason is that we are deeply rooted in two historical patterns of unipolar thinking:

1. Hierarchy was the norm in relationships, and we had little awareness of the importance of its opposite value, partnership.

2. The nature of practice was seen as a list of tasks to be done, while we lost sight of its interdependent pole, scope of practice, the very reason why most of us became healers. The absence of the skill of polarity management, the ability to balance opposites or very different values, prevented us from reaching a higher purpose or seeing new possibilities (Wesorick, 1995; Wesorick, 2002; Johnson, 1996).

As a result of history and our fast-paced cultures, we have not lived, known, or maybe even dared to believe interdisciplinary partnership at the point of care is possible.

Lessons Learned

Interdisciplinary partnership is the joining of hearts, hands, and minds around what matters most. It calls for the courage to lead a new way of thinking, practice, and relationships. It begins with a shared purpose or clarity on what matters most to those involved. For the last 30 years, the Clinical Practice Model (CPM) International Consortium has done core belief work to uncover what matters most to providers and recipients of care (Wesorick, 2008). The essence of the ongoing review consistently speaks to these beliefs:

- Each person has the right to safe, individualized health care that promotes wholeness of body, mind, and spirit.

- A healthy culture begins with each person and is enhanced by self-work, healthy relationships, and system supports.

- Continuous learning, diverse thinking, and evidence-based actions are essential to maintain and improve health.

- Partnerships are essential to plan, coordinate, integrate, deliver, and evaluate health care across the continuum.

- Each person is accountable to communicate and integrate his or her contribution to health care.

- Quality exists where shared purpose, vision, values, and healthy relationships are lived.

Principles of Partnership

Principle of Intention: A personal choice to connect with another at a deeper level of humanness.

- Is not just about doing, but also becoming.
- Requires going within, so one can reach out.
- Connects at a place where purpose and meaning of life emerge.
- Connects with others, not to control, but to deepen insights into oneself and others.
- Requires vulnerability and starts with personal work of becoming a partner.

Principle of Mission: A call to live out something that matters or is meaningful.

- Centers around shared purpose, principles, and core beliefs—not just position, policy/procedure, personal needs, bottom line, or power.
- Requires work of synchronizing personal and professional mission.
- Envisions work as an opportunity to make visible a person's purpose.

Principle of Equal Accountability: A relationship driven by ownership of mission, not power-over or fear.

- Holds each person to his or her choice: one is not the boss, one is not the subordinate.
- Knows competition and judgment interfere with individual and collective accountability to mission.
- Honors another's choice of role, responsibility, and contribution.
- Is accountable to support others in achieving mission.
- Is not in relationship to evaluate or judge the other's work or worth.
- Knows credibility relates to quality of work, not type of work.
- Does not feed the ego, but nourishes the spirit.

Principle of Potential: An inherent capacity within oneself and others to continuously learn, grow, and create.

- Sees self and others as continuous learners with untapped potential.
- Pursues clarity on others' role and responsibility, not to judge but to integrate and potentiate one another.
- Taps others' expertise related to mission.
- Enhances choices, options, creativity, and the imagination of others.
- Helps others recognize and tap personal wisdom.
- Seeks different perspectives but maintains common mission.
- Respects the individuality, uniqueness and diversity of self and others.
- Does not spend time molding others to be what he or she thinks they should be.

Principles of Partnership (*continued*)

- Supports others as they evolve and change to achieve the mission.
- Explores self and others' assumptions so to deepen wisdom.
- Knows when to ask for help.
- Requires compassion, forgiveness, and ability to learn from and see beyond vulnerability.

Principle of Balance: A harmony of relationships with self and others necessary to achieve mission.

- Understands that personal stability deters being controlled by external forces.
- Accountable for personal balance, choice, and competency.
- Cares for self and others.
- Knows that harmony in work relationships, as the mission, is not optional.
- Addresses imbalance in work relationships.
- Helps others self-organize.
- Knows the source of energy is not in the tasks alone, but in the relationships.
- Works on continuous learning and shifting to improve relationships.

Principle of Trust: A sense of synchrony on important issues or things that matter.

- Starts with self, must trust self first before trusting others.
- Knows personal trustworthiness precedes a trusting relationship with another.
- Recognizes that fear is a barrier to trust.
- Values the power that is within, not outside self.
- Does not have secrets, but shares information openly.
- Does not defend thinking, but shares it.
- Does not speak for the other, but seeks to hear the voice of the other.
- Does not try to get "buy-in" but dialogues to discover what is best for shared mission.
- Does not focus on who gets to make the decision, but what is the best decision.
- Does not blame, withdraw, instill guilt, rescue, fix, criticize or perpetrate.
- Focuses on quality of time together, not amount of time.

Wesorick, B. (1996). The Closing and Opening of a Millennium: A Journey From Old to New Relationships in the Work Setting. *Michigan: Practice Field Publishing.*

In the last 18 months, we asked more than 4,000 colleagues from diverse settings to evaluate their beliefs and their ability to clinically live each of their core beliefs. The results showed a deep value, but an inability to live out that value. The gap between what is believed and what is lived is statistically significant at the 0.001 level for every core belief. Only 10% of clinicians were able to consistently live what they believe (Wesorick, 2008). The challenge of transformation work is to bridge that gap. Shared purpose gives direction and a strong common ground to do this.

We have learned many lessons, but we have discovered three fundamental factors are essential to achieve interdisciplinary partnership: clarity on the principles of partnership, clarity on each discipline's scope of practice to support interdisciplinary integration, and an infrastructure that consistently brings the team together to do their work.

Principles of Partnership

Partnership is important because you cannot achieve standardization and the elimination of waste, fragmentation and "never events" (preventable complications, for example, bed sores experienced by patients in hospitals, which are no longer reimbursed by insurance companies in the U.S.) unless you stop the traditional patterns of disciplinary silos and task-driven practice. Partnership starts with compassion for each team member because compassionate care for those seeking health care can exist only when the workforce healers have a culture in which they can compassionately care for each other.

Talking about partnership and living it are very different. We have captured the lessons learned within the International Consortium in the Principles of Partnership sidebar. The principles provide insights into partnership, but it begins with respect. Respect is not a one-time act; it is a way of life. It is not just about what we do together, but how we are together. Theodore Roosevelt knew this when he said, "This country will not be a good place for any of us to live in unless we make it a good place for all of us to live in."

Clarity on Scope of Practice

No interdisciplinary partnership can exist unless each discipline is clear on its scope of practice and the scope of all its team members. Achieving that clarity is difficult because the health care culture has been historically focused on tasks, often those ordered by physicians. To deliver and advance a scope of practice that is different from the physicians' but equally important to the essence of quality care is challenging. It begins with the hard work to clearly articulate scope. Benjamin Disraeli noted, "The greatest good you can do for another is not just to share your riches, but to reveal to him his own." Foundational work to achieve interdisciplinary partnership begins with a commitment to do the work to strengthen each discipline's clarity on its unique scope of practice.

When disciplines are clear on scope, its memebers can teach each other about their scope and clarify how each impact the others. The conversation ignites the passion that brought them to their respective professions. It makes the wisdom of the famous poet Rumi come alive: "Everyone has been made for some particular work and the desire for that work has been put in his or her heart." When you invite colleagues to bring their hearts to the table, it brings an energy to the work that sparks creativity and innovation and unleashes a capacity that sits in the souls of healers.

Partnership Infrastructure

Interdisciplinary partnership is often lead by nurses because their scope calls for them to coordinate care. No one discipline, role, department, or unit determines quality of care. It is up to all of us, and we must be integrated. When the CPMRC International Consortium was formed, it came together with a clear mission to create the best places to give and receive care. It became obvious within the first year of the consortium's work that without an infrastructure in place that brings interdisciplinary healers together in dialogue and respect, the mission could not be achieved. The name given to the structure 30 years ago was Partnership Councils. The purpose: to take accountability to explore, innovate, and make decisions that ensure that the practice setting is the best place to give and receive care (Wesorick et al., 1998).

The next section contains the wisdom in the words of a mentee who is leading interdisciplinary partnership work and can take this work to the next level.

The Mentee's Perspective

When the hospital decided to focus on improving the care of seniors, the question was this: "Where should we start?" For me, the answer lay in the fundamental factors needed to achieve interdisciplinary partnership. Our hospital has an established and supported partnership council, which has allowed us to realize the benefits of bringing interdisciplinary teams together at the point of care. With this structure in place, it was easy to gather representatives from all disciplines. From here, disciplines had a chance to share what we each believed our own scope of practice to be. Disciplines also had a chance to show honor and respect for each other by stating what the scope of practice of other disciplines meant to them. Clinicians heard stories about what other disciplines had witnessed them doing to improve patient care. When we turned our discussion to seniors, we quickly realized that we shared a common ground: We all wanted to enhance the care of seniors and had already started in our own unique way. The sense of respect and purpose we shared with each other allowed us a break from the hierarchy, allowed us to not feel ordered around. We had a connection, felt a sense of direction, and could openly share ideas about how we could have a greater impact working together rather than in silos.

Shaping a New Culture

Interdisciplinary partnership often begins with a leader who is vulnerable enough to sit together with a team and admit that living the principles of partnership is new to him or her, but he or she is willing to learn. When colleagues are strong enough to be vulnerable with one another, it is the beginning of shaping a new culture. Where are we today? The words of Winston Churchill are true, "This is not the end, this is not even the beginning of the end, but perhaps it is the end of the beginning."

Self-Reflective Questions

1. What collective work have you done to clarify the core beliefs/values held by your interdisciplinary teams that solidify shared purpose?

2. In what ways have you assessed the gap that exists between what is believed and what is lived at the point of care?

3. How have you gained a clear picture of the point-of-care reality related to the nature of interdisciplinary partnerships within your teams?

4. In what ways have you assessed your ability to live the principles of partnership in your daily accountabilities?

5. Can each of the nurses articulate the difference between task-dominated practice and scope of professional nursing practice?

6. In what ways have you identified the barriers being faced by clinicians in the delivery of their professional scope of practice?

Self-Reflective Questions *(continued)*

7. How have the disciplines come together to clarify and integrate their scope of practice?

8. Can each of the disciplines articulate what they need to integrate their services at the point of care?

9. Have you put a partnership infrastructure in place that brings interdisciplinary colleagues together at the point of care on a continuous basis in every department?

10. What resources have you received that are necessary to support a partnership infrastructure? Are they enough?

Listening with Purpose

51

"Interruptions are inevitable, but you can manage them."

—Katherine Vestal

Mentor
Nancy Rollins Gantz, MSN, RN,
  PhD, MBA, NE-BC, MRCNA
President, CAPPS International
Sydney, Australia

Mentee
Susan Nardelli, RN, BSN,
  MSN/MHA
Charge Nurse for the
  Intensive Care Center
St. Mary's Hospital
Leonardtown, Maryland, USA

It is not often that we are taught something of value by a younger sibling, and a male sibling at that. The difficult part was admitting he was correct. At 25 years old, I (Nancy) began a new journey in a senior nursing leadership position. Shortly thereafter, people claimed that when in conversation I would stare through them or look away while they were still speaking. It was said to me that I appeared to be disinterested or distracted in what they were saying or was not listening. It was a younger brother who said to me, "It appears as if what I am saying to you is not of interest to you." That hit home and was never forgotten. Listening became a skill I was always cognizant of during communication. I have since developed the skill to an unconscious competence level (*see* Chapter 42, "Growing in Lifelong Learning" for a detailed discussion of competence levels).

Communication is one of the most critical components for the success of a leader. Global nursing health care leaders must commit to and consistently demonstrate superior listening with active hearing.

What Is Listening with Purpose? (Mentor)

From the early ages to the present day, listening has been a key characteristic for successful nursing leaders as well as global icons. Mother Theresa of Calcutta, who founded the Missionaries of Charity, spent her life caring for the dying and the poorest people in the world, and her endeavors will never be forgotten. Mother Theresa could not have accomplished her unselfish and humbling accomplishments if she did not listen with purpose. Mother Theresa listened to the dying, the hungry, the homeless, the crippled, the naked, and the poorest of the poor throughout the world while providing them shelter, food, clothing, words of comfort, and medical assistance. If she had not listened with purpose, Mother Theresa could not have provided these people with what they needed.

The same year that the world lost the beloved Mother Theresa, it sadly lost another individual that epitomized the quality of listening with purpose. In contrast to Mother Theresa, Diana, Princess of Wales, was not only famous for her humanitarian efforts but also her extraordinary listening. When watching Princess Diana on television or in person, it appeared that those around her were the only one with her and that her eyes were absorbing each word said to her. Listening with purpose was as natural for her as it was for Mother Theresa. Nelson Mandela, Gandhi, and the Dalai Lama are other examples of exemplary leadership and listening; their influence could not have been actualized without this quality. Being famous does not qualify one to be effective and purposeful in the practice of listening; the actions (and reactions) that come from being effective and purposeful in listening contributes to success.

The momentous day that I had the honor of meeting (then) South African President Nelson Mandela—a man who engages his whole being into what is being said to him—is etched in my memory. I was an American in a foreign country, yet President Mandela spoke to me as though we had been friends for years; and after every question he asked me, he then listened to me with genuine and sincere interest.

Getting in the Listening Paradigm and Staying There!

Talented and successful leaders know how to "stay in the zone" when it comes to listening with the outcome of purpose and action. These accomplished leaders know that effective listening is the foundation to strategic planning, development, and implementation of successful communication, relationship management, critical thinking and problem recognition, customer satisfaction, and community connections.

Listening as an essential leadership skill is assumed present, yet leaders tend not to emphasize listening when building teams and enhancing staff commitment and retention. However, the development of listening skills begins through education, grows to conscious competence, and eventually develops into unconscious competence. After a skill is repeatedly performed correctly, it is considered a conscious decision, or conscious competence. Once a leader demonstrates and uses this skill to a point of "second nature," it is unconscious competence.

Strategies and tools for the continual development and application of listening with purpose are not to be taken lightly. A leader must be aware and conscious of always being "in the zone." That is, being in a position where one is listening to the individual with their eyes, ears, mind, and a sincere willfulness to ignore all other distractions. This is where leaders inspire and lead others by projecting honest and earnest intent, verbally and nonverbally. While the environment may be chaotic, loud, or distracting, the leaders consistently stay in the zone even though sources of disruptions are all around.

Comparatively, the elements below simply identify the essential qualities basic to consistent and effective listening with purpose.

- **Stop, take a deep breath, and focus.**

- **Listen to the speaker.**

- **Listen with your whole body.** Make eye contact and lean in toward the speaker.

- **Let the other person do the talking.** Don't interrupt, offer an opinion, advise, or interpret.

- **Use reflective listening techniques.** In reflective listening, paraphrase what you just heard the person say and demonstrate your understanding of what you heard by restating the speaker's message.

- **Occasionally ask open-ended questions.** Asking questions shows that you are listening and helps you gather information.

- **Observe the speaker's body language to "hear" what they are not saying.** Emotions often leak out despite best efforts to control nonverbal expression. Notice facial expressions, gestures, and posture. Tight, closed posture indicates defensiveness and close-mindedness. Note discrepancies between what the person says and how he or she acts.

- **Use responsive silence.** Most listeners talk too much. When we become superior listeners, we not only improve our own productivity but we increase our ability to resolve conflict, work with and through people, and create a positive, respected influence on others.

Mentee Reflections

Good leaders must accept the individuality and autonomy of each person and treat them as one living and growing personally and professionally. That is how I want to be treated and how I aspire to treat others because of the potential growth that various interactions and experiences possess. My experience informs me that it all starts with effective communication founded on active listening. It's unfortunate to see managers preoccupied with tasks and innocently neglect the reason they are performing their duties—for a person.

Often, the human aspect is neglected, and leaders need to have zero tolerance for this behavior. I have been a victim of ignorance from people in a position of power. As a novice, I had no support. I was expected to perform, which I did thanks to the nursing training I received. Although, it was more like a boot camp: make it or get out. However, I did find a person here and there to guide me. My second nursing instructor gave me all the time in the world to express myself, used direct eye contact, and listened attentively. I knew she cared because her nonverbal communication— nodding her head at key moments, verbal acknowledgements, a gentle smile—reinforced that she was listening to me.

Smiling goes a long way as Mother Theresa, the Dalai Lama, and Nelson Mandela so eloquently showed us in their lives. Treating people with dignity and respect goes very far. For example, my parents juggled full-time jobs, cared for my frail grandfather, and raised six children. I knew they heard my concerns because they reflected my actions. My mother, a retired nurse, ingrained in me the motto, "Actions speak louder than words." She greatly influenced my growth and development, and gave me the strength that I share with others. This strength started as a seedling and was tended to over the years so now it gives back nourishment to those who seek it in the form of effective communication, active listening, and hearing with purpose to connect and support each other as successful nurse leaders and mentors.

Art of Listening (Mentor)

Encarta (2009) defines listening as "to concentrate on hearing somebody or something" and "to pay attention to something and take it into account." Leaders demonstrate best practice through their ability to master and consistently reveal this simple yet critical skill. They know the critical importance of acting appropriately to what is heard. Listening with purpose is an art, as is leadership. The art is validating through practice, day-in and day-out, that leaders are there to listen and hear from the team they work with (and work for), and to integrate those exchanges with the organizational vision. Mother Theresa, Princess Diana, and Nelson Mandela, all dedicated their lives to humankind in many significant ways. However, they each demonstrated purposeful listening. Their actions set the benchmark, and they serve as great role models of effective leadership for leaders today.

Self-Reflective Questions

1. How can you train yourself to maintain eye contact at all times?

2. How can you better "hear" what people are saying to you?

3. How do you provide undivided attention?

4. How can you better listen with facial and body expressions of being interested, accepting, and valued?

5. How can you condition yourself to form your response or opinion only after "hearing" what is said?

6. How can you train yourself to listen in group environments with the same attributes as in one-on-one conversation?

7. What are ways to request feedback from peer and staff on how you listen with purpose?

8. What are ways to seek help from a speaker if you are unclear about the message?

9. How can you mentor staff on the importance of listening with the purpose of "hearing and learning?"

10. Do colleagues consider you a role model for listening with the purpose of "hearing?"

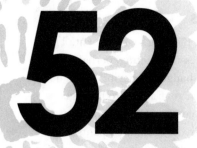

52 Meeting Management

"An effective meeting is 80 percent planning, 20 percent execution. Too often people spend most of their time in the meeting and the least amount of time getting ready for it. Plan better meetings. They don't just happen."

—Tim A. Lewis

Mentor

Sharon Lou Strutz Norton, RN, MSN
Independent Contractor
  Project Director
University of Fairbanks Center
  for Alaska Native Health Research
Examination and Skills Testing
  Administrator, Alaska Board of
  Nursing
Alaska, uSA

Mentee

Leah Gillham, RN, BSN
Public Health Nurse
  Graduate Student
Alaska, USA

Nurse leaders seek to increase the knowledge, quality, and performance of health care through effective management of meetings. They seek to engage and inspire others to become active participants in meetings. The major divisions of meeting management itself are as follows:

1. Initial planning.

2. Preparation before the meeting.

3. The meeting itself.

4. The actions following a meeting.

Rationale for Meeting Designs

Figure 1 displays the necessary steps to effective meeting management. The elimination of a necessary step can defeat a successful meeting, perhaps causing delays, disruption, and distraction; affecting budgets; delaying outcomes; defeating the purpose; and causing loss of faith in your ability to manage. Without appropriate management of meetings, you face the possibility of meeting chaos. Additionally, mismanagement discourages participants from attending future meetings needed to accomplish objectives to increase satisfaction, quality, and performance.

> "Effective meetings don't happen by accident, they happen by design"
> [unknown author]

Initial Planning

- Purpose/Objectives of the meeting.
- Prioritize issues to be addressed.
- Type of meeting.
- Number & make-up of participants.

Prior to the Meeting

- Identify the specific participants.
- Decide on date, time, & location.
- Equipment availability & hook-ups.
- Refreshments [if appropriate].
- Notify participants of upcoming meeting.
- Prepare and disseminate agenda & timeframe for meeting.
- Remind oneself to facilitate & not dominate meetings.

The Meeting

- Start on time.
- Assign note taker and timekeeper.
- Clarify agenda issues.
- Provide time for & encourage participant input—yet keep the meeting focused.
- Agree on priorities including: setting deadlines & delegation of responsibilities.
- Set timeframe for follow-up meetings.
- Critique the meeting, noting changes to be considered for future meetings.
- End the meeting on time.

Following the Meeting

- Provide minutes of meeting to participants.
- Follow-up on tasks/actions.
- Disseminate action progress updates to participants.
- Encourage & recognize task/action completions.
- Send out reminder of follow-up meeting.

Figure 1   Design for Meeting Management.

Meeting Tasks

In addition to those tasks listed in Figure 1, the meeting manager performs tasks that provide for meaningful interactions, respectful sharing, and movement towards accomplishment of the purpose. Some of those tasks include the following:

Before the meeting:

- Providing the agenda and educational materials before meetings and encouraging their pre-meeting review.

- Having discussions with selected participants to access their understanding of the purpose, their knowledge of the facts, and initial opinions.

- Encouraging attendance of selected participants.

At the meeting:

- Encouraging participation by all parties.

- Encouraging respect, clarity, and understanding.

- Keeping the group focused on the objectives.

- Clarifying areas of agreement and disagreement.

- Assisting the participants in finding effective solutions to meet the objectives.

- Summarizing the purpose, objectives, and the plan for achieving the individual/team tasks, including the timeline.

The participants must be able to trust that the manager can conduct meetings. As you model meeting management, besides the actual content of the meeting, the manager is like a mentor and those attending are like mentees. In this respect, meeting management leaders have a level of responsibility that should not be ignored.

Shared Meeting Management Experiences: Leah Gillham

I sit today and contemplate the meetings I have attended and those I will attend in the future. It is with thoughts of those meetings that I share some positive and negative feedback and experiences.

Sitting in this chair, my body hurts. I'm stiff. I feel like I could run a mile and then some and still not loosen up. I have spent the last four days sitting at a table listening to someone teach me how to chart correctly, using the correct form, the correct abbreviations, and the correct wording. The only thing going through my mind is that the facilitator for the first two days at least had plenty of energy. Perhaps, though, she should have ended the conference then, because by day four, my mind is a full sponge in a sink of water, and the person in front of me, with the monotone voice, sounds more like Charlie Brown's teacher from the Peanuts animated cartoons than an experienced instructor. I'm done. I can't handle another PowerPoint slide, another example, or another practice round. But we made it through more quickly than we had planned because of the pre-meeting work done by the facilitators. With as much information as we had to cover, we could have been sitting in meetings for weeks. Those in charge, however, did well in keeping us all focused and on track.

I also sit in weekly four-hour meetings. I can handle these. If at some point my mind decides to wander to what's for dinner or what I need from the grocery store, I know I can count on the minutes to catch me up. If, as a group, we get off track, someone, appointed at the beginning of the meeting, gets us back on topic so we aren't sitting at the table all day. If we need a break, because our coffee cups are empty or our bladders are full, we just step out and try to be as discreet as possible. We are all required to bring topics to the table that need to be addressed and to participate in the discussion. Our team leaders create the agenda, but each of us may add items as we go along. We recap last week's meeting at the start of the new meeting. Structure and organization is what makes it possible to come back, week after week, to the same room, knowing we have hours to go.

In my short career as a registered nurse, I have yet to attend a meeting that didn't have some sort of structure. Some meetings I have attended seemed as though they didn't pertain to me, so my interest might have been elsewhere; but still, it was not a complete disaster. Hopefully, with the information and guidance provided to me from my mentor I can manage my own meetings based on evidence, the kind of meeting where people can tolerate coming back, the kind with a point—the kind where something is accomplished by the end.

Comments Regarding the Mentor/Mentee Experience: Sharon Lou Strutz Norton

Leah has completed her first step in her registered nursing education and looks forward to continuing her education. From this experience, she takes notice of the negatives and positives of meeting management. She realizes what can make or break a meeting and how she might alter meetings she herself will lead. Leah now has a reference guide (this text) and me as a contact should she have questions now or in the future as she takes the lead in managing meetings herself.

Self-Reflective Questions

1. How is the meeting purpose/outcome made clear to all participants?

2. How are the objectives prioritized?

3. How can you ensure the agenda and educational materials are received and reviewed by participants prior to the meeting?

4. How can you make sure all the participant's opinions are treated with respect?

5. In what ways can you either dominate or facilitate the meeting?

6. How can you make sure the meeting starts and ends on time?

7. How can you inspire the participants to discuss and define objectives?

8. What approaches can you use to ensure participants are delegated appropriate tasks and timelines?

9. How can you identify and recognize completed tasks?

10 .How can you evaluate outcomes to ensure they meet the purpose?

Moral Courage

53

"Doing the right thing is, more often than not, not the easiest option in the short term and often requires more time and energy than doing the easy thing. In the long term, of course, it's the right decision."

—Jo Ann Love

Mentor
Vicki D. Lachman, PhD, APRN, MBE
Drexel University, College of Nursing and Health Professions
Philadelphia, Pennsylvania, USA

Mentee
Lisa Johnson-Ford, MSN, CRNP
Drexel University
College of Nursing and Health Professions
Philadelphia,Pennsylvania, USA

Being a leader requires the moral courage to speak out and do the right thing by first overcoming fear and then standing for one's core personal and professional values (Lachman, 2007). A leader puts principles into action, even in the face of the possible risks of humiliation, rejection, ridicule, unemployment, and loss of social standing. Bravery requires the audacity to speak the truth when others cower. Aristotle believed that virtue of courage was the balance (mean) between extremes of cowardice and rashness. This definition means a courageous nurse does not rush headfirst into danger because she is blinded by her anger, nor is she oblivious to the hazards that lie ahead. The space between knowing what is the right action and then acting is bridged by moral courage.

Evolution of Moral Courage

The initial writings of the Socrates, Plato, and Aristotle focused on the courage necessary in the battlefield. Plato was the first to define courage as one of the four cardinal virtues in the tradition of moral character development (*Stanford Encyclopedia of Philosophy*, 2007). The other qualities are temperance, justice, and wisdom. Socrates and Plato both believed that management of mind over body was the *only* way in which human actions could become good. Temperance, through self-control, contained the appetites with good judgment (wisdom) and a focus on justice (fairness for all, not self-centeredness). Nursing leaders need to be guided by wisdom and justice in situations requiring moral courage when advocating for patients or nurses. Courage manifests itself as the skill to manage the hardship that conflicts bring and an ability to endure adversity. So, what makes the difference between a coward and a courageous person?

Aristotle's view of courage further informs our present understanding of courage. His focus was not on cardinal virtues, but on two types of virtues: virtue of thought and virtue of character. Virtue of thought is increased through education and virtue of character is advanced through habit. Aristotle suggested both deficient and excess virtue could be catastrophic. He writes "he is courageous who endures and fears the right things, for the right motive, in the right manner, and at the right time and who displays confidence in a similar way" (*Nichomachean Ethics* (NE) III 7.1115b15–20). Aristotle steadfastly believed that a virtue, like courage, be used only for admirable ends. Aristotle's focus was on importance of acting, not just on reasoning. He said that "one must not only know what to do, but he must also be able to act accordingly" (NE VII 1152a5–10). Aristotle would agree with Albert Einstein, who said, "The world is a dangerous place, not because of those who do evil, but because of those who look on and do nothing."

That Florence Nightingale was acquainted with the lives of the ancient Greeks and read and translated the works of Plato is established fact. Nightingale equates doing what is right with happiness (Dossey et al., 2004). Letters depicting Florence Nightingale as an ambitious meddler who went over doctors' heads show a spirit the profession still needs, say nurse leaders (Nursing Standard, 2007). Nightingale would agree with Robert Green Ingersoll when he said, "The greatest test of courage on earth is to bear defeat without losing heart." What follows is an example of mentee Lisa Johnson-Ford demonstrating moral courage.

A Lesson in Moral Courage (Mentee)

As a novice nurse practitioner, I faced the challenge of managing critically ill bone marrow transplant patients along with a diverse group of physicians. An experimental protocol for leukemia was being offered to patients who did not respond to previous transplants. John, a 38-year-old man who failed in two previous bone marrow transplants, was offered the protocol. John cherished his quality of life and stated he wanted to live out his remaining days at home rather than in a hospital. This experimental protocol was given a high survival rate, but I became more uncertain of its validity because seasoned staff nurses told me that no one had survived the procedure beyond 3 months. I urged John to reconsider the procedure as he was unaware of the poor survival rate. When the transplant physicians became aware of my conversation with John, my employment was threatened. Later, after I was questioned by nursing, medical, and administrative leaders, the protocol was quietly placed back on the shelf, but not before John had decided to proceed. Within two weeks of the treatment, he became intensely ill and died. When reflecting back on this patient, I feel saddened by his untimely death but reassured that I had the moral courage to question the status quo. As patient advocates, we have an obligation to do what is right for our patients. When faced with conflict, we must cope and persist as our profession's founder, Florence Nightingale, envisioned.

Moral Courage as a Virtue

Moral courage is a virtue; a virtue that puts into action reasoning and wisdom harvested through education and experience. We need to ask the incisive questions Socrates would ask. We need to be aware of our fears, but not allow them to stop us from being the patient advocates we are duty-bound to be as nursing professionals.

We want to end with a quote by Eleanor Roosevelt that speaks to the task of all nursing leaders who want to demonstrate moral courage: "You gain strength, courage, and confidence by every experience in which you really stop to look fear in the face. You must do the thing which you think you cannot do."

Self-Reflective Questions

The following questions can assist you in reflecting on your moral courage in the workplace.

1. In what situations would you speak up, even at the risk of being ridiculed?

2. What sorts of illegal actions in the organization would cause you to speak up, even if it cost you your job?

3. What sort of unfair treatment from your supervisor might cause you to speak up?

4. In what situations would you admit mistakes to a supervisor, even when it could result in disciplinary action?

5. What approaches would you take to apologize and disclose an error to a patient?

6. In what context would you refuse a patient assignment that was beyond your ability, even if it created a major problem?

7. In what situations have you presented your ideas, even though they were ridiculed or rejected in the past?

8. In what ways do you speak up to peers, even when you are afraid of negative consequences?

9. When have you spoken up to physicians, even though they have a reputation for being abusive?

10. In what situations would you speak up if you saw actions that could harm a patient?

Management: Growth Through Goals

54

"Motivation is the art of getting people to do what you want them to do because they want to do it."

—Dwight D. Eisenhower

Mentor
Claudia Kam Yuk Lai, PhD, RN
Associate Professor
School of Nursing, The Hong
  Kong Polytechnic University
Hong Kong SAR, China

Mentee
Shirley K L Lo, RN, MSN, LL.B
Clinical Associate
School of Nursing, The Hong
  Kong Polytechnic University,
Hong Kong SAR, China

Shirley (Mentee): Having worked in acute care hospitals for years, I have seen how my superiors managed to get their tasks done by simply adopting an autocratic manner. Many times, those in power implement new policies or instructions from the top down, failing to reveal the rationale for such changes and largely neglecting potential differing opinions. This approach can be frustrating for frontline nurses.

When I entered my current academic career, I realized a very different kind of nursing leadership could exist. Claudia Lai, the associate head of the school and leader of the Ageing and Health Research Group, sets an example of influential and efficient leadership by motivating her colleagues to reach out for their individual and collective goals. I enjoy and am proud to be a member of this research team. It is amazing and rewarding to observe how Claudia leads.

Motivational Strategies—Points of View

Claudia (Mentor): Mentorship can either be formal or informal. It does not need to be formalized or highly structured to be effective.

Shirley and I are more like friends as opposed to a mentor-mentee pair. Motivation is about relationships. One cannot motivate another person unless there is a positive, or at least neutral, relationship between the two parties. It is only when each holds the other in positive regard that communication can be effective. I like Shirley because she is conscientious, personable, intelligent, and has a good sense of humor.

Showing the Way Ahead

Shirley: The mentee will not be effectively motivated when she or he does not know where to go and what to do. Claudia leads her team by helping them to visualize the way ahead and by engaging in good planning. For example, take the starting up of a collaborative project with a local long-term care facility: Claudia advocated a framework embracing both the strategic direction and the directions for formulating detailed action plans. In this way, she made the team aware of what needed to be done and where they were headed. This forethought motivated the team to pursue the project effectively and efficiently. In particular, this type of collaboration was a first in Hong Kong, and such a well-drawn roadmap served as an important guideline to colleagues (including me) who were too inexperienced to imagine the landscape ahead.

Calculating a Mentee's Ability and Creating Opportunities for Meeting Their Needs

Shirley: In spite of being such a learned scholar and a leader in the field, Claudia is always humble and treats others with empathy and respect. And even more important to her subordinates is that despite her tight schedule, she often makes time to keep up-to-date with how her colleagues are doing. This attitude of holistic concern means a lot to others, and she sends a clear message to all of us: You are not left alone with the task. This gives me, and others, the motivation to progress with no fear, because I know I can get help when necessary from a trustworthy superior.

Claudia: In fact, Shirley, I don't think much of superior-subordinate relationships. I think our positions are different, but we are each professionals in our own right and, therefore, equal in that sense. One of us is embracing and experiencing the novice-to-expert journey whereas the other has reached the expert goal.

Shirley: Understanding that I have some basic training in law and a great interest in legal and nursing aspects, Claudia makes sure that I do not miss the opportunity to attend relevant conferences, both locally and internationally, meet peers, and take part in relevant training courses or workshops. That said, she never applies undo pressure if I do not live up to her expectations. Her comment, "only we know exactly what we need," demonstrates her empathy and respect for others, including her subordinates. Her aptitude at creating opportunities for others to become aware of their own expectations and responsibilities makes her a distinctive leader of the day. In this, she is making use of her inner drive to motivate people, and it works.

Claudia: To motivate someone, the mentor must show the mentee the big picture. The mentor must introduce his or her perspective, likely coming from a broader angle as a result of more experience that the mentee might not see as yet, to the mentee to encourage him or her onward. The big picture might be the analysis of current situations, the mapping of necessary strategies, or the dream that the mentor envisions for the mentee.

Patience is required of a mentor when he or she is motivating someone. When Shirley first joined the university, she wanted to finish her master's degree and then move on to her doctorate. Later on, considering her life circumstances, she decided to further her study at a later time. The communication between us is open and honest. A person has his or her own time and tempo in life. That time to move ahead will come, but the person's choice must be respected.

Being Accessible and Constantly Providing Positive Feedback

Shirley: Young colleagues who are launching their careers face obstacles and may fall sometimes. As a learner, I can count on Claudia for her accessibility in providing timely feedback. Better yet, most feedback Claudia provides embraces a positive message, which is like a powerful fuel that provides ongoing energy from within to foster my progression. Having tasted that, I imitate this approach and practice it in my clinical supervision. The result is encouraging. I see the students on clinical placement who receive the positive feedback building up their confidence in the seemingly unfamiliar clinical setting and implementing newly learned nursing care more assertively.

Claudia: Continual feedback to mentees is crucial, so that they know how far they have come. When I recognize Shirley's potential and relay my observations about what I see in her capabilities, she appears to be energized. I did not do these things on purpose. But Shirley lets me know that these small acts boost her morale. It makes me feel good to know this.

Role-Modeling

Shirley: Believing that it would be a waste of others' time if someone were late, Claudia sets a good example by always being on time. Moreover, although she is at a management level, she remains kind and courteous and treats all staff members with due respect. What strikes me most is her never-shrinking courage to accept responsibility. Should a team action turn out to be less than successful, she never passes any blame to her colleagues. Similarly, she does not take credit for others' work. Such real-life conduct renders her an outstanding role model for her students and colleagues.

Claudia: Nobody is expected to be a saint, but at least the mentor must have certain qualities that the mentee would like to acquire. When a nurse leader takes up the role of a mentor, his or her integrity is being called upon.

Working Together

Claudia: The mentee needs to work hard on his or her goals. Shirley is one of the most diligent people I work with at our school. And, of course, the mentor has to work as well. When a mentor and a mentee work together on a project, such as co-authoring a manuscript or co-writing a grant proposal, it allows a mentor to show the mentee in more ways than mere words; it allows for hands-on training and experience. I helped Shirley to gain some hands-on experience writing a small survey on elder abuse, which is her area of interest, and obtaining ethics approval. Routinely, we discuss her ideas about possible study topics. I also try to look out for networking opportunities for her and introduce her to contacts.

One cannot motivate without mutual respect. Both the mentor and the mentee should operate on a level playing field. Mentoring is nurturing, but it must never be patronizing. The mentee might be in need of some advice as to how to advance his or her career, but he or she is not a lesser person because of his or her wants or needs. A power differential naturally exists in a mentor-mentee relationship. Power can easily be abused, leading to exploitation, which must be avoided. Trying to sweet talk someone into getting a job done is not motivation; it is only persuasion. Whereas persuasion might or might not have effects in the long run, motivation is usually expected to be transformational. A person whose potential has not been fully realized in the past is motivated to achieve and to aim higher in his or her pursuits. The mentor must be authentic, must have faith in the mentee (I have a lot of that for Shirley), and must believe in the goodness of people.

Final Thoughts on Motivation

Shirley: Unlike traditional autocratic leaders, Claudia motivates the team to move forward by calculating team members' limitations and abilities, by working together with members with mutual respect, and by providing juniors the opportunities to grow both personally and professionally. I am grateful to have the opportunity to realize my internal need to move forward.

Claudia: Motivation must be based on a genuine relationship with mutual respect between a mentor and a mentee. A mentor uses role modeling, collaborative projects, and continuous honesty as the essential means of motivating. Showing the big picture to the mentee is a good approach to motivating a person.

Self-Reflective Questions

1. Is your mentoring formal or informal? What are your and the mentee's expectations in this relationship?

2. Do you hold each other in positive regard?

3. What, if any, special interest or personal gain do you have in mentoring? Does the mentee know about it?

4. How do you treat the mentee? Do you treat him or her as an individual, a colleague in his or her own right? Are the two of you operating on a level playing field?

5. What are your mentee's capabilities, potential, and aspirations?

6. How willing are you to commit to developing your mentee over time?

7. In what ways can you be a good role model?

8. In what ways do you work together with your mentee? Or do you leave him or her on his or her own?

9. How can you display patience when the mentee doesn't seem to be moving along the way you think he or she should?

10. In what ways do you approach giving honest feedback, both good and bad?

55 Multisystem, Organization-Wide Mentoring

"None of us comes into the world fully formed. We would not know how to think, or walk, or speak, or behave as human beings unless we learned it from other human beings. We need other human beings in order to be human. I am because other people are."

—Desmond Tutu

Mentor
Karlene M. Kerfoot, PhD, RN, NEA-BC, FAAN
Vice President and Chief Clinical Officer
Aurora Health Care
Milwaukee, Wisconsin, USA

Mentee
Kristine Mohr, MSN, RN
Nurse Manager
Aurora Sinai Medical Center
Milwaukee, Wisconsin, USA

Systems are large, usually matrixed organizations that are not easy to navigate alone. It is a huge jump from the work at the bedside to chairing a system-wide team. Unfortunately, we have an inadequate supply of people interested in moving into leadership positions, such as nurse manager or chief nursing officer, at a site or a system. Mentoring has been researched as an important way to create the next generation of leaders. And, because systems are complex, it is important to use mentoring as a way to help people navigate through them to create that next generation of leaders. This chapter explores the authors' experiences with mentorship within a system.

Kristine's Background

Multi-hospital systems and integrated delivery networks provide interest-ing challenges for the nurses and leaders. It was within this framework of an integrated system that Kristine Mohr was elected to be the third president of the newly formed Aurora Health Care System's Shared Governance system that encompasses the entire system, including 13 hospitals and other settings, and approximately 6,000 nurses. Kristine learned shared governance from her home hospital in Sheboygan, Wisconsin, and chose to take the leap to the system leadership position after representing her facility at a system level. Un-der the mentoring of Sue Ela, MSN, RN, executive vice president for Aurora Health Care, Kristine created a viable governance structure and left an impor-tant legacy from her term in office.

During her four years at the system level, Kristine had the opportunity not only to grow the governance structure, but also to frequently interact with nursing leaders throughout the system. She also became a mentor to many nurses through her far-ranging influence as the system president. When her tenure was over, the experience of being mentored by impressive leaders in-spired Kristine to return to school to pursue her graduate degree in health care systems leadership from Marquette University.

Karlene's Background

In October 2007, Karlene Kerfoot joined Aurora Health Care as the chief clinical officer for the system. The mentorship began in the final semester of Kristine's master's program as she sought out a mentor for her final leadership course. The mentoring experience was negotiated to be several-faceted:

1. Completing a redesign of the system's shared governance structure based on the new Magnet model.

2. Experiencing new and varied leadership activities as preparation for a multistage leadership role for Kristine in the future, preferably at Aurora.

The Mentorship Begins

Was the experience successful? Yes, the activities of the mentorship were completed, and the redesign of the shared governance under Kristine's leader-ship was agreed upon and is well on the way to success. This redesign had to be "sold" to the multitude of nurses who were enthusiastic about the change, as well as those who were reluctant, and it was successful. The exciting finale occurred when Kristine was notified that she had been invited to deliver a podium presentation at the national Magnet Conference about the project in October 2009, but the most important part of the mentorship was the opportunity to complete a project that not only served as a valuable learning experience, but also has the potential to become a truly innovative, shared governance model to promote professional nursing and drive quality patient outcomes.

The Mentor/Mentee Experience

Desmond Tutu (2007) so eloquently stated, "I am because other people are" (p. 34). The mentor often receives more value from the relationship than the mentee. In this case, Karlene, new to the system, was privy to Kristine's historical knowledge of the Aurora system, and she learned many things that helped directly with her orientation to the complex system. Kristine also was far better at redesigning the shared governance structure because she saw it through the eyes of the stakeholders—the nurse and the nurse's ability to provide better care to patients. Therefore, Karlene would say that she was changed and humanized by the relationship because she had the opportunity of many individual sessions with Kristine that drew her closer to the voice of the nurse through Kristine.

Learning to work in a complex environment requires mentorship. Moving from local site-based thinking and perceptions into systems thinking that simultaneously holds what is best for all patients in the system with what is best for patients at a site/unit is difficult. The mentorship received from Karlene gave Kristine the foundation and support to navigate throughout the system. Great mentors also give autonomy. Kristine was given the latitude to work throughout the system to accomplish the best possible outcome and to learn from experience. From Kristine's view, working at the system level of an integrated system afforded her the opportunity to leverage a diverse pool of expertise into a functioning whole of shared governance for the system. Orchestrating the convergence of collective wisdom from staff nurses and nurse leaders from across the system proved to be complicated at times, but was necessary to obtain the best possible outcome.

Kristine also had the opportunity to work with Tim Porter-O'Grady, an international speaker and consultant on issues of governance and leadership, as he was invited to an all-day session to critique the work of the committees. This took mentorship to a completely new level. Not only was Kristine mentored by a highly respected executive within the organization, but was now being recognized, supported, and mentored by an internationally renowned expert she had held in high esteem for many years. Throughout the process of being a mentee, Kristine has grown in her leadership capacity and is now a mentor to others in their shared governance journeys. And through her future publications and presentations, she will be a mentor to many nurses who are striving to grow professionally and who are learning systems thinking and the skills necessary to leading in an integrated healthcare environment.

Lessons Learned

This journey provided many lessons for Kristine that were also lessons for Karlene. First, never underestimate your abilities. With the right guidance and support, mountains can be moved. Second, never doubt the enthusiasm and support from very diverse groups across a system. In spite of the fact that nurses come from every family background imaginable and work in diversified settings across many miles, we are more alike than we are different. In the words of Desmond Tutu: "Instead of separation and division, all distinctions make for a rich diversity to be celebrated for the sake of the unity that underlies them. We are different so that we can know our need of one another. (2007, p. 92)

Finally, when working in a complex system, ensure that the message intended for the entire diverse body is in a language and format that can be translated and understood by all its constituents. The development of the Aurora model of shared governance for the system that Kristine developed with the work of many others is an exemplar of how an organizing framework of shared governance can synergize 6,000 nurses who work in 13 hospitals, more than 100 clinics, and other sites throughout the system in the eastern third of Wisconsin into a professional body aligned around the values of professional nursing.

On Her Way

Kristine has accepted her first formal leadership position as a nurse manager in one of the Milwaukee hospitals where she can work at the unit level but continue to be involved at the system level. She comes to this position with a broad systems view because she has learned so much from so many. It is the hope of her mentor that Kristine will be able to move on to progressively more complex positions within Aurora and to further advance her education to prepare her to pursue her passion of shared governance at an even higher level and to help many more nurses become all they can be. Finally, in the words of Desmond, TuTu, "A person is a person through other persons" (2007, p.33). This is the experience of a mentor and a mentee-growing through others.

Self-Reflective Questions

1. What are three experiences that have accelerated your thinking from site-based to system thinking?

2. What was common in these experiences?

3. What was the tipping point when you knew you were permanently changed as a system-thinking person?

4. What prevents you now from losing that growth and reverting to unit/site based thinking?

5. When have you replicated that acceleration to system thinking when you have worked with others?

6. Did you modify the experience for others, or did you try to replicate your experience exactly—and why?

7. What experiences do you wish for that will accelerate your transitions to even greater ability to work in an integrated system in the next three months?

8. Will you wait for the learning to happen, or will you go forward and seek it out?

9. What are three missed opportunities in the last month where you failed to reach out to someone and help them in their journey to system thinking?

10. What will you do to make sure you don't have the opportunity to miss learning and growth in the next three months?

Needs Assessment: From the Bedside to the C-Suite

56

"A woman who thinks to herself: 'Now I am a full Nurse, a skilled Nurse, I have learnt all that there is to be learnt': take my word for it, she does not know what a Nurse is, and she never will know; she is gone back already. Conceit and Nursing cannot exist in the same person, any more than new patches on an old garment."

—Florence Nightingale

Mentor
Joy Gorzeman, MSN, RN, MBA
Former Senior Vice President,
  for Patient Care Services, and
  Chief Nursing Officer
Trinity Health
Novi, Michigan, USA
Interim Chief Nursing Officer
Tri-City Medical Center
Oceanside, California, USA

Mentee
Gay Landstrom, MS, RN
Senior Vice President, Patient
  Care Services, and Chief
  Nursing Officer
Trinity Health
Novi, Michigan, USA
and
Karen Hodge, RN, BBA, MSN
Interim Chief Nursing Officer
 St. Alphonsus Regional Medical
   Center
Boise, Idaho, USA

One of the first things nursing students learn before going into the clinical practice arena is how to do a needs assessment on a patient, which then leads to designing the plan of care. Therefore, this is the first thing that comes to my mind in considering a discussion about needs assessment. However, when you consider needs assessment from the bedside to the C-suite (which includes the chief nursing officer, chief executive officer, and other "chiefs"), you realize that the basics of needs assessment can be and are applied in numerous situations. Performing a needs assessment of a patient's physical, emotional, and spiritual needs is at the root of nursing practice, nurses at the bedside and nurse leaders perform other types of needs assessments on a daily basis. These might include the following:

1. **Self-assessment of learning needs:** what competencies do we need more information about?

2. **Assessment of what our leader needs:** at all levels—we are working for someone who is relying on us to perform.

3. **Assessment of what our community needs.**

4. **Aassessment of what our colleagues need from us.**

In doing a needs assessment in any area, the work of Patricia Benner, *From Novice to Expert: Excellence and Power in Clinical Nursing Practice* (2001), provides an excellent framework. Throughout our careers as nurse leaders, we find ourselves in varying roles, organizations, and new experiences. With each change or new responsibility, we move in and out of the levels of expertise that Benner describes. Consequently, because we shift in and out of these various roles, we find ourselves moving in and out of both mentor and mentee roles throughout our career, if we are open to that.

Mentor

In a recent leadership position as the chief nurse executive for a large national system, I experienced many levels of mentoring. I had the wonderful opportunity of working with 23 chief nursing officers (CNOs). These phenomenal leaders were already mentors within their organizations. As the leader of this group, I had the responsibility and privilege of providing guidance and direction, mentoring these leaders in the transformational work we were doing on creating excellence in the care experience and calling out the important role that nurses play in this work. These leaders had varying needs, depending on how much experience they had, what was going on in their particular organization, what career goals they had, and so on.

As the chief nurse executive of the system, I not only interacted with the CNOs, but also with other nurse leaders and staff nurses providing direct care in our organizations. I found the mentor/mentee relationship to be very much a two-way street. When I was open to it, I found the staff nurses I interacted with at our congresses to be my best mentors, even though I had been in the profession for more than 30 years and in leadership well over 15 years. They were the ones doing the work and provided a wonderful reminder of my role and their need for me to call out the very special work and role of nurses as the integrators of care and coordinators and leaders of the interdisciplinary caring team.

This essay provides two examples of the valuable mentor/mentee relationships I experienced when I served as chief nurse executive. In the first example discussed in this essay, one of the CNOs wanted to pursue her PhD and needed more flexibility in her schedule than her CNO position allowed. This individual was one of the brightest and best in the field. We discussed the possibilities, and she became a part of the corporate office team, which put her in a position that called for a new relationship with her colleagues. She went from running all of nursing in a hospital to being part of a team with responsibility for getting 23 CNO colleagues onboard with some of the key work we were doing.

In the second example, I was asked to coach and mentor a director in one of our organizations as part of our succession planning for CNO positions, a director who was placed in the role she was to assume sooner than anticipated.

These two examples reflect the varying levels of expertise and need throughout the changes in our roles and careers. By listening to the mentee and doing a "needs assessment" of her needs and questions, I am also being mentored into how to do this better, especially with insightful mentees who ask probing and insightful questions, as I have had.

Reflections from Gay Landstrom

I was in a role where I needed to work with all of the CNOs in my corporation. These were highly expert leaders, many of whom have taught me valuable lessons over the years. The challenge before me was to design and implement a shared governance structure for our whole corporation. With some decisions being made at the corporate level that would affect nursing practice, it was critical that staff nurses guide those decisions. Though I was very comfortable with shared governance and had implemented structures and processes many times, working with our CNOs to develop a structure at the system level was something quite different for me. I also had to be sensitive to the individual CNOs, who varied in their experience and understanding of shared governance.

My mentor asked me some very pointed questions to determine if I needed guidance in this work. She valued and recognized my own experience and expertise, but understood that I might still benefit from mentoring. She asked what made this shared governance development the same or different from others

I had worked with. She also assessed if I could strategically see the outcome I was trying to achieve or if I was buried in the details. Based on my answers, she asked if I would like to have some mentoring, an offer I heartily accepted. She was sensitive to the magnitude of the task and had known it was time to assess for a "mentoring opportunity."

Reflections from Karen Hodge

I have been a nursing director in the same organization for approximately 15 years. Over those years, I have managed many nursing and non-nursing areas, developed and implemented new services, and mentored nurse managers. As a nursing director, I would place myself on the expert end of the spectrum in the novice to expert continuum.

However, when asked to step into the CNO role, I am once again a novice. The hardest part of any new role is understanding the scope and nuance of the role and how these differ from a previous role. My mentor is helping me identify the nuances between the old and the new perspective. I am at a stage where I don't know what I don't know, and my mentor asks gentle, but probing questions. What is going well for you? Why do you think it is going well? What are your challenges? Why do you think this is a challenge? So, what do you think you should do about it? What help do you think you need? How or where can you get assistance? In other words, we are engaging in my needs assessment. Every coaching session is a learning and discovery session. Sometimes the discovery is how to solve a problem or handle a situation; other times the discovery is affirming that I am doing a good job, which helps me develop a new sense of confidence in a new role. In my situation, my mentor helps me use the critical thinking skills I have to adapt to this new situation.

Self-Reflective Questions

1. In what ways has the mentee experienced a change in role or responsibilities?

2. How experienced (or not) is the mentee novice or inexperienced in the work they are focused upon?

3. What changes in the environment of the work have made it new and challenging?

4. How complex is the cultural context of the mentee's work?

5. What possible conflicting priorities does the mentee have?

Self-Reflective Questions *(continued)*

6. What changes in organizational level of focus (for example, unit leadership versus organizational) has the mentee made?

7. In what ways is the mentee ready to focus on broader issues in the nursing community (for example, public policy, regional collaboration, and state or national professional leadership)?

8. What difficult barriers is the mentee struggling with?

9. In what ways are you open to being mentored as well?

10. How much time do you have to invest in the mentee and any necessary follow-up?

57

Needs-Based Resource Development and Allocation

"When resources are limited, the dilemma for nurses is how to fulfil their ethical duty to assist persons to achieve their optimum level of health in situations of normal health, illness, injury, or in the process of dying."

—Canadian Nurses Association

Mentor
Marga Thome, PhD, MS,
  Diploma of Advanced
  Nursing Studies, RN, RNM
University of Iceland, School
  of Health Science, Faculty of
  Nursing
Eirberg, Eiriksgata 34, 101
Reykjavik, Iceland

Mentee
Arna Skuladottir, MS, BSN, RN
Landspitali University Hospital,
  Pediatric Unit
Reykjavik, Iceland

An example of an innovative service in nursing will help illustrate resource development. A service for sleep-disturbed infants was started in January 1997 at the Reykjavik City Hospital, which later became part of the Landspitala University Hospital in Reykjavik, Iceland. The project, which began with a pilot study of sleep-disturbed infants, evolved into a research program focusing on interventions for sleep-disturbed infants and on the study of outcomes for infants and parents. Subsequently, several types of services evolved, starting with a service for inpatients that was followed by a service for outpatients and a telephone-based public education service in the form of courses and lectures for parents or specialized groups, and finally an Internet site or Web-based parenting school.

The demand for this service has been steadily rising. The number of those parents who sought services rose from 43 children in 1997 to about 800 in 2007. Ninety-five percent of the children receiving service are aged 6 weeks to 3 years. Parents pay for the telephone counseling, but outpatient service is free. Both types of services are accessible to the public and run by a pediatric advanced practice nurse (APN) who is licensed in the management of pediatric sleep problems.

Vision

Nurses hold visions of how they would like to assist persons to achieve an optimal level of health in different situations. The beginning of the afore-mentioned program can be traced to the mentors' experience of "a lack of services dealing with infants' difficulties such as crying, sleeping, feeding, and so on" and help "for distressed parents" (Thome and Alder, 1999). A motivating force behind establishing such a service was the rapidly increasing body of knowledge on infant and perinatal mental health disseminated by various scientific societies around the world (e.g., World Association for Infant Mental Health, Marcé Society, Society for Reproductive and Infant Psychology). The envisioned project was based on the belief that nursing and midwifery can contribute substantially to knowledge and service in the promotion of the mental health of this population.

Resources

Innovative services require resources on the individual, institutional, and societal level, all of which are important to fulfil the ethical duty of caring (Canadian Nurses Association, 2008). Resource allocation is the distribution of immaterial and material goods and services to programs and people. Resources may be neither obvious nor known in advance. They are to be discovered, and their use depends on many factors. These preconditions all apply to the program that is described here.

The first resource identified in our example is "the sharing of a vision" and establishing of dialog. In institutions of higher learning, mentor, and mentee frequently enter into dialog and inspire each other, as happened in our case. Higher education and dialog are considered immaterial resources that can lead to recognition of each other's ideas, values, and resources.

A precious resource of the mentee was a longstanding professional experience in pediatric nursing with the desire to advance her professional development within this field. The mentee had learned from experience that children's sleeping problems were not considered to be of particular interest and were of negligible concern in the pediatric service provided in a traditional hospital setting; this constituted a challenge to the vision and witness of the mentor. Little attention to (and obscure aims regarding) the management of children's sleep problems were related to a lack of evidence-based knowledge for this group in all types of pediatric health services.

Recognition and Use of Resources within Education, Hospital Service, and Social Context

The development of the service started with an educational pilot project exploring the feasibility of a nurse-led, systematic treatment for hospitalized, sleep-disturbed children. This exploration opened the establishment and evaluation of a nurse-led service in the management of all sleep-disturbed, inpatient children and their parents (Skuladottir and Thome, 2003; Thome and Skuladottir, 2005a). Evaluation of the new service was initiated and showed positive results. The evaluation's results encouraged development in the form of a research program aimed to describe and classify sleep problems and to test and evaluate interventions with all sleep-disturbed young children (in- and outpatient) and their parents (Skuladottir, Thome and Ramel, 2005; Thome and Skuladottir, 2005b).

Research and improved outcomes for children and parents assured the support of the nursing management, colleagues, and other disciplines in the hospital. The evidence base for the service proved to be an important resource in the maintenance and development of the service. Collaboration between mentor and mentee, which started during the mentee's graduate studies, continued afterward. The collaboration was influenced by several events that coincided with the project and influenced its development, as listed in Table 1.

Table 1   Events impacting collaborative research.

Events	Impact
Promotion of the Landspitali to University Hospital and of Department of Nursing to Faculty of Nursing, University of Iceland, both in 2000.	Sharpening common goals of both Institutions.

Table 1 **Events impacting collaborative research.**
(continued)

Events	Impact
Regulation of licenses of advanced practice nurses by Ministry of Health and Social Security in 2003.	Endorsing specialization in nursing and official recognition.
Treaty, regulating the collaboration between the Landspitala University Hospital and the University of Iceland, faculty of nursing (2001, 2006).	Facilitating collaborative research and service development. Recognizing nursing as an academic discipline within a traditional service setting.
Establishment of fields of science, that are related to fields of service, within the faculty of nursing at the University of Iceland (2001, 2006).	Attaching responsibilities for research and service development to a named academic head of the field and collaborating nurse manager.
Establishment of the Nursing Research Center in 1997, within the faculty of nursing at the University of Iceland. The research center is run collaboratively with the Landspitali University Hospital since 2002.	Facilitating collaborative research and the sharing of resources.
Establishment of postgraduate programs within the faculty of nursing, University of Iceland—master of science (1998) and doctoral studies (2004)	Facilitating collaborative scholarly work; development and dissemination of knowledge and clinical research.

Recognition and Use of Resources of the Service Setting and the Clientele

Services in the hospital setting are usually based on medical needs of its clients, and the patient is generally conceptualized as an individual, as opposed to a family member or part of a family. Ground was broken when a pediatric nursing service was established with the Landspitala University Hospital based on the specific developmental needs of infants arising from disorders of emotional and behavioral regulation, such as sleeping, feeding, communicating, and so on, conceptualizing the patient as a family (Papousek, Schieche, and Wurmser, 2007; Wright and Leahey, 1994).

The theoretical framework for the service consists of knowledge related to the individuality of the child, empowerment of parents, and individualized care within a family context. The relationship of the nurse with individual members of the family is viewed as a partnership in which each person contributes to the treatment protocol. Parents receive education on the individuality and developmental needs of the child; how to support its self-soothing capacity; and instruction of how to regulate rhythmic daily activities, such as feeding and sleeping.

Parents are listened to actively and empathetically, and the sleep problem that is causing their distress is recognized as real. Sensitive topics that emerge during interviews are discussed, such as intention to harm the child, depression of parent, relationship problems, and so forth. Of key importance in the treatment protocol is the infant's individuality, which can make a huge difference in the conception and execution of the treatment plan. Treatment can be most different for individual children in the same family for example, with temperamentally different twins.

The mentee learned to introduce change in the traditional system of a hospital health service by using the research process, which provides a rigorous and structured approach and a means to disseminate the work among the professional and scientific community. The high grading of research among professionals and recognition of the service by the public helped the mentee recognize her role in research as an immaterial resource. The change ensuing from the initial project escalated beyond the expectations of the mentor, mentee, and management of the hospital, leading to the establishment of a new specialization in pediatric nursing, which taught the mentee to be open for the unexpected to happen within a traditional setting and with her own professional development.

Advanced Nursing Practice in Iceland

The International Council of Nurses' International NP/APN network, in their Frequently Asked Questions section, defines advanced practice nurses (APNs) as registered nurses who have acquired the expert knowledge base, complex decision-making skills, and clinical competencies for expanded practice, the characteristics of which are shaped by the context or country in which they are licensed to practice (icn-apnetwork.org). In Iceland, development of advanced nursing practice is facilitated by access to academic education for nurses (from bachelor to doctoral degrees), by legal regulation of the practice (Ministry of Health, 2003), and by an increasing demand for highly specialized nurses at the Landspitala University Hospital (LUH, 2006).

The nursing management at the hospital has supported the project materially by providing staff, office space, finances, and secretarial service, and not least immaterially through recognition, praise, and valuing of this service. It also supports dissemination of knowledge through the mentee's participation at national and international conferences and through enabling her to devote time to writing and to public education.

The role of the APN entails practice, teaching, research, and counseling. Besides developing research and service, the mentee assumes teaching responsibilities at the University of Iceland, Faculty of Nursing, and her role in public education is growing steadily. A landmark in public education in this field is the publication of a book for parents and families on the sleep of young children and the management of sleep problems, the running of a parenting school, and the establishment of a Web site (Skuladottir, 2006; Foreldraskoli, n.d.). The service, regularly featured in mass media, has shown continued interest through the years. The interest of parents and the wider public into a particular kind of health service is considered an immaterial resource that helps to maintain and to develop it.

The mentee learned that her role as an advanced practitioner was first recognized by the public, the mass media, and parents; and subsequently, by the nursing and medical profession. Recognition—supported by collaboration in research with the mentor—helped the mentee obtain power for development of professional practice. Belief in the value of the service for parents and children, in evidence-based practice and in own expertise, were of key importance to maintain and to develop this specialized service, and proved basic to ensure resources.

Conclusions

An absence or lack of a health care or nursing service that assists persons in achieving their optimum level of health can be related to the lack of immaterial and material resources that are located at an individual, an institutional, and a societal level. Immaterial resources are equally important as material ones in realizing innovations. Through the interaction of knowledge and vision, innovations are conceived; and through dialog, they may become the driving force behind new developments. Dialog, professional collaboration, support seeking, and communication can be avenues in finding and using the resources required for execution of new endeavors.

Self-Reflective Questions

1. How do you reflect on the absence of important services in nursing/midwifery, and how could you respond to the situation?

2. How do you envision progressing from an idea to its realization? Describe your approach.

3. How do you seek to enhance health care and professionalism in nursing/midwifery through knowledge-based service?

4. How can you introduce change within existing traditional systems? For example, through knowledge of the research process or of the change process, and so on.

5. How can you communicate and argue your case in assuring material and immaterial resources with superiors?

6. How can you ready yourself to experience conflict and to seek conflict resolutions by dialog during the change process?

7. How can you become better aware of your personal qualities to facilitate the change process and resource allocation: for example, people trusting in you and in your way of working professionally, as well as your dialog, collaboration, and communication skills?

8. How does your attitude on patient/client advocacy impact how you argue with superiors about allocation of resources?

9. How do you seek support for your work and recognition of advanced practice by the public, your profession, other disciplines, and by the scientific community of which you are a part?

10. How can you be in a position to ensure financial and other material resources: for example, space, equipment, and staff?

Negotiating I: Principles and Practices

58

"Creating an atmosphere for winning negotiations can be compared to preparing to cook a meal. . . . Selecting the right 'recipe' for effective negotiations mandates the correct proportion of basic ingredients. These ingredients are fundamental to building successful relationships."

—Nancy Shendell-Falik

Mentor
Leslie Furlow, PhD, RN, MSN,
  MPH
Certified Family Nurse
  Practitioner
President and Founder of
  AchieveMentors
Cleburne, Texas, USA

Mentee
Wendy Hein, RN, BSN
Childbirth Educator for
  Women's Health Services
Baylor Medical Center
Waxahachie, Texas, USA

Negotiation is an essential skill for managing and leadership. The ability to negotiate well requires all the finesse, creativity, and practice that preparing a gourmet meal does. Whether negotiating with staff to cover the schedule, negotiating with administration for additional full-time equivalent employees (FTE), or negotiating with a physician to move or discharge a patient, the nurse leader is constantly negotiating—always ensuring that all the ingredients required are available and in the right proportions.

The ability to negotiate successfully requires understanding principles and practicing a skill set. The lists of principles and skills that follow are a compilation of concepts from years of reading books and articles and attending seminars. The principles include the following:

- Understanding the values of the parties in the negotiation.

- Determining the desired outcome.

- Articulating clearly the reasons for the negotiation.

- Separating "musts" from "wants."

- Seeking to preserve relationships.

Skills include the following:

- Identifying the emotional impact.

- Facing potential responses in advance.

- Crafting language and using the right words effectively.

- Checking for understanding by restatement.

- Role-playing interactions until you are comfortable and can retain composure.

- Maintaining focus.

Some negotiations are relatively straightforward, are not emotionally charged, and can be accomplished with a minimum of preparation. However, many negotiations are wrought with fear, especially for novice negotiators.

One negotiation that can create fear is working with a physician to move a stable patient out of the intensive care unit (ICU) to free a bed for a critical patient being held in the emergency department (ED). At issue is that some physicians are more volatile, and the fear of an outburst or caustic interaction leads some nurse leaders to passivity. This type of negotiation requires that you recognize the values of the physician and why that physician argues for quality care for his or her patient versus your facility's value in freeing the ED from holding patients and providing the best care for all patients.

An example of a negotiation that might be less fearful is the one you conduct with staff to cover vacancies in the unit. This might involve discussions with part-time personnel who aren't interested in full-time work. The negotiation might include pointing out the overall needs of the unit, the hardship created on coworkers, or the potential harm to patients. In this negotiation, the level of emotion is relatively low and can be approached from a win-win perspective without much preparation. However, if the negotiations move to the level of requesting additional staff in the form of registry or travelling nurses with administration, the level of emotional stress increases.

The interaction with a superior can be emotionally taxing, especially when the interaction includes requesting a variance to the budget. This type of negotiation requires preparation of budgetary information: what the cost of the agency is, how that fits into the budget, how long the engagement is necessary, and what the plans are to replace the position and eliminate the premium staff. The patient care aspect needs to be determined and articulated in a non-emotional, business-oriented manner. If this is a new type of negotiation to you, practice through role-playing can be of great benefit.

Another emotionally charged negotiation might occur when too many projects or priorities have been assigned by administration. This frequently happens to new managers. The level of frustration for those managers can be overwhelming as the number of tasks or projects escalates. This frustration can also lead to inactivity. The manager's resulting lack of production can lead to disciplinary action and the loss of a potentially great future leader.

The negotiation needs to be planned out with the precision of a surgery. Develop a list of all the tasks and expectations and then prioritize them from the perspective of most important to least important. Then develop a second list of what can be delegated and which tasks are essential for you, the manager, to complete personally. You should next prioritize the tasks based on which are enjoyable versus which are drudgery. This prioritizing and reprioritizing helps you identify and clarify the jobs by making clear needs versus wants and determining the emotional impact of the individual tasks.

Your next steps include planning the interaction with the nurse director or executive to ensure that the relationship is maintained and potentially strengthened and that the needs are achieved by both parties. This planning is best done through role-play. By role-playing, first in the mirror and then with a trusted colleague or mentor, you have a chance to craft the language you need and can work on limiting your emotion.

The role of the colleague or mentor is to help the manager face in advance any potentially difficult interaction, thus preparing her to negotiate from a position of strength and authority. The mentor should incorporate asking hard questions, challenging assumptions, and testing resolve as part of the role-play. Mentors who create this level of negotiation in practice sessions help the manager to develop critical skills including the ability to think "on his or her feet."

This type of interaction is exemplified in the following case study by my mentee, Wendy Hein.

Case Study with Mentee

As a new nurse employee in a supervisory role, I felt as anyone might in a new job—overwhelmed. To add spice to the punch, I also happened to be only 26 years old in a facility where most of the nurses had worked in their positions for the full amount of time I had been on the face of this earth. Furthermore, I had taken a position on a medical/surgical/telemetry floor, when my experience to that point had been working on a women's floor at a local county hospital. I'm really not crazy (if that's what you're thinking). However, I do enjoy a good challenge and decided to go for it, just as I've done with other challenges I've faced.

In transitioning to my new position at a different facility, I had to work with our facility's director. She also was new to the facility in a newly created position, which led her to be inquisitive and somewhat impatient in waiting for responses. She would make rounds on our floor and approach me with problems she noticed that needed to be fixed or with questions on policy and procedures and whatever else came to her mind. Normally, I am happy to answer and help with questions whenever I can, but given that I was still in "orientation" while working a full load on the floor due to the hospital being short staffed at the time, I was overworked, stressed, and didn't feel like I had time at every impromptu moment to engage with my new director. I was struggling just trying to learn the floor staff, learn how to be charge nurse on a medical/surgical/telemetry floor, learn the doctors, and learn how to care for post-op patients in a different setting than what I was used to, and all of this while also having to learn the office side of my position, which included payroll, reports, scheduling, work orders, and different computer systems. Because I was still in the process of learning my every day duties, I thought it was unfair for the director to give me more projects, assignments, and errands when I was still in the early stages of learning my position.

When I discussed with my mentors how I should handle this situation, their recommendation was for me to simply tell the director that I did not have time to deal with training her too. However, I did not feel comfortable with that approach. In the past, I had tried to be open with managers and communicate when the workload became too overwhelming. I never lived it down when I tried to communicate being overworked and faced a lot of criticism in doing so. Naturally, I was hesitant to say anything; I did not want to jeopardize my new position, or get off on the wrong foot with the new director either. I was beginning to feel burnt out and overworked; my head was swirling from all the new experiences and obligations coming at me all at once. Something had to be done, or I would have to find another position elsewhere.

After I opened up to my mentors, together we trudged through the process to help find a solution to my dilemma. We discussed the issues I was having and my dilemma in dealing with my director. My mentors reviewed with me the "how-to's" of negotiating, and then we role-played several scenarios. I believe that the most successful factor in effective negotiations is role-playing. I was nervous about what could be said or done to me by speaking up to my director. By role-playing with several different people, I was exposed to different perspectives on the possible conversation that needed to take place. After role-playing through the scenarios, my mentors and I decided what areas I needed to focus on to get my point across while still being helpful to my director. We developed a plan, and I developed the conversation with my mentors. I cannot begin to describe the boost of confidence I felt after knowing that I finally had the tools to be effective in communicating my desperate needs to my director. With my plan in hand, I scheduled a meeting with my director and my chief nursing officer (CNO).

I arrived early to the hospital for my meeting, but spent some of my time in the car getting myself jazzed up and running through the different scenarios in my mind. I wanted to be heard and find some common ground with my director, and not be put in yet another situation of getting more work or assignments pushed on me. I made sure all my points were written down on my notepad and that all my key subjects and refutations were all accounted for. I went in and did my best to exude the utmost of confidence and professionalism so that I could be taken as seriously as possible. I dressed appropriately, kept my posture straight and firm, and kept my hands in front and still by firmly holding my notepad. I engaged in a precisely planned conversation and stuck to my notepad of bullet points for guidance when I felt like I was losing control in the conversation. It was hard, and I was nervous, but I made it through the conversation and felt like we negotiated things in a more workable atmosphere for me. I felt like it was a success, but role-playing or practicing the conversation and spending time and energy on what was important to me instead of brushing it off again gave me that light at the end of the tunnel I so desperately needed to see. My director and I agreed to change my schedule so that I could spend time in the office and then schedule and spend time on the floor as well. We then agreed that when I was on the floor immediate topics could be brought to my attention, but other topics and assignments could wait for a scheduled office day.

This conversation did a lot for my confidence and my workload. I now believe I have the tools to communicate and am not timid about doing so. By being prepared and ready to communicate to my director and CNO, I gained their trust, and we are more open to discuss things now than before. I suggest that if you have a dilemma or obstacle that you are not sure about, role-play it with peers and mentors and come up with a plan. You will never solve anything by doing nothing!

Master the Skill

Wendy was able to negotiate with confidence and resolve a situation that could well have resulted in her leaving management and robbing the nursing field of a potentially great future leader. The ability to negotiate effectively is not an option but a necessity. Every day, every nurse must negotiate in some form or fashion. Those who master this skill are destined to lead others and advance the practice of nursing.

Self-Reflective Questions

1. Why are you entering into this negotiation?

2. How have you prepared and do you adequately know the issues?

3. In what ways can you articulate your position effectively?

4. How well do you know the person with whom you will be negotiating?

5. What values do you have in conflict with the issues you are negotiating?

6. Have you distinguished between your musts and wants?

7. How have you identified and faced your emotional attachment to the issues?

8. How much have you practiced your presentation with others?

9. In what ways do you display the confidence you now feel?

10. What sort of win-win situation do you want?

Negotiation II: Strategies to Reach Desired Outcomes

59

"Do not be fettered by too many rules at first. Try different things and see what answers best. Look for the ideal, but put it into the actual. Everything which succeeds is not the production of a scheme of rules and regulations, made beforehand, but of a mind observing and adapting itself to wants and events."

—Florence Nightingale

Mentor
Charles Krozek, MN, RN, FAAN
President and Managing
   Director
Versant Advantage
Los Angeles, California, USA

Mentee
Cherilyn Ashlock, RN, MSN
Implementation and Analytics
   Specialist
Versant Advantage
Atlanta, Georgia, USA

Effective negotiation is a key skill for the emerging nurse leader. The following is an example from personal experience that reinforced how paramount the ability to negotiate successfully was in the development of an interdepartmental new graduate registered nurse (RN) transition program that eventually became the Versant RN Residency.

A New Idea: The Mentor's Perspective

In 1998, as executive director of education and research at Children's Hospital Los Angeles (CHLA), I recognized that something had to be done to resolve the dire RN shortage problem facing the hospital.

If not, the common goal was at risk—CHLA's primary mission: quality patient care. Driven by a dwindling number of experienced pediatric nurses available for hire and an aging RN population staged to retire, the new graduate RN was fast becoming the major pipeline of new nurses joining the organization.

Historically, CHLA had hired a few new graduates into lower risk medical/surgical units. Now, with climbing RN vacancy rates, CHLA had an urgent need to hire greater numbers of new graduates and fast track them into high-risk areas such as critical care. This new approach to staffing required a dramatic change in the way new graduates were on-boarded (oriented); clearly a new, innovative approach was needed. This new approach required the cooperation of all key stakeholders, from the staff nurse to the hospital CEO.

Successful negotiation with key stakeholders was essential if this new transition program, or residency, was to be successful. In 1999, with everyone working toward a common goal, the pilot program was launched. Ten years later, the initial pilot program has graduated 450 residents at CHLA, and via the non-profit corporation Versant created in 2004, the new graduate RN residency has been implemented in more than 65 hospitals nationwide and has graduated more than 5900 new residents. The same negotiation skills needed to drive the development of the initial pilot program at CHLA are now used every time the Versant residency is replicated at a new hospital.

As the president and managing director of Versant, I've had the opportunity to mentor many of Versant's nurse leadership team members in the skill of negotiation. One pivotal role within Versant, the implementation specialist, is responsible for implementation and management support for each new hospital implementing the RN residency. I first recommend choosing a negotiation "model." Using a model provides a structured approach and ensures essential components of negotiation are not missed. Many excellent models exist, and I recommend a few be explored before deciding on one, or on a blend of two or three. For the purpose of this discussion, we use a model adapted from *Getting to Yes: Negotiating Agreement Without Giving In* by Roger Fisher and William Ury.

Fisher and Ury believe that strong communication and relationship-building skills are fundamental in all negotiations. Using these fundamental skills allows you to:

1. Understand the other's interest.

2. Create credibility.

3. Set mutual goals and share success.

This all leads to a shared commitment to the result (Fisher and Ury 1981).

The Mentee's Perspective

As an implementation specialist at Versant, I find negotiation a necessary skill. Building skills as a negotiator began early in my nursing career. It's then I realized that I would have to do a lot of bargaining. I had to negotiate with patients, families, physicians, coworkers, managers, other units, and myself. As my skills grew and others served as a role model in negotiation, I was able to determine some key factors in negotiating that almost always resulted in success. Those factors included effective communication, relationship building, and commitment to common goals. After spending seven years at the bedside, I chose to move into my current position at Versant. I now had to carry my knowledge and framework of negotiating out of my comfort zone and into my new consultant role.

I had a pivotal moment almost two years into my current role at Versant when at a company meeting Charles asked a very fundamental question, "Who is your customer?" At the bedside, the answer is simple—it's the patient. In this role, we all found the answer not so obvious. The conclusion that we all came to however, shapes how I approach my work everyday. With a little convincing from Charles, we all agreed that the Versant customer was actually the chief nursing officer (CNO) or nursing executive at each of our respective clients. After we identified the customer, I realized I had very little interaction with the true customer, but I nevertheless had a major impact on the work that goes on between initiation of the project and measurement of its outcomes. My role as negotiator with various players in our client organization was a key link to success for both Versant and for our customer, the CNO.

Learning to Communicate

One of the first steps in negotiation is learning to communicate. When you perform the consulting role, speaking the language of the client is important. Knowing the lingo of the facility, for example, knowing common terminology, titles, and responsibilities, gives you an instant mechanism of credibility. Making an initial effort to learn the corporate structure of the client allows me to use their terminology and communicate with them more effectively. In addition, this assessment allows identification of key players. With a broad view of the organizational structure, I can quickly identify the key players necessary for successful implementation and sustainability of the project.

Another key in effective communication is finding methods of communication that work for both you and the client. To accommodate unique needs of my clients, I use multiple modes of communication, ranging from simple handwritten notes to published data reports. Most of my more technologically savvy clients prefer electronic communication through email and instant messaging.

Building a Relationship

Another crucial step in successful negotiation is to quickly build a relationship with clients. To do this, I begin by seeking commonalities with people I know are pivotal to the process. When presenting to a large group, I share personal stories from the frontlines of my nursing experience at the bedside. This immediately makes me relatable to the audience, typically made up of beside nurses and clinical-based practitioners. Then I hone in on the skeptics. They are easy to spot. Their body language and activity during class make them obvious. They ask questions like, "How do you know this is going to work here?" or "Do you have any idea how much work I have to do already?" I know that I have to win this group over on a personal level by first finding common ground. I ask them about how long they have been in their current role, if they have kids, a husband, pets—anything to get a little conversation going. Then, at the next meeting we have together, during that awkward time when all the managers are shuffling in late in front of the CNO, I can break the tension by asking something like, "How did taking your son off to college go?" This strategy personalizes communication and often sets the tone for a very positive interaction.

Most importantly, I follow through on my promises. A good relationship finds its foundation in integrity. A relationship with integrity encourages accountability and ultimately forges success. After these relationships are established, setting common goals is easy.

Committing to the Result

Organizations engage in the Versant RN residency because they share or see the value in the four primary goals of the residency. The goals of the residency are to bridge the gap between nursing school and acute setting practice, to facilitate transition of the new graduate to professional nurse, to increase organizational commitment, and to increase retention of excellent nurses.

To achieve the proven results of the Versant RN residency, we provide a strategic methodology and architecture to attain the four goals. As an organization, Versant provides wisdom from our industry partner experiences and resources in our client facilities to help new participants achieve success. Getting clients to commit to the results often requires helping them break down organizational walls so that the players involved are not working in silos.

Getting everyone working together in that way is often the hardest part of the negotiation process. An example of this process occurs with the Versant RN residency task force. The purpose of the task force is to oversee residency development, evaluation, and modification within Versant standards. With many of my clients, the establishment of this task force is the first time that all of the key players that impact the new graduate sit down at the same table with the same goals in mind. This working body, a shared governance model, is critical to the outcomes of the residency because it serves as a reporting mechanism for the accountability necessary to achieve the residency goals.

Validating Success

After all the work of negotiation, take the time to reflect on achievement. Encouraging clients to look retrospectively helps them to acknowledge the impact they have made on processes, systems, policies, and most importantly, on individuals. This reflection is the basis for continued negotiation. The utmost acknowledgment of successful negotiation is evidenced by the achievement of those involved in the process.

Self-Reflective Questions

1. In what ways have you assessed the organization/project so that you can communicate effectively?

2. What do you understand of the interest of all involved parties?

3. How have you established credibility with all involved parties?

4. In what ways have you identified key stakeholders, skeptics, and champions and built a relationship?

5. What mutual goals have been agreed upon with all involved parties?

6. What steps have you taken to ensure you have a clear plan to achieve the mutually desired outcomes?

7. How are you maximizing communication by use of technology and in what ways are you communicating regularly with all involved parties?

8. What evidence do you have that everyone is committed to achieving the agreed upon outcomes?

9. In what ways have you reflected on achievements?

10. What strategies do you have for presenting the successes of the endeavor?

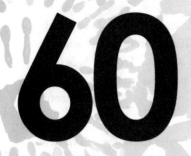

60 (From) Novice to Expert: A Journey

"A leader's role is to raise people's aspirations for what they can become and to release their energies so they will try to get there."

—David Gergen

Mentor
Susan Smith, DBA, MBA, BSc
 Hons, RN, RM, RHV, FWT
Management Consultant,
Choice Dynamic International
England, United Kingdom

Mentee
Michelle Clark, BSc, DipN, RN
Ward Sister, Neonatal Unit
Doncaster and Bassetlaw
 Hospitals
National Health Service Foun-
 dation Trust (NHS)
England, United Kingdom

This case study emphasizes the importance of creating a partnership between a novice and an expert leader. It presents the reflections of a staff nurse, Michelle, who works as a neonatal nurse in a National Health Service (NHS) hospital in the United Kingdom and her mentor, Susan, an independent nurse management consultant. The organization created a large change project that emphasized valuing the staff nurse, increasing efficiency and effectiveness, and releasing time to give more compassionate care to patient and families. This was linked in to a wider national initiative called "the Productive Ward" (www.institute.nhs.uk).

Background

This case study reinforces the value of a mentor using coaching and reflection as tools for developing effective leadership. Support for this approach is found in two books. In *Quiet Leadership*, David Rock

(2006) suggests these tools can help individuals do their own thinking by asking good questions, clarifying, listening, paraphrasing, and using intuition. In *The Reflective Practitioner: How Professionals Think in Action*, Donald A. Schon (1983), suggests reflection is a way of identifying personal expertise. Reflection exposes the thinking behind what you are doing and helps you to learn from your experience.

Coaching also provides the opportunity for a leader to address his or her commitment, autonomy, participative style, assertiveness, self-esteem, integrity, and sociability (Conger and Kanungo, 1988; Manojlovich and Laschinger, 2003; and Kanter, 1993).

The Beginning of the Journey: An Organisational Change Project

Michelle was asked to take on a new role called "ambassador" as a lead champion of the Productive Ward programme and to lead the initiative with the senior leadership team consisting of the deputy director of nursing and a group of matrons. She requested mentorship and coaching from Susan.

Michelle: There I was, arriving at a meeting in the boardroom, wondering what on earth I was doing there; I had been told by my manager to go. I didn't know what it was about or who it was with. It was a mystery! Staff nurses like me didn't attend meetings in the boardroom. That was usually reserved for people who didn't wear uniforms, or so I thought! This, I believe, was where my journey began. I was introduced to senior managerial members of the Trust. Also in attendance were eight or nine other staff nurses from across the Trust, and all of these people have become truly instrumental in my journey. We quickly formed a bond and developed friendships both professionally and personally. On reflection, this, I believe, was instrumental in building my confidence. I was delighted that people who were as passionate and dedicated to their profession as I am could actually do and make things happen, and that they were actually interested in spending time listening and nurturing my ideas and thoughts.

Supporting Change: The Role of the Coach/ Mentor and Top Team

Jean Faugier and Helen Woolnough make clear in their 2002 article the vital role of senior managers in supporting and empowering front line staff nurses. Two key elements provided the staff nurses with confidence they needed: the coaching relationship between the novice leaders and expert leaders and the leadership and support by senior nurse leaders.

The Coaching Relationship

An effective coach does not give advice; he or she simply supports the coached in their journey to achieve clarity of goals and provide genuine support to thinking and the decision making process. Figure 1 is a diagramme of the nine core stages used by Susan in her coaching sessions. The stages are set within a circle as 1-9. These stages help explain the leadership coaching journey experienced by Michelle and her personal reflections of that journey.

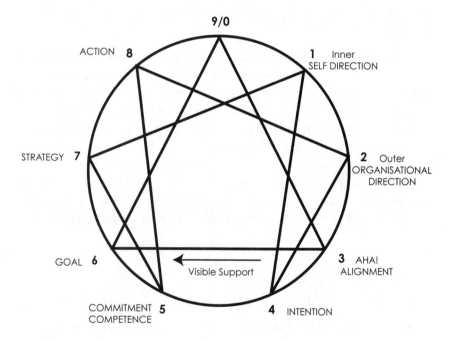

Dr Susan Smith 2008 © Based on the work of George Ivanovitch Gurdjieff (1866-1949)

Figure 1   Coaching Enneagramme.

The following are the stages of coaching/mentoring conversation:

1. Thinking about self, personal values, and beliefs.

2. Thinking about the expectations of the organization.

3. This is the moment the coached has a creative idea to take forward. This is called the "AHA" moment.

4. Exploration of intentions associated with the creative goal or idea.

5. Identification of commitment and competence to achieve a goal.

6. Formulation of clear memorable goals.

7. Defining strategies to achieve the goal.

8. Clarification of actions and timelines.

9. Creating an outcome or result.

Note that coaching is dynamic, not linear. As an example, sometimes the coached prefers to take action immediately (8) and develop strategies (7) before having thought through their intention (4) and commitment and competence (5).

The coach provides the visible support (questions, listening, and paraphrasing) during the process and helps the individual adopt a future and solution orientation in relation to his or her goals (6), strategies (7), and actions (8). The thinking process is dynamic and is depicted in the figure by the use of lines inside the circle (hexagon and triangle) showing the potential flow of energy and lines of discussion. Capturing the truly dynamic nature of the coaching relationship is impossible; the lines in the inner circle are based on the dynamic nature of the Enneagramme, which is based on the work of George Ivanovitch Gurdjieff (Webb, 1980). An example of one coaching session is simplified in the following list to illustrate the sequence of coaching by the expert leader with a novice using the model.

1. Inner—Self direction

Here the coach assists Michelle to explore her inner beliefs and feelings.

Michelle: Being able to facilitate at the summits is a joy! I feel more equipped to make a greater contribution because of my boosted confidence through support from my leaders.

Michelle values her senior leaders in giving her confidence to be creative. In an article by A.R Falk-Rafael (2001), the exposure of the novice to senior leaders is important in order to translate their experience into empowered caring.

2. Outer—Organisational Direction

Michelle is encouraged to explore her understanding of the direction of the leadership organisation, assessing the politics and dynamic nature of the change agenda. Here, she reflects on a leadership symposium trip to the Unites States.

Michelle: May 2008 was a fantastic moment in my journey—exploring culturally based healing traditions and practices in Minnesota. I found myself completely immersed in the most fantastic experience, surrounded by people who have truly made a difference in the world, not just through nursing but by being the people that they are: warm, inviting, knowledgeable, the list is endless! And here were Jo and I, embraced into this impressive circle of people; we just couldn't believe it, two little old staff nurses from the UK. Wow!

3. AHA! Moment—Coming to a Moment of Knowing

Michelle praises the leaders, and the coach asks an intuitive question; "What do you see in yourself that you see in them?" This question revealed a multitude of affirmations and future hope and visions.

Michelle: In October 2008, I was successful in applying for a ward sister post on the neonatal unit where I work. I feel very proud of this and hope that this will allow me to continue to grow as I still don't feel that this is where it all ends. I still hope to embrace new challenges and be involved in many new adventures.

4. & 5. Intention, Competence, and Confidence

Michelle explored her intentions for becoming a ward manager and spent many hours identifying the competence required. This process built her confidence to prepare for the position and go to the interview confident that she could do it.

6., 7. & 8. Goal, Strategy, and Action

As a new leader, Michelle was now in danger of disempowering her team. This tendency is common in a novice leader. If not corrected; it can lead to an egocentric leadership style.

Michelle: On my return I was desperate to tell everybody about our amazing experience! I seem to have taken ownership of the summit. I can't imagine a summit going ahead without me being there. Of course it will, but I don't want it to! America: I know it would be fantastic for others to attend the symposium in 2009, but I can't help thinking that I don't want them too (not sure why). I must deal with this!

Michelle reflected on the 10 most important things the senior leadership team had achieved and given to her on her leadership journey.

Leadership by Senior Nurses

1. **Create a champion leadership team**: The deputy director and matrons inspired the staff nurses and gave strong leadership, empowerment, and enthusiasm for change.

2. **Engage all staff nurses in the project, not just a few**: All 1,000 nurses were included and involved.

3. **Create a nurturing caring environment for the lead change agents**: Allow your change leaders (ambassadors) to practice their new skills in a safe environment. Michelle notes, "Give them time out to train as facilitators of change."

4. **Provide the opportunity to go to other countries, network, and share best practice**: Michelle notes, "We sought out healing environments to visit."

5. **Create opportunities for staff to move out of their comfort zone**: Michelle notes, "All 15 ambassadors were given wider organisational projects."

6. **Resource the project fully**: Michelle notes, "Give the spending power to the ward."

7. **Show active symbolic reward:** Michelle notes, "At the workshops, an award was given to the area demonstrating best practice in that month. This award—a small knitted "nurse doll" given by the chairman and known as the "chairman's award"—symbolised success to the winning ward."

8. **Assess the new behaviours**: Michelle notes, "Ensure that leadership behaviour change is going in a positive direction and not disempowering others."

9. **Involve the wider organisation so that elitist groups do not form**: Michelle notes, "Other disciplines were involved in the whole project."

10. **Celebrate success**: Michelle notes, "Reflect on your work daily. Write and talk about the changes widely, and be enthusiastic!"

Creating an Empowered Leader

This case study has illustrated the techniques and approaches of mentorship and coaching to support the development of effective, empowering leaders and achieve lasting change.

Michelle reflects the five personality factors associated with effective leadership: openness to experience, dependability and conscientiousness, agreeableness, extroversion, and emotional stability (Stogdill, 1948). The outcome is a productive and efficient group of health professionals who have now released time to care through their own efforts, offering better patient care that is compassionate and caring. Michelle has achieved her current goal of becoming a ward manager and has illustrated this through her coaching journey and reflections through helping people discover their own way.

Self-Reflective Questions

(Based on Michelle's Ten Top Tips)

1. How do I lead my team as an empowering example?

2. In what ways do I engage with a wide range of expertise in change projects?

3. How can I create a safe environment for leaders to practice their skills as leaders?

4. What opportunities exist to visit different leadership environments regularly to compare myself with others in their leadership roles?

5. How can I stretch myself as a leader and take on projects that are outside of my comfort zone?

6. In what ways do I delegate authority for finance to the lowest possible level within the organisation?

7. What approaches do I use to celebrate the success of staff and how often do we celebrate?

8. In what ways can I or do I take stock at regular intervals of the behaviours of staff and myself during a change project?

9. How can I encourage multiprofessional working practices?

10. How often do I reflect on my work and then write about it, to share best practices and enthusiasm with others?

(The) Nursing Process and Leadership Influence

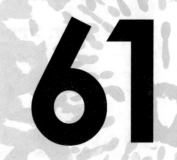

61

"The nursing process is the tool by which nurses contin-ue the human tradition of caring. It enables the nurse to use scientific advances, not to make nursing cold and impersonally scientific."

—Patricia W. Hickey

Mentor
Alžbeta Hanzlíková, PhD, RN
Associate Professor
St. Elizabeth Univerzity College
  of Health and Social Work
Bratislava, Slovakia

Mentee
Drahomíra Vatehová, PhD, RN,
  MSN
Adjunct Lecturer
Institute of Health and Social
  Sciences
St.Elizabeth University of Health
  and Social sciences
Bratislava, Slovakia

The nursing process as a method of care delivered to patients dates back many years. In Slovakia, after 1989, implementing the process into the profession became a need. In Europe, as well as in our coun-try, nursing developed under some influences of social, economic, and political issues (WHO Regional Office for Europe, 1977). In our coun-try, nursing was carried out in many ways, but the nursing process was not included. In this chapter, we discuss the importance of mentors in working with mentees to implement the nursing process in Slovakia.

Bringing the Nursing Process to Slovakia

After the Iron Curtain was pulled down in 1989, many nurses saw the opportunity for the change they had always desired, even with limited exposure to the nursing process as practiced in other countries. Leaders in nursing researched the nursing process thoroughly. They studied publications on nursing, understanding that responsible and independent decisions are made within the process.

Nursing leaders faced difficulties in introducing the process, including resistance from those in other medical fields. For example, doctors considered themselves as nurses' supervisors. In addition, nursing care was based on a biomedical model. Nurses did not have enough nursing competencies, they did not have any responsibilities for their profession, and they did not have any rights to make their own decisions.

Nursing leaders used their knowledge to persuade people to trust the nursing process and its effectiveness. In 2002, their efforts resulted in the passing of an act that mandates nursing care be delivered via the nursing process.

However, difficulties in applying the nursing process in practice remain. Mentors and mentees, such as the authors of this chapter, are key to advance implementation. Mentors use their leadership skills with mentees. Leadership is an ability or a process of influencing people in which leaders try to make the people who work under them achieve their goals willingly and voluntarily so that their needs can be met. Leadership in nursing transforms possible things into real ones (Grohar, Murray, & DiCroce, 2003).

What is the Nursing Process?

The first step in advancing the nursing process is to understand what it is. The process dates back to 1952 when Peplau defined four phases of interpersonal relationships. In 1955, Hall introduced the term "nursing process" (George, 1985). Since that time, the method has appeared in models made by many theorists.

The nursing process can be defined as a systematic, goal-oriented activity consisting of assessing the situation, patient's needs, diagnosis of human response needs that nurses can deal with, planning of patient care, and evaluation of the success of the implemented care. The care is aimed at achieving short-term and long-term goals and feedback (Aggleton & Chalmers, 2000).

Mentor's View of Teaching the Nursing Process

The definition of nursing developed by nursing specialists supervised by the Royal College of Nursing in Great Britain states as follows: "Nursing means applying clinical decisions in nursing care delivery (Royal College of Nursing, 2003). Based on this, one must admit that the need to teach how to diagnose has become a key point—a starting point for making clinical decisions. Nursing diagnosis is considered to be the trickiest part of an activity. Diagnosing requires much knowledge, experience, and practice. As a student of nursing, the mentee does not possess any of these, so individuals who are more experienced must be patient. If the diagnosis is wrong, the process creates many failures, mistakes, and errors that may result in problem-resolving taking a long time and may be unsuccessful, resulting in tragic consequences.

Leaders, as teachers or mentors, start their nursing jobs with background reading in science as well as other fields affiliated with nursing necessary to become proficient in nursing diagnosis. Nursing curricula are aimed at teaching how to work out a nursing diagnosis and mastering nursing care via the nursing process.

It is important for a mentee to see and feel a mentor's enthusiasm and skills at understanding problems.

Mentors' activities can be divided into two groups:

Impact upon the mentee's intellectual level:

- Forwarding knowledge.
- Developing skills.
- Gaining experience.
- Showing the ability to gather data.

Impact on relationships and attitudes based upon the mentee's qualities:

- Promoting enthusiasm.
- Promoting confidence for the job.
- Promoting patience.
- Developing understanding.
- Revealing kindness in themselves.
- Doing the job resolutely.

Mentee's View of the Nursing Process

The nursing process is a systematic, rational method of planning and delivering nursing care. The process objectives are to assess patients' needs, health conditions, and real or potential needs in health care to plan patient care and to plan nursing care so that patient needs can be met.

Before the nursing process was developed, nurses had delivered their care in line with a doctor's written instructions. The instructions stated the patient's conditions but not the patient's needs. Nursing care delivered by nurses independently of doctors was based upon intuition and not upon scientific methods. Applying and delivering the nursing process requires nurses' skills in interpersonal relations as well as for technological and intellectual issues (Kozierová, 1996). Not only must a nurse have requisite specialized knowledge and skills in interpersonal relations, technological, and intellectual issues, but the nurse must transform them into practice to deliver nursing care in the most effective way.

The mentor plays an important role in the process in which nurses gain theoretical and practical skills. The mentor's characteristics are influenced by their professional abilities, life experiences, personal qualities, behavior, and ability to be empathetic. Mentors serve as an example in the process of teaching nursing; they guide mentees to overcome problems and to cope with stress and frustration. They motivate mentees and guide their learning process (Závodná, 2005).

Possible Problems in Introducing Nursing Process

Introducing the nursing process is not always easy.

Mentor's point of view: After many years of fulfilling a mentor role, I know that neither mentees' understanding nor their lack of enthusiasm is a problem. The problems are unorganized labor, excessive workloads, no collaboration with doctors, and improper teaching in educational institutions.

Problems exist within the realm of nursing, too: a shortage of applicants for the job with little judgment regarding an applicant's ability to learn new skills or their personal qualities. Also, there has been a need for suitable mentors who can trigger an interest in the nursing career for nursing students.

Many mentees who have adopted the nursing process and its meaning cannot imagine any other method of delivering nursing care.

Mentee's point of view: Barriers that exist in nursing process implementation can be divided into internal and external.

Internal barriers include

- A nurse does not understand the nursing process and is not informed about it.

- A nurse does not realize that nursing care can be carried out through the nursing process. Nursing is oriented to the patient needs that must be met.

- A nurse identifies the nursing process with written nursing documentation and not with a method of thought about the nursing care.

- A nurse considers changes made in nursing, for example, to use the nursing process, to add to his or her workload.

External barriers can be:

- A doctor or manager in nursing does not believe in the nursing process.

- A nurse is not evaluated precisely whether she does his or her job by using nursing process or if he or she is working in the routine way.

- A nurse is not motivated.

The mentor's role is making nurses understand that nursing care can be delivered to patients only by a nursing process and that it is a method based upon careful thought. Mentors are advised to motivate nurses to be open and receptive to change (Hanzlikova, unpublished lecture, 2009).

Enthusiasm

The nursing process, a method of delivering care proven in practice, is the most suitable one for quality patient-centered nursing. The method can be learned, particularly under the supervision of enthusiastic leaders.

Self-Reflective Questions

1. What would convince you that care delivered via the nursing process method is effective?

2. How can you become confident about your abilities to lead others to reach goals you have set?

3. How can you best influence others, using proper reasons you are persuaded about?

4. Are your needs of self-realization met when you share with others who have achieved the desired goal? If not, why?

5. How can you make sure that you have abilities, proven in practice, to make clinical decisions within the nursing science?

6. Are you persuaded that the nursing diagnosis is the starting point in making clinical decisions? If not, why?

7. How can you improve your patience enough to lead others who are younger and less experienced than you?

8. Do you think that you are kind and have feelings and can forward your qualities to your young colleagues?

9. What are your thoughts on whether humanism can become an attitude in your future career or the future of younger nurses while doing their jobs?

10. What experiences have shown you that when different external barriers are removed, the quality of nursing care will be improved?

Organizational Development for Professional Autonomy

62

"I don't think it is possible for anybody to become over-prepared in communication skills. You have to be able to organize what you need to deliver, and to deliver it in a way that people are going to get it and remember it."

—Margaret McClure

Mentor
Dragica Šimunec, RN
President of Croatian Nursing
  Council
Zagreb, Croatia

Mentee
Adriano Friganović, RN, BSN
University Hospital ICU Unit
Zagreb, Croatia

Croatia (population 4.5 million), located in central Europe, gained its independence from the former Yugoslavia, a communist state, in 1991. With the fall of the Berlin Wall, a wave of political movements went through the socialistic bloc of central European countries, and most of them managed to change political and economic systems through a "Velvet Revolution." Croatia had to survive acts of aggression and an extremely cruel war that lasted five years.

The Yugoslavian Nursing Legacy: Mentor

In spite of more than 50 years of communism within former Yugoslavia, nursing has a long tradition, although nursing had no professional autonomy during that time. All nursing curriculum had been medically oriented, with a domination of medical doctors. Nursing education and practice were carried out in a socialistic philosophy, defined by collective responsibility, nurses following doctors' instruction, with no autonomy in decision making and no nursing research.

Establishing the new state meant the need to change almost all parts of life. In spite of a difficult situation, it appeared as a historic opportunity for serious intervention in nursing education and practice. In 1992, the Croatian Nursing Association (CNA) was established, which gave us the opportunity to speak up in the name of nurses and nursing. Through the association, a nursing magazine was established as well as a Code of Ethics and Scope of Practice (albeit only on a level of recommendation). It was soon obvious, though, that a professional organization with no authority is simply not strong enough to have influence on a political level.

Most nurses did not really want change. The fear of taking personal responsibility had roots in the educational system they went through. It was hard to identify a critical number of influential people who were ready to support change. In Croatia, it had to be medical doctors and politicians. I decided (at that time, I was president of CNA) that taking the position of chief nursing officer at Ministry of Health, which was offered to me, might give me completely different possibilities. At the time, being the only nurse in state administration was a challenge and a risk for possible personal and professional disappointment. As a hospital nurse with 20 years of experience, I did not understand much of what was expected from me, but my employer did not know, either. So what do you do when you face public work with your ideas and philosophy and no practical knowledge of how a political administration really functions? There is no possibility other than to try to make yourself visible and aggressive enough so that "important people" realize that you will not give up.

Being the president of the CNA and working for government was, in my point of view, not a usual situation. However, at this particular time the situation was very useful for nursing. Being the chief nursing officer gave me additional strength and credibility in front of the government. The CNA was becoming a serious professional organization with a clear vision and mission. Using all opportunities to work with the International Council of Nurses (ICN—the CNA joined ICN in 1993) with the World Health Organization (WHO) and other international organizations gave me enough determination and confidence to represent the need of fundamental changes in education and practice. In 1994, nursing became part of regulation, an important step forward that signaled this was the time to take further steps.

We saw significant changes to nursing education on the university level in 1999: A three-year professional study with a completely nursing-oriented curriculum, followed with implementation of the first and second cycles of the Bologna Process, brought Croatian nursing to European Union standards.

The Bologna Declaration was signed in Bologna in 1999 by most European ministers of education. The purpose was to make academic degree and quality assurance standards more comparable and compatible throughout Europe. The basic framework is three cycles of higher education qualifications. The first cycle leads to a bachelor's degree, the second a master's degree, and the third, the doctoral degree.

The Nursing Act was introduced to the government in 1999 with examples of good practice from the United Kingdom and Spain. Changes of government slowed us, but with systematic lobbying on a political level, the Croatian Parliament adopted the Nursing Act, which gave us a legal basis for self-regulation. In 2003, the Nursing Council was established as an independent regulatory body with public authority for nursing in Croatia. Today, nursing in Croatia is a profession based on professional standards, a register (a list of all authorized nurses), an obligatory continuing education, a licensing system, a Code of Ethics, Fitness to Practice Rules, and so on.

The Croatian experience proves the thesis that strong commitment, persistence, self-determination—and above all, using passion to follow the goal you believe in—can make the difference. Representing the profession with a clear vision in a basic aim to protect the public through responsible and accountable nursing professionals who practice according to clear rules is a new value of the Croatian health system. Working for so many years in different settings, I consider myself a lucky and person. Winning in impossible situations and winning over the unbeatable people—specifically, one from your own profession—does not make you a popular person at the time. But building and developing an organization is necessary because without a strong organization, it would be quite impossible to create changes.

The structural organization and function of the Nursing Council today represents the strength of the nursing profession and the work to guarantee patient safety. It also gives the opportunity to and motive for nurses to cooperate with Council through informal specialist groups and organizations to improve quality of care and to create new roles for nurses and nursing.

Reflections from Adriano Friganović, Mentee

When I speak about nursing in Croatia, I stress that I am proud because I belong to a nursing profession, and because I had the opportunity to watch and learn from senior nurses such as Mrs. Dragica Šimunec and to implement that experience in my future practice. Here is a short story about how her mentoring has made a significant impact on my nursing practice and development.

During my nursing education, I was disappointed because I didn't feel any reason to stay in this practice. There were several reasons. At that time, nurses were not autonomous and education was on a basic level. Further, it was limited, and nursing wasn't a respected profession. Our teachers tried to facilitate our movement in the right direction and give us as much as possible, but it wasn't enough. When I finished my education, I started to work in an intensive care unit for cardiac surgery patients. I enjoyed the nursing care of critically ill patients, to assist in different procedures, and to learn new things.

In 1999, I started to work for the central office of the CNA (in my free time), and I met many nurses from all parts of Croatia. All of them wanted to improve nursing in Croatia. The key person at that time was my mentor for this text—Mrs. Šimunec—who did many positive things for nurses. She never gave up. We had many problems at that time, but despite everything, my attitude toward my profession started to change. I decided to try to do all that I could to help in this struggle.

The CNA has become a respectable (and at the time, the only) professional nursing association in the country with a membership of the majority of active nurses. It was exciting to see the development of the organization. An important effort was applying for membership in relevant European and world nursing federations.

At that time, we had nurse representatives in the Ministry of Health and Social Welfare as chief nursing officer, which was crucial for lobbying and requesting legal regulation of nursing practice. We did a lot, but it wasn't enough. Every document was only a recommendation. But Mrs. Dragica Šimunec was relentless in pushing through all the significant processes that our profession needed to move forward.

The adoption of the Nursing Act by the Croatian Parliament was a breakthrough in Croatian nursing. The Nursing Act was a result of long-time fighting of our leaders with politicians. This was our victory. After that time, the Croatian Nursing Council was soon established. Croatian nursing became a regulated profession, with obligatory membership and an obligatory long-term educational system. The council became our instrument for influencing all relevant institutions and preserving our independence in nursing care. The council made sure that every nurse had a license to practice, that all nurses attended educational courses as a long-term education, and that the council had the ability to control nursing care quality.

After a few years, we started to develop professional associations as independent organizations with their vision and mission. Five independent organizations have established the Croatian National Nurses Federation as a platform for mutual agreement and cooperation.

In the past 18 years, Croatian nurses have come a long way from being dependent practitioners to becoming independent professional nurses. Thanks to our leaders, we gained professional regulation, a Code of Ethics, and nursing documentation. We succeeded in making changes in the educational system and implementing all recommendations of the Bologna Process. Our educational programs in the nursing college are applicable to every country in the European Union, and we made all adaptations to EU directives.

As I mentioned earlier, I am proud to be a nurse. In the past 12 years, I have gained a lot of experience in the fields of intensive care and nursing politics, and I learned how to build an organization through the mentoring of Mrs. Dragica Šimunec. Her positive way of thinking was a stimulant for us, the young potential nurse leaders of the future.

Right now, I am studying for my master's degree in nursing management, and I have my way determined by my vision. It was a very exciting journey from then to now. Despite our gains, we are still at the beginning. Many battles are in front of us, and we have to be prepared for every situation. We need to work together to create a better future and to achieve more.

Self-Reflective Questions

1. How do you define the process of organizational development?

2. What are the differences of organizational development when it relates to the nursing profession?

3. How would you define organizational development in your environment?

4. What are the differences between the nursing organizations in Croatia compared with your nursing organization?

5. What are the steps in the process of organizational development?

6. Of the problems in the Croatian nursing organization, what would you do to solve those problems?

7. What experiences have you gleaned from senior nurses and implemented in your work?

8. How have you learned to use professional knowledge in the process of political lobbying?

9. What are the key issues in organizational development?

10. How have you shared your experience to become a positive example to other nurses?

Outcomes: An Old Language With New Meaning

63

"Effective leaders help others to understand the necessity of change and to accept a common vision of the desired outcome."

—John Kotter

Mentor
Julita Sansoni RN, MNS,
   Dr, Prof.
Nursing Associate Professor
Sapienza University of Rome
Rome, Italy

Mentee
Cristiana Luciani RN, MSN
Quality Coordinator
Saint Andrea Hospital of Rome
Rome, Italy

The most advanced way to design and organize health trusts in countries where health care is designed by tasks is through processes (process management). This method, applied to an organization, works best when care is planned and delivered by using processes instead of a structure of functions and task assignment. Through this way of service delivery planning, we can actively involve those responsible for the care and their collaborators. In the arena of health, the introduction of a new reasoning and organization creates an intrinsic value and meaning because it will require workers and professionals to change or modify their way of thinking—and, consequently, their way of performing.

To think in this manner, one must look at health care activities not only as a single act, but as several steps that make up the diagnostic/therapeutic process that involve other competencies.

We define *process* as a sequence of coordinated activities that culminate in the creation of an outcome that is recognized and valued by someone, typically the patient. The process receives an input (that is, client's need); interventions are carried out, and they result in the required output (performance/product).

After carrying out an intervention, health professionals assume that the task is completed; it is equivalent to a final result (output) without considering the impact of its performance. In this way, we start to introduce the concept of a patient's outcome resulting from goods or performance that produces an effect on a condition, or a state, or behavior (for example, mortality after surgery of aortocoronary bypass; clients' dissatisfaction).

To facilitate the process, the outcome classification is usually considered from three diverse analytic visions, depending upon what part is taken into consideration at that moment for the involvement. As considered by Donabedian (1986, 1990), this entails structure, process, and outcomes. A vision of the structure (organizational quality) takes into consideration all aspects of the structure and logistic. It includes topics related to educational programs. Also, structure can be considered what materials are necessary from a practical standpoint. Process (professional quality) considers health care professionals' acts and performances. Results/outcomes (percept quality) are measured on receivers and clients of given care.

For an intervention project on people/clients to be contemporary and distinctive, it must be evaluated from performances given by health professionals (intermediate results) via specific output indicators and final results. These final results are measured on clients as the effect and result of a given performance (improvement of health or prevention pathology's grade), using specific outcome indicators.

It is important to differentiate between these two levels of evaluation. Output indicators consider the evaluation of efficiency of a given performance, and of productivity capacity throughout concrete actions and activities carried out by professionals. Although outcome indicators refer to efficacy, they consider real utility and benefit from interventions.

Having stated the differences, clearly it is impossible to evaluate interventions exclusively considering the quantity and volume of performances, but rather they must be evaluated by measuring real effects on clients' wellness status.

If we think about a process as nurses, we can recall the nursing process. Thus, we can compare that with the quality method. The nursing process is a series of systematic steps—a representation of the application of a scientific method. It is represented by a series of planned phases and actions with the aim to satisfy patients' needs and solve their problems by using the application of the scientific method throughout the problem solving. This process itself uses the scientific method process.

Mentee Perspective

The quality control system's aim is to organize and provide better health care for patients. Health care professionals, especially nurses, need a structured tool based on specific knowledge to help facilitate the delivery of services in the work place.

In this view, it is important to emphasize that the quality system is operating according to the problem solving process Plan-Do-Check-Act (PDCA) when it faces the resolution of a precise problem. In this process, a shift from a traditional model—which puts the focus on blame and punishes the guilty professional—to a model that focuses on finding out causes behind the practitioner's error. This method would follow the actions taken before an error has occurred so as to provide us with answers to learn and prevent future incidents. The main focus here is not to blame, but to learn from mistakes and correct them where necessary.

Mentor Perspective

The nursing process is a series of defined actions carried out to reach nursing care objectives, to maintain wealth, and/or furnish necessary and qualified care based upon a specific situation to allow clients to recover their health as well as participate and/or contribute to his or her quality of life, therefore solving the client's problems. The nursing process also serves as a facilitator to understand what steps to take to deliver high quality health care. Therefore, it also helps patients to achieve their health and maximum functional potential (see Figure 1).

In some sectors of hospital field activities, outcome is clearly defined, specific, and not to be discussed; for example, to reach a statement of a diagnosis, healing after surgery, say, or an emergency act in a temporary but serious pathology situation. For other occasions, though, it is difficult to state. Additionally, in many other clinical situations, it is difficult to demonstrate a result although a culture of objective measurement has been implemented as the foundation of care, and as an expected behavior.

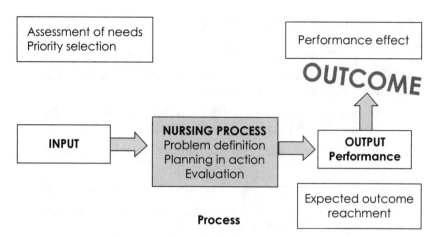

Figure 1   Nursing process and quality system outcome process.

Joint Perspective

Mentee: Outcomes research studies do exist—both subjective and objective. They pay particular attention to treatment effects that are considered and perceived by clients as more important; for example, a modification in activities of daily living (ADLs), or satisfaction and/or quality of life and mortality in the case of chronic illnesses. We are referring to so-called "patient-oriented measures."

Of course, by a methodological point of view, the debate on the topic is rich and intricate: What are the outcomes to study? Do they have to be referred to an organ or to an apparatus? Have they considered the person's autonomy? Or, are they to be studied on generic criteria of quality of life?

Mentor: As a mentor, I think that one of the most important characteristics of a good nursing leader ought to be the capacity to make decisions (strategic, operational, and clinical decisions). The realization that the overall activities of clinical governance are the continuous success of decisions and related actions based on concrete factors that we call outcome indicators (Waltz & Strickland, 1988).

In addition, to be a leader, it is necessary to be a self-confident, modest, open-minded, and competent professional. A leader has to be able to involve colleagues and be participative.

Mentee: From a coordinator's point of view, process management is a key factor in order to improve clients' outcomes. The process needs to be re-evaluated by professionals to suit their expectations so a higher grade of acceptance can be achieved.

Self-Reflective Questions

1. Would this process be suitable for your work place?

2. If you tried to implement a new decision-making process at your unit, how would you start doing so?

3. Are you currently working with this process? If not, do you think that this process could improve clients' outcomes? How?

4. What methods would you use to evaluate client's outcomes in your work place?

5. Do you think that this method would reduce nursing errors? Why?

6. How can quality control methods be compared with the nursing process?

7. What decision-making process do you currently use in your practice?

8. Do you think patient's outcomes should be evaluated by more than one method? If so, which ones, and why?

9. Do you think that quality of health care overrides quantity of health care? Why?

10. How would you compare the nursing process with the new method?

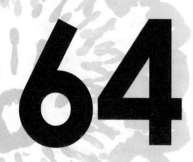

64 Paradoxical Role Models: Positive and Negative

"I learned so much from her about what not to do—whom not to be—that it influenced my career and my development as a leader. We learn—I think—as much sometimes from negative experiences as we do from positive mentors."

—Esther Green

Mentor

Joy Richards, RN, BScN, MN, PhD
Vice-President, Collaborative Practice and Quality, and Chief Nursing Executive
Baycrest Geriatric Health Care System
Toronto, Canada

Mentee

Gina Peragine, RN, BScN, MN
Program Director
Baycrest Geriatric Health System
Toronto, Canada

Many eminent nursing leaders might say they are who they are and where they are, personally and professionally, because they have been blessed to have strong role models—women and men who willingly shared learnings, triumphs, and challenges to encourage them to find their voice, speak truth to power, and grow and develop. By bearing witness to others entering into courageous and difficult situations, while others turn away, we begin to understand what strong, courageous leadership truly requires. To go, to enter, and to become fully engaged in a fearful and uncertain time lays bare their humanness to us.

It is indeed fortunate—although often rare—when we can talk about these precious teaching moments together. Indeed, many leaders choose to maintain a strong façade to protect themselves or shield others from pain. By bearing witness to strong role models in action, we learn the importance of creating life patterns of speaking or acting that might open up others to act who might not have done so otherwise. Strong role models build legacy by seizing every opportunity to model the behavior they hope to see in others. To that end, this chapter explores the importance of both positive and negative role models in our lives.

The Power of Positive Role Models

We have all drawn support or learned powerful lessons by watching the actions and outcomes of our mothers and fathers—those older and insightful role models and mentors whom we have looked up to and who have similar values and passions to our own. Positive mentors and role models have the ability to recognize our potential, help us to grow, advocate for us, give us confidence and voice, and model what courageous leadership looks and feels like. The best role models recognize our skills and abilities and take an interest in seeing us succeed and find happiness. We are drawn to these individuals: We want to be like them, to emulate them.

The Power of Negative Role Models

Although both the literature and experience speak to the value of positive role models, something much less talked or written about is that negative role models also provide strong resources for leadership development (Richards, 2008; Rilke, 1993). Strong leadership skills and courage can develop and emerge from encountering people we do not particularly like.

Do not underestimate the value of what negative role models and their styles teach us: We often learn more about our comfort zones and tolerance levels when we experience moments of conflict and disagreement. For example, when someone confronts us directly or indirectly—about what we believe in or what we are trying to do—it forces us to think about an issue or a decision differently.

Although we strive to be like positive role models, we also strive to understand negative role models. Either such reflection makes us stronger or we become less confident or less self-assured about our direction. The importance of embracing conflict with negative role models is that it allows someone to push up against our firmly held ideas, values, or opinions. We either validate our thinking or appropriately move into a new frame of mind that we might not have gotten to on our own. This is equally inspiring and phenomenal for our personal and professional growth. The paradox of negative role models is that they teach us what not to do and who not to be.

Our First Role Models

When we mature and gain work experience, our articulation of what we are looking for in mentorship and role models changes. Initially, our mentors or role models might be chosen for us, say, in a clinical placement or project work during school. In this setting, our admiration and respect for those modeling excellence in care most often reflects our lack of knowledge and therefore focuses on clinical soundness, therapeutic responses to client questions, proactive care, and clients' feedback about their care.

The role models we remember and cherish from those early days reflect more than just sound clinical skills. More likely, their values and strong sense of self resonate—how they stayed loyal, upfront, and honest about what they felt was important, no matter what walls or ways of being confronted them. Demonstrated through their words and actions, staying true to their self-identity was simply non-negotiable.

Choosing Later Role Models

Most often, we find our first mentors and role models within our places of employment. Thus, finding supportive bosses and work environments is equally important in thinking about mentorship because they foster trust and courageous actions, particularly when they are connected and aligned with our own values and visions. In such environments, one is allowed to safely speak, challenge, and disagree with others respectfully without fear of retribution. It is important to report to and work with people in environments that are aligned with our own values who stimulate, challenge, and encourage us to speak about what we believe is right.

Up-and-coming leaders desperately need role models who willingly share their vulnerability in times of struggle, not just the lessons learned after the fact. Young leaders may briefly see the pain, frustration, or anger on their role model's faces before the mask slips back on, but fledgling leaders desperately need to know that they are not alone in their moments of struggle, loneliness, and failure. Rather, all successful leaders struggle and fail, yet learn from those lessons.

What Makes a Strong Nursing Role Model

Strong nursing role models and mentors speak the truth, as best they can, to make a significant difference. They put time and energy into investing in activities that improve the lives of others, often in the most selfless of ways. However, the most influential role models and mentors show not only their strengths but also their weaknesses and failures so that others can learn. They have the exceptional ability to share these moments with others in a way that paradoxically demonstrates their power. We don't think less of them; rather, we feel empowered and less alone in our own missteps and foibles.

Positive and negative role models enter our lives through many chosen or assigned paths. Life changing experiences happen in both. The most important factor is how we choose to act within these relationships because we play a strong role in the eventual outcome. The deeper our own sense of self, the more someone can influence us on multiple and meaningful levels. We need to take the time to step back, think about, and ask ourselves two important questions: "Who has influenced my life?" and "How?" The purpose of intentionally engaging with negative role models and mentors is to influence and challenge ourselves to not only think or react but also to transform and become better people, nurses, and leaders. We may disdain these paradoxical role models, but we will remember them, learn from them, be thankful for them, and, in our turn, pay it forward.

Self-Reflective Questions

1. Who are the strong, positive role models in your life?

2. If this positive mentorship relationship is informal, how can you formalize this relationship?

3. Describe a specific situation in which you have been able to bear witness to this role model in action.

4. Have you had deliberate conversations with this mentor or positive role model about this specific experience? If not, why?

5. How has this experience changed you or affected your professional growth and development?

6. Who is a person in your personal or professional life who acts as a negative role model?

7. Describe an experience in which this negative role model confronted you directly or indirectly.

8. How did this experience influence you? Did it force you to think about an issue or a decision differently?

9. How can you be a formal or an informal positive mentor for others?

10. Consider a time when your behavior might have been a negative role model for others. What did it feel like? How might it have felt for the other person?

(Zero Defect) Patient Safety

65

"If you are dreaming about it, you can do it."

—Chihiro Nakao

Mentor
Patti Crome, RN, MN, CNA, FACMPE
Rona Consulting Group
Seattle, Washington, USA

Mentee
Becky Dotson, RN, BSN
Saint Joseph's Hospital
Signature Corporation
Parkersburg, West Virginia, USA

You may wonder why a chapter on patient safety opens with a quote from one of the world's foremost experts on the Toyota Management System or "Lean manufacturing"—until you reflect upon the power of using Lean methods to support the pursuit of perfection that is desperately needed in health care today. Using the scientific method and focusing on the customer—the patient—significant gains in patient safety can be accomplished.

Pursuing perfection or "zero defects" is one of the fundamental principles in the Toyota Management System. One may ask whether zero defects are possible in health care. Consider a 99.9% perfection rate - That would mean a wrong surgery 500 times per week. Now consider that the error rate in hospitals is 3%. Zero defects are an imperative goal and an achievable one.

Whether you agree with the preceding statement or not, you can't ignore that health care as a whole is at a critical juncture. It is estimated that 80% of medical errors are system derived (Frankel, Simmons, & Vega, 2004). The old ways of doing things won't work. External pressures for transparency, outcomes measurement, and safety will only increase.

In *To Err is Human* (Kohn, et al, 2000) the Institute of Medicine suggested that building a safer health system includes

- A center for patient safety.

- Mandatory reporting.

- Performance standards.

- A culture of safety.

Performance standards and culture are two areas that individual leaders can impact.

"Organizations with a positive safety culture are characterized by communications founded on mutual trust, by shared perceptions of the importance of safety, and by confidence in the efficacy of preventive measures" (Reason, 1997). A safety culture is an *informed culture*, "one in which those who manage and operate the system have current knowledge about the human, technical, organizational, and environmental factors that determine the safety of a system as a whole" (Reason, 1998).

This is where the Toyota Management System fits, namely, that it was founded upon two key elements: respect for people and continuous improvement. Respect for people includes not only the patient and eliminating the waste or nonvalue-added work (or what patients are willing to pay for); but also respect for the employees. Employees are the ones who know the opportunities for improvement and, given the authority and support, have the ability to design the necessary changes. Leaders must support the improvements and hold people accountable for the standard work.

Standard work and accountability are key to creating a safe patient environment; unfortunately, however, both are often lacking in health care. Standard work is a set of repeatable processes that assures the patient that the system is free of waste and inefficiencies that often allow defects to occur.

In a Lean organization that uses the Toyota Management System, standard work is designed by using the Deming improvement cycle of Plan-Do-Check-Act (PDCA). Often, the PDCA cycle is used in a workshop that is based on fast cycles of education and application (learn/do).

So how does one create a safety culture? That is, a climate where people feel safe to question assumptions and to report problems candidly? The phrase *care and concern* comes from crisis researcher Nick Pidgeon's description of what it takes to create a good safety culture: "senior management's commitment to safety; shared concern for hazards and a solicitude over their impact on people; realistic and flexible norms and rules about hazards; and continual reflection upon practice through monitoring, analysis, and feedback systems" (Turner & Pidgeon, 1997). If a company truly wants to change the culture, it must develop Lean leaders who can reinforce and lead that cultural change.

Leaders must be involved at the "gemba" (translated as "the real place," or where the work actually occurs) so they can learn to see inefficiencies that can cause errors.

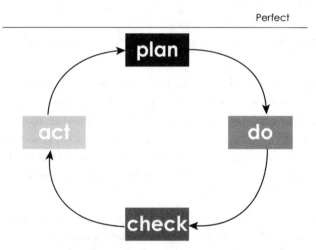

Figure 1   In a Lean organization that uses the Toyota Management System, the standard work is designed using the Deming improvement cycle of Plan, Do, Check, and Act (PDCA.)

It starts with a goal—a commitment to the patient, with a major focus on creating a culture of safety through the following:

- Recognize and reward behaviors and activities that improve patient safety.

- Recognize and reward reporting of errors and near misses.

- Increase executive leadership interactions with staff on safety issues.

- Enhance workforce knowledge about zero defects.

- Enhance skill set in communication of unanticipated outcomes.

- Increase the amount and quality of feedback to staff regarding changes made after reporting.

- Ensure communication and understanding of the organization's critical policies and implications for failure to comply.

- Implement processes that are convenient for broad staff participation.

- Engage patients and families—distribute a patient safety brochure encouraging them to be more involved in their care.

- Identify a validated culture of safety survey instrument; monitor progress.

- Provide tools to assist managers and staff with the expectations for improvement.

- Report results throughout the organization with the goal of transparency.

- Create an audit/monitoring plan; report progress to the board, executive leadership team, and throughout the organization.

- Adopt "Executive Patient Safety Walk Rounds" asking staff to call out safety concerns or near misses.

- Create an annual "Patient Safety Award" to recognize outstanding teamwork in making patient care safer.

Patients and families continue to entrust their care to a health care system that remains imperfect. With the right tools and leaders willing to join in the pursuit of perfection, there is the hope that health care can be transformed into a quality, defect-free product.

The mentee's application that follows demonstrates that pursuit with the use of *Kaizen*, which is the Japanese term for continuous improvement. A *Kaizen* event is a 3-to-5 day workshop focusing on specific targets in which the staff working in the area of opportunity use the tools of the Toyota Management System to implement improvements.

Mentee's Application

Saint Joseph's Hospital, Signature Corporation, Parkersburg, West Virginia began its journey to implement Lean starting with seminars, led by my mentor, which focused on the key principles of the Toyota Management System. Initially, there was resistance to using an automobile system in a hospital setting. With doubt, we studied the readings provided by our mentor.

During our first *Kaizen* event led by my mentor, we were determined to improve patient safety. Just a few months before, the corporation rolled out a new proprietary software reporting system, The Insights Engine. The system gave management the ability to more readily identify the root cause of various patient safety issues. One safety factor identified through using The Insights

Engine was specimen labeling. The team went to the Gemba (the workplace) and created a Value Stream Map of the actual steps of a specimen starting from the physician's order thru collection, testing, and reporting. A value stream is a map of the sequential steps in any process, including the waits between the steps and the waste within the steps. Through the *Kaizen* the team identified that five employees handled either the order or the specimen and the specimens were not always being labeled upon collection.

Therefore, the focus of the *Kaizen* became ensuring that specimens were labeled at the bedside in the presence of the patient. Staff designed the new process, creating a step-by-step standard work document that they used to teach the new process and to hold each other accountable. Over a 9-month period, a dramatic decrease in mislabeled specimens was documented via The Insights Engine, and zero defects were noted during the 10-month period—a fundamental principle of Lean and certainly our goal.

Self-Reflective Questions

1. How are employees involved in your improvement work?

2. Do you work in a culture of safety? Does staff feel safe discussing problems and reporting errors, and are they rewarded for doing so?

3. How could you shift to using a validated culture including safety-survey instruments, and then monitor progress?

4. What standard work is in place to support defect-free processes?

5. How do you monitor/audit and hold people accountable for standard work?

6. If you do not currently share information with all staff about actual or potential defects in systems or behaviors that need to be corrected immediately, why not?

7. What tools do you provide to assist managers and staff with the expectations for improvement?

8. Do you have a patient safety brochure available that encourages patients and their families to be more involved in their health care and to act as "safety inspectors"?

9. How could you benefit from doing "Executive Patient Safety Walk Rounds" in which staff are asked to call out safety concerns or near misses?

10. How could you benefit from implementing a monitoring report used to report to staff, leadership, and the Board of Directors?

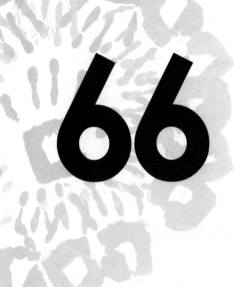

66 Peer-to-Peer Mentoring Around the Globe

"Many people have gone farther than they thought they could because someone else thought they could."

—Author Unknown

Mentor
Lynda Law Wilson, RN, PhD
Professor, School of Nursing
University of Alabama at
  Birmingham
Alabama, USA

Mentees
Debora Falleiros de Mello, RN, PhD
Professor, University of São
  Paulo Ribeirao Preto School of
  Nursing
Ribeirao Preto, Brazil
and
Maria de La Ó Ramallo
  Veríssimo, RN, PhD
Professor, University of São Paulo
  School of Nursing
São Paulo, Brazil

Collaborating across global boundaries offers unlimited opportunities for professional growth and leadership development as well as improving global nursing education and practice. This chapter describes the development of a collaborative research and leadership development partnership between a nursing professor in the United States and two nursing professors from Brazil. The partnership developed during an International Nursing Leadership Institute that was offered by the Pan American Health Organization (PAHO)/World Health Organization

Collaborating Center (WHOCC) on International Nursing at the School of Nursing at the University of Alabama at Birmingham (UAB) in January 2008. The chapter first presents a description of the leadership institute followed by a brief description of the use of mentoring and collaborative projects as a strategy for nursing leadership development. The chapter continues with a description of the two collaborative projects that were initiated during the Leadership Institute and concludes with thoughts on benefits and challenges to mentoring and collaboration across national boundaries.

Objectives of the International Nursing Leadership Institute

In January 2008, the WHOCC at UAB offered a 3-week International Nursing Leadership Institute for 18 nurses from Brazil, Chile, Colombia, and Honduras.

Participants lived with volunteer host families, which provided an opportunity to learn first-hand about local culture; studied English for health professionals; and participated in a leadership course that was co-taught by the deputy director of the WHOCC (Dr. Wilson) and by Reina Lidylia Grogan, the director of the school of nursing at the University of Honduras. In addition, each participant collaborated with a nursing faculty collaborator/mentor at UAB to develop a proposal for a project that participants would implement in their host countries to enhance family or child health in their respective countries. Initial planning for these collaborative projects began during the three-week institute and then continued by e-mail and Internet chat technologies after the participants returned home.

Mentoring and Collaboration as a Leadership Development Strategy

Collaborative mentoring partnerships can address the lack of support from colleagues with similar interests and expertise that has been cited as a challenge to developing nursing scholarship (Cumbie, Weinert, Luparell, Conley, & Smith, 2005). As International mentoring partnerships have increased, the nursing profession has become more "globally focused" (Byrne & Keefe, 2002). The term "E-mentoring" refers to use of electronic mail, Internet communication, fax, and other technologies to facilitate mentoring, and are essential to sustaining international mentoring relationships. However, Byrne and Keefe noted that opportunities for periodic face-to-face meetings are critical to the success of such mentoring relationships and should be planned and supported whenever possible. The opportunity to initiate the collaborative projects through face-to-face meetings during the International Nursing Leadership Institute provided the authors of this chapter with a chance to develop personal connections that are critical to the success of our partnerships.

Mentors teach, guide, sponsor, validate, and communicate with mentees to encourage their professional growth and development. Many different models of mentoring have been proposed, including traditional hierarchical models as well as more horizontal peer-mentoring models in which the more experienced mentor shares knowledge and expertise with colleagues but also learns and grows from the relationship. Our partnership reflects a peer-mentoring model in which all members of the partners contribute and benefit. The success of the collaborative mentoring partnership is influenced by characteristics and contributions of all partners in the relationship. Positive responses to the questions listed in the self-reflective checklist at the end of this chapter will increase the success of any collaborative partnership.

Description of Collaborative Projects

The collaborative project developed by Debora Falleiros de Mello focused on evaluating the effectiveness of teaching undergraduate nursing students at the University of São Paulo in Ribeirao Preto, Brazil about the principles of Integrated Management of Childhood Illness (IMCI). IMCI is a strategy promoted by WHO to enhance provision of holistic health care for children under 5 years of age to improve their growth and development, and to reduce childhood morbidity and mortality (World Health Organization, 2007).

The specific goals of the project are to

- Describe the level of knowledge and confidence related to IMCI principles among students in the beginning and end of the second year public health nursing course

- Compare changes in levels of knowledge and confidence related to IMCI principles of students who have had only the didactic content related to IMCI with students who have had both didactic and clinical experiences related to IMCI

Initial plans for this project were developed during the Leadership Institute, and the proposal and data collection instruments were developed following the Institute through ongoing discussions between Dr. Mello, Dr. Wilson, and other colleagues via e-mail as well as Internet chat technologies. The content validity of the instrument was assessed by five nurses with expertise in pediatric nursing. The project was initiated after it was approved by the Ethics Committee at the University of São Paulo and by the National Research Ethics Committee of the Brazilian Ministry of Health.

At the end of the course in December 2008, students were asked to complete a post-test. Data analysis involved comparison of pre- and post-test scores for the entire sample, and comparison of change scores for 20 students who had clinical experience using IMCI principles in addition to the didactic course content, with the remaining students who had didactic content only, without associated clinical experiences in the use of IMCI. Dr. Wilson has continued to work with Dr. Mello in analyzing and developing publications related to this research. This project reflects a peer-mentoring approach, in which both partners contributed to and learned from one another.

The objective of the collaborative project developed by Maria de La Ó R. Veríssimo was to evaluate the implementation of a new program designed to improve parents' abilities to care for children in a primary care center in São Paulo, Brazil. The program, Our Children: Windows of Opportunities (OCWO), was developed in São Paulo in 2003. The program is based on a conceptual framework that addresses health promotion, family and social networks, strengthening family competencies, and child development. The program provides a systematic framework for assessment and health promotion during well-child health visits for children under the age of 5 years. The program also includes educational materials to orient members of the health care team to developmental issues and suggestions for emancipator education, educational information for parents about childcare and development, and a record-keeping system for documenting the child evaluations and agreements between health professional and family.

During the Institute, Dr. Wilson worked with Dr. Veríssimo to plan the studies, design, and methodology, including identification of study instruments and plans for data analysis. The objectives of the project are to:

- Describe nurses' and physicians' activities in implementing the OCWO program in a community health center

- Describe nurses' and physicians' perceptions and levels of satisfaction with the OCWO program

- Describe perceptions and levels of satisfaction of parents/caregivers with the OCWO program

When Dr. Veríssimo returned to Brazil after the institute, she presented a report about her experience and project to faculty in the school of nursing and to the financial agency that supported her trip.

A unique benefit of our collaborative experience was the simultaneous mentoring of two different mentees while they developed different-yet-related projects. During the institute, each mentee met individually with Dr. Wilson, but we also scheduled joint meetings during the institute as well as joint meetings using Internet chat technology following the institute. In this way, Drs. Mello and Veríssimo were able to share information with one another, and the three-way partnership contributed to the growth of all three participants because of shared information about the research projects and about teaching and clinical practice.

Benefits and Challenges

Our experience in developing this collaborative partnership has provided us with many personal and professional benefits, including the opportunity to learn new ideas and to identify literature and other resources to support our collaborative project and to enhance other professional roles, including teaching and professional service roles. We have also been able to identify other resources for funding our research, and other experts who have similar interests whose expertise can enhance our work. The collaborative projects that we developed grew from the initial interests of the Institute participants (Mello and Veríssimo), but complemented the expertise and professional interests of the Institute organizer (Wilson).

Despite these many benefits, we acknowledge that our collaborative partnership has presented us with ongoing challenges. The primary challenge has related to multiple competing demands and responsibilities that have made it difficult for us to devote the time we would like to implement our collaborative projects. Another challenge has been the change in the health system in São Paulo that delayed the implementation of the project initially proposed by Dr. Veríssimo. Language differences also present special challenges because all research proposals and instruments have had to be translated from Portuguese to English, and such translation is time-consuming and often cumbersome.

Despite these challenges, our partnership is beneficial, and we look forward to working together on this and other projects.

Self-Reflective Questions

1. How can you establish clear goals for your collaborative partnership?

2. How can you devote time to maintain communication and implement your collaborative project?

3. What can you do to maintain open and honest communication with your partner?

4. How can you become flexible and able to make changes as needed as your partnership and project develops?

5. How willing are you to share your knowledge and expertise?

6. How open are you to learning new ideas from your collaborative partnership experience?

7. How willing are you to seek and accept feedback from your partner?

8. How can you define your collaborative project based on mutual interests and areas of expertise of all partners?

9. How can you establish clear guidelines for co-authorship of presentations and publications that arise from the collaborative project?

10. How committed are you to the success of your collaborative partnership?

67 People Skills and People First: Walk the Talk

"The staff must feel that you understand what the front line looks like, and active listening is the key to this end."

—Margaret McClure

Mentor

Chua Gek Choo, RN, BHSN,
 Grad. Dip (Higher Education)
Deputy Director of Nursing
 (Alexandra and Khoo Teck
 Puat Hospitals)
Adjunct Lecturer at the Nan-
 yang Polytechnic (School of
 Health Sciences)
Singapore

Mentee

Eunice Nah Swee Lin, MSc HRM
 BHSN
Senior Staff Nurse
SingHealth Polyclinics
Singapore

Caring for our patients is a natural or trained inclination that comes with the job of nursing. However, more often than not, we display more care toward our patients than each other. If we cannot start caring for our own, we will fail ourselves as nurses in walking the talk of care. We require people skills to successfully engage and energize our team so they will be better motivated to do their best for our patients and each other.

People skills are key to people management and development. People skills are learned skills; part of people skills is learning to meet people's needs.

Abraham Maslow's 1943 paper, "A Theory of Human Motivation" succinctly described the steps to meeting human needs. Our people (the backbone of our institution) require us to understand, encourage, and engage them to believe that they are working in a caring environment that will nurture them to reach their maximum potential for peak performance.

Mentoring Conversation 1

Eunice (Mentee)

We often take for granted what is the most obvious and easiest in human relations. Smiles can start conversations between strangers and warm the heart. A smiling leader begets a smiling nurse. A heartfelt smile is the first people skill.

The spoken or written word is one of the most frequently employed mediums of communication. However, because of cross-cultures and varied family upbringing (where we are taught different ways of interpreting the meanings of words), we may not always fully understand the messages sent by others as accurately as what they had intended them to be.

Chua (Mentor)

We also need to think positively by believing in ourselves and believing in our people. Only when we start believing in the best of our people can our people start believing that they are capable of greater things. Affirmation is a free motivational tool. Use it.

Learning to communicate effectively by choosing the right words is another key to people skills. Words can give or sap life. After they are spoken or written, we can seldom change the effect that words have on the recipient. So, consider the destiny of your leadership legacy through the impact of what you say. Seek wisdom to guide the expressions of your heart.

Clear and open communication is the first step toward building trust. Leaders who choose to openly communicate their vision, core values, and plans (with a forum for discussion input and participation) invite their people to join them in the ownership of the goals and plans for a joint future. Without a clear, communicated vision and core values, people will wonder and wander.

Clear communication building blocks should

- Be jargon-free to promote understanding.

- Be frequent enough to engage people. Make each encounter count.

- Discard assumptions, and explain rationale and benefit to all.

- Include straight talk from a sincere heart.

- Be inviting of clarifications and suggestions. ("What do you think?")

To build trust with people, you need to earn it by walking the talk through spending time with them and sharing, listening, and encouraging. Trust is also built through acting honorably as well as being accountable and principle-centered.

Mentoring Conversation 2

Chua

In my tour of duty at a local specialty institution in Singapore, I met a nurse leader who was different from the usual stern and demanding nursing administrators. The senior staff describes her as such: "We call Ms. C. 'Boss.' She is very strict, but the thing that is different about her is that unlike others, she will listen; and if what you say makes sense, she will consider changes. If you talk to her, she will stop to listen and not tell you that she has no time. If necessary, she will also fight for your rights."

It was a huge relief to me to know that my leader is someone who can see reason. I felt a sense of trust and pride in a nursing leader who is accessible, humble enough to listen, and compassionate enough to stand up for us.

Eunice

A leader's role is a position of vested power, and with it comes an authority of representation that the ordinary person does not have. Having the courage to represent our people is not enough. We need to expand our network and extend our influence—to be effective in representing them.

Within the leadership mantle is also the mandate of reconciliation. It is hard work and requires much wisdom. Without reconciliation, there is no harmony. Without harmony, it is difficult to perform in peak condition. Reconciliation is a necessary people-skills tool if you intend to build a people-focused culture.

Chua

People skills are not meant for leaders alone. The possession of people skills can ease the rigors of the technical aspect of the caring profession. People skills translate into core service skills that help in our interactions with each other, patients, and society. Grow your team's people skills so that they, too, can benefit from putting people first. Acquire strong people skills and build a positive culture of placing people first, and almost everything else will find a way to fall into place thereafter.

Mentoring Conversation 3

Eunice

When I worked in HR, I had the privilege of conducting a scholar retention interview to discover why an extremely talented staff member wanted to resign suddenly. He related an incident (among others) of how he had made an application to take a day's urgent leave. When asked why, he related that it was so he could be at his dying godfather's bedside. He related how his nurse manager broke into furious rhetoric about how leave application should not be abused, that he should have made the projected application in advance last month when the godfather was very ill, and because it was his "God-father," "God" could take his place—and she laughed. He told me that he had no intention to abuse the use of his leave because there should have been no problem with staffing that week with extra personnel. He could not understand why his supervisor, a nurse, could not be compassionate about such matters and joke inappropriately about something that was so dear to his heart. He could not see how he could continue in such a culture of hypocrisy where there is only a public display of care toward patients yet no compassion for our own when behind closed doors.

Chua

Organizational skills are essential for work effectiveness, and we are taught to build a rapport with our patients. However, the majority of nurses do not employ people nor communication skills to build rapport with each other. In my mentee's story, we see evidence of inflexibility for the wrong reasons, a lack of compassion, and a poor sense of humor that dampens the spirit.

The manager should have understood the bond that the staff member had with his godfather even though he was not a blood relative. She should have been more flexible about such exigent matters. We cannot take each other for granted, and we need to practice emotional intelligence as leaders when relating to our staff. Yes, having a sense of humor and being able to laugh at ourselves is an important people skill, but it should never be used at other's expense. Rather, humor should be used to lighten the day, be of cheer, and, in the case of leadership, motivate colleagues. Compassion cannot be taught, but we can learn to be flexible. Humor when used appropriately, can be a very powerful, energizing motivational tool in a stressful health care environment.

Developing People Skills

If we are to affect our world, we need to develop our people in skills sets beyond nursing, management, and teaching. In this day and age of constant change, we need to equip ourselves with the one skill that will never be obsolete and always be for the betterment of people everywhere—people skills that create a synergistic team.

Author Fredrick Collins (1967) wrote, "There are two types of people. Those we who come into a room and say, 'Well, here *I* am!' and those who come in and say, 'Ah, there *you* are.'" Which will you choose to become?

Self-Reflective Questions

1. How do you make the effort to walk the talk by putting people first through people skills?

2. Do you smile when you meet people along your way? If not, why not?

3. How can you shift your mindset to try to think positively and speak words of affirmation?

4. How do you invite clarifications to check whether what others hear you say is what you really mean?

5. How can you make the time to build sincere and strong relationships with those around you?

6. What results have you gotten when trying to use humor to motivate and ease another's workday?

7. What steps can you take for your team to defend and represent them?

8. How can you become a better agent of peace through reconciliation to promote harmony?

9. How do you help your team learn and practice new people skills?

10. Are you a life-time learner of effective people skills? How do you accomplish this?

Performance and Improvement Evaluation:
Policy and Procedure

68

"For there is a proper time and procedure for every matter."

—Ecclesiastes 8:6

Mentor
Marion Eulene Francis Howard,
   PhD, MSN, BA, SCM, SRN
Lecturer
Barbados Community
   College
St. Michael, Barbados

Mentee
Mellon Nsingu Manyonga-
   Jordan, MSc, BA, RN
Registered Nurse
Queen Elizabeth Hospital
St. Michael, Barbados

Every organization has set goals and objectives that its leaders expect to achieve. Usually, these goals are clearly expressed in the organization's philosophy, charter, mission statement, and strategic plans; and such goals form the basis of the organization's policies as well as the review of the employee's performance or evaluation. Vestal (1995) notes that in health care the goal is service and that in nursing the goal is bringing people to the highest level of health care, self-care, or helping them to die with dignity. Therefore, the goal of a hospital is to produce quality patient care. It naturally follows that employee performance is measured against the organization's set goals and objectives.

Performance and Improvement Evaluation

Performance and improvement evaluations add to the developmental nature of the review process. Employee performance is reviewed in a positive manner to correct any shortfalls that the employee might exhibit; hence, it should not be punitive in nature (Marquis & Huston 2003). Performance is measured against predetermined standards, and action is taken to correct discrepancies between these standards and actual performance. Thus, measuring performance is impossible if standards have not been clearly established.

How Policies and Procedures Help Achieve Goals and Objectives

To achieve the overall goals and objectives of the institution, health care settings use clearly established policies and procedures that guide employees in carrying out their daily functions. Policies, which are the defined courses of action that guide and determine present and future decisions, include standards. Standards are the desirable and achievable level of performance against which practice is compared. A complete job description defines and outlines overall role tasks to be accomplished. Specific procedural policy outlines those standards of care that define quality patient care.

In nursing, performance standards may be measured against skills checklists or other tools that explain each skill in measurable and behavioral terms. Such standards can also suggest resources for learning. More than 20 American Nurses Association (ANA) Standards for Nursing Practice exist. These clinical practice or standardized guidelines reflect areas of specialty nursing practice and provide step-by-step interventions for individual nurses to follow in clinical practice (ANA, 2001). The guidelines have been developed to promote quality care. However, having guidelines and policies in place in an institution for evaluation of care and performance is not enough. The human touch of the nurse leader is most important.

A Case in Point: Mentee's Story

I was excited at the end of my 10-day orientation programme at the General Hospital, where I landed my first job as a registered nurse. It was heartening to know that the hospital had policies and procedures that would guide my day-to-day practice as a nurse on the ward where I was assigned. I was given a copy of my job description and the terms and conditions of Service document for my employment. It was a good feeling to know that my hospital was adhering to international standards. Since the early 1990s, The Joint Commission has advocated the use of employee job descriptions as the standard for performance appraisal.

The terms and conditions of service document included a chapter on the performance management system, which outlined that a performance appraisal would be conducted for all employees. The document noted that the appraisal would help the hospital relate a person's performance with the organization's goals; encourage and assess competencies; provide an opportunity for communication between employees, supervisors, and managers; promote a fair and open appraisal; resolve performance problems; and recognize good performance.

Further, the performance appraisal would evaluate achievement of the duties and responsibilities in the job description, and of departmental level objectives; identify training needs; and encourage behavior that best reflects the institution's values. The document also stated that an appraisal form for each employee would be discussed and completed in accordance with the Performance Review and Development System (PRDS).

However, soon after starting my job, I became concerned about the performance management system. At no time had my ward manager spoken to me about my evaluation, and I often wondered whether my performance was measuring up enough to secure my permanent appointment at the end of my probation period.

My concerns would have been alleviated if, at the beginning of my job, management had outlined the contents of the PRDS and furnished me with a copy of the appraisal form. I expected management to talk with me and set the objectives and criteria for measuring my job performance for specified periods, in keeping with the intended purpose of the PRDS. In this case, the performance appraisal policy document was not enough; something more was needed from the procedure.

The Importance of the Human Touch for Employees

The human touch was missing. For example, my supervisor and I had no meeting to set individual goals and objectives and to clarify understanding of my roles and function. Supervisors must observe staff members carrying out their duties, offer words of encouragement, demonstrate techniques, reinforce teaching, lead by example, and give positive and negative feedback. Showing staff members that you value and care about them and making them feel comfortable in their job—that is the human touch.

The message to nurse leaders is that a leader's role is to set specific performance goals for each important aspect of a subordinate's job, measure progress toward the goal, and provide feedback. Not only must standards exist, but also leaders must ascertain that subordinates know and understand them. Standards vary among institutions, so employees must know the organization's expectations of them and be aware that their performance will be measured by their ability to meet the established standards.

Many performance methods dominate, and all have important criteria to be met (Plunkett, Attner, & Allen, 2005). Whatever method is used, the manager and subordinate need to meet periodically to agree upon specific performance goals for the subordinate over a fixed period. At the end of the period, the subordinate is evaluated. For example, measuring how many goals were met, how effectively and efficiently each one was achieved, and the growth that occurred.

Takeaway: How My Mentor Exemplifies the Human Touch

I feel privileged that my former lecturer is now my mentor. I am inspired by her academic achievement in nursing, which I hope to achieve someday. I am impressed with her presentation and oratory abilities, and I hope I can sharpen mine similarly. I admire her simplicity and ability to explain complex health processes so that students can understand. I admire her level of organization. Her method of teaching is facilitation not "handing it down." I admire her calmness. She is always approachable and humorous. She cares for students and takes extra time to clarify any misunderstandings.

I also admire her leadership abilities as chief nursing officer and other capacities in which she has served. I admire her spirit. She is hardworking, determined, and motivated. Above all else, she is selfless and encourages others to grow and participate at higher levels.

My experiences with my performance appraisals and my ward supervisor are a constant reminder to me about how *not* to treat my subordinates. I learned the importance of helpfulness and a human touch from my former lecturer's selfless caring and mentoring. She has touched me through our interactions and will always be a source of inspiration to me, an aspiring nurse leader. A mentor is not a work supervisor who evaluates only job performance, but someone who demonstrates the human touch that nurse leaders need to learn and practice. That is what makes the difference!

Self-Reflective Questions

1. How can you make your subordinates feel welcome, important, needed, and comfortable?

2. What can you do to make sure that your subordinates understand the organization's goals, objectives, and the effect specific roles play?

3. How can you clearly outline specific tasks and functions (who, when, where, what, how)?

4. How do you meet with your subordinates to specify the criteria on which their performance is evaluated?

5. How can you make available all necessary resources and materials to get the job done?

6. How can you better observe your subordinates on the job and work alongside them?

7. How can you offer better feedback sessions with your subordinates on their performance?

8. How can you best give praise and/or constructive criticism to your subordinates in an appropriate and timely manner?

9. How can you best identify areas of growth for your subordinates?

10. How have weak areas been identified and remedial action recommended, such as further training?

69 Perseverance, Persistence, and Hard Work

"When there is more insecurity and more danger, the only way to respond to it is by awareness."

—Osho

Mentor
Gladys Mouro, RN, MSN
Assistant Hospital Director for
  Nursing Services
American University of Beirut,
  Medical Center
Beirut, Lebanon

Mentee
Zeina Kassem, RN
Oncology Unit
American University of Beirut,
  Medical Center
Beirut, Lebanon

During the past 30 years of my life at the American University of Beirut Medical Center (AUBMC) in Lebanon, I've often wondered why I was so stubborn about achieving my dreams. Although everything around me was falling apart and hopeless, and I would go to bed fed up with the miseries and difficulties I encountered, but somehow wake the next morning energetic to begin again and to strive for the impossible.

My story is of leadership throughout 30 years of war that has not ended, the destruction of nursing infrastructures, the rebuilding of standards, and my dream—against all odds—to join the American Nurses Credentialing Center's Magnet Recognition Program, which recognizes health care organizations that provide nursing excellence. It is the story of my persistence, perseverance, and determination to work hard to achieve when everything around me was hopeless and frightening. How did I refuse to give up in spite of the odds against me? The leader and the nurse inside made it happen.

War in Lebanon and the Survival of Nursing

Lebanon is a Middle Eastern country located in southwest Asia. It faces the Mediterranean Sea on the west and has a coastline of 150 miles. The capital of Beirut has a population of around 2 million. For almost two decades, every possible form of brutality and terror known to humankind has besieged Lebanon. The magnitude cannot be described unless you actually live it. About 170,000 people have perished; twice as many have been wounded or handicapped. Almost two-thirds of the population has experienced some form of dislocation from their homes and communities. For two decades, Lebanon has been subjected to every conceivable form of collective terror. The incidents of humiliation, insult, intimidation, and harassment are high. The scars and scares of war surface repeatedly.

Impact of War on the American University of Beirut Medical Center

The American University of Beirut, established in 1886, is one of 20 universities in Lebanon and is the first of higher education. This great institution is where I work. In 1978, I witnessed the war creep in from all sides until it engulfed AUBMC in a wave of anarchy and violence. When the war began, the necessities of life slowly disappeared. The air conditioning, ventilation, and electricity were cut off in most areas of the medical center. Water was a rare commodity. Often, there was no fuel or fresh food. Bombs fell, houses were destroyed, and one by one, people left, including our medical and nursing staff. The medical center was transformed from a teaching hospital to a disaster area, and the educational links with the outside world were cut off.

My Journey

From 1976 to 1991, the medical center suffered and had to survive with no tools to meet the basic needs of patients. I was determined not to leave my nurses, no matter what. I became a head nurse in 1978, a supervisor in 1980, and a director in 1982. An American who should have packed and left, I stayed to support the medical center's staff and not give up because they were worth the pain and suffering.

Staff believed in me, and had they felt I was giving up, they would have left. I knew that if I were there for them, they would stay with me to keep the medical center open. I rounded on our staff regularly and was visible at all times. I listened to their stories and the sad encounters that they faced because of the war. I tried to instill a sense of security within them that someone would protect them, no matter what. Seeing their faces smile provided so much strength and energy.

There were times when I thought that I would be kidnapped—I received many threats telling me to leave the country. I refused because I knew that the work was, and continues to be, important. Leadership required my perseverance, persistence, and hard work. I was not afraid to face the challenges of the war, fall down, or fail. I was determined. As Peter Drucker says, good leaders learn from failures, try again, sometimes in a different way (Hesselbein, Goldsmith, & Beckhard, 1996).

From 2002 to 2007, I found myself facing a different struggle—a fight to change attitudes. After so many years of war, rebuilding an atmosphere of credibility and trust among patients, visitors, and medical staff was difficult. When technology in the world was improving and nurses in other countries were on the journey to Magnet, I was figuring out how to survive. It required strong passion and drive to make the changes and achieve. There were times I wanted to give up, and times I hated myself for trying.

In leadership, however, you make a decision to go on or surrender. Your passion spreads to those around you and keeps the flame alive. Your eyes talk, your heart bounces, people around you feel it, and together you experience the satisfaction of not giving up. People, including nurses, left the country, but my determination and perseverance to achieve excellence never died. There is an opportunity for all who want to lead. Be determined and passionate about what you do as well as what you say you will do. Be credible so that those who follow you will put their life in your hands. The challenges of the 21st century will bring greater and more complex demands than ever before. You need to be a visionary and believe you can do anything you want in order to persevere. "When there is more insecurity and more danger, the only way to respond to it is by awareness" (Osho, 1999).

I believed in the strength of all the staff members and did not give up trying to make them believe in themselves and our abilities as a team. When you feel down, depressed, and helpless, your enthusiasm and persistence can be contagious, and motivation spreads. You can make a difference in the life of a patient, a nurse, the profession, and the country.

I have been privileged and blessed to mentor people like Zeina and see them grow and succeed. While I do that, the pain and discouragement turns into joy and happiness to have been part of their lives. Many people do not achieve their goals because they give up too soon. Be patient, and understand that great triumphs take weeks, months, and sometimes even decades of hard work. Keep your faith alive when things are not working. Work harder, and never give up or look back at the dark days. When I began my career as a nurse, I was shy, timid, and afraid of being in the real world of nursing. I learned a lot from falling down and picking myself up. I learned from the pain I faced, and every time, I became a better, wiser, and more determined person.

Reflections from Zeina Kassem, Mentee

When I finished school, the expectation from my family was that I would pursue a technology career, but I wanted to do something that required courage and that I enjoyed. I saw the nursing program offered, and many friends were applying. Initially, I liked being a nurse because I had the tolerance and passion to help people. With time, I realized how fulfilling my job was and how much self-satisfaction I received by helping others.

My family was against my nursing education in the beginning and never thought that I could advance in such a career. I proved them wrong. I believed in my abilities, and because of the integrity, determination, perseverance, and passion I have, I do something special in my life that I am interested in and enjoy. Our society (especially Arab countries) still considers nursing to be a nonprofessional occupation. This view undermines nursing education, autonomy, competency, retention, recruitment, and regulation, further indicating that nursing has not yet achieved the power and status that it works so hard to achieve.

My Mentor

My adventure continued when I joined the nursing service team at AUMBC. My practice started, and being a nurse, I dedicated my life to the sick and needy. It is inspiring that there are people in this world who can care for someone they don't know and do their best at it.

AUMBC was always supportive. I am in awe of the team I work with at AUBMC. My mentor, Ms. Gladys Mouro, has empowered me, guided my professional growth, supported me, and discovered the best in me. This team has taught me to persevere, work hard to achieve excellence, and always aim high. As a nurse, I am proud that I have acquired the knowledge, skills, and attitude that allow me to cross many roads and overcome many obstacles.

Self-Reflective Questions

1. How are you persistent during difficult times?

2. How do you persevere when times are difficult?

3. How do you define hard work and determination in health care?

4. How do you equate survival with persistence in health care situations?

5. What drives you to retain the commitment to continue to mentor and coach during difficult times?

6. Should you sacrifice personal needs in times that require persistence, perseverance, and hard work?

7. What do you look for to see strength and energy in others?

8. How do you learn from your failures?

9. How do you try new, innovative ways to approach the challenge to persevere in times of failure?

10. What do you do when you find it difficult to face new and unknown challenges?

(Building a) Person-Centered Model of Care

70

"We have to radically change the way nursing care is delivered in the hospital and develop our care giving around the role versus just throwing another position onto the practice site."

—Jolene Tornabeni

Mentor
Kathleen Collins-Ruiz, RN, MSN, CNA
Associate Director for Nursing Services
VA Caribbean Healthcare System
Puerto Rico

Mentee
Gladys Navarro, RN, MSN
Associate Chief Nursing Service for Geriatrics and Extended Care
VA Caribbean Healthcare System
Puerto Rico

The health care delivery system in the United States is facing a crisis as health care spending increases and the shortage of health care professionals continues. Many organizations are looking toward new models that can deliver care in a safe, effective way while also promoting the autonomy and retention of nurses.

The model of delivery of nursing care in the nursing home setting is facing many challenges due to a national initiative to transform the culture of the nursing homes. The Veterans Healthcare Administration (VHA) is transforming the culture of the nursing home. Spotswood (2006) states that according to Dr. Christa Hojlo, chief nurse for Geriatrics and Extended Care in the Veterans Administration Central Office, if you over-focus upon the medical piece, you miss the fact that people are in nursing homes because of the impact of a chronic or a recently acute medical condition upon the person's ability to function. Considering these aspects, we have used primary and team nursing and are now designing a new model of care delivery that is person-centered.

Innovative Care Delivery Models: Mentor

Each care delivery model has pros and cons, with an all-professional staff in primary nursing being costly; and team nursing seeing care fragmentation, shared responsibility without accountability, and complex communication channels (Pontin, 1999). Therefore, it is not surprising that efforts continue to identify innovative care delivery models.

One such effort is the identification of 24 innovative and successful care delivery models as part of a research project to profile new models of care that could be widely replicated. The research was funded by the Robert Wood Johnson Foundation and published in 2008 by Joynt and Kimball of Health Workforce Solutions, LLC (HWS), using a set of criteria that included:

- Innovation.

- Increased continuity, including transitional care to the home setting.

- Improvement in quality, safety, cost, and/or patient or caregiver satisfaction.

- Replicability.

- Sustainability.

The models would primarily serve adult patients. The criteria were applied to 60 models selected from among 171 leads, narrowing these to 24 that were further assessed.

Many of the organizations that have developed or sponsored these models have used similar approaches, and Joynt & Kimball (2008) describe elements common to many including:

- New roles for nurses as integrators of care.

- A move toward an interdisciplinary team approach.

- Models that extend to the home, outpatient clinic, or long-term care.

- Use of technology.

- The active participation of the patient in the plan of care.

- A focus on patient satisfaction and outcomes.

As of July 2008, many of the models had been replicated externally and/or internally (Joynt & Kimball, 2008). It is expected that others will be encouraged to innovate in their own institutions.

Our Road: Mentee

We learned from the work on innovative delivery models as we created our person-centered model.

Our vision is to instill a feeling of community where the long-term care resident is the center of the health care team. We are creating an interdisciplinary person-centered care model where staff is empowered and are assigned to permanent units, known as "neighborhoods."

When you want to foster a sense of community, everyone has to be involved, from the administrator to the housekeeper. For example, say you have a resident who is dependent upon the staff for feeding and his meal arrives when the social worker was going to interview him. Why should the social worker leave and come back when the nurse finishes feeding the resident? Wouldn't the social worker be able to get a more accurate estimate if he or she sits down, helps feed the resident, and chats with him/her? This small task could create an environment of trust in which the resident will be able to talk openly with the social worker about many subjects that would otherwise might have been too hard for him/her to talk about. Although you may have only one social worker for the entire community, you will have him or her be a member of a particular neighborhood, thus creating a sense of belonging. The social worker will be able to make more contributions as a human being to one neighborhood and thus improve his or her overall performance as a social worker for the entire community.

In the person-centered model of delivery of care, the nurses know the residents and their life-long preferences. They do not have to wait for the nurse manager to give them their assignment; instead, they arrive to their shift, take the report with the outgoing nurse, give rounds, and immediately become engaged with the resident. As everyone gets involved, we are promoting continuity of care, quality, safety, and cost-effectiveness. Evidence of this is a two-thirds decrease in the time the nurse spends taking the report, thus being more cost effective and a decrease in the residents with little or no activity engagement which has decreased from 8.2% (lower is better) in 2007 to 3.8%.

Change Management: Mentor

Of importance in developing and implementing a care delivery model is the process that is followed to bring about change. Allen and Vitale-Nolen (2005) describe the increase in nurse satisfaction when a relation-based nursing model was implemented in an acute psychiatric setting. In this instance, nurses were part of the design, the whole organization supported the project, and nurses were given time to visualize the ideal system and reflect on theory. The transition occurred in stages, and both formal and informal methods of communication were used. In other words, the orderly and participative change process itself contributed to an increase in nurse satisfaction as much or more than the model chosen (Allen & Vitale-Nolen, 2005).

Boynton and Rothman (1995) describe the process used to move from an all-RN staff to a patient-focused care model in which an RN leads a team and assumes the day-to-day responsibility for care. The use of specific change management strategies involving communication, training, and measurement and monitoring of quality of services along with the management of the emotions involved led to a successful transition.

The Importance of Input: Mentee

When you are implementing a change, such as the model of delivery of care, it pays to have everyone's input and contributions. It is also satisfying for the staff to be empowered and to be able to make decisions. For example, our staff distributes the tasks among themselves and can consider their preferences. You may have a nurse that doesn't like to administer medications but enjoys bathing residents and taking them out of bed. This can be a topic of discussion in their neighborhood meetings, and they may all agree that this nurse can do the tasks of preference, but when needed, will administer medications on enough occasions to validate her competencies. Each neighborhood team has a leader that may be any member of the health care team. Neighborhood meetings are held once every two weeks during which neighborhood life is discussed. Group educations can also be given during these neighborhood meetings.

The Continuing Evolvement of Delivery Models: Mentor

Patient care delivery models continue evolving as nursing knowledge grows, especially those related to the impact that care delivery models can have upon patient outcomes. The desire alone to implement a new model is not enough to bring this about; use of effective change management strategies is essential.

Nurse leaders as mentors must model these behaviors as well as provide an environment in which the mentee feels supported as he or she strives for excellence in patient care.

Be Creative, Flexible: Mentee

As we implement models of delivery of patient care, it is important to be creative and flexible while ensuring that the staff is fully engaged in all changes. As leaders, we must listen to our staff and always know that our main role is to serve them in what they need. Also, always have an experienced mentor to guide you in your journey.

Self-Reflective Questions

1. How does your patient care delivery model reflect your vision for patient care?

2. How does your model improve quality, safety, and cost?

3. How does your model promote continuity of care?

4. How can your model promote professional development?

5. Does your model have an interdisciplinary approach? If not, why?

6. Does your model have nurses in the role of care coordinator? If not, why?

7. How does your model make use of available technology?

8. How could your model better promote staff satisfaction?

9. How could your model better promote patient/family satisfaction?

10. How have you implemented your model, using change principles and strategies?

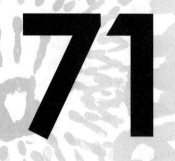

71

(What's Your) Philosophy: Own It, Live It

"I think I've always done things differently than others, and usually, as a younger child, I'd be punished. I remember trying to create and engage things, but I didn't do it like everybody else. I've just not been afraid to take the plunge; I didn't, and I don't, think, 'should I' or 'shouldn't I'?"

—Gail Mitchell

Mentor
Joy Richards, RN, BScN,
  MN, PhD
Vice-President, Collaborative
  Practice and Quality, and
  Chief Nursing Executive
Baycrest Geriatric Health Care
  System
Toronto, Canada

Mentee
Penelope Minor, RN, BScN, MN
Manager/Professional Practice
  Leader, Nursing
Baycrest Geriatric Health Care
  System
Toronto, Canada

Do you ever wonder why some nursing leaders only scratch the surface of an issue or turn away from it while others choose to act? In those moments of choosing, something—courage, passion, or commitment—comes from within and is realized suddenly and intensely. It is a deliberate, thoughtful choosing—given the risk—to engage and take action. Such leaders are cognizant of the choice and the risk, but are willing to, and feel obliged to, act in spite of the risk. Why? Some say it's because they could not live with themselves if they did not take action. But where does this sense of obligation come from?

The Risk Takers

A published study (Richards, 2008) noted that courageous Canadian female nursing leaders described themselves as making different choices, not quite fitting in, and playing outside the standard rulebook typically used by many women in Western society. For example, study participants discussed things like *swimming in a different direction, working against the flow, reinventing things, not being afraid to dive in, breaking the mold, finding different ways of getting there, walking as close to the edge as possible without falling off the cliff,* and *going under the radar screen.* It is also interesting to note that they described themselves as *trouble-makers, risk takers,* as *getting kicked out of places, differentiating themselves, doing their own thing, not quite fitting in, introverted,* and *rebellious.* They also felt *absolutely confident, independent, no need to please others,* and *a bit apart.* Another way of looking at it is that they all "owned" their own philosophy, and they are living it. This often means making counterintuitive choices and often taking different directions than others.

Embracing Risk

For those of us who can relate to these words, we know that this type of stance is not only energizing but also provides new opportunities to solve current profession/work related problems and supports achieving our goals. However, we can also find ourselves on the margins and not fitting in. In fact, it can be a rather lonely journey. We don't like following traditional rules or asking permission, nor do we like being told how we should think or what we should do. We often learn how, and then choose to work outside the system to break existing paradigms. We become good at finding different or alternative ways of getting to our goals and often walk as close to the edge as possible—hopefully without falling off the cliff.

The Freedom of Risk

As a senior nursing leader, I embrace innovation, trust, freedom, ambiguity, creativity, and confidence. I find that more and more, while gaining experience, I don't worry as much about the consequences, but rather trust the process of innovation, taking huge leaps of faith into the unknown. I have developed a tremendous sense of freedom to invite the impossible. In doing so, I experience an enthusiasm and openness to what could be. I have learned to not only tolerate but also embrace ambiguity. I hate to admit it, but sometimes it is just taking my best guess and going for it. Life is too complex to do otherwise. A colleague of mine once said that a lack of total clarity is a gift, and I have learned that she is right. By plunging into the pure unknown with a freedom to invite the impossible, you can transform and creatively fill up that space. How do we, as mature leaders, impart these gifts to up-and-coming leaders who follow in our footsteps?

Enlisting a Mentor: A Mentee's Perspective

Young leaders gain comfort in walking that fine line or challenging the status quo by first identifying with someone in their organization who they feel demonstrates these abilities. When linked with a mentor, up-and-coming leaders establish a relationship in which there is comfort knowing that someone will answer questions, steer you in the right direction, and always be there to keep a watchful eye on you. This does not mean that someone will make decisions for you or tell you which path is the right one to take. However, a mentor will also not let you fall flat on your face, either, unless it is done within a safe and trustful situation to promote learning.

When reflecting on how I, as a young leader, have moved to a place where I now have comfort in working within the fog of ambiguity, I can recall not only experiences and challenges that were placed in my path as learning opportunities, but also key individuals that I purposely surrounded myself with. All these factors have played an integral part in my ability to find comfort in doing things differently. An important part of gaining this kind of confidence has grown from exposure to various avenues, such as exposure to senior leadership meetings, participating in political nursing organizations, being a key player in research implementation, gaining exposure to academic writing, and presenting my work at conferences and workshops. Each experience provided opportunities for others to provide me constructive criticism and feedback in a supportive and nurturing way. Although the feedback you obtain might not be what you always wish to hear, these venues are safe environments to learn and grow in as well as develop important skills.

Changing Your Comfort Zone: A Mentor's Perspective

Choosing your work environment also contributes to such confidence. It wasn't until I left working in an academic environment—with an established sense of comfort and several mentors in key leadership positions—that I truly began to find my voice. Having no choice but to advocate for my patients and myself, I began to experience and understand the development of my philosophy. Upon leaving my comfort zone and working at a facility where I had no support, I had to prove to others and myself that I had acquired the leadership skills to allow me to take chances. Being a novice practitioner in an environment where your mentor is not physically located can be a frightening experience. It leaves you with a sense of abandonment and fear of the unknown. However, it is through this sense of fear and excitement that the process of courage began—with the realization that I could act, take risks, and succeed.

Ensuring that you surround yourself with more than one leader who will mentor you is key—and, ideally, not all from within your discipline. This helps you as a young leader to gain confidence in various interdisciplinary discussions. The ability to look through another discipline's eyes has helped me create outside-the-box thinking. I believe that if I had surrounded myself only with leaders in nursing, I would not have developed the ability and skills to communicate and gain trust of others working in the complex environments in which we all find ourselves in health care. This can be quite a fearful area to challenge. For example, I had always wondered how I, as a young nurse leader, could ever disagree or challenge the thoughts of a physician. Did I have the right to comment on the practice of other discipline's team members?

Take Time to Reflect

Leaders have always encouraged me to reflect upon these situations. If I, as a mentor, must challenge others, I must ensure I always view the current situation through the lenses of my patients. This means that you should address the issue at hand by asking, "What is in the best interest of your patients?" This question is always my guiding principle for difficult situations in which, and for which, I don't initially see the path forward. To date, it has served me well and has been one of the most powerful tools that established nursing leaders gave me.

Establishing your guiding principles does not always provide you with all you need to challenge systems and individuals. How many times have you heard comments similar to *you have not been around long enough to understand the full picture, you don't have enough experience, we have tried that before,* and *this is the way we have always done it.* These types of statements are demeaning and often leave you feeling frustrated. I have learned to use these situations by leveraging the energy from my frustration to walk that fine line that pushes me out of my comfort zone toward action. A mentor of mine who I often turn to when deciding how close I am willing to walk to that line advised me to remember to take a step back and decide whether this is the hill I am willing to die on. Interestingly enough, when I am at the point of asking myself this question, the answer is usually, "Yes!"

Self-Reflective Questions

1. What is your leadership philosophy?

2. What is the interconnectedness between your philosophy and the actions that it generates?

3. How would you describe yourself? As making different choices, not quite fitting in, and playing outside the standard rulebook?

4. How would others describe you? Is this description similar or different from your description above?

5. How comfortable are you at taking huge leaps of faith into the unknown? Why?

6. How well do you tolerate ambiguity in any given situation?

7. Who is a mentor/role model in your life that demonstrates the traits outlined in this chapter?

8. What do you need to make sure that you provide opportunities for others to provide constructive criticism and feedback in a supportive and nurturing way?

9. How does your organization allow you to take risks and leaps of faith? Are you supported when you fail?

10. What is the lens through which you view the world or that helps guide your decision making? How close to the line are you willing to walk?

Presentation: Personal and Public

72

"Two roads diverged in a wood, and I took the one less traveled by, and that has made all the difference."

—Robert Frost

Mentor
Lourdes Casao Salandanan, MSN, RN-BC, FNP
Director of Education Department at Citrus Valley Medical Center
Covina, California, USA

Mentee
Maria Aurora Rebultan-Suarez, BSN, RN, CCRN
From the Philippines and now practicing as a Nurse Educator at Citrus Valley Medical Center
Covina, California, USA

I remember how excited I (Lourdes) was when I was hired into the role of nurse educator at Citrus Valley Medical Center in Covina, California. I had 10 years of experience as a clinical nurse in the adult critical care services, and felt that I could make a difference as an educator. I also remember how surprised some of my associates were when they realized that I had made the decision to step away from my specialty and into nursing education. I received my fair share of criticism about my decision. Sadly, much of the criticism came from Filipino nurses.

I recall several individuals commenting on how boring nursing education was. I also recall nurses saying the first department an organization eliminates during a financial crisis is the education department, and I should stay at the bedside where my position would always be safe. Amidst the skepticism and criticism that my Filipino colleagues provided, I still decided to take this path. I felt it was a calling and knew that I would be satisfied with my career choice.

The Road Less Traveled

One of the greatest surprises I had was when I walked into my first health care educator's meeting. The meeting room was filled with San Gabriel Valley educators from both academia and service. To my surprise, I was the only educator who was both a Filipino and in her early 30s. I immediately thought of Robert Frost's poem about the road less traveled. My thoughts later were of my Filipino colleagues who criticized my career choice. Perhaps they had already decided to take the well-traveled road. Perhaps they thought that nursing education was not a road that Filipino nurses usually took, and neither they nor I should be the first ones to take it. I thought of Robert Frost's poem again. Because I had already taken the road less traveled, I decided I should also make a conscious effort to make a difference on my journey.

My Road

I strive to make our education department more visible and accessible to staff members. Our team members ndeavor to develop and present educational offerings that are both entertaining and enlightening, thus increasing program participation and attendance. Our team members promote our services and represent the commitment we have toward professional growth and our organization's mission. In the beginning, I speculated that our nursing staff, many of whom are Filipino, believed that nursing education was not a career option for them. I thus made extra efforts to engage staff members into the processes and programs we have in our department. In so doing, we promoted nursing education as a viable career choice for all staff members, including the Filipino nurses. In our zeal to engage staff members, we came upon Maria Aurora Rebultan-Suarez.

Although Maria and I had both worked in critical care services, I never had the opportunity to work closely with her before she became our nurse educator. She had just transferred to the coronary care unit when I was preparing to transfer to the education department, but I knew of her. She was well respected by her colleagues. Many of her colleagues commented on the self-motivation and the professionalism she consistently displayed. I was not surprised when one of our educators gave her a brilliant recommendation for the position of nurse educator. By this time, I was the director of the education department and the responsibility to interview and eventually hire Maria was mine.

When I interviewed her for the position, I immediately saw her willingness to learn a new craft and her commitment to excellence. I have now worked alongside Maria for more than four years and have had the privilege of watching her grow into the nurse educator and professional she is today. I was delighted when she received two awards in 2008: the Excellence in Education Award from the Iota Sigma Chapter of Sigma Theta Tau International and the Nurse of the Year Award from Citrus Valley Medical Center. It is an honor to know that I influenced who she is today.

Mentee (Maria)

"Begin with the end in mind." I think this statement encompasses everything that Lourdes has shown me on our mentorship journey. A continuing education offering does not start with the speaker's presentation; it begins way before that. I witnessed this during our Annual Citrus Valley Health Partners Critical Care Symposium where tedious efforts are taken in preparation for the day. I vividly remember when Lourdes called me in her office the day before one of our events and said, "Our emcee cannot make it tomorrow. I will have to cover for her, and I need you to coordinate the event in the background." I was terrified, but at the same time honored to take on the challenge. We were expecting 310 critical care nurses at the event. She gave me the list of details to manage, including the key people to contact for technical concerns. She also instructed me to make sure that bathrooms were clean before the breaks and that the water pitchers were replenished during break time. Although the symposium was held in a prominent hotel, Lourdes was concerned about the small details to ensure the program ran smoothly and ultimately satisfied the participants.

Looking back, Lourdes taught me two phases that need to be addressed to ensure a successful presentation:

- **Preparation of the venue:** Follows the adult learning principles— refreshments; room temperature; clean, functioning restrooms; and comfortable chairs and tables.

- **Preparation of self:** Includes master the contents of your presentation; practice; know and understand that you possess information that others do not have; and build your confidence with the knowledge that you prepared your venue and yourself.

Other key strategies that I have observed in working with Lourdes during her presentations include

- Dress professionally because this gives the speaker a sense of confidence and leaves a strong impression on the audience.

- Pause and wait for responses to questions addressed to the participants.

- Walk around the room and engage participants in the discussion.

- Gracefully move from a topic a participant is lingering on.

- Return to unresolved issues after the program and send follow-up notices to participants if necessary.

One of the struggles I have in presentations is the use of English as a medium. My struggle may not be apparent to English speakers, but when conversing in English, I have to translate my Tagalog thoughts in my mind before actually speaking in English. In some cases, this might be a blessing in disguise; but in public speaking, it sometimes results in "ums" and "ahs" that are distracting to the audience. Lourdes recognized this during the early stages of my presentation skills development. She referred me to an article titled, "Are You the Invisible Employee?" I've kept a copy of the article to this very day, occasionally referring to it to make sure I am not slowly slipping back to my old habits.

Lourdes further guided me to improve my presentation skills when we were invited to facilitate our organization's customer service program, Class ACT (Attitude, Courtesy, Teamwork). In preparation for the program, Lourdes coached several other educators and directors with presentation skills. Seeing her apply the techniques that she has taught me throughout the 4 years that I have worked with her reaffirmed how effective they are.

I realize that I have chosen a lengthy and fulfilling career path. I am glad my mentor has equipped me with principles that I can apply throughout my journey. After all, she always begins with the end goal in mind.

Lourdes' Conclusion

Nursing education—oral presentations, in particular—can be frightening to many people. There is a universal fear of public speaking that is not limited to those of us who speak English as a second language. The mastery of presentation skills is important to all of us who wish to either excel or advance in our career paths. I have several challenges for all nurse leaders: master your personal presentation skills, test your presentation skills in other countries, and mentor someone along the way.

While meeting the challenges, you will witness your continuous growth and enjoy the satisfaction of seeing others grow with you.

Self-Reflective Questions

1. How can you train yourself to maintain eye contact at all times?

2. How can you better "hear" what people are saying to you?

3. How do you provide undivided attention?

4. How can you better listen with facial and body expressions thay portray interest, acceptance, and value?

5. How can you condition yourself to form your response or opinion only *after* "hearing" what is said?

6. How can you train yourself to listen in group environments with the same attributes as in one-on-one conversation?

7. What are ways to request feedback from peer and staff on how you listen with purpose?

8. What are ways to seek help from a speaker if you are unclear about the message?

9. How can you mentor staff on the importance of listening with the purpose of "hearing and learning?"

10. How would colleagues consider you as a role model for listening with the purpose of "hearing?"

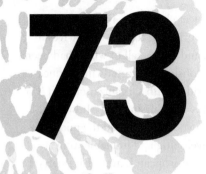

73

Program Project Management

"Of all the things I've done, the most vital is coordinating the talents of those who work for us and pointing them toward a certain goal."

—Walt Disney

Mentor
Valerie Fleming, RN,
  RM, MA, PhD
Professor and Head of
  Division, Women's and
  Children's Health
Glasgow Caledonian
  University
Scotland

Mentee
Teja Zaksek, RM, Msc Midwifery,
  BSc (rad)
Head of Teaching and Learn-
  ing, Midwifery Department
University of Ljubljana,
  Ljubljana, Slovenia

The International Confederation of Midwives' Young Midwifery Leaders' Programme began in April 2003. The goal of this prestigious program was to create a small group of midwives, intensively educated in leadership skills, who can network at national and international levels and have a good understanding of current and emerging issues in women's and reproductive health. Those who complete the program can act as role models and disseminate what they learned.

Invited to become a mentor in the program in 2003, I was honored to join a small group of six mentor/mentee pairs from around the world. Although the initial program covered aspects common to all leadership roles, the major part of the program focused on a project designed by and led by the mentees under the guidance of their respective (and at times, the other) mentors.

In this chapter, we outline the ambitious project chosen by Teja and how that project was managed. This project involved bringing together midwives in three countries—Croatia, Bosnia Herzegovina, and Serbia, all of which had been at war with each other in the recent past—to reconsider their midwifery education programs. As Secretary General of the World Health Organization (WHO) Global Network of WHO Collaborating Centres for Nursing and Midwifery, I was leading a three-year project in nearby Kosovo when I joined the midwives confederation. The Kosovo project involved developing and implementing a three-year program for nursing and midwifery to European Union (EU) standards (EU, 2005). Some of the lessons learned from that experience, as well as data collected for a WHO Europe project (Fleming & Holmes, 2004), were applicable to the midwives project, along with the negotiating, networking, and advocacy skills learned by the mentees during the first 18 months of the program.

The Project and the Rationale

The approach to do something for midwives in Bosnia first came from a midwife in a small town who had been instrumental in setting up a woman-centered birth center. She believed the next step should be to ensure better education for midwives throughout the country. Rather than repeat the Kosovo experience, I suggested to Teja that she might consider something a bit wider for her project.

My mentee and I decided to establish an education system in Bosnia that would provide midwifery education to the bachelor's degree level. Our intent was to offer 30 midwives of Bosnia who have a diploma from higher-level medical colleges the opportunity to build upon their existing qualifications and study for a BSc in Glasgow Caledonian University in collaboration with the University of Ljubljana. This opportunity would allow midwives from Bosnia not just to participate in interventions, treatments, and procedures directed by the physicians (as they do now), and also to offer an individual, holistic approach to pregnant women and new mothers and their families.

Slovenia (where I, Valerie, am from) and Bosnia were once part of the same country. In 1991, Slovenia was the first country that with 10 days' war gained independence from Yugoslavia. Croatia and Bosnia followed. Bosnia had a most devastating war, perhaps because Bosnia is very culturally and ethnically diverse. At the end of the war, the Dayton Agreement was signed, which split Bosnia into two provinces—the Federation of Bosnia and Herzegovina (BH), and the Bosnian Serb Republic—as well as a special area called the Brčko District, which was too diverse to join any of the provinces. The Federation of BH now has a complex set of ministries with no clear picture of their roles.

Project Process

I knew that careful selection of partners in this project was of great importance. First, we needed to decide on a local coordinator to act as program organizer and liaison between project leaders, midwives, higher education institutions, midwifery associations, and other relevant bodies. Our initial contact organized and led a meeting in Sarajevo. She invited midwives from all districts in Bosnia, and representatives from the newly established Association of Bosnian Midwives also attended. In the meeting, we identified the partners who needed to be involved and agreed on the core principles for the project. The meeting attracted considerable publicity, and we presented the project on prime-time television news.

We also assessed the commitment of the Bosnian midwives by contacting one of the two government chief nursing officers and Sarajevo cantonal Ministry of Health, both of whom gave positive feedback and support. Partnership was not formalized, but appropriate objectives were set. Approximately six months after the meeting in Sarajevo, I was contacted by the Croatian and Serbian midwives who also wanted to take part in this project. My mentee and I held a meeting in Zagreb, and invited key people from Serbia as well as Bosnia and Croatia. At that stage, we appointed local coordinators for each of the countries. The task of the local coordinators was to establish a link between the universities, midwifery associations, and the project team.

Miller et al. (2008) recognize that the more stakeholders involved, the greater the levels of complexity for decision makers who have to try to satisfy a number of often-conflicting interests. We expected this with our stakeholders because it is often thought that countries once at war with each other are unlikely to collaborate without hesitation. However, this potential problem was openly discussed at a meeting, and we were assured by all that it was not a problem. A good example of collaboration between these countries would increase the possibilities for EU funding from one of their core budgets.

Progress

It soon became evident that the midwives acting as local coordinators did not have the right contacts with the universities to ensure their involvement. I tried to contact universities later, but got little response. This might take a while, we realised, because these universities are preparing midwifery programs by themselves or because they do not intend to collaborate with each other. Perhaps it was too much done too quickly, or perhaps it was too demanding of a job for the local coordinators to act as advocate agents.

I also think now that many midwives lack the skills needed to encourage policy change among government officials, health system administrators and personnel, and other decision makers, and that perhaps the expectations on our local coordinators were too high. With this insight it would have been more useful for the approach to have been made concurrently to both senior midwives and university deans to have ensured the engagement of all stakeholders.

Preparation for Change

During the preparation of this project, Teja gained a considerable amount of confidence and competence in dealing with high-level personnel in the midwifery world, ministries of health, and education and universities. There were many negative moments, but every time we believe that this project will not materialize, a positive step is taken. We have every confidence that although we are not yet reporting on a completed project, with time and continued effort, we will eventually be able to launch the project because the program has equipped Teja with the knowledge and skills, as well as support, to advocate for policy change.

The Mentee's Perspective

The project was conducted in the last year of Young Midwifery Leaders' Programme. The program changed me a lot, mostly in the last year when I worked closely with my mentor on this project. I well remember the first meeting with high-level midwifery educational personnel: I had no confidence to speak, and my mentor had to take over the conversation. At the last meeting, though, I confidently led the discussion. During this project, I have developed a broader understanding of current and emerging issues and respect for different cultures, thinking, and ways of conducting practices. I have also been able to share the experiences with fellow mentees and other regional nursing and midwifery leaders, and, through conference presentations and publications in local, regional, and international journals.

Self-Reflective Questions

1. What do you suspect could have been done to improve this project?

2. What problems have you encountered that are solvable?

3. How can you present yourself well when meeting people for the first time?

4. How can you differentiate priorities as well as short- and long-term needs?

5. How do you use your leadership ability to gain support for what initially has strong opposition?

6. How have your values and beliefs influenced your relationships with others?

7. In a work experience where you had to work closely with others, how did you overcome difficulties?

8. What are the ways that you could become involved in a project such as this in the future?

9. What would you do differently from the authors of this chapter?

10. How would such an experience aid you in the future?

Public Policy, Health Care Reform, and Legislation

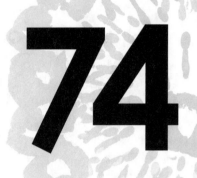

74

"One of the messages of nursing caring theory today is a call for the restoration of basic values, commitment, and informed moral action that leads to social and political action."

—Jean Watson

Mentor
Joyce C. Clifford, PhD, RN, FAAN
President, CEO, and Founder of The Institute for Nursing Healthcare Leadership
Boston, Massachusetts, USA

Mentee
Stephanie Wilkie Ahmed, DNP, FNP-BC
Associate, The Institute for Nursing Healthcare Leadership
Boston, Massachusetts, USA

At its most basic level, leadership is a process through which people, systems, or organizations may be influenced to accomplish specific objectives. While leadership, is an expectation of the C-suite members (the executive staff of an organization including the chief nursing officer) there should be no question that whether at the patient's side or in the board room, all nurses need to demonstrate leadership to effect meaningful change within the organization as well as for the greater health care system. Leadership occurs at all levels of an organization and no matter the organizational position held, every nurse has an obligation to engage in acts that demonstrate leadership. An integral component of leadership is the art of mentorship, which may be described as a developmental relationship that forms between an experienced individual, the mentor, and a person usually of less experience—known as the mentee. From such an exchange, both parties derive meaning, as was the case when a mentoring relationship blossomed between a well-established national nursing leader often described as the architect of the professional nursing practice model (Joyce Clifford), and myself, a nurse practitioner (NP) enrolled in a doctor of nursing practice program.

Nurse Practitioners and Change: The Mentee

Striving to define the organizational structure necessary to optimize NP practice in an academic medical center, this relationship afforded me the opportunity to gain a better understanding of organizational frameworks that support practice, and the opportunity to explore the inter-relatedness of this topic with those of broader national agendas including physician shortages, the national need for health care reform, and the role of the nurse practitioner within such a movement.

Through the mentoring relationship I established with Joyce, I was able to discuss my concerns about the limitations some NPs face in organizations. In such settings, the opportunity for individual nurses to identify a means by which they can influence practice in a way that impacts broader health care agendas, including health care reform, is at risk of being overlooked. How do actions in the clinical environment translate to what is happening in our communities? How can the individual nurse practitioner create a broader meaning for practice?

The Nurse Practitioner Political Role

These areas initially became central to many of our mentoring discussions because of high legislative interest in our state to mandate staffing ratios for nurses. The actions taken by nursing and health care organizations as well as those of the state legislative body brought public policy to the forefront as an area in which nurses need to become informed. This is due in part to the eventual impact on their practice and ultimately on the patient and family. In addition, this was the time of the presidential election in the United States, guaranteeing that a new administration would be elected to lead the country. Once again, it was apparent that health reform, a central part of each of the presidential candidates' agenda for the future, could have a strong impact on the role of nurses and the way their practice might be shaped as a result of change. Thus, the interest in public policy was reinforced as a major discussion in this mentoring relationship.

When possible, I was invited to attend the same meetings where Joyce would be speaking, furthering the opportunities to advance the public policy discussions. Exposure to policy makers who were not necessarily well versed on some aspects of the health care system became a strong learning experience for me as I recognized the opportunities that existed to educate those involved in drafting and moving forward legislative policy.

In light of the change in administration in the USA, there has been much hope that health care reform will take place as well. Access to care for example, has been a pressing problem for generations and a growing physician shortage in primary care has evolved from policies instituted over recent years. Understanding how national policy changes, such as reducing resident work hours, impacts at the local level of practice as well as at the national level, is an example of understanding the relationship of practice and policy. Essential to the leadership role is developing a greater appreciation of how nurse leaders affect change in policy by becoming influential as a result of their competence, communication, and collaborative skills, as well as through their advocacy skills.

The moral obligation of the nurse to serve as the patient advocate is inextricably woven into the fabric of the nursing profession. Transforming that obligation from the locus of the bedside to include the broader arena of health care reform, including legislative and policy development activities that address how resources are accessed and allocated, require that nurses re-engage with their roots in social justice. Promoting collaborative relationships between physicians and nurse practitioners will create a foundation upon which we can collectively begin to address the broader issues that affect the health care system and establish a spirit of inter-disciplinary teamwork. Participation in professional organizations to move an agenda for the development of competency based standards for credentialing and scope of practice can be effective in ensuring quality and safety. With respect to political action, NPs can lobby for legislation that revises restrictive nurse-practice acts that limit professional scope of practice, particularly in the areas of prescriptive authority, reimbursement for services, and mandated physician oversight.

The Mentor Role

Making a commitment to the next generation of nurse leaders is the role of all nurse professionals, especially those of us who have been afforded many opportunities to lead and make change. As the mentor in this relationship, I became aware once again of how narrowly leadership, policy, and politics can be defined. As indicated earlier, leadership should not be confined only to those who have organizational titles of "leader," but must become an inherent part of the professional's being. When this occurs, the "Ah-Ha" moments are experienced in many different ways. My own experience suggests that understanding the importance of gaining organizational influence often leads nurses to become active in community and professional advocacy. In this mentoring relationship, my mentee had already experienced some success in community activities not directly related to her work. Our relationship and discussions brought to the mentee a greater understanding of the connection of her external community work together with the organizational and professional responsibilities she holds. For me, as the mentor, one outcome of this mentoring interaction included an opportunity to gain insight from a practicing nurse practitioner of the current issues, practice barriers, and successful outcomes experienced.

Self-Reflective Questions

1. How is leadership connected to your work?

2. What qualities would you want to have in a mentor?

3. Where do you believe that politics takes place?

4. What are the special activities that you feel nurses should engage in to influence policy development and politics?

5. What are some methods you use to keep up with the broader issues of the health care system?

6. How can nurse practitioners create broader meaning for their practice beyond the exam room?

7. What are the global issues that impair the ability of the nurse practitioner to meet patient care needs—and how can meaningful change be created to improve in these areas?

8. How can activities with professional organizations strengthen our cause and our ability to serve our patients better?

9. How can we strengthen the role and the next generation of nurse practitioners, specifically through mentorship, scholarship, and preceptorship?

10. How can we strengthen the nurse practitioner role organizationally and politically?

Qualities of Leadership: Career Planning

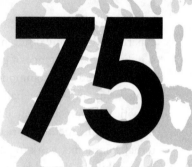

75

"I can invest in moderate potential and make a difference. But I can invest in strong potential and make a miracle."

—Gail Wolf

Mentor

Gail A. Wolf, RN, DNS, FAAN
Clinical Professor at the
   University of Pittsburgh School
   of Nursing
Pittsburgh, Pennsylvania, USA

Mentee

Anu Thomas, RN, BSN
Student in the MSN Administra-
   tion & Leadership Program,
   University of Pittsburgh
Pittsburgh, Pennsylvania, USA
   (from India)

As a nursing leader for more than 30 years, and now as a professor teaching nursing leadership, I am always searching for "leadership gems"— those bright, shiny, energetic souls who have what it takes to serve as pathfinders for our profession. I believe it is our job as experienced leaders to help nurture and develop them, for they are rare. Developing a leader does not happen by accident, nor is it easy. Given limited time and energy, I have found my efforts bear fruit if the person I am developing has three essential qualities:

- *Hardiness*: being committed, seeing problems as challenges, taking responsibility for successes as well as failures.

- *Motivation*: being willing to learn and not letting obstacles defeat you.

- *Insight*: learning from mistakes and seeking self-understanding.

My mentee, Anu Thomas, has all three. Listen to her story, and you will see what I mean:

1999 was an eventful, foundational year for my career. In India, nurses often do not have as many financial and professional growth opportunities as those in other careers. However, I felt that in nursing, I had found my true calling. I remember when my father heard my decision, he asked me, "Are you sure you want to do nursing? It is a tough job, and we don't have any nurses in this family." My unexpected answer, "If I walk in another person's tracks, I will leave no footprints of my own," silenced the room. After a few more discussions, my parents supported my decision. I went on to join one of the oldest and finest universities in India to complete my bachelor of science in nursing.

2003 was also a decisive year, and a significant turning point in my career. During my interaction with a college alumna, I realized that better prospects for nursing existed in the United States (U.S.). I was determined, and with my sights firmly set on transitioning to the U.S., I juggled my full-time job, studying for three international qualifying exams, and completing all the necessary procedural requirements.

My first year as a nurse in the U.S. was both exciting and trying. I was becoming familiar with a new country, attempting to understand a diverse culture, and learning to practice in a very different health care environment. The desire to do my best, made me eager for greater responsibilities. In time, my hard work and enthusiasm paid off, and I was recognized as a diligent and valuable employee.

Spring 2007 presented a great educational opportunity for me. I realized that nurses needed to take a much more dominant leadership role to meet the challenges of health care for the future. Additionally, I came to believe that the future of health care lies in education and empowering nurses for evidence-based practice. Therefore, I embarked on a quest for a master of science in nursing degree in administration and leadership.

I take great pride in the journey I began 9 years ago. At present, as an RN in one of the most prestigious hospitals in the U.S., I am a confident team player and a leader. In addition to performing my core functions and taking care of patients, as a charge nurse I am also responsible for taking a leadership role, managing resources, and handling tough situations.

I have benefited greatly from the depth of knowledge my esteemed teachers have helped me build. The interaction in my classes and the wealth of experience of the nurses has provided many perspectives from a diverse set of people. Learning from them has inspired me to continuously strive to improve personally and professionally.

My journey has just begun; I still have miles to go. The knowledge I gain from the wisdom of my nursing leaders and my efforts will provide me the necessary tools to make the journey—expanding my horizons, helping me learn, inspiring me to make a difference—and maybe someday to make my own footprints.

Core Elements of Leadership

Hardiness, motivation, and insight are the core elements of leadership. They are difficult, if not impossible, to teach. For example, the hardiness Anu demonstrated in overcoming the challenges of multiple qualifying exams and moving to a new country where she knew no one speaks to her commitment to achieve her goals and not let obstacles get in her way. Her motivation to become an excellent practitioner led her to take a job in a major academic medical center where the expectations and challenges go beyond the norm. Her insight in recognizing that she needed additional knowledge in order to be as good as she could possibly be led her back for her master's degree. With these characteristics in place, providing Anu with the knowledge, skills, and competencies needed to become a nursing leader became easy. With experience, learning, and coaching, Anu's passion and willingness to do whatever it takes will continue to amaze. Watch for her footsteps.

Self-Reflective Questions

1. Do I have a focused goal that I want to accomplish? If so, what is it? If not, spend time thinking about developing a focused goal.

2. Do I have a strategy for accomplishing that goal? If so, what is that strategy?

3. What are the ways I can overcome obstacles in the way of achieving my goal?

4. How can I overcome disappointments and keep going?

5. How hard am I willing to work to accomplish my dream?

6. What are my strengths and weaknesses?

7. Am I able to learn from my mistakes? Think about at least one instance of a mistake that presents you with a valuable learning experience.

8. How can I maximize my strengths and minimize my weaknesses?

9. Who is my mentor or coach that can help me?

10. How can I best capitalize on my mentor or coach's tutelage and best put his or her recommendations into action?

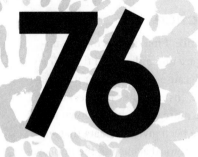

76

(In Pursuit of) Quality Outcomes

"Let's face it, pursuit of quality outcomes is consuming a significant amount of hospital resources and showing no sign of slowing."

—Cindy Rohman

Mentor
Carol A. Reineck, PhD, FAAN, NEA-BC
Chair and Associate Professor, Department of Acute Nursing Care, and the Amy Shelton and V.H. McNutt Professor
University of Texas Health Science Center
San Antonio, Texas, USA

Mentee
Charles C. Reed, MSN, RN, CNRN
Patient Care Coordinator for the Surgical Trauma Intensive Care Unit
University Hospital
San Antonio, Texas, USA

Improving patient outcomes by process improvement to bring evidence into practice can be painstaking and lengthy. Girard (2009, p. 299) stated that "Although there are various methods used in quality improvement, one of the most common methods is a process that plans, collects data, analyzes the findings, evaluates the outcomes and acts to implement a new or revised tool or procedure." This lengthy process is especially the case when you take into consideration that improvements require collaboration among the nurse, patient, physician, and sometimes the entire health care organization. What issues surround changing clinical practice toward improving patient outcomes? In this chapter, we share insights gathered in dialogue between Carol Reineck as mentor from academe, and Charles Reed as mentee from expert clinical leadership practice.

Challenges of Changing Practice

Various factors affect the ability to change practice. First, nurses may be unwilling to adopt practice changes because they are unfamiliar with them or have received little or no education on them. Because of insufficient information, they may not see the value in the initiative. Instead, they may feel the initiative increases their workload or is just one more thing driven down from management. Additionally, staff may never have been given the data that support the change nor informed of progress made toward achieving the improvement goal.

Second, physicians often lack the time and/or the desire to participate in the development and implementation of an initiative if it is not of perceived value. In some cases, the initiative may be viewed simply as a process to improve regulatory compliance rather than a substantial improvement to patient outcomes. Personal preferences, beliefs, and current literature may influence their decision making.

Third, although patients desire the best outcomes possible and are typically willing to cooperate, the disease process or other physiological issues may be a challenge. Let's look at the example of a patient in the ICU who is receiving mechanical ventilation after a motor vehicle collision. Evidence supports a number of initiatives to reduce the incidence of ventilator-associated pneumonia such as elevating the head of the bed 30 degrees.

Depending on the size of the patient, injuries, and neurological status, elevating him or her to a 30-degree angle may not be easy. The patient may become restless and slide down in bed, requiring the busy nurse to pull the patient back up in bed, just to have the patient slide back down again. This can become frustrating and physically draining. Although the nurse knows the literature supports elevating the head of the bed, the perceived lack of patient cooperation, along with other factors such as fatigue, may reduce the nurse's enthusiasm to ensure compliance.

The 4 Cs of Process Improvement

Four crucial insights have emerged for successful implementation of process improvement. These concepts are

1. **Champions:** Individuals willing to own the process and put in the extra effort needed to bring about change.

2. **Communication:** Dissemination of information by any method (verbal, e-mail, bulletin board) toward the goal of understanding.

3. **Collection:** Systematic method of obtaining and compiling data.

4. **Comparisons:** Examining how the data relate to benchmarks.

Champions

The primary champions should not be the hospital administrators. Successful implementation means champions at the front line. The empowered nurses driving change at the bedside, for example. Of course, there will always be those who hold out, or do not become invested in the process. Remember it only takes a few champions to make a project successful.

Communication

Communication is not only the exchange of information but also the means to achieve an understanding of the whys and hows of the initiative. Poor communication and lack of understanding lead to poor adherence, lack of commitment, and failure of the program. Champions are key to communicating the importance of the initiative to the frontline staff to ensure the new practice becomes ingrained into the workflow. Having staff speak to other staff regarding quality initiatives is important because it helps to demonstrate that staff understand the process as well as indicate ownership and support of the initiative. Moreover, regulators no longer are interested in talking to administrators or managers; they want the bedside staff to be able to explain the processes. Therefore, because nurse and physician positions change, on-going education and communication is also imperative. In communicating with a diverse group of people of varying education levels and of different generations, data can be posted in the break room on bulletin boards, graphs e-mailed to the staff, and information can be shared verbally on rounds and in staff meetings.

Collection

Collecting data before and/or after the process improvement can be challenging and time consuming. Transparency—that is, letting staff know the nature of and reasons for the process improvement effort—may not be part of the culture. Therefore, access to data may be limited to managers and executives. A lack of an electronic medical record, budgetary restraints, manual collection, and few available personnel may further hamper data collection. However, if manual collection of data is the only option, inter-rater reliability should be estimated to ensure accuracy of the data. Timely reporting of data is crucial. End of month reports only tell practitioners where they have been. Real time data allow the clinicians as well as managers the ability to influence the care and outcomes of patients in the unit *now* versus telling us what happened last month.

Comparisons

Comparing our outcomes with others demonstrates success and highlights opportunities for improvement. However, teams may not always be able to compare themselves against other organizations. Appropriate benchmarks may not even exist. In these situations, a hospital in a multi-hospital system may try to compare itself against others in the system. A single hospital may compare data from one unit to another or a single unit may only be able to compare the before and after results across time.

A Process Improvement Case Study

One example of such a clinical practice improvement is achieving tight glycemic control (TGC) (Malesker, Foral, McPhillips, Christensen, Chang, & Hilleman, 2007). Tight glycemic control is the vigilant observation and management of glucose levels. Researchers are still studying how "tight" control should be. Although TGC in ICU patients has been reported to decrease morbidity and mortality, other studies have shown that glycemic control can be too "tight," causing hypoglycemic episodes (Solylemez Wiener, Wiener, Larson, 2008). It is important to carefully look at national standards, for example, the consensus statement from the American Association of Clinical Endocrinologists and American Diabetes Association (Moghissi, 2009), when determining controls goals.

As glycemic control (GC) has been more closely analyzed as a standard of care in ICUs, nurses and physicians find it challenging to implement this into practice successfully. Champions, communication, collection, and comparisons will be described to illustrate this process improvement. The term TGC will be used because that was the focus of the original project.

When the Surgical Trauma Intensive Care Unit (STICU) at an academic medical center first started working on TGC, there was minimal initial success. Implementing TGC meant something different to everyone. No protocol existed, the team had no idea what the base line data were, and the commitment to implement TGC varied based on the doctor and the nurse.

When the team organized faculty, physicians, nurses, unit management, and pharmacy champions to support the initiative, the team was able to make progress. Champions made the process improvement move forward through their collective, focused efforts. The team was dedicated to applying the evidence about the benefits of TGC. One nurse team member suggested that the 4 Cs would be a useful framework to drive the evidence into practice and provided guidance. The team met weekly, communicated the agreed upon target range for blood glucose to the staff, and developed the protocols and order sets. Constant communication with and education of the nurses and physicians were required in order to achieve the improvement goals. Over time, the number of champions increased. Effort necessary to sustain the initiative decreased.

However, it wasn't until the TGC team went from end of the month data collection reports to daily access to the data that the team of champions made the most substantial improvement in the new program. Access to real-time data allowed the team to make changes to treatment. Additionally, the software program that afforded the team access to real-time data also provided the mechanism for data comparison over time and across units. This feature allowed the unit to track improvement efforts over time and comparison data of other units.

The champions provided the leadership and vision for the improvement in TGC practices. The team communicated on an intentional basis, to provide the guidance and information needed. Data collection made it possible for staff to see the effects of their changes in real time, making a positive change for patient care in the STICU. Finally, comparing data with benchmarks allowed patterns to emerge and further improvements to be planned.

Mentee Reflections

I was fortunate during my graduate studies to have Dr. Reineck as my instructor, advisor, and mentor and now as my colleague and friend. It was through this relationship that I was able to become successful. Dr. Reineck offered support and insight when I was faced with challenges I had never dealt with. She offered encouragement and enthusiasm—characteristics so valuable to a mentee—when I felt overwhelmed attempting to implement a hospital-wide project.

During a subsequent project, and in my effort to improve communication between ventilated patients and health care workers, Dr. Reineck mentored me through the process of developing, designing, and piloting a research study that examined perceptions of communication in the ICU between the patient and nursing staff. Specific mentoring behaviors were active listening, directing me to resources, and helping me realize I had been working at a higher plane, with health system-level concepts including accreditation standards and workforce empowerment. Finally, Dr. Reineck helped me with the dissemination of findings. She helped me prepare abstracts for my project, titled, "Effects of communication techniques in a STICU unit with mechanically ventilated patients." I presented at the American Association of Critical-Care Nurses' National Teaching Institute; a manuscript has been accepted for publication; and I presented this work for our local Delta Alpha Chapter of Sigma Theta Tau International and at my own hospital, University Hospital.

Clinical practice improves patient outcomes if systematic processes are employed. A mentoring relationship optimizes the liklihood that the processes will be sustained and will lead to professional growth.

Self-Reflective Questions

1. Have you identified the specific clinical practice that will be changed to improve patient outcomes?

2. Are champions identified and ready?

3. Do the champions represent all involved professions?

4. Are communication efforts aimed at explaining not only the *what*, but also the *why* and *how*?

5. Are communication modes diverse to match varied learning styles?

6. Are data collected in real-time as well as retrospectively?

7. Have champions displayed data where staff can readily access and understand?

8. If data were collected manually, were inter-rater reliability techniques present to ensure data can be trusted?

9. When comparing the data, were the comparisons based on like populations in like facilities?

10. If no comparison unit is available, can comparisons be made across time?

77

Reciprocal and Supportive Mentoring

"Nursing in contemporary health care systems faces many barriers; yet in these challenging times, there are many opportunities. . . . Investing in an effective mentoring relationship is crucial in supporting nursing leadership."

—Patricia M. Davidson

Mentor

John Daly, RN, PhD, FRCNA
Dean and Professor, Faculty of
  Nursing, Midwifery & Health
University of Technology
Sydney, New South Wales,
  Australia

Mentee

Patricia M. Davidson, RN, PhD,
  FRCNA
Professor and Director of the
  Centre Cardiovascular and
  Chronic Care Research
Curtin University of Technology
Sydney, New South Wales,
  Australia

Good and effective leadership is a prized commodity in contemporary organizations and a resource that is often in short supply. The issues facing societies globally underscore the importance of leadership in focusing on a shared vision. This poses leadership capacity building challenges for many areas of industry, from academic settings to health care and the broader world of business. We need to grow new leaders if organizations are to maximise and sustain their performance. Leaders play a critical role in setting the pace and establishing a values-based vision and agenda in an organization (Daly, Speedy, & Jackson, 2004; Heifetz, 1994; Kouzes & Posner, 2002). They are able to influence its direction in profound and meaningful ways (Cummings, Lee, MacGregor, Davey, Wong, & Paul, 2008). In many instances where organizations are challenged to change and adapt, leadership is crucial to the success of organizations in achieving their goals.

Many sources in the literature note the complexity of leadership as a construct underscoring the multifaceted elements. Cummings et al., note that, "although leadership has been conceptualized in many ways in the literature, the following elements are central to the definition of leadership: leadership (a) is a process; (b) entails influence; (c) occurs within a group setting or context; and (d) involves achieving goals that reflect a common vision (Cummings et al., 2008, p. 240).

In the complex world of nursing and health care, leadership is often regarded as an ingredient that can influence quality of care in positive ways (Davidson, Elliott & Daly, 2006; Firth-Cozens & Mowbray, 2001). "Effective nursing leadership provides guidance for solving complex problems related to nursing care delivery. Nurse leaders create structure, implement processes for nursing care, and facilitate positive outcomes" (Cummings et al., 2008, p. 241). Hence, the challenges of leadership are great. It is also important to note that these positive outcomes are not only for patients and their families but for organizations and the nursing profession as well.

In the leadership journey, the process of learning and growth can be greatly enhanced through effective partnerships that are guided by mentorship principles. Developing effective mentoring relationships cannot be dependent upon a chance encounter. As in most successful undertakings, they require planning, structure, reflection, and evaluation. Working together to achieve a common goal and understanding is dependent on honest and transparent communication and mutual respect.

Mentee Thoughts

The relationship between mentor and mentee is one of mutual respect and reciprocity. John has provided me with direction and opportunities to carve an academic career and clinical leadership role. The mentor-mentee relationship is a partnership where each party takes on roles and responsibilities where they work to achieve mutually negotiated goals. Commonly, it is about sharing information and the reflections and expertise of the mentor. This is also a relationship where individuals look beyond themselves, not only in regards to their relationship, but also to factors that influence their goals. In respect of nursing leadership, this is commonly the social, political, and cultural factors in which we work. In contemporary health and education systems, these are commonly complex and dynamic organizations where assistance, advice, and expertise are necessary to help in negotiating these challenging issues. John has provided me with sage advice, direction, and expertise. He has also empowered me and given me the inspiration and belief in myself to work toward my personal and professional goals.

In the initial stages of a mentor-mentee relationship, it is often useful to negotiate the goals and purposes of the relationship through asking the following questions:

- What are the factors you personally want to achieve from the relationship?

- What are the skills and expertise you require from the mentor?

It is also important that you value the mentor relationship and identify the boundaries and scope of the relationship. For example, it is not appropriate to ask for favours or special treatment that may place the mentor in a position of conflict of interest. Many of the values of the mentor-mentee relationship span far beyond conversation to observation and reflection of your mentor's activities and performance. Taking the time to observe the mentor in the leadership role, to reflect on the performance, and to ask pertinent questions is also a valuable and crucial step.

Undeniably, the mentoring relationship is based on trust and shared values. As a mentee, you expose your vulnerabilities and insecurities, and place trust in your mentor to respect your confidences and be both constructive and instructive. Often the mentor will tell you things you do not feel entirely comfortable with. For example, that you have been too emotionally invested in a situation. Unambiguous and direct communication is an important aspect of the mentoring relationship. Therefore, the mentoring relationship is a critical and reflective relationship where you work to achieve a desired goal. It is not about necessarily making the mentee feel better all the time. Building a trusting relationship can take time and is an investment of your time and self.

Effective mentoring relationships can span many decades and in some cases evolve into a deep and sincere friendship and mutual regard. As this evolves, it is also important to be mindful of the mentoring relationship boundaries. It is important not to take advantage of your mentor or take them for granted.

Sharing relationships, opportunities, and networks is often a product of effective mentoring. Generous mentors often experience great satisfaction from observing their mentee's achievements and growth. On reflection of both my own mentoring relationships and those of others, I recognise that generosity and an open and engaging style and spirit are the characteristics of effective mentors. Generally, those with effective and professional networks are keen to engage and bring people together to achieve influence and impact.

Constructive and enabling mentoring is crucial in leadership development. These valuable relationships allow opportunities for reflection, negotiating solutions, and sharing expertise, networks, and experiences. Sharing the highs and lows of your professional life is a key factor. Mentors and mentees alike should be committed to information sharing as well as sharing their expectations of the relationship.

I have been privileged to be in a mentoring relationship with John for many decades where each of us has carved our professional niche. I have learned considerable lessons from his astute and constructive advice. I have also taken great delight in seeing his career develop and his recognition internationally as a nurse leader. I have learned just as much from observing his career and performance as through our conversations. As a mentee, it is important to be receptive and open, to observe and critique, and to engage in self-reflection.

Nursing in contemporary health care systems faces many barriers. Yet in these challenging times, there are many opportunities. Investing in an effective mentoring relationship is crucial in supporting nursing leadership. In my experience, preparing yourself to engage in these opportunities is dependent on professional support and collegial advice. Developing an effective mentoring relationship is crucial in preparing yourself for the nursing leadership journey. Looking for and embracing opportunities is integral in leadership development.

Final Thoughts From the Mentor

We have worked together in reciprocal ways based on expertise and experience. Hence, context has required Trish and me to embrace both roles in our professional relationship. At times, I have been in the position of mentee and at other times in the position of mentor. We both have individual expertise, so roles have switched depending on the context. My professional relationship with Trish has greatly enriched my career. She is an outstanding research leader, and she has taught me to expand my research repertoire in many ways. While I am an accomplished nurse scientist and researcher, my major passion is for the challenges of academic leadership and governance. Somehow, when we engage on a project or leadership journey, an energy is created that propels us forward. This is exciting, inspiring, and sustaining. We both have a strong sense of social justice and a keen awareness of the power of good nursing—important ingredients, too. Trish is very generous in her appraisal of me. I thank her for this, and I have to say that this is consistent with her character. Our working relationship started 32 years ago. We are always there for each other, which is special.

Self-Reflective Questions

1. What roles and skills are required of a mentor?
2. What are the mutual expectations of the mentoring relationship?
3. What are the boundaries of the mentoring relationship?
4. What areas do you need to develop?
5. Where do you want your career to be in 5 years?
6. What are your strengths?
7. What are your weaknesses?
8. What specific leadership skills do you need to develop?
9. How do you assess the value of your mentoring relationship?
10. What are the strategies to ensure that the mentoring relationship is effective and productive?

Regulating Advanced Practice Nursing

78

"God grant me the serenity to accept the things I cannot change, the courage to change the things I can, and the wisdom to know the difference."

—Reinhold Niebuhr

Mentor
James L. Raper, DSN, CRNP, JD, FAANP
Associate Professor of Medicine & Nursing
Director, 1917 HIV/AIDS Outpatient, Research and Dental Clinics
University of Alabama at Birmingham
Birmingham, Alabama, USA

Mentee
Gina C. Dobbs, RN, MSN, CRNP
Certified Family Nurse Practitioner, 1917 Outpatient Clinic
University of Alabama at Birmingham
Birmingham, Alabama, USA

Regulatory and organizational standards for advanced practice nursing embody the governmental provisions to protect public safety, assure that practitioners are skilled to practice, and discipline those who are immoral and unprincipled (Poe, 2008). Oddly, the regulation of advanced practice registered nursing (APRN) practice is diverse and sometimes limits scope of practice and patient access, and also restricts APRNs' abilities to work across jurisdictions. In this chapter, we examine similarities and differences of APRN practice on the global level, explore APRN regulation, introduce the tenets of the Census Model for APRN Regulation, and consider a path toward unencumbered APRN scope of practice.

APRNs include certified registered nurse anesthetists (CRNAs), certified nurse-midwifes (CNMs), clinical nurse specialists (CNSs), and certified nurse practitioners (CNPs). APRNs proliferated and evolved to meet the health care demands in societies worldwide. The International Council of Nurses (ICN) created the International Nurse Practitioner and Advanced Practice Nursing Network (INP/APNN) in 2000 (Sheer & Wong, 2008) to promote the exchange of advance practice nursing concerns and issues. Information sharing and research about advanced nursing practice are major issues of IPN/APNN interest.

Regulation of APRNs

The IPN/APNN supports professional self-regulation by boards of nursing, not by medical councils (ICN, 2005). In addition to self-regulation, the IPN/APNN supports broadening scope of practice and reimbursement for advanced practice nursing. In New Zealand, the NP role is relatively new, and struggles for prescriptive authority persists (O'Connor, 2008; Sheer & Wong, 2008). Although RNs in Canada have the ability to move freely between provinces or territories, NPs do not have the same ability (Robinson, 2008). Challenges related to reimbursement for services, prescriptive privileges, and unencumbered practice autonomy are universally problematic (Ketefian, Redman, Hanucharurnkul, Masterson & Neves, 2001).

Licensure: A Key Element of Practice Regulation

As a newcomer, the transitioning APRN is busy developing work skills and abilities while establishing an identity. Unfortunately, it is far too common that frustration and stress occur when professional needs for practice autonomy cannot be met because of state licensing constraints on the breadth of the scope of practice for APRNs within their jurisdiction—even though there is a nationally recognized scope and accepted standards. Although APRN education, accreditation, certification, and practice standards are established and maintained at a national level, licensing privileges that define the scope of practice are determined within each state, a power left to state legislative initiative by the fourth Amendment of the U.S. Constitution.

In a comprehensive review of states' regulations, three major barriers to NPs were identified (Safriet, 1994). It seems reasonable to say the same barriers remain today and equally affect other APRN groups. The barriers are the lack of:

1. Third-party reimbursement.

2. Prescriptive authority.

3. Hospital admission privileges.

It is these practice barriers that are responsible for much of the stress encountered during newcomer APRN socialization. Challenges of meeting increased costs generated by physician supervision requirements, complex billing arrangements, and lack of autonomy in decision-making without direct third-party reimbursement serve to disadvantage NPs in providing direct services. NPs unable to prescribe medications delay necessary treatment and require unnecessary complexity, such as pre-signed prescription pads, telephone call-in services, and prescription writing by duly licensed providers who have not themselves assessed the patient's needs in order to provide for prescriptions. Lastly, the goal of continuity of care is thwarted when NPs and CNMs are denied the ability to

- Admit patients to a hospital.

- Follow a patient during the hospitalization.

- Obtain referral information when the patient is discharged.

These barriers not only hinder the delivery of health care, in both collaborative practice and independent health care models, but they can eventually lead the APRN newcomer to dissatisfaction, lack of professional fulfillment, and a sense of feeling disenfranchised.

Disappointingly, the stress-evoking realization of constrained practice by APRN newcomers will not be alleviated until APRNs everywhere achieve uniform state licensure as independent practitioners with full prescriptive authority and no regulatory requirements for mandated collaboration, direction, or supervision by physicians. This vision for APRN practice is set forth in the work of the APRN Consensus Work Group and the APRN Advisory Committee of the National Council of State Boards of Nursing, a Consensus Model for APRN Regulation: Licensure, Accreditation, Certification & Education (2008).

However, until such time as APRNs achieve an unrestricted scope of practice, an integrative approach to the socialization process, facilitated by a strong mentor, can moderate the degree of role-strain that APRN newcomers encounter. A strong mentor can guide and reinforce agendas that occur in the daily experiences of the new APRN as well as clarify why practice restrictions exist and how to advance APRN scope of practice. Similarly, peer support needs to be available to foster the professional growth and development of APRNs.

Reflections from Gina Dobbs, the Newcomer

During graduate school, one learns about APRN regulation. However, the real education begins after the tassel crosses the mortarboard. The light at the end of the proverbial regulatory tunnel is but a speck in the distance. The transition from student to APRN necessitates tolerance and patience. Following graduation, the wait to be eligible to write the certification examination takes at least six weeks. This wait can yield anxiety for the new graduate in need of employment. The road toward credentialing can be bumpy and filled with seemingly unnecessary obstacles.

When the degree is awarded, certification attained, and paperwork for practice submitted, the false sense of relief is temporarily welcomed. One's ability to practice to the fullest degree of preparation remains under the jurisdiction of the state practice act and scrutiny by the licensing board. The requirement for mandated collaboration or supervision can lead the new APRN to feel like a permanent "apprentice."

The newcomer, with an idealized scope of practice and evidenced-based patient care, quickly confronts the realities of practice and prescriptive restrictions. At this point, it is important to remember one's personal desires for becoming an APRN: to make a positive difference in patient outcomes, provide preventive health care, serve the disadvantaged, and promote the profession. Understanding and abiding by the regulations of APRN practice is imperative but is not to be passively accepted. While developing confidence in providing advance practice nursing, the newcomer must similarly become a voice for changing the status quo—a champion for an optimistic future where APRNs will practice unrestricted to their fullest potential. Membership with APRN organizations is essential. Through the collective work of these organizations, APRNs will achieve self-regulation, a broadened scope of practice, third-party reimbursement, and the ability to manage patient care from hospital admission to the outpatient setting. Newcomers must:

- Learn the process and key issues for revising APRN regulation.

- Become active in organizational meetings.

- Write and meet with legislators who control the nurse practice act.

Just like the seasoned APRN, the newcomer must help educate peers, colleagues, and the public about the need to revise APRN regulation to promote patient access to care. And, when in doubt concerning regulation and the potential for change, the mentee should always consult the mentor to glean a deeper understanding, explore alternatives, and plan strategically to meet goals. Mentor and mentee can combine their voices for positive change to ultimately improve patient outcomes and increase patient access to care around the globe.

Self-Reflective Questions

1. In what ways can you advocate for all APRNs to be reimbursed at 100%?

2. In what ways can you advocate for full prescriptive privileges?

3. What practice restriction, if any, pertains to your scope of practice?

4. What steps will you take to continue your professional development to ensure you maintain competence as an APRN?

5. How can you increase your familiarity with the nurse practice act that governs your practice?

6. What can you do to ensure that APRN practice is regulated/organized solely by the board of nursing and not the board of medical examiners or pharmacy?

7. How can you best remain abreast of pending legislative action that would revise your nurse practice act?

8. What steps would you need to take to belong to your state (country, providence, or territory) professional nursing association?

9. Through which professional organization(s) could you work to advocate for issues important to your practice?

10. Do you know how to contact your state legislators who ultimately control your nurse practice act?

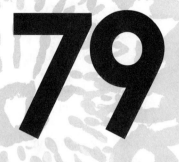

79 Regulatory and Organizational Standards

"Regulation is the point where the consumer and the health care provider meet within the health care system."

—Anne Morrison

Mentor

Jesmond Sharples, MBA, MMus (Comp) (Lond), BSc (Hons) (Nurs), Dip Ger, SRN, FLCM
Director of Nursing Standards and Services
Malta

Mentee

Thresanne Howland, RM, BSc (Midwifery) (Glasgow), MSc Midwifery
Directorate of Nursing Standards and Services
Malta

Standards of care have been defined as the desirable and achievable level of nurses' performance against which actual nursing practice is compared (International Council of Nursing, 1989). The setting of standards for the education and practice of nurses is pertinent to the public needs and to identify the cornerstone of professional scope and accountability (World Health Organization, 2002). Thus, standards of care are also the core of regulatory and organizational systems.

Jesmond Sharples (mentor) is the director of the nursing services standards department in Malta, and Thresanne Howland (mentee; a registered midwife) has recently joined the standards team within the same department to coordinate the formulation of midwifery care standards. The main focus of this department, which forms part of the public health regulation division, is the regulation of health care services in Malta and the licensing thereof. The department's mission statement is: *"To promote excellence in all aspects of nursing and midwifery services, to ensure the delivery of high quality care at a national level"* (Directorate Nursing Standards Services, 2009). The department is involved in research to produce evidence that will facilitate setting up necessary processes that will improve health outcomes, quality care, and access to health care. All this will lead to the betterment of clinical practice that is patient-centric. Tied to this process is the setting of benchmarks for quality patient-centered care services in conjunction with the relevant stakeholders as part of the health care licensing, credentialing, and regulatory mechanisms.

Mentoring for Leadership

During the process of mentoring, the mentor must demonstrate qualities of patience, enthusiasm, knowledge, a sense of humor, respect, and advocacy toward the mentee. These qualities are an integral part of a leader-mentor process. This chapter will demonstrate six essential lessons that the mentor and mentee had to go through for the professional development to set standards.

Mentee: My involvement in standard setting is a new role that is stimulating my professional growth and development. This has been possible to attain through adequate guidance to develop knowledge and expertise. Using the self-reflective questions at the end of this chapter, the mentor and mentee have identified and communicated their weaknesses and strengths for a better relationship as well as to define a way in which to work toward similar goals.

Lesson 1: If You Are in Love with Regulation, You Can Only Marry Integrity

During the standard setting process, integrity is one of the most important values that a person must possess. A good leader must believe in and seek to possess integrity. Integrity exists when a leader's personal inner values correspond with organizational values, which in turn reflect outward personal actions. Integrity involves three Rs: respect for self, respect for others, and responsibility for one's actions (Brown, 1991). Standards are, by their very nature, objective and should thus be evidence-based: They should not be based upon arbitrary criteria, such as who is providing health care services. Independence from certain stakeholders (such as health care associations, nongovernmental organizations, etc.) and service providers is of the utmost importance when devising regulation. This tenet is important to substantially reduce any possible conflict of interest and consolidate trust, which is requisite when setting up standards.

Mentee: Working with a person who deems integrity as an essential characteristic of a leader has motivated me to perform and accomplish the objectives set by the department and to build goals. Through professional experience with different leaders, I have learned that a failure of integrity within leadership will destroy trust between subordinates, thus obliterating respect and esteem—and, consequently, undermining an organization's cohesion. Conversely, being coached by a mentor who has integrity, I discovered that leading by example and by being honest, reliable, and consistent, the mentee's essence and character is enhanced.

Lesson 2: Patience and Perseverance Are a Regulator's Peace of Mind

Another aspect of setting organizational and health care systems standards are the values of patience and perseverance. "Slow but steady" is an apt adage when setting up health care standards. This important lesson has been discussed at length with the mentee, with particular reference to meticulous attention to detail and scientific evidence. Cultural relevance is also important, as is consultation, which is often one of the hardest tests of patience and perseverance. When a leader attains these values, he or she can attain peace of mind.

Mentee: Although leadership can be described as an art, my mentor has reinforced that leadership is an art that can be learned and is not necessarily something you have to be born with. Perseverance, he reminds me, is not just an attribute of your character. Rather, it is an attitude that you develop in conjunction with a mental prowess that also requires vision and determination to realize that vision. Both can be practiced to help build a stronger and more resilient character. Perseverance entails practice as well as hard work, commitment, and patience with yourself and others. It is only through personal growth and patience that you can learn to tell the difference in knowing when to stop and when to continue trying to overcome failures and disappointment. Working hard no matter what the task, giving it your best shot at all times, and being able to maximize the use of limited resources will definitely lead to success. Dr J.N. Reddy (2008) aptly stated, "Success is sweet. Its secret is sweat."

Lesson 3: Communication, Consistency, Commitment, and Control Are Important in the Process of Quality Improvement

Communication, consistency, commitment, and control are the four Cs of an organization that is setting up standards. These aspects all tie in well with the previous vaalues of integrity, patience, and perseverance. If passion does not steer such wheels, setting standards and enforcing regulation falters or is ineffective.

Mentee: These four mentor characteristics are the main reason why I have been motivated to step forward to join the standards team and be guided by the steps of Jesmond. His vision of what can and has to be done to improve midwifery practice by standards setting has been inspiring. The passion to reach this vision and improve the quality of clients' care is strongly shared by me, and such passion could turn any challenge into a tremendous opportunity.

Lesson 4: Humor Is the Humerus of the Regulatory Arm

This may be a strange notion in connection with regulation, but I always insist that on top of this commitment to standards, humor is what keeps such an organization going. It helps people get together in achieving their objective.

Mentee: With the stress of everyday life in an office and the strain throughout the process of formulating standards, you can easily lose your sense of humor. However, Jesmond focuses on his humor to ease communication through a combination of three mechanisms: by conveying information, generating effect, and drawing attention to the speaker. Thus, I comprehend that humor is one of the prime means enabling leaders to achieve their various transactional as well as relational objectives (Schnurr, 2008).

Lesson 5: Standards of Care and Resource Rationalization Should Go Hand in Hand

From experience, I learned that in spite of all good intentions, setting excessively high standards would probably have the opposite desired effect. Standards have to be reasonably achievable and be established within the context of resources rationalization without compromising patient safety.

Mentee: This lesson came to a shock for me initially. I used to think that standards should be driven to produce the best possible care. However, after reviewing various standards and discussing this issue with Jesmond, I understood that standards should be written to be achievable, without compromising patient care, while ensuring continuous improvement in the process of care delivery.

Lesson 6: The Patient is Our Focus, and We Are the Lens through Which Society Perceives the Delivery of Patient-Centered Care

The ultimate and most important lesson I tried to convey is that ultimately the patient is the raison d'être of all standards' setting and enforcement.

Mentee: Women-centered care is the focus of midwifery practice and education. This has always been my notion while practicing and when setting midwifery standards.

Self-Reflective Questions

Based on Hakala, 2008

1. **Vision.** How can you have a clear vision of where to go, as well a firm grasp on what is a successful outcome and how to achieve it?

2. **Integrity.** How do your outward actions and inner values correspond? How can you become trusted by your followers as being true to your own values in whatever you do and decide?

3. **Honesty.** How can you convey being honest in your dealings, as well as predictable and approachable?

4. **Perseverance.** How can you commit yourself to spend whatever time or energy is necessary to accomplish the task and persevere in spite of sometimes-insurmountable difficulties?

5. **Magnanimity.** How can you improve in giving credit where it is due in instances where success is visible and even when success is not so evident? Do you take personal responsibility for failure?

6. **Humility.** How can you best recognize that you are no better or worse than other members of the team?

7. **Openness.** How can you become more open to new ideas, even if they do not conform to the usual way of thinking?

8. **Creativity.** How can you try to think differently, to think "out of the box," which can confine solutions?

9. **Fairness.** How can you better deal with others consistently and justly, checking all the facts and hearing everyone before passing a judgment?

10. **Assertiveness.** How can you best clearly state what you expect to prevent misunderstandings and get the desired results?

11. **Humor.** How can you employ a sense of humor to relieve tension and boredom, as well as to defuse hostility at the work place?

Retention Starts With Recruitment

80

"Retention starts with recruitment. Clearly understanding your group's culture and pursuing the candidate who fits, can ensure a longer, more productive relationship and can help to sustain an environment that attracts new candidates to support the growth of your practice over the long term."

—Carol Westfall

Mentor
Franklin A. Shaffer, EdD, RN, FAAN
Executive Vice President and Chief Nursing Officer, Cross Country Healthcare Inc.
Chief Learning Officer, Cross Country University
Boca Raton, Florida, USA

Mentee
Jean S. Shinners, PhD, MSN, RN, CCRN
Director for Collaborative Learning and Career Enrichment
Cross Country University
Boca Raton, Florida, USA

Today, probably more than ever before, corporations are concerned with talent management. Their concerns embody all phases and components from recruitment, engagement, and performance management to succession planning, and their goal is to retain the best and brightest. The ability to recognize potential employees' unique talents and what they can offer to the organization takes skill in communication and the ability to visualize how these individuals will mesh with other prospective and current employees in creating a positive, productive work environment.

The Challenge of Integrating Into a New Environment

Once the applicant has been selected, onboarding begins. Onboarding refers to the process of obtaining, familiarizing, and assimilating applicants into their roles. It includes all aspects of orientation as well as an introduction to corporate attitudes, values, and beliefs that provides new hires direction in navigating their new positions. To be successful, onboarding must be structured carefully to introduce the employee to company strategies and departmental processes. Properly designed, onboarding goes far to ensure that the new employee will be a success in her or his new position. Onboarding reinforces mutual expectations and reinforces the culture, vision, and mission of the organization and the impact each employee has on the organization's success. During this time, the employee is creating internal network connections that should help in job performance and is also developing a rudimentary understanding of the corporate culture.

A few basic principles of engagement support employee development—and job satisfaction—during this time:

- Recognize an employee for his or her expertise.

- Express appreciation and respect for a job well done.

- Encourage autonomy.

- Provide ongoing coaching.

The Transition Challenge of Moving from a Nonprofit to a Corporate Health Care Environment: Mentor

Cross Country Staffing is a division of a large, publicly traded company, and Cross Country University (CCU) is its corporate university. CCU was created in 1996 by me (Franklin Shaffer) as a learning community and to ensure employee competence, which in turn helps our clients achieve positive patient outcomes. Since then, CCU has been responsible for the development and implantation of company standards as well as providing lifelong-learning opportunities for our mobile healthcare providers and other professionals. CCU developed assessment methods and tools that have been adopted by some of our leading clients to ensure competence of their own staff.

When meeting Jean Shinners (mentee) for the first interview, I had to consider her knowledge, attitude, and skill mix as well as her potential skill development. She had a strong clinical background, a good work ethic, and considerable clinical knowledge and experience, but she was moving from a not-for-profit clinical setting to a for-profit corporate setting. I had no doubt that she could develop the skills she needed, so my main concern was whether she would find the job satisfying. Moving from the clinical/caregiver role to managerial/educational role is, in itself, a challenge, and one compounded by moving from a clinical to a corporate setting—all of which takes significant adjustment.

Joining and Thriving in a Corporate Environment: Mentee

In 2004, I was working in the heart lab of a large hospital in south Florida. I had 28 years of strong clinical and education experience, with periods of management and supervision that provided opportunities to exercise my managerial skills. I enjoyed being at the bedside, but I was looking for something different where I would be encouraged to use the educational and administrative talents I had acquired during my masters program and work experiences. It was during this time that I was offered an opportunity to apply at Cross Country Staffing (CCS) for a director position within its corporate university. Cross Country provides contracted staff nurses to health care facilities across the country, and although I had worked as a contract staff nurse in the past, the concept of corporate nursing—and a corporate university—was new to me. After careful review of the job description and role expectations, which stressed education and professional development, I applied for the position.

The interview consisted of a meeting with Dr. Franklin Shaffer. We met in the hallway, with me in professional business attire and he in shorts, t-shirt, and sandals! While I appreciated the casual work environment and the many employee benefits Cross Country offered, I was a bit concerned. Dr. Shaffer quickly explained it was "dress-down Friday." The dress-down day was something special since the employees voted to receive this as a token of management's appreciation for employees achieving the week's production goals. His attire and demeanor set the tone for a relaxed and engaging interview. While we discussed the performance expectations of the position, and Dr. Shaffer reviewed my curriculum vitae, I assessed Dr. Shaffer. His "reach for the stars—anything is possible" attitude reminded me why I wanted to pursue nursing in the first place. Dr. Shaffer identified the character traits that he recognized in me that would contribute to the further development of professional skills as well as presented a spirit that I was sure would provide the support and direction needed to obtain these skills. I knew then that I wanted the job.

As my mentor, Dr. Shaffer developed an onboarding program designed to help me make the transition from hospital-based nursing. He introduced me to the particulars of the corporate culture, including dress-down Fridays. He spent one-on-one time with me to be sure I was clear about the mission, values, and vision of the company, and he expected me to reflect upon them and consider how they would be incorporated into my practice role. In fact, the foundations for our early mentor-mentee relationship occurred during our discussions and reflections about how the work of Cross Country contributed to the goals of nursing—to provide safe and competent patient care.

As a mentor, Dr. Shaffer helped create a welcoming environment in which I knew that my nursing knowledge was appreciated, and I was comfortable as I met a world in which nursing practice met "the corporation." Early onboarding consisted of meeting with key corporate stakeholders—many of whom come from a non-nursing background. I was armed with a list of questions that encouraged investigation into their role and in identifying the common ground we shared in the delivery of quality, professional staff to health care facilities. At the time, it seemed very practical, but what was really being orchestrated was more than an orientation—it was an opportunity to develop the relationships I needed to make my role successful. Without realizing it, I was developing an invaluable internal corporate network. It was rewarding to take responsibility for what I knew, and humbling to recognize what I had yet to learn.

Integration Promotes Retention and Rewards

Over the years, my position has offered both rewards and challenges. After my initial onboarding was completed and the "honeymoon phase" over, it was even more important that my relationship with Dr. Shaffer remain active as mentor-mentee-colleague. It's common to have a "decline in engagement" with a new job as the day-to-day job responsibilities make the most demands for time and effort. It is during this period that a mentor's abilities are most critical for ongoing successful integration and professional development. It is the professional possibilities that are envisioned and encouraged that ensure retention.

Now that I have been at Cross Country for five years, I have learned that retention is not always rewarded by bonuses or large salary increases, but rather in a multitude of ways that have encouraged my professional growth. I have always enjoyed school and am committed to life-long learning. Cross Country's culture supports ongoing education, and the company has provided financial support while I complete my doctoral degree. This has been a long-term goal of mine which Dr. Shaffer fully supported. I started on the PhD journey in 2006, and defended my dissertation in September 2009. Dr. Shaffer proved to be an invaluable mentor and friend while I was working through the often demanding scholarly requirements.

In addition, Dr. Shaffer continues to encourage me to look beyond the confines of Cross Country Health Care to examine the challenges facing the profession as a whole. About a year after joining the CCU team, and after I was well enmeshed in the fine points of providing continuing education, I was encouraged by Dr. Shaffer to apply to the American Nurses Credentialing Center (ANCC) to become an appraiser in their continuing education accreditation program. I was accepted. Over the years, I've had the good fortune of being mentored by nationally recognized nurse educators as part of my appraiser role. This has resulted in opening new doors that I never knew existed. I continue in the ANCC role where I now mentor others in their appraiser roles, and I have progressed to an Accreditation Review Committee (ARC) position.

I have always considered my strengths to be in clinical practice and have been certified as a critical care registered nurse (CCRN) since the early 1990s. Dr. Shaffer has encouraged me to maintain clinical competence, and I continue to work in the cardio-vascular intensive care unit (CVICU) of our local hospital. In this role, I am able to keep active in clinical nursing and maintain a clinical connection that is helpful when dealing with the daily concerns of the contracted staff nurses. I am currently on the American Association of Critical-Care Nurses Exam Development Committee, where my connection to clinical practice and competence is maintained while challenging my abilities as an item writer.

For me, retention has meant being offered opportunities to learn in a multitude of ways in safe, nonthreatening environments; to achieve new levels of satisfaction in my work; and to recognize the unlimited potential for the further development of my role. What is most important to me is that the values and vision of Cross Country that were presented during my onboarding almost five years ago have been constantly reinforced in both words and actions by all members of the executive leadership team. I have been consistently encouraged to challenge myself to identify and meet new professional goals. Through it all, Dr. Shaffer helped me to become an integral part of the team.

Self-Reflective Questions

1. How will taking this position encourage me to further develop prior interests and areas that I have received educational preparation for?

2. What do I have to offer this position?

3. What are the goals and objectives of the role?

4. How am I comfortable this is a good fit as far as corporate/organizational values and work ethics and my own values?

5. How will I obtain support and internal relationships that I need to learn a new role and grow within it?

6. What kind of support do I need to identify and achieve my goals?

7. How does the organization demonstrate characteristics that allow me to effectively use my knowledge and expertise?

8. How does the organization demonstrate qualities as far as a supportive management style?

9. How does this position encourage autonomy and accountability?

10. What is the extent of emphasis on professional development?

Risk Management and Safety

81

> "It may seem a strange principle to enunciate as the very first requirement in a hospital that it should do the sick no harm."
>
> —Florence Nightingale

Mentor
Anna Margherita T. Bork, RN,
  MSN, MBA
Albert Einstein Jewish Hospital
São Paulo, Brazil

Mentee
Cristina Satoko Mizoi, RN, MSN
Albert Einstein Jewish Hospital
São Paulo, Brazil

Risk management, a specific approach to improving safety and quality in organizations, emphasizes situations where users or professionals suffer damage or are exposed to potential damage. A risk management system has a set of instruments to identify, analyze, prevent, and correct risks. In healthcare organizations, safety must be a priority. A safety system includes:

- Patient safety.
- Worker safety.
- Environmental safety.

Why Risk Management Is Important

When we identify risks, we can act upon them to reduce the injuries caused to people and organizations. J. Williams showed that many conditions that predispose to human errors should be considered to properly manage risks (Reason, 2001). Notably, three of the best-researched factors—sleep disturbance, hostile environment, and boredom—carry the least penalty. Additionally, those errors producing factors at the top of the list are those that lie squarely within the organization's sphere of influence. This is a central element in the present view of organizational accidents. Leaders rarely, if ever, have the opportunity to jeopardize a system's safety directly. Their influence is more indirect—top-level decisions create conditions that promote unsafe acts (Reason, 2001). Effective risk management essentially depends upon a confidential (and possibly anonymous) system of monitoring that records the factors associated with accidents and potential incidents that are individual factors, linked to the task, situation, and/or organization. Risk management should focus more on damage prevention than on simply reducing errors. Table 1 presents explanations for some of the main concepts related to risk management and safety.

Table 1   Main concepts of risk management and safety.

What is a hazard?	A hazard is anything with the potential to cause harm. Example: working at height on scaffolding.
What is risk?	A risk is the likelihood that a hazard will cause a specified harm to someone or something. Example: if there are no guard rails on the scaffolding, it is likely that a construction worker will fall and break a bone.
What is risk management?	Risk management is a process that involves assessing the risks that arise in your workplace, putting sensible health and safety measures in place to control them, and then making sure they work in practice.
What is risk assessment?	A risk assessment is nothing more than a careful examination of what in the work could cause harm to people, so that you can weigh whether or not you have taken enough precautions or should do more to prevent harm.
What do ALARP and SFAIRP mean?	You may come across these abbreviations. ALARP stands for *As Low As Reasonably Practicable*, and SFAIRP stands for *So Far As Is Reasonably Practicable*. In essence, these are the same; however, SFAIRP is the term most often used in health and safety at work and in regulations. ALARP is the term used by risk practitioners.

Table 1 *(continued)*

What does "reasonably practicable" mean?	This means that you have to take action to control the health and safety risks in your workplace except where the cost (in terms of time and effort as well as money) of doing so is "grossly disproportionate" to the reduction in the risk. You can work this out for yourself, or you can simply apply accepted good practice.

Classification of Risk

A common and very effective method that involves working out a risk level is categorizing the likelihood of harm and the potential severity of harm and then plotting these two risk-determining factors against each other in a risk matrix, as shown in Figure 1. However, it does require a fair degree of expertise and experience to accurately judge the likelihood of harm. The risk level determines which risks should be tackled first (see Table 2). Like with any other method of risk assessment, you should not overcomplicate the process, for example, by having too many categories.

		Potential severity of harm		
		Slightly Harmful	**Harmful**	**Extremely Harmful**
Likelihood of harm occurring	Highly unlikely 1	Trivial 1	Tolerable 2	Moderate 3
	Unlikely 2	Tolerable 2	Moderate 4	Substantial 6
	Likely 3	Moderate 3	Substantial 6	Intolerable 0

Figure 1   Risk management scale matrix.

Table 2   Summary of error-producing conditions ranked in order of known effect.

Condition	Risk Factor
Unfamiliarity with the task	(x 17)
Time shortage	(x 11)
Poor signal noise ratio	(x10)
Poor human system interface	(x 8)
Designer user mismatch	(x 8)
Irreversibility of errors	(x 8)
Information overload	(x 6)
Negative transfer between task	(x 5)
Misperception of risk	(x 4)
Poor feedback from system	(x 4)
Inexperience not lack of training	(x 3)
Poor instructions or procedures	(x 3)
Inadequate checking	(x 3)
Educational mismatch of person with task	(x 2)
Disturbed sleep patterns	(x 1.6)
Hostile environment	(x 1.2)
Monotony and boredom	(x 1.1)

Mentee Case Report: Administration of High Electrolyte Concentration for the Wrong Patient

Drug administration is a multiple-step process that involves many professionals, meaning it is vulnerable to errors and adverse events (Brennan, Leape, Laird, Hebert, Localio et al, 1991). At least 10% of the patients admitted in tertiary hospitals suffer injuries related to medication use, and almost half of these adverse events could have been prevented with the implementation of safer processes (Cousins, 1998).

In an intensive care unit (ICU), administration of critical drugs occurs all the time for unstable cases, in which quick therapeutic interventions are necessary (time shortage). It is important to highlight the environmental disturbances in areas, such as an ICU, in which there are frequent monitor alarms, many professionals from different specialties, and family members all in close proximity which can contribute to error (noise ratio).

For example, a nursing staff member was providing care in the ICU, and the physician gave a verbal order to administer electrolyte replacement to a patient under his care—however, not to the patient he was caring for at that time. The physician gave the name of the patient and bed number, and reported that he had already prescribed it in the medical prescription. The professional nurse had the pharmaceutical prescription filled by the pharmacist. When it came time to administer the medication, the nurse failed to check the patient identification and administered the drug to the wrong patient. Instead, the nurse started the IV solution in the patient the physician had been caring for when he gave the verbal order for the medication. Many causes and contributing factors were found in this event. First, the nurse was focused on another activity when he received the verbal order (interruption). Second, there was a short time to start the IV drug, given that it was electrolyte replacement. Third, an interference occurred during the delivery of care to another patient. Fourth, there was noncompliance with the patient-identification process—namely, check five elements: right patient, right drug, right dose, right route, and right time.

After this occurrence, we implemented actions to minimize the risk of new events: a critical drug list that has to be double-checked by nursing staff before administration (after following the patient identification process); preparation of drugs inside the room (proper place); and medical orders executed only when the medical prescription is readily available, with a nurse reading the prescription back when the physician asks for a new prescription.

In nursing practice, it is essential to know our responsibilities to promote safe delivery of care. Recognizing that human beings may make mistakes and that the healthcare process involves risks to patient safety is the first step to transform the care setting into a safer place, for both patients and professionals.

Risk Assessment Checklist

These five steps support you when assessing risks at your organization.

Step 1: Identify the hazards.

To spot hazards, ask yourself these questions:

- Am I walking around my workplace paying attention to possible risks?
- Am I asking my employees what they think?
- Am I visiting and asking patients and families what they see and think?
- Am I aware of the root causes of accidents or adverse events reported?
- Am I contacting other healthcare organizations, associations, and industries to get good information?
- Am I checking laws for healthcare industry and general safety regulations?
- Am I checking manufacturers' instructions for the equipment and materials used?

Step 2: Identify who might be harmed and how.

Identify groups of people. Remember the following:

- Am I focusing on patients?
- Am I focusing on workers?
- Am I thinking about members of the public?
- Am I thinking about how to address other sites (if you share your workplace)?
- Am I paying attention to all the processes and systems that affect others present?
- Am I identifying how the hazard could cause harm?

Step 3: Identify what you are already doing.

Ask yourself whether you have documented what is already in place to eliminate the likelihood of harm or to make any harm less serious. You need to make sure that you have reduced risks "so far as is reasonably practicable." For example, are you comparing what you have already done with good practice?

Step 4: Determine how you will put the assessment into action.

Prioritize. Deal with those hazards that are high-risk and have serious consequences first. (See the risk matrix in Figure 1). Have you built an action-done table that delineates by whom and by when?

Step 5: Monitor progress.

Review your assessment to make sure you are still improving, or at least not sliding back. If there is a significant change in your workplace or processes, remember to check your risk assessment—and, where necessary, amend it.

Self-Reflective Questions

1. How can I better educate those in my institution/department about the potential workplace hazards for patients and staff?

2. How can I better learn the root causes of accidents or adverse events reported?

3. How can I focus a plan of corrective and preventive actions for patients?

4. How can I focus a plan of corrective and preventive actions for workers?

5. How can I focus a plan of corrective and preventive actions for members of the public?

6. How can I best stay current with laws for healthcare industry and general safe regulations?

7. To make sure that I have reduced risks "so far as is reasonably practicable," how can I make a complete list about what is already in place to eliminate the likelihood of harm or make any harm less serious?

8. How can I put into place an Action-Done table, citing owner and deadline?

9. How can I best compare what I have already done with good practice?

10. How can I plan to review my assessment to make sure that I am still improving, or at least not sliding back?

82 Self Leadership

"Mastering others is strength. Mastering yourself is true power."

—Lao Tzu

Mentor
Karien Jooste, PHD, RN
Professor, Health Sciences,
   University of Johannesburg
Johannesburg, South Africa

Mentee
Elsa Jordaan, RN, BSN
Lecturer, George Hospital
   Training School
Johannesburg, South Africa

As a nurse leader, you can do anything when you believe you are capable of doing it. All successful actions start with a good self-image. Therefore, you should craft a self-image capable of sustained acts of greatness. Preparation, conditioning, persuasion, and training precede leadership actions. Invest adequate time in developing and becoming the nurse leader you know you should and can be, by acquiring the skills you know you must have. You should not hesitate to start today. Only you can decide what you become in your career path and in life. Self-leadership is:

- The process of influencing yourself to establish the self-direction and self-motivation needed for effective performance or to accomplish desirable outcomes (Politis, 2006).

- The process in which people direct and motivate themselves to behave and perform in a desired way, to take responsibility for creating the conditions that help them to achieve set goals (Georgianna, 2007).

- A personal philosophy to follow a systematic set of actions and mental strategies to achieve higher performance and to be effective.

- The ability to communicate clearly your worth and potential to yourself so that you can create your life for who you really are.

- Knowing and understanding yourself, leading followers to exceed their own expectations, and being that person who leads others to lead themselves (Elloy, 2008).

Not Looking Back—Being Visionary and Focused

From the perspective of a mentor, you should know that the notion of a sense of progress persists among upcoming nurse leaders. Individuals do not just seek their own subjective markers of success, but want some form of objective criteria by which they and others can judge their ongoing progress. Knowing where you are going is part of your success. Visions help to transform possibilities into realities. You have to want something badly enough to let nothing stand in your way of achieving it. A successful leader helps the mentee to let things happen. The main thing is to keep the main thing the main thing; in other words, stay focused. Success is the result of consistently concentrated energy focused on your vision.

As the mentee, many lessons are learned from the mentor. No matter who you are or where you come from, at some point in your career you will believe you have hit a dead end. You might lose hope. That is when the real learning takes place and your character is re-formed. The mentor makes it clear—that it is the end of the past (mistakes) and the beginning of the future (new possibilities). Do not look back, but set realistic goals to obtain at specific time frames to measure your success. View every experience as a gift to increase your personal and positional power. Commit to a decision and concentrate all your resources on achieving your dream. You have it within you to handle work-related problems and to stretch and grow by being given tasks that might initially seem impossible.

Doing a SWOT on Yourself

The mentor guides the mentee to analyze *strengths*, *weaknesses*, *opportunities*, and *threats* (SWOT) in her or his career path. Self-leadership is a life-long personal journey in self-management, one in which you develop your strong qualities and address your weaknesses. The SWOT is a useful way to assist the mentee in gaining access to self-knowledge, self-remembering, and self-honoring.

As the mentee, the first step is to list your strengths and accomplishments followed by your weaknesses, areas for improvement, doubts, anxieties, fears, and worries. Next, list all the opportunities you have available. Lastly, jot down the threats (obstacles) that are stumbling blocks in achieving your goals. After doing this, you can better understand yourself and the situation. The better you know yourself, the better you can apply your strengths to those opportunities you encounter. Success comes to those who have self-knowledge of their strengths and how to use them.

Treasuring Humility—That Is Where Self-Leadership Starts

As a mentoring leader, you must be humble and willing to serve others. People do not want to follow someone who is arrogant. The leader should always strive to acquire more knowledge, to better him- or herself, to improve and grow.

From the perspective of the mentee, when the leader is humble, that leader becomes genuinely interested in the mentee because he or she wants to learn from you. The leader becomes a far more effective listener because he or she is open to what you have to offer. This open listening is a powerful communication tool of an effective leader. If mentees sense that mentors are truly interested in them and listen to them, they will in turn naturally listen to what is said.

Following Your Passion

Successful leaders as mentors follow their passions. However, passions can become blurred early in your career, when you decide to pursue goals that are expected rather than those that are personally meaningful. Leaders who want to be successful mentors should foster an atmosphere that supports mentees who are gifted at certain tasks and passionate about results.

As a mentee, you can use this principle. You will always have opportunities to uncover and retrieve meaning in your work environment and personal life. Every individual has special gifts, and he or she doesn't have to be a genius to inspire management and to find work-related roles that fit those talents in mutually beneficial ways. However, when you depend on external standards and rewards such as compensation and security, it is easy to lose sight of who you are and what you care about. Reflect on your life and work achievements to find evidence of your passions. You might remember certain life events in great detail and hardly recall others. By reflecting on these events, you can recognize the powerful themes of passion in your life. Performing work that engages your passions is the best path to finding a meaningful life.

Honoring Your Word

A mentor should never break his or her word. It makes you lose power (Holcomb, 2005). A mentor should reflect personal power. Personality characteristics relate to personal power. Effective and honest communication serves to enhance personal power. To break your word, therefore, negatively affects your personal power (Jooste, 2009).

The mentee views how the leader walks his or her talk. You treasure the words of the leader as gold and honor it. Through a mentor's keeping his or her word, you learn that your core values should drive you and that you are willing to stand by them without compromising them. Your mentor should be someone who sets an example and who acts according to what he or she says and believes in.

General Self-Leadership Qualities

Courage

Mentor: You only really fail when you stop trying. Setbacks should merely be viewed as feedback to help you chart your course.

Mentee: Courage is a special personal quality that helps you distinguish between what ought to be feared and what need not be feared. Never back away from any encounter that threatens you.

Excellence

Mentor: Excellence comes from striving higher, maintaining the highest standards, looking after the smallest detail, and going the extra mile. Successful leaders never compromise their standards.

Mentee: You cannot reach your goals unless you commit yourself fully to the outcome. You cannot inspire others if you are not prepared to take a stand for quality. No one is more powerful than a person who is decisive and committed to a desired outcome.

Self-Development

Mentor: Successful leaders believe in themselves and are confident in the knowledge that they can achieve what they set out to do.

Mentor: First know yourself so you head in the right direction in your career. Everyone has a predisposition toward a particular direction in their career that fits their personality. The trick is to know yourself well enough to find that direction.

Creativity

Mentor: All creativity depends on optimism and imagination. You have to see the opportunities in all the different and difficult situations around you.

Mentee: The mentor guides you to view problems as opportunities that should be uncovered. The only thing you need is insight into how the solutions to problems can benefit a particular situation.

Focus on Positive Thoughts

Your openness to opportunities ensures effective self-leadership. Focus on positive thoughts and get the most out of your networking. Successful leaders know that setting specific goals with the mentee helps to provide the necessary focus and direction for personal and professional growth.

Self-Reflective Questions

1. How can you influence others to establish the self-direction and self-motivation needed for effective performance?

2. In what ways do you take responsibility for creating the conditions that help you achieve your set goals?

3. What personal philosophy or systematic set of actions and mental strategies do you follow to achieve higher performance?

4. How can you communicate clearly to yourself your own worth and potential so that you create the life for which you really are suited?

5. How can you lead followers to exceed their own expectations?

6. How do you remain focused on a clear vision for your future?

7. In what ways can you determine the strengths, weaknesses, opportunities, and threats (SWOT) of your leadership style?

Self-Reflective Questions (continued)

7. In what ways can you determine the strengths, weaknesses, opportunities, and threats of your leadership style?

8. How can you stay humble and willing to serve others?

9. What tasks do you perform that engage your passions?

10. How do you act according to your beliefs?

83 Self Recovery and Renewal

"That no man can sincerely help another without helping himself. . . . It is one of the most beautiful compensations in life."

—Ralph Waldo Emerson

Mentor

Kimberly Richards, RN
President, Kim Richards and
  Associates, Inc.
President, NurseFit
Littleton, Colorado, USA

Mentee

Jennifer Campbell, BSN, RN
Staff Nurse, ICU
University of Wisconsin Medical
  Center
Madison, Wisconsin, USA
and
Katie Flaherty, BSN, RN
Staff Nurse, ICU
Aspen Medical Center
Aspen, Colorado, USA

In the continuing search for my higher purpose, I (Kimberly) decided that after 20 years of nonclinical practice, I wanted to be part of a greater medical mission in Africa. After a career of pouring my efforts into building my own businesses, I needed to be jolted out of my everyday life as a nurse entrepreneur to re-experience the satisfaction of caring for those in need. To most, I was successful, but I felt mentally and emotionally drained. I was desperate to escape my comfortable and predictable surroundings and get outside of myself. Little did I know that in testing my courage I would actually meet myself again in the eyes of these young nurses.

Sometimes Caring Comes with a Cost

My two co-authors, Katie and Jen, are nurses whom I had the honor and privilege of working with on a mission, and their perspective on nursing and on their own lives affected me profoundly. Their maturity, eloquence, and insight were reflective of women with much more life experience, and I was in awe. I had never met any of the women on the trip before, and as happens when 8 nurses live, work, and play in very close quarters 24 hours a day, every day, for two weeks in a Third World country, there are no secrets that aren't exposed by the end of the trip!

Certainly, we were different in age, career paths, and history, yet there was a common thread that ran through our lives—the awareness of a mandatory need to practice self-care and allow ourselves time to renew our caregiver spirit. The most inspiring, passionate, and well-balanced nurses incorporate consistent self-care practices into their lifestyle, knowing that they must take personal responsibility for nurturing their care-giving spirit. They are fully aware that physical activity, stress reduction, and mental/emotional "refueling" are mandatory to creating an authentic, abundant life, one in which they continually fill their reservoirs so that they in return can give the very best of themselves to others.

That awareness proved to be our lifeline to our sense of sanity during the two weeks, and we were thankful that each of us had honed our personal arsenal to combat and transition the effects of compassion fatigue. Compassion fatigue, a common condition that afflicts caregivers, is described as a debilitating weariness brought about by the repetitive, empathetic responses to pain and suffering. Compassion fatigue is a result of absorbing and internalizing the emotions of patients, and sometimes co-workers. It's an occupational hazard that can affect any professional who works with those who are challenged physically, mentally, or emotionally or who have been traumatized, whether by illness, violence, or other tragedies.

At times, our experiences were incredibly raw and overwhelming—almost too much for the mind and heart to comprehend. We agreed that even beyond our two weeks together, our individual practices of self-care had proven to be a lifesaver for each of us even though our career journeys' were vastly different.

A mission trip is an extreme example, yet over the course of a nurse's career, the accumulated emotional residue of caring for others without making self-care a priority is a recipe for concocting a toxic life. Without implementing healthy avenues in our daily lives to release the accumulation of trauma and stress, we travel a path that eventually forces us to face our own demons.

Barbra Stanny (2004) says, "An empty vessel has little to offer. Obligatory or guilt driven self-denial is always undermining, leading to anger, resentment and pain. Without taking care of ourselves, we engage in self sabotage."

Here are some very personal experiences shared by my friends and me.

Katie

Many times in my six years as a nurse, I said to a patient's family member, "Go home. Get some rest. You can't be there for your loved one, and you certainly can't absorb any information the doctor gives you if you don't rest and take care of yourself." Such perfectly sound advice I gave, but I was a hypocrite!

My hard-knocks lesson all started with a series of unfortunate events: the death of a close relative, a break-up, a challenging mission trip to a third world country, a physical problem that caused small hormonal changes, and the death of another relative. When it rains, it pours, but then there is usually a rainbow, right? Day after day, month after month, the sun never seemed to come back out. As soon as I felt I was coping with one issue, another thunder-cloud would show up.

Eventually, these stressors started to manifest themselves. First, I was ir-ritable. Then I started losing sleep. I was working the night shift and sleep-ing about 3-4 hours per day between shifts. I would lie down to sleep, and thoughts would consume me. With the lack of sleep, I predisposed myself to a multitude of viruses. I must have gone to the doctor a handful of times in a few months for sore throats, swollen glands, ear infections, and chest colds. In addition, I began noticing a low level of anxiety at all times.

I had a nervous stomach, and I felt a tingling in my veins almost constantly. I also had a loss of appetite. I craved only sweets and McDonald's hamburgers, and somehow still dropped 10 pounds without trying. I started crying at the drop of a hat—me, the person I would self-describe as jolly! I was, as my gen-eration likes to call it, "a hot mess"!

All the while, I was still working 36 to 40 hours weekly in the intensive care unit (ICN). I can pretty much guarantee that my patients were suffering. I told myself that I was leaving my problems at home instead of bringing them to work. I was still safe in practice. After all, I wasn't physically neglecting my patients, making med errors, or compromising their safety. However, I am *positive* that the quality of care I was providing, along with the emotional sup-port at the bedside I pride myself on, was not there. How could it be? I was an irritable, malnourished, distracted insomniac!

With some insight from friends, co-workers, and family—and at the persuasion of the ones I love the most—I made some changes. Fitting in better with the younger staff and enjoying the extra money, I had convinced myself that I was a night nurse. I finally realized the vampire-like hours were working against me, and moved to the day shift. What a difference the day made! Next, I decided to focus a little more on what I was neglecting—myself. I surrounded myself with loved ones who could evoke even the smallest chuckle from the depths of my darkness. Then, at the persuasion of one of those special angels, I began therapy to work through my sadness and anxiety head-on. I confronted my biggest fears and began developing new coping strategies. I also made a flight home for the holidays to surround myself with the people who would unconditionally love me.

To elicit some endorphins (those little happy chemicals in the brain), I relied heavily on yoga and snowboarding. Although a social drinker, I knew that even one sip of alcohol could deplete my little "happy" friends, so I took a hiatus from drinking altogether. As a spiritual person, I did pray and recite my mom's mantra, "God doesn't close a door without opening a window." After months of work with myself, I began seeing glimpses of light. I still didn't feel quite back to myself and did start on a low-dose of an anti-depressant. The combination of all of these disciplines eventually started working. Within six months, I finally felt better.

I eventually reached a point where I was sick of thinking about myself. I was tired of my self-pity and self-loathing. I wanted to focus on something and someone else! I *wanted* to go to work and help others the way I had been helped. The excitement of feeling better soon began showing up in my work. I felt focused again. Co-workers even noticed a positive change and commented. Laughter and teamwork seemed to reappear where there was a void for so long! Most importantly, though, my patients were getting my full, undivided attention again. I received a couple of compliments in the period of my reawakening, like, "You are the perfect example of what a nurse should be." I can't think of a better compliment!

I have learned to balance my work with measures that keep me healthy. I continue to exercise 3-4 days per week. I get outside as much as possible. I maintain close contact with the positively influential people around me. At work, I take my allotted breaks. When I come home from work, I spend about an hour alone to decompress from the physical and emotional exhaustion of the day. Essentially, I embrace the coping strategies I have had to learn to take care of myself.

I honestly believe that my patients benefit from my being in this healthy place. I may have never been in a hospital gown or stuck in an ICU bed during my difficult time, but I was suffering still the same. I had to go through the healing process to be able to help heal others.

Jen

I think I lost myself somewhere between Africa and the ICU, or maybe it was the lavish ski lodges juxtaposed with the shantytown of cardboard boxes. Or perhaps the obese versus the starving, or simply the realization that no matter how much I could give, it would never be enough to overcome the massive discrepancies of our world. I started looking for more ways to fund missions overseas; working extra shifts; applying to jobs in unstable countries; and looking for units serving the homeless, forgotten, and underserved. The joyful hobbies that once consumed my life, I packed up in boxes. My experiences— my worldly, raw encounters with life and death and health and humankind— overwhelmed my ability to just simply be a nurse and enjoy life.

Luckily, I have wonderful friends, people who hold me to my center. If the world were flat, I was certainly very close to falling over the edge, but my friends reeled me in from oblivion. As clarity set in, I realized that the line between work and self had obscured, and my ability to give to myself had vanished. This is hard to believe as I had initially turned to nursing as a lifestyle career. Now I practice life with more awareness, knowing that the slippery slope always seems to be in a blind spot.

Learning my own tendency to losing myself in intense work was unfortunately something I couldn't learn from a class, academic reasoning, or even common sense. Like most of my career, it's been experiential learning. While I still continue to seek intense work, I also work with an intense awareness of myself—how work affects my life, where energy is drained and restored, how much I give to work versus to myself and my loved ones, and what activities fill my reserve of self.

Those who are drawn to nursing have an affinity to giving, but selflessness allows us to give to another in a sustainable manner. I have found in my own practice to draw lines, set boundaries, say "no," and not lose sight of myself. Health is simply more than absence of disease: It is an enriching vitality of a balanced life.

Kimberly

I have the opportunity every day, by my words and actions, to demonstrate the grace of goodness, generosity, and purposeful living. I honor my purpose by allowing myself to be used as a vessel through which a higher power can flow. When lives are changed through my words, actions, or focused energy, it is very rewarding. The "self talk" I provide myself is vital to my productivity and success, but I am a brutal self-critic. My mind is my most powerful weapon in the entrepreneurial arsenal. I find it mandatory to incorporate daily activities as well as lots of humor into my life to help me deal with the frustration of business and the resultant impatience that is always just below the surface of most entrepreneurs.

My day starts with a little meditation, just quiet stillness the moment I awaken. I start *every* morning by expressing gratitude for my abundant life.

I find great stress relief in being outdoors in my beautiful state of Colorado. I feel fully alive hiking, biking, or skiing, and find if I don't make those activities a priority, I don't perform my best work. Yoga creates a much-needed mind/body connection and allows me to naturally flow into centering my breath and my thoughts, and strengthening my body. Music has the capability to relax and de-stress me almost instantly, so I self-medicate with music *prn* (as needed).

I love to travel and feel my mind opening to new possibilities as I interact with different cultures. I often reaffirm my life/business purpose and have time to develop new avenues of exploration. I also have time to reconnect with my family and friends, which can often be difficult in our fast-paced world.

There was a time when I experienced a very personal and debilitating crisis that hit me like a ton of bricks. Up to that point, I thought I had all the resources to "just shake it off" and "gut it out." I was wrong. I waited too long to reach out and get professional help while sliding down the slippery slope of depression, and almost lost it all. Well-meaning friends and family tried their best to help, but I was in agony and didn't know how to climb out of what seemed like a steep, black hole. I could not work, I could not sleep, and I could not smile. I was numb.

While this had nothing to do with being an entrepreneur, it had everything to do with the "inner work" needed. With the aid of a wonderful counselor, short-term medication, and renewal of my dormant spiritual faith, I was able to rebuild my life and my courage. "One day at a time" did not always work for me. There were times when I literally had to take it one minute or one hour at a time.

After much personal discovery, meditation, and prayer, I was able to pull myself out of that black hole and get on with life. What I had learned about myself during those painful and difficult times fueled my resolve to start a new life. I was committed to building an authentic, purposeful life and didn't really know how to start. This defining, pivotal point in my life has proven to be the best gift I could ever have given myself. I finally learned that I must love, accept, and respect myself more than anyone. I learned that *I* am the most important person in my life and that by doing things that make me happy, my soul is genuinely free. The abundance of love, energy, and possibility is endless and infectious when you allow yourself to actively participate in your own life. My level of happiness is my responsibility.

I am now aware of triggers that can diminish my sense of self and will not hesitate to stop myself dead in my tracks, preventing any situation or any person from ever defining my direction or intent. I don't allow others to set my standards. Yes, I work intensely, but I make the time I need to fill up my soul and look around at the amazing life with which I have been blessed.

Self-Reflective Questions

1. What do you do when you feel depressed and estranged from others?

2. How do you cope when you have difficulty falling or staying asleep?

3. What makes you have outbursts of anger or irritability with little provocation?

4. Could you benefit from having more close friends and someone to talk with about highly stressful experiences?

5. How can you counteract periods of excessive work?

6. How have you coped when you thought you might have been "infected" by the traumatic stress of your patients?

7. How can you successfully separate work from personal life?

8. How much compassion do you have for most of your co-workers?

9. How do you combat a sense of worthlessness/disillusionment/resentment associated with your work?

10. What do you do when you worry that you are not succeeding at achieving your life goals?

Self-Image and Self-Esteem

84

"An individual's self-concept is the core of his personality. It affects every aspect of human behaviour: the ability to learn, the capacity to grow and change. ... A strong self-image is the best possible preparation for success in life."

—Joyce Brothers

Mentor

Debra Thoms, RN, RM, BA
Chief Nursing and Midwifery
    Officer New South Wales
    Department of Health
Advance Professor, University of
    Technology, Sidney,
New South Wales, Sydney,
    Australia

Mentee

Alison Zecchin, RN
  Director of Nursing and
    Midwifery Royal Northshore
    Hospital
New South Wales, Sydney,
    Australia

Psychology tells us that self-esteem is a powerful force in our personalities and that its development is a response to both internal and external factors. Our self-esteem influences our self-image. Given this, though, our perceptions of ourselves are not always congruent with how we are viewed by others and those we manage and lead. At times, we may allow ourselves to be defined by the views of others, and this should be questioned when it occurs. Further complicating our understanding of ourselves is that nursing, as a profession, at times is not well understood by the public. There is often a belief by the public that they know what nursing entails, but this is often a limited and narrow view based on history rather than the reality of modern day. This, though, can influence our self-image both as members of the profession and as individuals. Additionally, the self-image and self-esteem nurses express can reinforce the publicly held views, whether intentionally or not. If we are to develop and practice effectively as leaders, it is necessary to understand ourselves. Self-reflection is critical to the ongoing development of leadership capacity and in enabling nurses themselves to grow and reach a clearer understanding of both themselves and their profession.

Reflecting on Self-Reflection: Mentee

Self-reflection can be undertaken in a variety of ways. Originally, I had thought that self reflection is molded through life experiences, until I encountered nurses who had been traversing the health system in a variety of roles. Self-reflection, I have learned, shouldn't be seen as being introspective. In fact, through the open self-reflection of mentorship you gain a greater self-awareness and develop a stronger self-image. This mentorship need not be formal; it can be accomplished through a brief e-mail, phone call, or face-to-face conversation. Part of this willingness and openness to accept and move forward is integral to how I develop and see myself from others' perspectives or how I impact those around me.

Looking Inward: Self-Reflective Steps for Nurses

Bernice Buresh and Suzanne Gordon (2000) outline steps that nurses need to take to help the broader community understand what truly describes and reflects nursing. It is critical as leaders to not only have an understanding and ability to describe nursing, but also to have an understanding and a confidence in our abilities. The image we have of ourselves affects how we communicate, how we work with others, the expectations that we have of ourselves and others, and the level of confidence with which we approach challenges. Self-image also impacts our ability to enable and empower others to achieve, as well as our effectiveness as leaders.

Self-image and self-esteem can be both positive and negative. Those who have an overly positive self-image will perhaps be unwilling to seek and take advice. Their ability to empower and enable others and to inspire staff to embrace their vision may be limited. Those who have negative or low self-esteem may find themselves experiencing more stress in their work. Gaining an accurate understanding of how you are performing as a leader while identifying the level of congruence with your perceptions can be difficult. I have at times undertaken discussions with trusted colleagues and tested my perceptions of myself with my colleagues to gain a clearer picture of how I could develop further as a leader. Although this approach can be useful, Covey advises that it is important not to let yourself be defined by the perceptions of others (1992). An understanding of yourself—your strengths and weaknesses—is key to leading successfully.

Weighing Perceptions: Mentee

As a learner-leader, sometimes it is hard not to let others' perceptions of you color how you feel or how you think you may/may not be achieving goals you set (or even goals that others have set for you). In forums where nurse leaders speak, you take away a variety of messages. The messages that ring true to you may challenge you to think, but the messages that don't ring true may be the very ones that you need to take on, develop, and explore further. This is where I think Covey is challenging us as leaders.

Self-image fluctuates and can be very dependent upon the culture and team that you work within, although this could be indicative of professional experience. I have had to work hard to fight against a negative self-image, knowing that it is imperative in my position to portray positivity. Through professional connections and support, I can attain this attitude and utilize it to refocus my efforts. Support, guidance, and someone to vent to can never be underestimated.

Developing Confidence

Through an understanding of self, and from an outward demonstration of our self-image and self-esteem, is the development of confidence—an important behavior for those in leadership positions. Confidence is the belief that you have in your abilities and the reliance or trust you have in yourself. Without this, it is difficult to grow and develop (Yoder-Wise & Kowalski, 2006). When a leader lacks confidence, he or she may be unwilling to take some of the risks that leadership sometimes requires. Alternatively, confidence enables us to recognize when we need assistance and seek advice to assist us in moving forward.

Goleman (1998) states that those who are self-confident do three things:

- Present themselves with self-assurance, and have a "presence."

- Voice views that are unpopular, and go out on a limb for what is right,

- Make decisive, sound decisions despite uncertainties and pressures.

In demanding and complex work environments, successful leaders need these critical behaviors to provide leadership for their staff and to function effectively within the management team. When self-confidence is lacking, it makes it more difficult to take on and make the sometimes-tough decisions required of leaders. A lack of self-confidence may mean that when a plan does not go entirely as anticipated, we may take only the negative aspects and concentrate on these instead of seeing what components worked well and how other less successful aspects could have been done differently to achieve the desired outcome. Not everything we undertake will be completely successful the first time we implement it, but as leaders, it is important that we reflect and learn from every occasion and build our capabilities. To reflect, it is also necessary to have a high level of self-awareness and capacity to evaluate our actions realistically.

A positive self-image grounded in an understanding of self, coupled with positive self-esteem, provides us with the confidence to tackle the complex and demanding leadership roles within nursing and the broader health care system.

Weaknesses as Strengths: Mentee

Self-confidence, self-image, and self-esteem can be wavelike for a learner-leader, but what has become evident to me through experience and guidance is that your ability to move through the ebb and flow is what sets you apart, allowing you to see these times for what they are and to learn from them yet not harbor the experience in a limiting or self-destructive way. Through times of self-reflection—reaffirming values and goals and understanding your weaknesses—as a leader, you move forward.

The informal and formal processes of mentorship have certainly afforded me the ability to continue to grow as a leader. I have found that having a number of mentors can afford you different perspectives on events, and they can walk you through a variety of aspects in your career. As a mentee and learner-leader, I have found it important to take those steps and risks so that I grow and challenge myself, and, in turn, offer the support and guidance to others in my profession.

Self-Reflective Questions

1. What are the values that you hold important in your role as leader?

2. What would you do if your values and those of an organisation were out of alignment?

3. How can you develop an understanding of your strengths and weaknesses?

4. How can you better make use of your strengths while seeking to develop your weaknesses into strengths?

5. How can you consistently display your values and beliefs in stressful situations?

6. How can you take and accept accountability for your actions?

7. How prepared are you to admit when you might be wrong?

8. How prepared are you to seek guidance and support when necessary?

9. How can you prepare yourself to take reasonable risks in order to improve or achieve desired goals?

10. How can you become able to withstand criticism instead of letting yourself be defined by the opinions of others?

85

Shared Governance:
Looking Back and Looking Forward

"If the infrastructure does not consciously bring the teams together on an ongoing basis to build their relationships and to integrate their practice, partnerships will not be created, and the duplication, repetition, and fragmentation of care will not stop."

—Bonnie Wesorick

Mentor
Laurie Shiparski, RN, BSN, MS
President, Edgework Institute, Inc.
Rockford, Michigan, USA

Mentee
Paula Payne, RN, BSN
Clinical Practice Manager
CPM Resource Center, an Elsevier Business
Grand Rapids, Michigan, USA

During the 1970s and 1980s in the United States and Canada, there was a strong trend toward initiating shared governance systems in health care settings. Shared governance can be described as a system within a health care organization that is an organized way to get direct care or bedside nurses involved in decision making with formal leaders. It included specific goals like better patient care, increased nurse satisfaction scores, and minimizing the need for labor unions. Over time, we as health care leaders have come to expect even more from our efforts in shared governance.

So what has been learned that will support us in evolving that work into the future? We have worked with hundreds of health care organizations as they have embarked upon advancing shared governance systems. Some have been more successful than others in their attempts. In this chapter, major transitions will be explored that have been occurring in shared governance, as well as effective ways to initiate and advance the work, and strategies to monitor success and course-correct.

The Five Transitions of Shared Governance

The five transitions that we will explore as part of the evolution of shared governance are

1. Changing the name from shared governance to partnership councils.

2. Expanding participation from nursing to include all disciplines and departments.

3. Aligning the hierarchical (vertical) system with a staff (horizontal) system.

4. Balancing staff engagement focus at unit level and central level.

5. Frontline engagement and leadership development.

The first notable change has been the movement away from calling this endeavor *shared governance* because it has evolved into implementing an effective staff-engagement system. For maximum acceptance, it should be called something that represents the intent of the effort. Some health care organizations have reported a negative association with shared governance because they have had negative experiences in the implementation. In particular, the formal leadership either removes themselves from the decision making which sets up staff decisions to fail or they say it is joint decision making but continue to control the decisions. The best practice is to have a partnership between formal leaders and staff where both can lend expertise in the decision-making process. After working with many health care settings, one organization called the Clinical Practice Model Resource Center (CPMRC), has published a practical book to implement a shared governance or staff engagement system (*Partnership Council Field book: Strategies and Tools for Co-Creating a Healthy Work Place*, 1997). In this book, the authors re-name this effort partnership councils which resonated positively with health care settings, and the practical strategies offered for success helped organizations avoid the old pitfalls associated with shared governance systems.

Secondly, expanding participation from nursing to include all disciplines and departments has been one of the most significant reasons for recent success in organizations. The nursing-specific councils or groups were productive and yet did not have enough bandwidth to address care issues in a complete, patient-centric way. Thus, the councils began to have more interdisciplinary participation. Rehabilitation and psychiatric units were often the leaders in interdisciplinary frontline engagement. Now, most health care organizations have interdisciplinary council structures, or they are transitioning to them. This impetus comes from national agencies in health care, such as the Institute of Medicine (IOM). Organizations, patients, and clinicians are all seeking coordinated, interdisciplinary health care.

Thirdly, staff engagement has been expanding from being only at the global organizational level to include local unit/department councils. The shift over the past two decades has been to have an infrastructure that includes all levels, from individuals at the point of care, to the unit level, and on to the system level.

The initial step is to have each unit develop an interdisciplinary partnership council whose membership mirrors the unit. The council would then identify "one-to-one" assignments for each council member, ensuring that every person on the unit has a representative. The goal of the one-to-one connection is to build relationships while providing an opportunity for each person to have a part in decision making within their organization. Councils can potentially become overwhelmed with work, so there should be the option to develop shared work teams to do ground work and report to the unit council. The chairperson is always a staff person or persons (co-chairs) who become the unit's representative to the central interdisciplinary council that connects units across the system. This model has been successful in many organizations because it offsets many predictable pitfalls including

- Burnout of council members.

- Isolated decisions being made by one unit or council without considering the implications to the bigger picture.

- Redundant work on issues.

- Lack of involvement of all staff.

- Staff representative feeling overwhelmed by communicating to large number of other staff.

- Staff feeling as if it is just another management meeting.

- Lack of a consistent structure that everyone knows how to use.

This design aligns the hierarchical (vertical) system with a staff (horizontal) system. It acknowledges that although the formal leadership structure is imperative and will continue to function, there is also a need for an engagement structure (or staff councils) to add breadth and lateral involvement of frontline care providers. The two systems intersect and complement each other with intentional points of intersection. On the councils, it is essential to have clinical, educational, and operational expertise present. It became apparent that having no management representation on councils was a mistake because the expertise of the operations resource was missing. Additionally, too much management was stifling, which usually resulted in low participation of staff.

The fifth transition focuses the intent of shared governance on frontline leadership development. Many clinical frontline care providers want to be leaders but wish to stay in their clinical roles. The focus of each person as a leader at the bedside has supported better care decisions. A council infrastructure offers formal leadership opportunities for staff to address system-, workforce-, and practice-related issues.

Strategies to Advance Shared Governance

With the major transitions in mind, how can a nurse leader intentionally design an interdisciplinary council system that reflects the shifts and offers consistency and flexibility? The best approach is to analyze what is in place because of previous shared governance work and then optimize to meet the new evolving needs. It is critical to honor the work done before as learning, build on successes and mistakes, understand this as an evolving process, and value it as a worthy endeavor.

According to the CPMRC Partnership Council Workbook (2008), when initiating or optimizing, it is imperative to be clear on the intended purpose and suggest that a council infrastructure should create a place to

- Develop and sustain leaders.
- Tap individual gifts and collective capacity.
- Enhance relationships and provide connections.
- Have meaningful conversations.
- Improve care and service.
- Achieve the shared mission and vision.
- Initiate and sustain large-scale change.
- Engage point-of-care providers to enhance communication, accountability, and decision making.

Additionally, to maximize optimization, there needs to be education on the structure and processes of a successful council to all members and leadership. It is helpful to do a session for managers to explore their changing role with councils and then invite them to attend with their staff chairs for the education. Additional strategies to support managers can be found in the article *Engaging in Shared Decision Making: Leveraging Staff and Management Expertise* (Shiparski, 2005).

Finally, a key success factor for advancing shared governance is to have ways to monitor progress and course-correct. Partnership councils should conduct a checkpoint on a quarterly basis, using tools that measure progress, stimulate self-evaluation, and provoke dialog and development of action steps. Table 1 offers a quick way for a council to assess its status and pulse. Using this tool, council members complete the four questions individually and then share results. They discuss differences in opinions, reasons, and possible course-corrections. Any rating less than 4 indicates a need to take action.

Table 1   State of the Council Tool ("Taking the Pulse")

Event	Rating
MOMENTUM: Level of forward progress exhibited by council at this time. Circle the number that best describes the current state.	1 2 3 4 1 = Stagnant 2 = Modest 3 = Moderate 4 = Fast-forward movement
RELEVANCY: Issues currently being addressed by council are pertinent and key to the success of the unit/department. Circle the number that best describes the current state.	1 2 3 4 1 = Not doing this 2 = Somewhat 3 = Mostly 4 = Of high priority
COUNCIL MEMBER INTERACTIONS: With trust and respect, members are supporting each other in their leadership roles and challenging one another to tackle tough issues.Circle the number that best describes the current state.	1 2 3 4 1 = Not doing this 2 = Somewhat 3 = Mostly 4 = Consistently
PERCEIVED IMPACT: Impact that non-council member in the unit/department feels the council is making in the unit/department and/or organization-wide. Circle the number that best describes the current state.	1 2 3 4 1 = No difference 2 = Modest 3 = Significant 4 = Consistently

(Modified from the CPMRC Workbook, 2008)

Whether initiating or optimizing a staff engagement structure, Table 2 offers key success strategies for effective councils. This can be turned into a self-evaluation tool for the councils as well.

Table 2 Partnership Council Success Factors

Achievements

MEMBERSHIP: Council membership reflects sustained and regular participation by all interdisciplinary roles and tracks that make up the unit/department (including physicians, managers, etc.) and community served (patients, family members, etc.).

LEADERSHIP: The council chairperson(s) is a staff member who exhibits resourcefulness in leading the unit council and is the one who links to the central council to represent the work of the unit/department within the global organization.

PARTICIPATION: All members attend monthly meetings or have someone present to cover for them and participate to represent the work of their role.

NEW MEMBER ORIENTATION: An established orientation process exists that ensures that all new members fully understand their role, as well as the function and promise of the council infrastructure.

ONE-ON-ONE ASSIGNMENTS: Through one-on-one assignments, *all* staff are connected through trusting and respectful relationships, heard in council discussions, and are fully informed regarding the outcomes of council work.

LOGISTICS AND CONTENT: Meeting minutes effectively communicate council work; agenda is designed to make best use of limited time available; and topics are balanced in addressing relationship, operational, and practice issues.

SKILL BUILDING: Council members routinely assess their skill sets and seek out additional training and learning opportunities to enhance these sets (e.g., dialog, polarity management, relationship skills).

GOAL SETTING: Annual goal setting stems from thoughtful consideration of unit/departmental needs, internal and external variables, and the organization's strategic plan and provides clarity regarding vision, action steps, and goals to guide council work.

MANAGING WORK FLOW: Effective use is made of long-term and short-term shared work teams to permit the efficient investigation of multiple issue areas, engage others from the unit/department to tap their expertise, and provide timely feedback to the council.

APPRECIATIVE INQUIRY: Regularly engage in highlighting the outstanding achievements of the council and drawing lessons from these to guide future work to the council.

Table 2   **Partnership Council Success Factors**

Achievements
MEASURING PERFORMANCE: Councils consistently engage in self-assessment activities and course-correction.
SHARING OF EXPERTISE: Council members present their work and achievements within the organization and to the community.

(Modified from the CPMRC Workbook, 2008)

A Journey and Vision

There have been many successes and failed attempts at creating shared governance systems in health care organizations over the past few decades. It is important to honor all experiences and embrace this as a journey. Nurse leaders need to have vision, commitment, and practical tools as well as the belief that growing interdisciplinary staff engagement is the right direction for the future of health care.

Lessons Learned: Mentee

Since beginning my work at the CPM Resource Center in 2006 with Laurie Shiparski and my colleagues there, I have had the opportunity to witness many impressive achievements at various organizations around the nation made possible only through shared governance. How each individual organization manages to get there is going to be different because no two are going to be the same or have the same needs.

However, I have noticed two essential ingredients make all the difference in the world: leadership support and a clear vision. Several challenges will be met along the way, and some might always be there. Some of the tools shared in this chapter have enabled organizations to quickly implement best practices and avoid known pitfalls. Laurie Shiparski was a primary leader and developer on many of these tools and processes for partnership councils which helped me guide clients more effectively.

It is imperative that we have a clear vision of where we want to be in the future and what we plan to do to get there. If people are going to invest themselves in the work, they need to know that they will be supported along the way. Just like most things in life, you get back what you put in, and very few shortcuts are worth taking.

Self-Reflective Questions

1. In your experiences with shared governance systems, what strategies worked well?

2. What are the pitfalls you would advise others to avoid in optimizing shared governance or council structures?

3. What wisdom have you gained about implementing staff-engagement structures?

4. What is the best advice you could give a new leader in a shared governance organization?

5. What is the greater purpose for putting the effort forward to advance staff engagement?

6. What are the pay-offs of engaging staff in interdisciplinary councils?

7. Is there a personal/professional story that you can tell that was a fulfilling experience with shared governance?

8. What is your greatest fear in advancing staff engagement?

9. What is your greatest hope in advancing staff engagement?

10. What are some steps that you can take to advance staff engagement in your workplace?

86

Staffing and Workforce Management: Is It a Numbers or a Bodies Game?

"If you add more nurses without also reorganizing the way they work, that simply results in more nurses not spending enough time with patients."

—Holly De Groot

Mentor
James F. Veronesi, RN, MSN,
  CNAA-BC, CHE
Director and Faculty Member
  of the Advisory Board
  Academies, a division of The
  Advisory Board Company
Washington, D.C., USA

Mentee
Pamela R. Dugle, RN, MSN
North Florida-South Georgia
  Veterans Healthcare
  Administration
Gainesville, Florida, USA

Ask any nursing leader from around the world to identify the issue that tends to keep them up at night, and more often than not, you will hear something related to staffing and workforce management. Many nursing leaders struggle to staff their departments effectively, leading to the traditional battle cry, "We need more staff!" Staffing any nursing enterprise need not be a difficult task. However, it does require that nursing leaders exert significant discipline and attention to what is really needed to drive patient care. It is not reasonable, nor is it acceptable, for nursing leaders to default to adding more nurse bodies when doing so isn't always the right fix for the underlying root cause of the staffing issue.

Jim's Underlying Theory: Mentor

Staffing and workforce management isn't about either numbers or bodies. At the core of any hospital or health system's success, regardless of whether publicly or privately funded, are financial performance, productivity, and quality. Hospitals must generate a profit from operations or risk financial instability—and ultimately, bankruptcy—leading to facility closure. In the United States, more than half of all hospitals are insolvent, and most do not generate a profit from providing care (Alvarez & Marsal, 2008). The largest expense in any hospital is the cost of labor. Thoughtlessly adding more nurses to what is typically an already financially strained system serves only to increase financial strain without necessarily improving actual productivity or outcomes.

As an example, initial results following implementation of mandatory nurse to patient ratios in California have not resulted in improved outcomes for those measures most impacted by nursing (CalNOC, 2008). Coupled with a shrinking workforce and continuing nursing shortage, it seems the nursing profession would be better served by working toward needing fewer nurses who provide higher quality care rather than focusing on "quantity nursing," which may add little to no value. Not inconsequentially, the U.S. Bureau of Labor Statistics projects a need for 233,000 nurses each year through 2016, against a supply of 200,000 each year (U.S. Bureau of Labor Statistics, 2009).

Cracking the staffing and workforce management nut must be centered on improving financial performance and productivity, which means close adherence to reasonable productivity metrics. Human resources must be used when needed, but must not be wasted. Nursing has a responsibility to ensure that resources are used effectively while reducing the cost of care—and at the same time, improving quality of care. This means that every nurse leader must work to have a clear understanding of how, logistically, nurses are executing work at the bedside, of patient acuity, and of how an individual nurse's work experience affects overall staffing and workforce needs. Nursing leaders must be prepared to support this analysis through effective data collection and analysis, which are skills rarely taught in baccalaureate and masters programs.

High-quality nursing care is not dependent upon, nor is it synonymous with, high-cost nursing care. It is quite possible to provide high-quality nursing care without breaking the financial back of the institution. High-quality nursing care occurs when nursing leaders are actively involved in designing and holding themselves and their direct reports accountable to a rational care-delivery model. Such models must be predicated on refined processes that eliminate wasted effort and unnecessary work rooted in tradition rather than in science.

Resolving ineffective process steps begins when nursing leaders start with a blank slate and an open mind. Leaders must listen to staff, hear their stated challenges to delivering high-quality care, and ask clarifying questions to make sure that the work is understood. Information obtained must then be used to collaboratively develop a rational staffing plan that takes into account patient acuity and the experience level of nurses. It is not reasonable to staff a work shift predominantly with a department's least experienced nurses. Leaders must thus work to achieve an experience balance on a shift-to-shift basis when scheduling staff to maximize the opportunity for quality care at the bedside. Creating a scheduling balance requires that the leader fully engage their staff in the design of the staffing plan. Staffing should be added when justified, but not before staffing and shift patterns are evaluated and adjusted to match actual workload.

Taking the steps outlined here will lead to a determination of the right number of staff required in any nursing enterprise. The result will be a collaboratively designed plan that addresses staff concerns, acuity, and staff experience levels, leading to high-quality nursing care without breaking the budget. Here is a real-life example of how these concepts have been put to work.

Pam's Experience: Mentee

An area of instruction that the education system has failed to provide for future nurses is the business aspect of management. My experience is that good nurses are placed in leadership roles without any formal business training. Being a good nurse does not mean a person will be a good business manager. The reality is that without successful business operations, a hospital will not succeed. This means that nursing leadership must learn to present departmental needs in an organized business format.

From the time student nurses are introduced to documentation, they are instructed to paint a picture of the patient's condition thoroughly in an organized head-to-toe fashion. Acquiring the tools, equipment, and staffing to perform the duties of nursing must follow the same process. The responsibility to paint a picture understood and recognized by senior leadership and the finance arm of an institution rests entirely with the nursing leaders attempting to obtain these resources.

What I have learned is that nurses historically have requested more staffing but met resistance from administration who did not understand the need being expressed. Meeting with the staff of the emergency department (ED) when I became the manager brought the same response from the existing staff. More nurses were needed. When asked to justify the need, the staff was unable to do so. The only justification the staff was able to offer was their "feeling" that they could use more staff on evenings and days.

The staff of the ED provided a great deal of grumbling when challenged to collect patient census data by shift and by hour. By following a 10-step approach shown in the following list, even the newest of nurse managers will likely be successful when seeking additional resources. My staff required reassurance that the future success of the department would depend upon their cooperation and hard work to collect the data, which would then be analyzed and presented in such a manner that senior leadership would recognize the need and support the request for additional full-time equivalents (FTEs), if needed. Charts, graphs, the data, and everything done to improve the current practice must be included in the request for additional resources. The request must also include how the change will benefit care quality and the larger organization.

Determining Resource Needs

1. Determine need.

2. Develop a data collection tool.

3. Perform retrospective data collection.

4. Perform prospective data collection.

5. Analyze the data.

6. Develop supporting charts and graphs.

7. Determine the impact of recommended changes.

8. Develop a formal business plan and secure approvals.

9. Implement a business plan.

10. Reassess and adjust as needed.

Developing a data collection tool to provide the data became necessary because nothing existed to provide the essential information. The tool would incorporate times of day, day of the week, and overtime usage. After a retrospective look for one to two years and a prospective look at the data for a period of six months, an analysis of the data was conducted to determine changes in workload and reorganization of duties. Additional tours of duty were established to facilitate the fluctuations in census at the various times throughout the 24-hour period. Based upon analysis, the staff had the correct instinct that more staff was needed during the day and evening shifts. Retrospective data had been collected for three years for comparison purposes.

The department consistently required 6.0 FTEs in overtime usage to meet the needs of patient care. The data demonstrated a 365% increase in census over a three-year period and justified an increase in staffing of 5.5 registered nurse (RN) FTEs. Reorganization of duties, reconfiguring the shift starting times within the department, and the additional RNs would reduce overtime and improve both the quality of patient care and patient safety.

Data to support the request for additional FTEs provided the senior leadership group with the information that they needed to make an informed decision regarding the appeal for additional staff. Talking in language that the senior leaders understood provided me with the ammunition needed to make the request and for senior leadership to make an informed decision. The request was approved for additional FTEs, not because the staff felt they needed more staff, but because emotion was removed from the request and replaced with facts and supporting data.

When the ED staff saw what their efforts had accomplished, they became believers of data collection. Their approach now is to ask what data they must collect to obtain needed resources. Data collection is no longer a disagreeable activity within the ED but a method to obtain resources. The staff recognizes the importance and continually has some form of data collection in process.

After results are tabulated and resources are obtained, data must continue to be collected. Constant assessing and reassessing of the situation must be completed to determine whether changes are required to adjust to the changing climate within the department. During the reassessment phase, data showed that census began to change at various times, and shifts were adjusted to meet the changing needs. Whereas the original plan added staff to the day and evening shift, the reassessment phase revealed that additional staff was needed on the night tours. Knowing additional staff was not justified based on the data, the shifts had to be reorganized and adjusted to meet the changing needs of the department.

This same approach can be used with any type of nursing department, and is not limited to just the ED. Demonstrating the need to increase staffing requires a serious look at current practice to determine whether the same outcome can be achieved by reorganization of current staffing patterns.

One important reminder is that while collecting data, outliers will invariably exist. A contingency plan for these outliers must be included in any business plan that is presented to executive leadership to exhibit one's ability to distinguish between the normal and the outliers. Thinking ahead and being prepared for the unexpected is an asset appreciated by the executive leadership.

Businesses are built on strong foundations, not emotions. Stepping back and looking at needs in an objective manner will help cement the foundation of the department's request for resources. Nursing leaders must react rationally and without emotion, which is the hallmark of a solid leader. Presenting staffing ideas in a concise data-driven format with a well-written business plan showing current practices and alternatives that have been attempted will paint the picture that senior leadership requires, allowing them to make the informed decisions to effectively support high-quality patient care at a reasonable cost.

Self-Reflective Questions

1. Do you have a strategic staffing and workforce plan?

2. Describe the strategic staffing and workforce plan.

3. How much collaboration and input do you receive from staff involved in day-to-day patient care?

4. What tool does your organization use to calculate staffing needs? Describe the process of analyzing staffing needs.

5. Do budget constraints mandate staffing ratios?

6. In what ways does your organization's nursing leaders take a strong stand on adequate staffing and nurse ratios?

7. How flexible are staffing ratios and workforce depending on the acuity and focus of the unit? Are decisions based on collective data analysis and trends in census or acuity?

8. Is data and trend analysis shared with staff at the point of care and managers continually?

9. How do nurse leaders assist units in requesting or re-adjusting staffing ratios if needed?

10. Are staffing plans and workforce requests presented to the C-Suite or appropriate individuals in a methodical, well-researched, and concrete data without emotions involved?

87

(Taking One) Step at a Time (*or* You Cannot Do Everything at Once, But You Can Do Something)

"The journey of a thousand miles begins with one step."

—Lao Tzu

Mentor

Christine Duffield, PhD, RN, MHP, FRCNA, FACHSE, FAICD
Director, Centre for Health Services Management and Deputy Head
World Health Organization (WHO) Collaborating Centre for Nursing, Midwifery, and Health Development
Faculty of Nursing, Midwifery & Health,
University of Technology
Sydney, New South Wales, Australia

Mentee

Katherine Becker, MN, RN, BN, NP
Nurse Practitioner Neurosurgery
Royal North Shore Hospital
Sydney, New South Wales, Australia

It takes one step at a time to reach a significant goal or milestone. The components to get there are defined here.

The introduction of the nurse practitioner (NP) role in Australia has been slow. Even now, its value in enhancing the quality of patient care is poorly understood by many in the medical and nursing professions. The complex process of gaining and maintaining authorization to practice is not for the faint-hearted. It requires professionals who are self-directed; passionate about their work; articulate; and sufficiently confident in their ability to demonstrate their preparedness to undertake what, at the outset, seems to be a daunting challenge. This is the story of one individual's journey to gain acceptance of the role—one step at a time.

Background: The Mentor

There has been extensive debate regarding the introduction of the NP role in Australia (Royal Australian College of General Practitioners, 1999). The Australian NP role is relatively new in comparison to the United Kingdom (UK), where the first NP was qualified in 1991 (Cross, 2009), and the United States, where NPs were first trained by the University of Colorado in 1965 (Hill, 1998).

While the introduction of NPs has been on the nursing profession's agenda in Australia—and, in particular, New South Wales (NSW)—since 1990 (The Australian Nurse Practitioners Association, 2008), these positions were not established until 2000 and only then within the context of ad hoc economic rationalist strategies, restructuring of the health workforce, staff shortages (medical), and the need to develop new models of care to deal with these issues (Furlong, & Smith, 2005).

Throughout the debate over the introduction of the role of the NP, ill-informed sectors of the medical profession generated a great deal of adverse publicity. However, perhaps most disappointing was the resistance from nursing managers, some of whom now oversee NPs. Strategies to overcome resistance from nursing colleagues and superiors form the basis of this mentee's journey.

The Road to NP Status: The Mentee

My journey commenced in 2003 when I applied for a case management role in neurosurgery. I had been a clinical nurse specialist and a nursing unit manager within the department of neurosurgery. Consequently, I was an established clinician and had well-defined relationships with the multidisciplinary team in my health facility. The Nurses Amendment (NP) Act was proclaimed in 1998, and after a very slow start, the NSW Government progressed the implementation of the Act. In 2003, the Minister for Health announced plans to advertise 92 NP positions in the public health sector. My case manager position was quickly targeted as a potential NP position, and I was approached by a nurse manager and asked whether I was prepared to consider authorization as an NP.

The NP role was one I had always wanted; however, the slow pace in which it was being introduced in NSW had made it appear to be an improbable career path. My authorization was granted eight months later after a very challenging process. At this stage, there were only 14 NPs in NSW, and only six were actually employed in dedicated positions. The authorization process was rigorous and required a great deal of preparation.

During this time, there were significant staff shortages within my neurosurgery unit, and there was no established nursing unit manager (NUM) leading the unit. The expectation was that I would supplement the poor nursing skill mix and mentor the acting NUM. The introduction of a new role is often challenging, and I was careful to consider my decision in the context of service needs, service deficits, and the potential threats and challenges to the change process. This required self-awareness, the use of change management theory, and the complexity of developing a new clinical role while mentoring the unit manager to whom I reported.

My longevity and experience in the unit also resulted in my position absorbing parts of many of the roles either not replaced or not being performed safely. This resulted in more confusion regarding role delineation because I was viewed as a solution—a "stopgap" in issues ranging from secretarial work, to bed management, to relief for junior medical staff during times of poor staffing. Nurse managers to whom I reported had lists of tasks that had been identified as potential projects for me to undertake. The neurosurgeons with whom I worked were very supportive because many had worked with NPs during their fellowship experiences in the United States and so more readily understood the role.

The Journey

Mentor: Mentoring has not been formed as a part of the nursing culture in Australia and therefore has not been well understood (Pelletier & Duffield, 1994). Providing encouragement as a mentor is important when potential has been recognized. This has been found to contribute to successful careers and promote leadership (Moran et al., 2002; Pelletier & Duffield, 1994). In the context described earlier, it was important for the mentee to develop skills to deal with colleagues and their incorrect perceptions about the role—and, more importantly, to be able to work with her immediate supervisor. It was also important to separate personal from professional issues and to network with others to further her career (Chyna, 2000).

Mentee: The first issue I tackled was the misinformation that circulated about the role of the NP: namely, that it was a cheap alternative to a physician, or a solution to shortages of junior medical officers and nursing staff. In addition, the media often portrays the role as a "Super Nurse." This interpretation significantly disenfranchises other nurses who are providing complex care and who are clinical leaders in their own right. Friction can result.

I surrounded myself with like-minded clinicians so we could draw strength from each other. I was fortunate that two NP positions had been introduced; I filled one position and a long-term colleague filled the other. This nurse shares the same philosophy in her nursing practice and conducts her care as a mirror image of mine. Together, as fellow NPs, we were always able to articulate a single vision that was transparent and consistent. For many NPs in NSW, the journey is lonely, and many speak of being disheartened and feel isolated from other NPs in practice.

I also realized that I needed to promote the role. To do this would require me to be present in the clinical setting so I took the initiative to present at clinical forums for both managers and clinicians. I looked at the referral teams with which I would be closely aligned, met with them, and took the opportunity to demystify the role and allow everyone to ask questions. This was an important step because waiting for the hospital to formally introduce this new paradigm of care would take a long time. More importantly, though, it was clear to others and me that managers and other clinicians were also unsure of the role's functions.

Mentor: As one of the first NPs appointed, it was important for the mentee to promote the position and assist others to walk the path. Mentors have been identified as having particular roles: teacher, sponsor, adviser, agent, role model, coach, and confidante (Tobin, 2004). It is hoped that a successfully mentored individual would eventually become a mentor to others.

Mentee: I realized that actions do speak louder than words. As one of the first NPs in NSW, I felt frustrated at many stages through this journey that I had not had time to submit a journal paper about the establishment of my role. However, my commitment to hands-on patient care will always inhibit my academic contribution. However, I find time for lecturing on- and off-campus as well as for mentoring and teaching interested new neurosurgical nurses. Meeting with mentors has helped me to pace myself on this journey, which I now know will be a marathon and not a sprint!

The team of clinicians with whom I work understands the extent and limitations of my role, seeks my advice, and uses my skills to ensure optimal patient care. Knowing that I do make a difference to the patient journey and have the respect of my colleagues for the work I perform and the care I provide is rewarding enough. It has taken time, but I eventually accepted that I could not do everything at once—and that as a relatively young NP, I have time on my side. This has allowed me to plot my journey more carefully and not feel that I need to accomplish everything at once.

Mentor: The mentee NP reports to a nurse manager, or sometimes directly to employing physicians. It is important, therefore, that managers understand the role and assist in transition process. However, one of the difficulties faced by the mentee was the instability in nursing leadership during the journey. There have been five divisional nurse managers since the implementation of this role in 2003. High turnover of nurse managers has been studied (Duffield, et al., 2001; Johnstone, 2003), but little has been written about how best to deal with this.

Mentee: The problem created for me by the continuous changes to senior staff was that most either did not support or understand the role. In an ideal world, it would be more productive for this position to report to a senior nursing clinician for supervision; however, this was not the case. I dealt with this by engaging in clinical supervision, which is essential for individuals working to challenge traditional practice and pursue new roles. It allows appropriate reflection and review of achievements and ongoing challenges. This has assisted me in maintaining motivation in the face of continual requests to justify my role or conform to traditional models of care.

Following several attempts to obtain a mentor as a clinical supervision relationship, I realized it was unlikely that one individual would materialize who possessed both clinical experience and the wisdom required. Therefore, I arranged for several professionals to assist me with this process, including a professor of psychology as well as the neurosurgeons with whom I work. Prior to this arrangement, my colleague (the other NP in neurosurgery) and I found that debriefing and reflecting upon challenging cases and situations with her was helpful. However, neither of us really had sufficient distance from the scenario or the skills to add optimal value to these debriefing discussions.

Mentor: It was difficult to maintain optimal working relationships with nurse managers who were constantly changing, and conflict often arose. Resolving this conflict required skills in negotiation; a capacity to deal with the issues and not the personalities, which at times means separating the person from the position; and maintaining open lines of communication, no matter how difficult. It was also important at times to maintain a physical separateness until sufficient time had passed that conversations could again be had. The mentee was encouraged to debrief regularly with respected and trusted colleagues and family.

Mentee: I have accepted that some working relationships will always be challenging even if I make a significant effort. The health profession attracts a variety of individuals, many of whom have a different work ethic than I do. Although I can be altruistic in my outlook at times, I believe it is essential to strive for a gold standard of patient care, even when it may seem that the institution is dysfunctional and lacking a patient-centered focus. I acknowledge that I am a challenge to manage because my commitment to quality care makes others uncomfortable, and I make managers accountable for the decisions they make that affect patient care.

Lessons Learned

When new roles were introduced into the NHS, Hyde et al. (2004; 2005) found that it worked best when introduced *locally*, when key stakeholders were involved, and where local willingness to hand over tasks existed and usually required local training programs. This implies that the introduction of a new role is more likely to succeed when it is understood and supported by all team members, and when team members are clear about their roles and have expectations of what the new position offers. This is particularly challenging as the NP role will often evolve as their skills and experiences develop (Alpert, Fjone & Candela, 2002; Kleinpell, 2005). The nature of the NP role is one that should be dynamic and change with the service need. Therefore, formal, regular communication opportunities with managers must be developed to discuss progress and problems that arise.

This mentee's experience indicates that the journey can be daunting, that it cannot be undertaken alone, and that it requires skills beyond those expected of a NP at a personal level, but certainly within the scope expected of future leaders. Persistence, resilience, endurance, and determination are required. This journey is not over. Today, NPs in Australia still face difficulties with explaining their role and its differences from other nursing and medical positions. Many still do not have rights to prescribe, and most importantly, NPs are not allowed to claim their services against Medicare even though other health professionals (such as physiotherapists and podiatrists) are able to do so.

It is important to realize when undertaking a new role not to take on responsibility for everyone who may follow in this role. Individuals cannot make this journey alone: They need a supportive network of colleagues, friends, and family. It is also important to realize that not all goals can be achieved, but someone has to take the first step!

Self-Reflective Questions

1. Why is this journey important to make?

2. How can you determine whether this is the right time for you?

3. How can you tell whether you are the right person to make this journey?

4. How can you assess whether you have the courage, determination, and persistence to commence this journey?

5. How can you best secure a supportive network of colleagues and friends?

6. Who can you trust to tell you when you lose perspective?

7. How can you prepare yourself to risk everything to pursue this dream?

8. For how long are you prepared to take this risk?

9. How will you know when you have succeeded?

10. What will you do if you fail?

Strategic Management

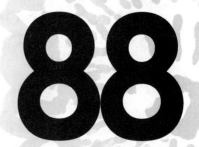

88

"The fellow that can only see a week ahead is always the popular fellow, for he is looking with the crowd. But the one that can see years ahead, he has a telescope, but he cannot make anyone believe he has it."

—Mark Twain

Mentor

Roxane Spitzer, RN, PHD, MBA, FAAN
Editor-in-Chief for *Nurse Leader*
Texas Tech University, Clinical Professor
Stuart, Florida, USA

Mentee

May E. Bennett, CPA, NHA
Managing Director in Healthcare Finance
Nashville, Tennessee, USA

Sun Tzu—one of the greatest strategists of all times—defined strategy through discourse, calling it the Art of War (Sawyer, 1994). Alexander the Great was also a great strategist, and his accomplishments in achieving results were carefully crafted through long-range vision and tactical implementation at the front line (Bose 2003). In the early days of business strategy, the focus was on planning, and implementation seemed to take a backseat. Frequently, strategic plans were heavy documents with reams of paper and materials relegated to the back of a file cabinet.

Although strategy today is based on data retrieval and analysis, it is more an art than a science because it encompasses a desired future—forecasting—which by itself is an inexact science and requires the input of many stakeholders. The purpose of strategy was originally a planning process, orchestrated to forecast changes in the external environment, including demographics that would influence the business. A primary purpose was to meet competitive challenges in response to the changing environment.

Health care is a newcomer to strategic planning and implementation because until relatively recently, we have practiced in a nonprofit environment, and the concept of competition was foreign to the basic notions about the provision of health care. My (Roxane) doctoral dissertation, completed in 1992, demonstrated that out of 10 southwest/west hospitals, if a strategic plan existed, it was unknown to many of the major stakeholders. Consequently, each executive had a different perspective on the direction and initiatives of the organization. Because this became a triangulated study, one outcome of the study showed a high correlation of lack of knowledge with operating losses (Spitzer 1994).

As part of strategy, it is critical to determine whether the strategy has been or is effective; therefore, control mechanisms must be put into place. The concept of control is basic to the practice of management and includes the four functions of planning, implementation, controlling, and evaluation. This is the framework used in open systems. That is, adaptability to adjust to incoming data to provide information about the effectiveness and efficiencies for any one of these processes, thereby affecting the strategic outcomes, either through necessary modification of the inputs and/or examining the results to determine whether these meet the organization's imperatives.

These controls are not about controlling people; rather, they are control systems designed to ensure accurate measurements and achievement of the desired outcomes. In the 1980s, the process was primarily financial, with the emphasis on financial statements including balance sheets, operating statements, and cash flow. Managerial outcomes such as productivity, variance analysis, and some patient quality measures were infrequently measured. Occasionally, physician satisfaction was measured because of the impact they have on admissions and ultimate success of the organization. Rarely did the control mechanism match strategic goals or initiatives.

These outcomes include satisfied stakeholders, delighted customers, efficient and effective processes, and a motivated and prepared workforce (Kaplan & Norton, 1996). All these elements were recognized as crucial to success first in the business world and then in the health care environment.

Development and Implementation of Strategic Management

Getting there, however, is another story, which requires the powerful and complex process of implementation. This is where strategic management transcends strategic planning.

I (Roxane) am frequently asked when I consult or speak on strategy whether I am a strategic planner, and my answer is emphatically, "No." My skill and the skill of nurse leaders must be in the realm of implementation. Planning, analysis, and talking do not meet the needs of the organization in achieving its objective. Often, that is a hard lesson to learn as a leader. This is particularly true when a new leader is hired, and the organization needs a great deal of change. Changing the table of organization (organizational chart) is probably the worst first step or even second step that any nurse leader could make. Form must follow function; therefore, understanding organizational strategy and how the areas that the nurse leader is accountable for should be prioritized. It is my experience and belief that whatever managers are in place must be given the opportunity to succeed under new management. This led me to believe that when a collaborative decision was made, if the manager said it would be done, I accepted it as a commitment. When I made rounds, asked questions, spoke with staff, and looked at the processes in place, it became evident that my beliefs weren't always accurate. This was a career epiphany for me.

Because managing to the organizational strategy requires operational expertise and experience, the importance of having a developed operational plan that includes key stakeholders is critical. At the CEO level, this includes the board, executive staff, and the organizations' management staff. This provides not only buy-in but also an opportunity for stakeholders to recognize and understand their individual and groups' role in achieving success. This same paradigm applies to the nursing department and others that interface continually with nursing. Therefore, it is critical that appropriate department managers be included in nursing's strategic sessions if nursing is to achieve their goals. Certainly, it is critical for managers to be included in the higher-level strategic process as well because the basic purpose and intent of strategic management is implementation. The management staffs are accountable for meeting the annual operational objectives.

Each manager, as well as each member of the executive staff, must think each day of the role they play in facilitating the accomplishments essential to meeting the strategic imperatives of the organization. At the very least, the organization's direction and strategic outcomes must be shared with the managers to ensure that an operational plan and resource allocation is defined at the unit level. The operational plan or business plan (which converts strategy into action planning) is tactical and provides the framework for the budgeting process at the level of delivery of care. Effective strategic management requires an inclusive process. The first time around, it makes sense to assure inclusion at the service level or unit level because reviewing the organization's mission, vision, and strategic direction is imperative. Using this framework provides the baseline mandate required to establish a unit based mission, goals, and objectives as well as tactical action plans that are consistent with the organization's direction.

The Framework of Strategic Management

Mission

The mission describes the business that the organization is in. Although the mission statement should not be lengthy, it must be specific enough that the external communities as well as internal participants know what the organization is about and what it deems important. For example:

> Health care system X provides inpatient services to the community inclusive of _____(e.g. cardiac care, oncology, surgery, etc.) In providing this, we ensure excellence in the delivery of care and fiscal responsibility to our community, employees, and physicians. Our values incorporate commitment to lifelong learning and the dignity of our staff, the highest quality of care to our patients, and an environment that exceeds expectations.

Vision

The vision is a desired future—generally, where the organization would like to be in 5 to 10 years. It is often measurable in the long term. For example

> Health care system X will be the premier choice of physicians and patients for the delivery of health care services in County A.

The outcomes, which are measurable through market research data, can inform the organization of their accomplishments. It seems fairly obvious that achieving this mission really requires operational implementation.

SWOT Analysis

The development of the organization's (or service line, unit level) strengths, weaknesses, opportunities, and threats (SWOT) require market research and input from the stakeholders at a strategy session. In my experience, it is at this level that an outside consultant becomes the most valuable. This is because stakeholders are more likely to provide honest input with a consultant, and the consultant is not biased by being a part of the organization.

A brief example of each one of these follows:

- **Strength:** *We are the only provider of cardiac surgery and intervention in the county area.*

- **Weakness:** *We do not have a second cardiac surgeon on staff.*

- **Opportunity:** *We provide training opportunity for the resident program located at B University.*

- **Threat:** *The health care system in the adjacent county is in the process of attempting an affiliation with B University.*

When the organization examines these parameters, it provides a framework for the establishment of strategic goals which should address both the marketplace and the internal issues. If, for example, a lack of ability to recruit and retain professional nurses is a weakness, an organizational goal designed to remedy that situation would be hammered out at the strategic level with the tactical steps to accomplish that done at an operational level.

Establishing Strategic Goals

Strategic goals in general should be specific and few; often a strategic goal in a plan can be identified as something to be accomplished in year 2, 3, or whatever the timeframe for the plan is. It is important that these goals can be and are measured both qualitatively and quantitatively. My recommendation is for no longer than five years because rapid change is a way of life, both globally and in the health care system. Usually, no more than five goals should be established because even one of them may take several years to accomplish.

Some examples of strategic goals for Hospital X might include the following:

- Ensure fiscal success through increasing our adjusted net revenue by 3% per year for the next five years.

- Increase productivity and quality through the recruitment and retention of professional staff; turnover should be reduced to no more than 10% for the next five years.

- Provide a continuous learning environment for our staff to improve skills and abilities in the delivery of patient care.

- Increase our market share through the development of viable programs that are needed by our community.

- Increase specialty physician recruitment in the area of cardiac surgery, interventional cardiology, oncology, and geriatrics by 10% for each specialty.

These are just a sample of what organizations might consider in establishing a five-year plan. They are all measurable, but they now must be put into operation by the management staff. Because part of the management process is control, it is important to recognize that control relates to information on a system and unit level. Again, control today as a management function is not about controlling people, but rather establishing mechanisms that measure outcomes against stated goals and objectives. This is where a dashboard mechanism and the balanced scorecard come into play.

Measurement Systems

The balanced scorecard is an internal control mechanism that measures four major measures of organizational performance. These incorporate data about financial performance, customer service, learning, and growth initiatives (motivated and prepared workforce) and efficient, effective internal processes (Kaplan & Norton 1996).

The measurement of outcomes against these indicators is the most effective way to ensure that strategy is managed to achieve the desired outcomes. The dashboard is no more than an internal tool that takes the information and correlates it to the previously established strategic goals. It is important to remember that the concept is predicated upon understanding that we are measuring performance at the operational level where the action happens.

Benchmarking is another performance measurement tool that also determines how our strategy is working generally in the competitive arena: that is, how we are doing compared with other organizations. The three types of benchmarking include competitive, cooperative, and collaborative (Kaplan & Norton 1996). These might be used in addition to internal performance indicators, particularly if the institution is in a very competitive market. If performance against other institutions is favorable, it becomes a valuable marketing tool.

Competitive Benchmarking

Competitive benchmarking determines how well we are doing against a known competitor. A particular program's performance, for example, is as follows: namely, the measure of market share and patient volume in a cardiac surgery program over a defined period as compared to a competitor.

Cooperative Benchmarking

Cooperative benchmarking is a truly exciting way to learn from outside the health care industry. Innovative health care organizations in the last decade have learned from other industries. An example of this is competing for the Baldridge award, which measures process and quality in business organizations. Another example is the application of ISO 9001 standards, which comprises a framework used in manufacturing to determine both efficiency and effectiveness.

Collaborative Benchmarking

Collaborative benchmarking occurs within the industry. For many years as both a chief nursing officer (CNO) and chief executive officer (CEO), I used the measurement system from the University Health Consortium, which allowed for comparisons between peer organizations on a national level. The organizations remain anonymous, but their demographics closely parallel your own organization.

Of most importance for all these measurement/control systems is determining those areas needing improvement on a cost-effectiveness basis. Not all can or should be benchmarked because the expense and use of resources would not be worth the effort, nor is this a realistic approach. In essence, if a strategic goal is identified to increase productivity, determination of those areas that appear to need improvement must be analyzed to ensure that it is worth the cost and effort to implement essential changes.

Mentoring in Strategic Management: Mentee

Investing adequate time and effort in strategic management can be challenging even during times of organizational stability; in the midst of organizational crisis, delaying such work can be easily justified. However, when I assumed responsibility as chief operating officer (COO) for a large, post-acute care facility where the board's imperative was to accomplish a turnaround, the CEO (Dr. Roxane Spitzer) guided implementation of a strategic management process that proved instrumental in accomplishing the desired outcome.

Despite the need to extinguish many organizational "fires" during the first two years, within the first six months, through collaboration with many stakeholders, we revised the mission, vision, and values and developed strategic goals as well as operational objectives that were assigned to organizational leaders. Much to the surprise of leaders whose previous exposure to strategic plans had been ethereal documents that, once developed, gathered dust on a shelf and were quickly ignored, we implemented quarterly progress reports for objectives to ensure that the plan continued to be updated and prioritized.

When faced with significant community concerns about changes in the organization, Dr. Spitzer's advice was to develop a community advisory board to include prominent community leaders, such as city councilpersons, who could become aware of the reasons for the changes and provide input. As a result, we were able to garner support from the community and the city council for major changes that would otherwise have been impossible.

Dr. Spitzer wisely cautioned all of us involved in the turnaround that changing the culture of an organization from being a safety-net provider (known as the health care provider of last resort) to a preferred provider of care known for quality and innovation required not only a well-developed plan, but more importantly, intense execution by organizational leaders. Often, inexperienced leaders were surprised when they learned that previously implemented changes "disappeared," after they moved forward to implement other changes. Developing a dashboard of key indicators helped ensure that improvements were monitored and stayed on-track over time and also served as a means of communicating with key constituencies, such as the board of directors, concerning progress and opportunities.

In this situation, the CEO was a leader with extensive experience in strategic management and turnarounds, so she was also able to continually impress upon all stakeholders the time commitment required for culture change. We talked about the rather odd combination of patience and impatience required to lead organizational change. Impatience and unwillingness to accept the status quo are required to establish the "burning platform" required to overcome inertia in an organization, especially one that has existed for many years.

However, patience is required to press forward, day after day, when it seems like the efforts that have been expended should have already achieved the desired outcomes. Dr. Spitzer reminded us often that culture change takes five to seven years in most organizations, and by using the principles of strategic management, she helped our leadership team regularly measure progress while remaining focused on the agreed-upon goals and interventions required to move closer to the desired outcomes.

Complex, Yet Systematic

Strategic management uses strategic planning as a baseline to initiate the framework for an organization's mission and vision. However, planning is just the initiation of the process, which includes establishing or reaffirming strategic goals, operational objectives, and tactics. The essence of strategic management is implementation; therefore, involvement, input, and buy-in of key stakeholders is essential to success.

The process must make provisions for all elements of the organization that are responsible for goal achievement to be involved. At the strategic level, this is usually the board and executive management. At the operational level, unit and departmental management have to determine what objectives will achieve the desired outcomes and what tactics must be implemented to support that direction. Of critical import is measurement of success against the defined organizational imperatives. A variety of mechanisms can be put in place. Whatever mechanisms are used, they must be valid, reliable, and timely as well as understood by all and used to determine modification and changes when necessary. A competent leader also ensures that the key staff can understand and direct the process and implementation, assuring continuity and success over the long term.

Strategic management is complex but systematic in approach. An outside consultant to facilitate the process, assist in data analysis, and goal and operational implementation may be a good use of an expert resource.

Self-Reflective Questions

1. What strategic planning model do you use?

2. What measurements are used for strategic planning?

3. How can you involve the entire health care team in strategic development?

4. How often is the strategic planning process re-evaluated?

5. Why would you choose to make the strategic planning process goal-driven?

6. How does the strategic planning process mirror the mission, vision, and values of the organization?

7. How can you use competitive and cooperative benchmarkng in the organization and in collaboration with strategic planning?

8. What are the steps you take to begin strategic planning?

9. What is a SWOT analysis and how does it complement strategic planning?

10. How can you use outside resources in the strategic planning process?

89

Stress Management: Starting a New Chapter in a Professional Nursing Life

"A scholar must be broad and resolute, for his responsibilities are burdensome and his path is long."

—Zengzi

Mentor
Loke Yuen Jean Tak Alice,
  (Prof.), RN, MN, PhD
School of Nursing, The Hong
  Kong Polytechnic University
Hong Kong SAR, China

Mentee
Lam Yuk Yin Winsome, RN, APN,
  MN
School of Nursing, The Hong
  Kong Polytechnic University
Hong Kong SAR, China

There are many crossroads in life. The decisions we make at these crossroads in our life often have significant impact and change the direction of our personal life. As such, career decisions may open up new chapters in our career path.

Having worked in hospitals as a registered nurse for more than 12 years, I (Winsome Yuk-Yin Lam) was accustomed to daily operations and patient care routine. I enjoyed caring for my patients, and the recovery of patients for whom I gave care provided me a strong sense of satisfaction and commitment to the nursing profession. I was, and am, proud and honored to be a member of this caring family.

However, I had been working in the same capacity in a hospital for a long time. At times, I had thoughts about my professional development—my inner-self told me to do more, and my passion for challenges crept in. I questioned whether I could transmit my knowledge and skills as an expert nurse clinician, entering the academic arena as a nurse educator, and whether my contribution to the nursing profession and the health of the people I served would multiply. These thoughts and questions became an inner fire and passion and gave me a direction and purpose even though I was apprehensive about change.

Change is not at all easy. I could not find a suitable time, hesitated to make the move because I was comfortable in my daily routine, and knew very well that changes can be stressful and demanding.

Career Change: A New Challenge

A year ago, I finally summoned enough courage to make the decision to enter the academic arena to begin my career as a nurse teacher, and moved from my long-comfortable job as a clinician into the world of academia.

My worries were not ungrounded. I expected a certain level of stress in the early stages of my new role as an academic, but I did not expect it to come from so many different directions, and I worried about my ability to adapt to my new role. I had to start almost everything anew; I had to learn the nature of the job as a nurse teacher and adjust to the difficulties that come with the new role. The culture of the academic arena and the work demands are entirely different. The job was no longer routine or something I was accustomed to and could easily handle.

Having to anticipate students' questions and meet their expectations, I found it stressful trying to find the best explanations for students so that they would learn. How to attract and maintain students' attention, arouse their interest in the subject matter, and listen attentively to presentations became a challenge.

Adding to my already stretched responsibilities, I then learned that if I stayed in the academic arena, I needed to further my studies for a doctoral degree; and if I wanted to excel, I needed to conduct research and publish in journals. There can be no doubt that I am in a different world and that the decision I made has repositioned me in a new chapter of my life, from being an expert nurse clinician to being a novice nurse academic.

This was stressful because I felt as though I was new in my career, and I sensed my limitations. Although I knew that feeling stressed in the early stages of a career change is normal, I was hoping desperately that someone would come along to rescue me.

Giving My First Lecture

I made an effort to mobilize my energy into preparing dynamic presentations to stimulate student learning. My mission was to facilitate students' learning by giving presentations that captivated them and aroused their awareness of the connectedness of their knowledge, the surrounding world, and nursing practice. How to prepare for teaching and the strategies for teaching was a challenge. All these require creativity and skill in teaching.

I still remember my first tutorial for a class of students. From their puzzled eyes, I was well aware of the need to provide clear explanations and to improve my teaching. This troubled me and shook me out of my comfort zone; I started to search for different strategies for making clear explanations in an effort to make my teaching interesting. It was taxing and mentally draining, but I knew that it was an important aspect and much needed in the academic world. I needed the reassurance that this was a common concern for new teachers and that I was not alone.

Initiation of the Mentoring Relationship

I would say I was fortunate that the school had arranged for me to co-teach a subject in a master's degree program on Health Concerns of Community with Professor Loke. Although I had elected to join the research group led by Professor Loke when I entered the school, I had not had a chance to work with her on teaching. The research group arrangement is intended to put staff members with similar research interests together to foster the development of nurse researchers through collaborative research opportunities. It also serves as a platform to provide a mentoring process that supports the development of new clinical researchers.

About a month before the term was to start, Professor Loke set up a meeting with me to discuss the teaching arrangements. At the first meeting, she provided me with her proposed subject outline and asked me whether I had any comments or suggestions for changes. She also openly acknowledged the fact that although she had been teaching the subject for a number of years, she would love to hear what I, as an experienced clinician, thought should be taught about the subject and suggestions for a more creative approach. She also welcomed creative ideas to make the subject interesting while meeting the learning needs of students.

Professor Loke reassured me that I did not have to worry about preparation or the appropriateness of the teaching content if I was not ready, and that she could always take over and help. She offered to teach the subject the first time around so that I could become familiar with it and get to know more about the subject and students' expectations. I had been told by other colleagues that in her previous experience in working with other new colleagues in a mentoring relationship, she always allowed time for newcomers to work with her until they felt comfortable and ready. I felt relieved because I had been anxious when I first learned that I was going to co-teach this subject at the master's level.

An Eye-Opening Lecture

A brief introduction to the subject was given in the first lecture. Professor Loke then asked the students whether they agreed that Hong Kong, a comparatively affluent society, nevertheless has a population with numerous health concerns in our community. Nearly three-fourths of the students disagreed with that suggestion. Professor Loke further explained that many health concerns surrounding us can be found in our daily newspapers. The students still looked puzzled and did not quite believe this suggestion. I was sitting quietly in the class, waiting to see how Professor Loke was going to handle the situation.

She then took out a stack of that day's newspapers that she had brought to the class, asking each student to take just one page to see whether they could find any news related to health issues. Students were asked to share with the whole class if they thought they had found any in the newspaper, albeit some with a little help from Professor Loke. As a result, students were surprised that many health issues were found. Professor Loke then concluded by saying that the public, including health professionals, often miss or overlook the health issues surrounding them in the news media. Students were encouraged to pay more attention to what is hampering us from achieving health and to societal issues that impede our health. She then concluded that in this subject, students are to learn to look at health from different perspectives and to be aware of the surroundings in our community.

Inspired and Relieved

This was the first time I had ever witnessed a teaching approach such as this. This approach to connecting the community and the nursing profession and pointing out the significance amazed me. I also realized then that teaching is not meant to be, and never should be, boring! The students were surprised that they could learn about the health of the community by simply reading daily newspapers, and also that nursing can be involved in the community as an advocate for and contributor to the health of the community.

Professor Loke's teaching skills in the use of probing questions kept students involved, leading them to think, allowing time for discussion, arousing interest, and at the same time developing critical thinking among students. Her skills impressed me. I was convinced that I, too, could arouse interest and a sense of curiosity and involvement in my other classes by adopting the same strategies that she had used in this class. I felt relieved and quickly realized that I could seek advice from her and that she would be my role model.

The Mentoring Relationship Is Formed

On that day, a mentor-mentee relationship was established between Professor Loke and me. I have found that even as an experienced teacher, she continues to reflect upon her own teaching and strives to find ways to improve. She even gave me advice on furthering my education and joining her in her research projects. I must say that this mentoring process has created a rich environment for role development and direction, enabling me to start to plan my teaching career in the certainty that I am going to grow in the near future.

I found that the co-teaching arrangement opened a wealth of experiences that I was not exposed to in the clinical arena and that I could not acquire on my own. It is what I was looking for, and I am now satisfied that my personal and professional growth is on the right track.

The energy and enthusiasm of Professor Loke impressed me. She inspired in me that I have to make use of my capacity to accept challenges in life; I am to make full use of my dynamic ability, grasp opportunities that come my way, and be able to face any possible adversity that arises. This new role as a nurse teacher no longer is a "stress" to me, but a welcomed challenge.

Self-Reflective Questions

1. How often do you imagine or dream about what can be achieved in your professional life?

2. How can you explore the different pathways that could lead you to what you want to achieve in your professional life?

3. How can you take challenges as opportunities? And face it from a positive perspective?

4. How do you find creative ways to deal with your stress and changes in professional life?

5. How do you deal with stress? A bit at a time? Do you break it down into small tasks and deal with it little by little?

6. How often do you talk to people who you think can help, or ask for advice?

7. How do you take time out when under stress?

8. How can you re-examine and identify the positive outcomes after you had tried your best?

9. How can you plan your next step with a vision in your careers?

10. How can you count your learning every day?

90

Student Mentoring at the International Doctoral Level

"Mentoring is beyond static role modeling—it is the cultivation of a continuing relationship. It is a relationship investment for future global collaboration and mutually satisfying professional work from the other side of the globe."

—Veronica Feeg

Mentor
Rita M. Carty, PhD, RN, FAAN
Professor and Dean Emerita,
  College of Health and Human
  Services
George Mason University
Fairfax, Virginia, USA

Mentee
Yanika Kowitlawakul, PhD, RN
Assistant Professor, School of
  Medicine and Health Sciences
Department of Nursing
  Education
The George Washington
  University
Washington, DC, USA
Native of Thailand

Hunt (2003) stated that the nature of the mentor relationship is expert/learner (senior/junior), and the quality of the relationship is professional development through expert guidance. According to Wellington and Spence (2001), the best mentorship involves a natural affinity between two individuals. In this case, the mentor relationship began formally between a doctoral student and a senior faculty member. After they worked together, the relationship became less formal, as they developed mutual respect and trust.

Mentoring for Leadership

Handing off the baton of leadership in a smooth transition is not only the way to win the race but is also a critical move to ensure that someone is coming up behind you who is fully able to sprint out in front and be a leader in the field. In our profession, individual accountability is not the only necessity. The profession also needs teamwork and the preparation of others to ultimately deliver quality care, to carry out research, to guide work, and to educate others to carry on the work. Nothing is as important as preparing that next generation of professionals and the next generation of leaders for this important work.

Volumes have been written about leadership. Many have researched the subject. Leadership books, plays, movies, songs, and autobiographies abound. Some people are described as born leaders. Others insist that leaders are made not born. Of the many paths to leadership, mentoring ranks among the tools and strategies proven to be successful throughout the ages.

Mentoring for leadership can take many forms: in government service, the military, the corporate world, the arts, and certainly in our profession. In nursing education, senior professors often mentor junior faculty, students, or other colleagues. Mentoring doctoral students can be as rewarding as it is challenging because these individuals are the next wave of potential leaders for our profession.

Mentoring international doctoral students can be even more rewarding because mentors know this budding leader is not only necessary for the profession but necessary for the profession in another country that might not have the human capital and resources for leadership that we have in the United States. One example of mentoring an international student took place at George Mason University. The student (Yanika) was enrolled in course work and has continued with the successful completion of the doctoral program and the start of a new career in nursing education. She was a foreign nurse and inexperienced researcher. Initially, this presented a challenge for her enrollment in the graduate program in nursing, but with determination, motivation, and career goals, Yanika found that the PhD program became a reality. Having an inspirational mentor who can provide opportunity, connections with others, advice, support, and role modeling is significant for career success and achievement. It's the passion of leadership and opportunities provided by a mentor that may help make the student's dreams come true.

Mentor's Goals

The mentor's goals must be reflective of the mentee's ultimate career goals. Yanika expressed a career goal of international professional work, either through teaching or research. Therefore, I carefully planned several goals to help her achieve this end by providing actual experience with international health care organizations through internship placements, one of which was an overseas experience as an intern with the assignment of carrying out a project for the host organization. I considered networking with other colleagues involved in international nursing activities an absolutely necessity. In addition, I arranged the opportunity to increase the mentee's knowledge of international issues and current and future initiatives to address these issues through attendance at international conferences and meetings. Finally, I modeled the role of a U.S. nurse educator involved in international nursing and health care activities.

Mentee's Goals

Defined career goals can serve as a compass for achieving the desired goals. Yanika has been interested in teaching, research, and international nursing since she started her PhD program in the college of nursing and health sciences at George Mason University. Her goal is to be an excellent professor, a qualified researcher, and work with an international organization to achieve a more interdisciplinary worldwide view of global health. Because of her interest and career goals, she always seeks opportunities to learn from her professors, to participant in research studies, and gain experience with international organizations.

Mentoring Experiences

I provided Yanika with the following opportunities throughout the PhD program and after she graduated. The following sections discuss the opportunities provided.

Research Assistant

Yanika served as a research assistant to assist in reviewing literature and analyzing data on the study "Building a Community of New Scholars." Yanika took this opportunity to practice her writing, statistical, and research skills. This opportunity helped her to learn more about the research process and teamwork in real life on top of the experience that she had in the classroom. She gained more confidence in her research knowledge, in her statistical knowledge, and in collaborating with others. When the article from this project, "Predictors of Success for Saudi Arabian Students Enrolled in an Accelerated Baccalaureate Degree Program in Nursing in the United States" (Carty,

Moss, Al-Zayyer, Kowitlawakul, and Arietti, 2007), was published, it made Yanika proud to be a part of the team and inspired her to hone her writing skills and to pursue more opportunities for professional and scholarly writing.

Internship at the Global Health Council (GHC), Washington D.C.

In a 30-hour internship for a public health policy course, Yanika was required to experience current health issues and the implementation process of health policy. I introduced her to the Global Health Council (GHC) and connected her with an administrator who was a deputy director of policy at the GHC at the time.

Even though it was a very short period of time, Yanika gained knowledge of the structure and culture within the GHC as an international organization of NGOs (non-governmental organizations). It was her first opportunity to broaden her view of health issues and health policies from the hospital level to the international level.

Internship at the World Health Organization (WHO), Geneva, Switzerland

An internship for her health care administration, policy, and ethics class was required for the PhD program. This internship allowed Yanika to pursue both research and professional development. The WHO has been her dream organization since she was very young. Together, we made a connection with the nursing and midwife chief scientist and arranged for Yanika to be at WHO headquarters, Geneva, Switzerland, for the internship semester.

While Yanika was at the WHO, she learned the structure, culture, dynamics, work environment, and processes associated with health policy, health care administration, and ethics within the WHO. Fortunately, she had the opportunity to attend two very important meetings: the ninth meeting of the Global Advisory Group Nursing Meeting (GAGNM) and the Regional Nursing Advisers Meeting. Attending these two meetings was unforgettable for her because she met many great leaders in nursing around the world, which inspired her to want to become one of them someday.

International Conferences

After Yanika came back from the WHO, I invited her to attend two more international conferences: "Building Global Alliance III: The Impact of Global

Nurse Migration on Health Service Delivery" by the commission on graduates of foreign nursing schools and the workshop on human resources for nursing by the Pan American Health Organization meeting in Washington D.C.

These conferences provided Yanika with more information on how the nursing community around the world and within the United States shares information, finds solutions, implements the solutions, and works together. Again, she had a chance to meet and interact with great leaders from the United States and from many countries around the world. This time, she gained more confidence to interact with and have discussions with those great leaders.

Lesson Learned

Mentoring is both challenging and rewarding for the mentor and the mentee. Whereas mentoring is a highly successful strategy with professional goals and outcomes, it may also become personal through compatibility, respect, and accomplishment. The mentor and mentee's goals must have common purposes, opportunities, and commitment. Though formal professional planning drives the process, planning is not enough without a good fit between mentor and mentee. Positive outcomes and success for the mentee are always at the forefront of the relationship. The mentor needs to be confident enough to allow the mentee to shine, not only now, but also in the future.

Self-Reflective Questions

1. How do you share your knowledge with others?
2. What personal and professional and life lessons do you have to share?
3. What professional network do you have to share?
4. In what ways can you have a positive attitude and inspire others?
5. How can you establish positive relationships?
6. In what ways do you communicate effectively?
7. How can you demonstrate that you trust and respect others?
8. In what ways do you give credit to others?
9. How can you share your success?
10. How can you demonstrate that you want others to succeed?

Succession Planning

91

"Succession planning ensures that there are highly qualified people in all positions, not just today, but tomorrow,
next year, and five years from now."

—The United States Office of Personnel Management

Mentor

Donna M. Herrin, MSN, RN,
  NEA-BC, CNEP, FACHE
2009 President of the American
  Organization of Nurse
  Executives
Clinical Associate Professor,
  The University of Alabama
  Huntsville
Senior Advisor/Nurse Executive
  and former Senior Vice Presi-
  dent/Chief Nurse Executive
Methodist Le Bonheur Health-
  care
Memphis, Tennessee, USA

Mentee

Anna L. Herrin, BSN, RN
Registered Nurse, Orthopedic
  Surgery and Sports Medicine
St. Vincent Hospital
Birmingham, Alabama, USA

Leadership is a phenomenal journey for the nurse professional and is essential for the nursing profession to be able to deliver care to those across
the world who need that care. Additionally, effective nursing leadership
is a main element for success of the profession overall. However, creating
interest in and guiding those early in their nursing career toward nursing
leadership can be challenging for those responsible for creating future
leaders. Without planning for the paths aspiring nurse leaders should
traverse, the journey can be haphazard and learned by trial and error. To
help nurse leaders, we offer some observations—from the perspective of
a leader in the profession with that of an aspiring nurse leader—offer basic principles to guide a leadership path and plan.

Need for Replacement Nurse Leaders

An aging workforce means that many nursing leaders will be leaving the profession over the next several years. This alone is a call to the profession to purposefully identify and move leadership-talented and interested professionals toward a leadership career. This succession-planning approach in nursing has historically been scarce if not nonexistent. Current programs to interest nurses in leadership and prepare them for those roles are emerging, but the vast majority of nurses in leadership positions were first appointed to their leadership post because of expert practice as a clinician even though the science and practice of nursing leadership is a specialty with its own knowledge base and competency definition. A more formalized approach to succession planning will benefit the profession long-term.

Myself as a Leader: Mentee

Even before entering the nursing program, I knew that leadership was in my future. Seeing my mentor pursue leadership roles, gain responsibility, and lead at the national and international level was a source of pride. I could see that she was making a difference for those she worked with as well as the patients she always had at the center of her leadership. Guided by my mentor, I studied with great interest the issues surrounding the nursing workforce shortage and realized that I could make a difference. I know that I must have a plan for my future path and that I need additional academic preparation. Most importantly, I need to surround myself with those who are positive about our profession and seek out opportunities now to lead in small ways.

So what is succession planning? What key elements should nurse leaders integrate into education and practice settings to interest novice nurses in a leadership path? What do new nurses need from nurse leaders when they set out on their leadership journey? What do nurses early in their careers need to inform their leadership aspirations?

Broadly viewed, succession planning is work by the leader to develop high-level competencies in a field of interest (in this case, nursing leadership) to prepare an individual for increased challenges and responsibilities. The steps in a formalized succession process within an organization may vary and range from an individual, person-by-person approach to a full scale, formalized program that includes talent mapping, creating a pool of candidates with high potential, and then tapping them for expanded training and experiential learning.

Organizations having such plans are investing in the future by ensuring that the company continues to be effective by retaining high-potential individuals, and continuing a company legacy with little to no disruption. Corporations, in general, use this approach in talent planning. Could our profession find a return on future generations if succession planning was more prevalent?

Concerning nursing, the first step leading to succession and developing an interest in a leadership path begins with nursing faculty in undergraduate education. It is essential that faculty at every level understand and explain the many forms of leadership and unlock that potential early on. Upon assuming the first professional role, a novice nurse must experience a leader's presence through a positive practice environment, seeing the leader as a positive, interesting, and influential leader.

Specifically, the nurse needs training programs, customized mentorship opportunities, and coaching by the leader, in accordance with his or her strengths. Focusing on confidence building, providing feedback on talents and improvements, promoting opportunities to serve in leadership positions to display individual and team talents, and ongoing goal alignment are strategies that nurse leaders must consider. While interrelated specifically with mentoring, succession planning brings intent to the process, with leaders positioning talented, aspiring nurses in a track to assume formal leadership positions in organizations and to lead the professional ranks of associations and boards.

Keeping an Eye on Leadership Principles: Mentee

Because of my relationship with my mentor, and the interest I have developed in leadership as a professional path, my practice is focused on leadership principles. Knowledge of how leadership "looks" guides my choices, and I believe that I am already influencing colleagues to think about leadership. I know I have a lot to do—graduate study, deciding what type of role within leadership I aspire to, refining my goals—but I know that I am on my way. What I have to do is complete these and identify the role, the mentors, and the organization that will help position me formally for the next steps of my career.

The Leader

- Learn about succession planning and your role in creating leaders for the future.
- Help your organization seek out best practices in succession planning and talent mapping and bring those to the organization.
- Create a positive practice environment, rich with positive encouragement and feedback .
- Identify high potential leaders on your clinical team. Help them identify their leadership characteristics, bringing them into view.
- Proactively schedule individuals for leadership development programs within and outside the organization.
- Promote involvement in a professional organization that focuses on leadership as a core value.
- Specifically identify two to three potential successors to your own position. Involve them in departmental operations and broaden their expertise through experiential assignments.

The Novice

- Become a student of leadership in nursing. Learn about the vast opportunities to develop in a leadership role. Learn about nurses who are pacesetters in nursing leadership and ask to be mentored by one identified.
- Demonstrate a leader "voice" across all aspects of your professional work. Focus on the positive of our profession and bring others along with you.
- Ask for assignments that provide opportunity to demonstrate team leadership skills and flexibility.
- Ask for feedback on performance, with a specific focus on leadership characteristics.
- Seek out opportunities to participate in formal learning programs and professional associations.
- Reflect upon long-term career goals. Commit them to writing and share with your leader. Ask to be considered as a future, aspiring leader.
- If your organization has a formalized, succession planning program, ask to be considered for placement in that plan.

Self-Reflective Questions

Mentor Questions

1. How do you embrace and honestly implement principles for a rewarding practice environment? How can you become versed on principles of coaching and mentoring?

2. How can you seek those new to the profession and appoint or encourage their involvement in initiatives of the organization to provide them the opportunity to demonstrate their capability and potential?

3. How can you become knowledgeable about and involved in your organization's formal succession planning process? How can you use the process to position future leaders?

4. Have you identified two or three individuals capable of replacing you in your leadership role? How can you maximize their leadership development through formal and experiential learning opportunities?

5. How can you encourage involvement in professional activities (association membership, attending conferences, and other development, for example) through active support, such as providing dues payment or flexible scheduling?

Mentee Questions

6. Have you completed a reflective process and identified your strengths and areas where you need additional growth? How can you become familiar with tools in the profession that can help you complete an assessment of your leadership strengths?

7. Have you identified a leadership mentor? Is this relationship formalized? Through this relationship, what do you contribute?

8. What is your written plan regarding your leadership aspirations and goals, with a detailed plan on how to achieve them? If your organization has a formalized succession planning process, how can you make your aspirations known and ask to be placed in the program?

9. How can you become a more active member of your professional association, participating in the work of the organization?

10. How can you share your knowledge and love of leadership? Even being new to the profession, how can you contribute to the understanding of leadership to those yet to come?

92

Synergy and Win-Win: The Goals of Effective Leadership

"You can't go somewhere without leaving somewhere."

—Marla Salmon

Mentor
Anna K. Karani, PhD, MA, RN, BScN
Registered Nurse, Midwife, and Community Health Nurse
Head Education Administrator, School of Nursing Sciences, College of Health Sciences
University of Nairobi
Nairobi, Kenya

Mentee
Patrick Kimani Wairiri, MA BScN
Lecturer
Kenya Methodist University
Meru, Kenya

Leadership is the means by which things get done in an organization. It is essential for the appropriate execution of plans, decisions, strategies, organizational structures and designs, and other processes that are the day-to-day concerns of a manager.

The overall purpose of leadership is goal accomplishment. When attempting to accomplish a goal that involves the contributions of others, the leader must stimulate release of the followers' efforts and then harness and focus these efforts so they are used effectively and efficiently in goal accomplishment. The more specific goals of leadership thus revolve around the themes of stimulating and focusing followers' efforts, and may vary from one perspective of leadership to another. The following is a generally agreed upon list of essential nurse leadership responsibilities.

Basic Nurse Leadership Responsibilities

- Set the moral tone and reinforce the values of service.

- Establish and reinforce a service-oriented morality through vision, goals, and values.

- Exercise flexibility and consideration in establishing legitimate courses of action.

- Take the main responsibility for setting service goals and strategies.

Communicating the Direction of the Organization

A leader must conceptualize the desired future of the organization and the path toward achieving that future vision, and state it in clear terms that are easily understood by all members of the organization. This often takes the form of organizational vision, mission, objectives, and strategies. Setting the direction of the organization helps people to understand what priorities are highest, how the organization's vision and values can be put into action, and where they should place their energies. The Association of University Programs in Health Affairs' (AUPHA) *Manual of Health Services Management* (AUPHA, 1994) notes that leadership in health care bears certain unique elements owing to the distinctive nature of health care businesses compared to other industries.

The first two leadership responsibilities serve to achieve the goal of communicating direction and roles. Initiating structure includes defining jobs of subordinates, initiating new ideas, planning, and giving feedback to subordinates—all of which serve to accomplish this goal (Graham & Bennett, 1998).

My Perspective: Mentee

An important aspect I have learned through interaction with my mentor is the value of setting personal goals for career development. Working with Professor Karani, I have experienced consistent vertical career and professional mobility since we began our mentorship relationship, essentially by remaining focused on goals and seizing opportunities. In addition to personal gain, I have also learned the value of supporting those working under me, and focusing students on priorities.

To reinforce a service orientation, my mentor has encouraged me to participate in a number of voluntary community activities—most notably, St. John Ambulance Community Care activities.

Direction of the Organization and the Roles of Team Members

Having communicated the organizational direction, the next goal for the leader is to motivate followers to buy into the new direction and perceive their new roles as useful in contributing to the identified organizational goal. This is usually achieved by demonstrating how the new direction will improve organizational performance and the welfare of members, as well as clarifying how the individual contributions shall add up to produce desired results. The classic Path-Goal Model of Robert House (1971 and 1996) presents the leader as using influence to increase the motivation of a follower attempting to accomplish a specific goal, in a particular context, over a specified period.

A follower's level of motivation is a result of his perceptions of expectancies, instrumentalities, and valences. *Expectancies* refer to the belief that a particular level of effort will result in a particular level of performance, and *instrumentalities* refer to the relationship of the various outcomes resulting from that effort. *Valence* refers to the individuals' preference, particularly in relation to rewards.

From this model, House and Baetz (1979) observe that the connection between effort, performance, and reward is often unclear to followers. Leadership behavior, therefore, should focus on clarifying the relationship between follower efforts and outcomes. People tend to resist change because they feel uncertain and insecure about what the outcome will be. If they perceive few benefits, they may reject the purpose behind the change (Jones, 2007).

My Perspective: Mentee

It is easy to assume that people will quickly understand the connection between their efforts or specific roles and your desired results. Having worked with my mentor in several ways, I have learned how motivating it can be to point out the importance of each person's role in achieving a group outcome. Indeed, one of the habits I have cultivated is to discuss with colleagues, subordinates, and even students the desired end states. Then, having appreciated such state is desirable, work with them to identify what contributions they need to make toward its achievement.

Ensuring Access to Requisite Knowledge, Skills, and Technologies

Despite the conviction that the direction taken is appropriate, and the efforts are useful to achieve the desired goal, team members will perform optimally only when they know how to perform the new roles and have the necessary tools to support their performance. Workplace changes are usually stressful to workers because they often involve changes in established task and role relationships. Jones (2007) observes that providing workers with training to help them learn how to perform new tasks (or providing them with time off from work to recuperate from the stressful effects of change) can be useful in facilitating change and innovation. He gives examples of companies, such as Microsoft and Apple, that give their talented programmers time off from ordinary job assignments to think about ways to create new kinds of products. In the Lead model of leadership, Hersey and Blanchard (1977), as quoted in Shortell & Kaluzny (2006), argue that the single most important contingency in selecting an effective leadership style is follower task-relevant maturity. Maturity in this model is a function of motivation, competence, responsibility and willingness to plan, organize, and complete the task.

Competence in this context connotes possessing the necessary knowledge, skills, or experience to perform the task proficiently. A mature follower is conceptualized as being highly motivated, willing, and able to assume responsibility for the task. AUPHA (1994) observes that health care organizations are values driven and that their leaders establish and nurture the appropriate values. One of the various ways identified for doing so is through their commitment to development of others, by encouraging and supporting subordinates to maximize their understanding and skills.

Facilitating followers as a goal of leadership can also be inferred from Goleman's Emotional Competence framework, which identifies two dimensions (personal and social competencies), five competency areas, and 25 attributes (Goleman, 1998). Within the social competencies dimension, four attributes (developing others, conflict management, building bonds, and team capabilities) may be seen as contributing to this goal.

My Perspective: Mentee

The relationship I have had with my mentor has gone beyond encouragement to include facilitation for me to achieve certain goals. Specific action from my mentor has included introduction to

- The professional association in which I have served several terms as a branch secretary, branch treasurer, and one-time member of the association's research committee through my mentor's encouragement.

- Introduction to and support for my participation in a two-year HIV/AIDS training and support program sponsored by Marquette University and USAID.

- Introduction to and support through the process of applying for the teaching job at Kenya Methodist University, where I now work and study.

To Show Support for Subordinates

An important goal of leadership is to convince the subordinates that the leader empathizes with the difficulties they are going through. Showing support through appreciation and empathy for subordinates requires a great deal of intellectual flexibility on the part of the leader. This goal is paramount among leaders in health care organizations that are typically characterized by highly autonomous roles and where the allegiance of the professionals is much more to the individual clients and the profession than to the organization. Shortell & Kaluzny (2006) observe that most work done in this area suggests that a style high in consideration, relationship orientation, and participation is most appropriate while leading professionals.

The path-goal model discussed earlier portends that in leading, the leader should appreciate that individual's preferences are varied. The leader should consequently understand what individual followers value, and thus create a reward system that responds to these preferences. Indeed, it is virtually impossible to lead effectively if you do not clearly understand your followers, on whom your effectiveness and success depends.

My Perspective: Mentee

In my opinion, this goal is about looking at, as well as appearing to look at, the people you are leading as just that—people—as opposed to viewing them as tools necessary only to get certain tasks accomplished. This is the hallmark of the mentorship relationship I have with Professor Karani. My mentor's concern about my progress is as much about, "You look stressed out," "How are the kids doing?" and "When do I get to see the family?" as it is about my career and professional development. I have found the same approach useful while dealing with the students for whom I am an academic advisor, and I must say that I have managed to break many barriers and establish relationships that are useful between us.

Focus Toward Achievement of Identified Goals

An important goal of leadership is to ensure that the efforts contributed by all the individuals in the organization are harnessed and directed toward achievement of organizational objectives. Individuals may be highly motivated and committed to performing their individual roles, but as long as these are not integrated and harmonized, they will most likely fail to produce the desired overall effect.

My Perspective: Mentee

One perspective from my observations of how my mentor works is, "It's okay to work very hard, but when you work, it is important to ensure that your efforts are not in vain. They need to be directed in the general direction you have chosen to follow." The achievements I have seen my mentor accomplish are immense, particularly considering the time span within which they happened. This has taught me the value of not only being motivated to work hard, but also ensuring that such work is relevant to the set goals.

Focus for Success

Leadership aims at stimulating and focusing the efforts of people for the accomplishment of the common goal. The exercise of leadership aims at achieving various goals, which include communicating direction and roles; demonstrating how that direction and the roles are useful; facilitating followers to acquire necessary knowledge, skills, and technologies; showing support for followers; and focusing the efforts of individuals toward accomplishment of group goal.

Self-Reflective Questions

1. How can you make your leadership goal clear?

2. How can you make the importance of leadership more clear?

3. How are authority and power for the leader important?

4. How can you make the overall goal of leadership clear?

5. How can you be sure that the specific goals of leadership revolving around the themes are understood?

6. How can you determine that the organization direction and team roles are necessary?

7. How can you best make leaders' and team members' relationships show clear outcomes?

8. What else can you do to facilitate followers to ensure that access to knowledge, skills, and technologies aid important quality outcomes?

9. How can you demonstrate as a leader that showing support to subordinates is a clear, important goal?

10. How can you best focus workers on achieving identified goals for the good of the individual and the institution?

Teams, Team Players, and Team Building

93

"Coming together is a beginning. Keeping together is progress. Working together is success."

—Henry Ford

Mentor
Marla E. Salmon, ScD, RN, FAAN
The Robert G. and Jean A. Reid
  Endowed Dean in Nursing
University of Washington School
  of Nursing
Seattle, Washington, USA

Mentee
Susan B. Hassmiller, PhD, RN
  FAAN
Robert Wood Johnson Founda-
  tion Senior Advisor for Nursing
Director, RWJF Initiative on
  the Future of Nursing at the
  Institute of Medicine
Princeton, New Jersey, USA

Marla Salmon: When it comes to nursing making a real difference in the lives of others, probably nothing is less productive, rewarding, or professional than "going it alone." Still, a lot is happening in our profession as we strive to demonstrate our independence, leadership, and creativity, and all too often, we act and reward the actions of individuals. However, we do this not only to our own detriment as nurses, but, most importantly, to those we purport to serve.

This chapter is about working together. Though the chapter is similar to other chapters in overall approach, it has one fundamental difference. Each of the authors for this chapter is both mentor and mentee to the other. Though each of us started in separate roles, our connection and work together across time has changed our relationship to that of partner. And, this partnership has taken on all of the best characteristics of a team.

Sue Hassmiller: I first spoke to Marla in 1991 when I called to ask her if she would be my sponsor for a mandatory policy internship for my PhD program. The program prided itself in giving its students an experience with real health policy experts, but we had to find our own experts to have that experience with. Having a background in public health, like Marla, and just having heard that she was going to be the new director for the Division of Nursing at the Health Resources and Services Administration, I thought she would be a perfect fit for me as a sponsor and a mentor. She immediately agreed, but when I showed up for work on the first day (also Marla's first week or so on the job), she steered me away from doing something that might have turned out to be more administrative and personally helpful to her towards an experience that would turn out to be one of the most substantial of my life.

Marla claimed that a new program being developed, the U.S. Public Health Service Primary Care Policy Fellowship, could use the input and expertise of a nurse. The fellowship was a 3-week, on-site Washington, D.C. policy experience for primary care leaders in the United States. (Although it successfully ran for more than 10 years and produced a few hundred graduates, the program has now ended because of lack of funding. However, the alumni association comprising physicians, dentists, nurses, social workers, and public health leaders lives on.)

I had mixed feelings about working with a team of leaders from other professions. After all, wasn't this supposed to be an experience with Marla and about nursing? However, Marla assured me that she was on the advisory team overseeing the fellowship and that her door would always be open for me. She also claimed that my experience with her (because she was so new in the position) would not be nearly as substantial as what the fellowship could offer. She also counseled me that one of the most important roles I could have as a nurse leader was to be part of a powerful interdisciplinary program made up of other health professionals, especially physicians. As director for the Division of Nursing within the Bureau of Health Professions, she, herself, would be part of a high-level government team that represented a number of disciplines including medicine, public health, and dentistry.

In asking me to work on this program, Marla did two things: she pushed me out of my immediate comfort zone which she knew would stretch me, and she gave me the opportunity to attend many meetings with her in her role as division director where she role modeled for me how a nurse could successfully be part of a high-level interdisciplinary team. I listened to how she spoke to her peers from other professions (she gave respect, but demanded it as well), watched her body language (confident and facilitative), and especially enjoyed our debriefing times when she told me what was "really" on her mind. In essence, she was helping me to understand how to be a successful leader on an interdisciplinary team through her role modeling and by my "practicing" through the fellowship experience.

Now in my current role as senior advisor for nursing for the Robert Wood Johnson Foundation (RWJF), I cannot imagine developing or being part of any programs that have not been conceived out of the unique perspectives of a host of individuals, preferably from an array of disciplines. My current work at the foundation has included incorporating the expertise and participation of businesses, consumers, economists, government, and philanthropies in advancing the nursing profession. Marla taught me early on that, although cumbersome and frustrating at times, the most successful and sustainable work comes from the engagement of many. I think I might have even surprised Marla, who now sits on our RWJF Board of Trustees, when we announced that a particularly important nursing program would *not* be headed by a nursing organization, but by one of the state chambers of commerce, an organization geared towards supporting business and industry. The organization has developed a "Business Coalition for Nursing" and will be bringing new dollars, fresh and powerful thinking, and strategies to the challenge of the nursing and nurse faculty shortage. Using business partners, consumer groups, economists, and our colleagues from other disciplines can surely bring us to heights and new solutions that alone we would never have been able to achieve. As author and organizational expert Ken Blanchard (2000) says, "None of us is as smart as all of us."

Marla Salmon: Being a part of a team is not unlike folk dancing in almost any culture. It is the beauty of living within a larger tapestry and understanding the connection among one another in the larger context of culture, music, and audience that makes folk dancing so much like nursing. Nursing is fundamentally about being connected with others in ways that make things better—with our patients, families, and communities, and with one another. For us, the team is truly across generations, occupations, traditions, cultures, time, and space. What ultimately brings us together is that fundamental human instinct to care for one another.

The following questions are but a lens or frame through which to see yourself relative to the larger team. They apply to much of life and are fundamentally important to our lives as nurses.

Self-Reflective Questions

1. Have you identified the vision of what can be done together?

2. Why is it worth being a part of this team? Articulate why it matters.

3. Why does it take a team to do this? What is the added value?

4. What roles can you play in the team now and play over time?

5. How will you follow and support the leader(s) and who might he/she/they be?

6. In what ways can you provide leadership and grow in this capacity?

7. How can you measure your performance now and in the future?

8. What attitude, knowledge, and skill gaps do you have and how can they be bridged?

9. What can you do to advance the well-being of the other group members?

10. Have you identified and celebrated the ways in which being a team member helps you grow?

Technology to Transform Practice at the Point-of-Care

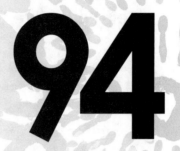

94

"We need to balance the wonders of technology with the spiritual dimensions of human nature."

—John Naisbett

Mentor
Bonnie Wesorick, RN, MSN, DPNAP, FAAN
Founder and Chair, Clinical Practice Model Resource Center
Grand Rapids, Michigan, USA

Mentee
Chad Fairfield, RN, BSN
Technology Implementation Director
Clinical Practice Model Resource Center
Grand Rapids, Michigan, USA

The implementation of technology will affect every caregiver and every recipient of care, but do not make the false assumption that it will improve the process or outcomes of care. Unless there is a strong nurse leader engaged in the process of bringing technology/automation to the point of care, ensuring it supports both those who give and receive care, the outcomes can be detrimental.

The Call for Technology

Globally, billions of dollars are spent annually on health care technology. An electronic health record mandate is being considered in the United States. This mandate is being driven by diverse stimuli. Most important among these are the growing cost of health care and the concern for patient safety (Eden et al., 2008; Institute of Medicine, 2004; Gillean, Shaha, & Sampanes, 2006;).

As the United States moves toward integrated health care systems through technology, open data sharing, and standardized evidence-based medicine, the danger we now face is that practice and the art of caring can take a backseat to the progress of technology. Unless the technology is designed using a professional practice model that integrates the whole of practice across disciplines, it has the potential to perpetuate "what is" and not "what can be" (Wesorick, Troseth, & Cato, 2004).

The Hope of Technology

Technology is only a tool. It must be designed with functionality that will enhance the work and patterns of thinking for the clinicians. Commitment of an organization to automate provides nurse leaders a rare opportunity to transform practice with the support of executive leadership. Because of the cost of automation, there are high expectations for practice and financial improvement, which provides an opening to have an organization commit to the work of point-of-care transformation.

Automation provides an opportunity to create a new reality at the bedside. This requires a nurse leader who is in touch with realities and can articulate the often unspoken truths that interfere with practice and patient safety (Wesorick, 2008; Troseth, 2009). One seldom articulated truth is the exhaustion occurring in health care that no day off or extra hours of sleep will make go away. This exhaustion is draining the passion from the souls of those who come to provide direct patient care every day but are met by the following common realities:

- The system has no infrastructure to bring clinicians together to make decisions about practice transformation—there is a lack of partnership infrastructures to bring clinicians' voices and wisdom to the decision-making table.

- The historical focus on tasks dominate services instead of professional scope of practice services.

- Inconsistencies in the delivery of care due to variance of scope of practice among nurses and interdisciplinary partners.

- Frequent fragmentation, duplication, and repetition of care because of the lack of integrated competency across the interdisciplinary team.

- Absence of a valued interdisciplinary plan of care to support individualized, integrated care.

- Lack of evidence-based tools.

- Documentation tools that interfere with care providers knowing the patient's story and providing integrated care that reflects wholeness of body, mind, and spirit

It is important that someone with clinical skill manage the polarities or dilemmas association with transformation of practice. Polarities are the presence of two or more values (called poles) that look different, appear as opposite or competitive, but are really *interdependent*. Interdependent means they need each other; each represents half the truth, and one is not more important than the other. A dynamic tension always exists between them. One of the key polarities that needs to be managed is the technology and practice polarity. Figure 1 shows the positive outcomes achieved when both poles/values are supported. It makes visible not only the positive outcomes of implementing technology but also clarifies what is needed to support practice as well.

Note the polarity map provides warning signs when one preferred pole is being focused on at the neglect of the other. That is important because the most common detrimental pattern of the past 10 years within the CPM International Consortium is that implementation of technology is often seen in the organization as an information technology (IT) project, not as a technology and practice polarity.

When the implementation of technology is seen as an IT project, as opposed to a practice and technology polarity, two common patterns interfere with the transformation and the desired clinical outcomes. The opportunity to transform practice at the point of care is lost because the technology is not seen as a tool to achieve a higher purpose and the technology is designed only as a documentation tool to replace the paper system (Belmont, 2003; Doebbeling, Chou, & Tierney 2006). When the focus and resources are on a quick implementation of technology, the underlying support needed to help clinicians transform practice at the point of care is absent. Without a strong partnership within nursing practice leadership and technology leadership, the functionality—and equally important, the clinical content—needed within technology to support clinicians in the transformation of practice will not happen.

Action Steps to enhance the Technology pole
A. Ensure users understand the design, purpose and functionality of technology tool.
B. Provide time for users to learn the technology tool properly

Action Steps to enhance the Practice pole
A. Create and support time for interdisciplinary team to do transformation work needed to integrate evidence-based professional practice
B. Provide process that assures what matters to both those who give & receive care is embedded into technology, scope, holistic pt. profile, individualized plan, education & professional exchange

Greater Purpose Statement (GPS)*-why balance this polarity?

Transform practice at point of care

Values = positive results from focusing on the left pole

Values = positive results from focusing on the right pole

• Innovative technologies bring information to the fingertips of clinicians at the point of care.

• Technology standardizes and integrates information for both patients and clinicians.

• Technology increases efficiency with easier access, retrieval and delivery of patient information.

• Organizational commitment to provide evidence-based information needed to support professional scope of practice and work flow.

• The organization provides opportunities to integrate practice across disciplines to stop isolation, fragmentation, and repetition.

• Actions demonstrate a Humanistic culture that supports professional practice/service.

Technology Focus   **and**   **Practice Focus**

• The lack of evidence-based information to support practice/service.

• Technology design interferes with integration of care across disciplines.

• Technology takes the "human touch" out of how we interact with others to give quality care.

• Unaware of the benefits of technology to provide information that enhances care.

• Quality of care being compromised because consistent integrated information is not available across disciplines.

• Lack of timely access to and retrieval of patient information needed for quality care.

Negative outcomes from focusing on technology to the neglect of practice

Negative outcomes from focusing on practice to the neglect of technology

Unable to transform practice at point of care

Deeper fear from lack of balance

Early Warnings when over focused on Technology Pole *
A. Timelines for "activation are all about technology, not practice transformation.
B. Having modification or deconstruction of evidence-based content integration.

Early Warnings when over focused on Practice Pole *
A. Users demand that technology not change what is known and familiar, i.e., documentation practices.
B. Comments about the fear that technology will dehumanize care and dictate practice.

PolarityMap™ 1992, 2008 Polarity Management Associates, LLC/ *Thanks to John Scherer, The Scherer Leadership Center/ ** Thanks to De Wit & Meyer BV/ ***Thanks to Todd Johnson, Rivertown Consultants

Figure 1   Polarity map showing the practice and technology poles and ways to balance the tension between them.

Historically, documentation has been seen as a dreaded task and not as a tool to support interdisciplinary colleagues and achieve individualized patient care. As an IT project, the focus is on making the actual act of documentation easier but not on shifting it to a higher purpose. A common approach is to make the technology screens look just like the present familiar forms, thinking this will decrease the stress. It does nothing more than perpetuate the present broken reality. The opportunity is lost and so is the hope.

The following tips should be considered by anyone facing technology implementation:

- Do not see the implementation of technology as another project. See it as a tool that will help the organization transform practice.

- Articulate the clinical outcomes that will be achieved from point-of-care transformation using intentionally designed automation and technology to achieve that end.

- Live the principles of partnership and discuss daily in every encounter, and ensure all disciplines giving care are invited to the table of planning, implementing, and evaluating.

- Be clear on the vision as to what an integrated, healthy, healing, healthcare system looks like.

- Be prepared and clear on the nature of the work needed to not just create but sustain the best places to give and receive care (e.g., work to clarify scope of practice across all disciplines, accountability to evidence-based practice, and changing the structure and process of care necessary to achieve clinical outcomes).

- Develop polarity management skills and use daily (Johnson, 1996).

- Ensure that no technology implemented increases barriers to best practice.

- Ensure that evidence-based content is embedded into each screen used by clinicians.

- Know the difference between referential content and executable evidence-based content delivered to the fingertips of the clinicians during care (Hanson, Hoss & Wesorick, 2008).

- Ensure adequate resources to attain evidence-based content.

Mentee

While working with numerous health care entities, it has become quickly apparent that many are ready to jump on the technology bandwagon for the sake of "getting it done." It is seen more as a task, not as an opportunity to transform practice. The importance of understanding the technology/practice polarity has been critical in my ability to improve the implementation process with the client. I frequently see many warning signs within organizations, and these signs guide me to ask questions that I might not have asked. For example, when the nurses are not talking about scope of practice, evidence-based practice, or integration of practice with other disciplines, it is a warning that the practice pole is very weak and needs strong nursing leadership. I often ask if the technology and practice leads are in partnership.

When I encounter a health care institution that has purchased an intentionally designed automation (IDA) tool that includes evidence-based content, and they deconstruct the evidence-based content to support the institution's old ways of practice and outdated paper tools—or intentionally create automated tasks to override professional accountability—I intervene. It is important to demonstrate the practice ramifications such as interfering with the delivery of evidence-based scope of practice and perpetuating non-evidence-based practice. Then I explore a different approach with the client.

Often, clients schedule classes to prepare for automation that are only focused on how to use the technology and do not include how the technology will influence the process and outcomes of their care. This is another warning sign. It is often easy to show care providers how to click and open an icon or a flow sheet row, but it is a whole other situation to give practitioners the knowledge to use the tools in symphony with a solid scope of practice definition and interdisciplinary collaboration. That guidance is fundamental to transforming practice in order to reach best clinical outcomes.

Keeper of the Legacy

Nursing, because of the essence of its practice, is the keeper of the legacy to implement technology that enhances every step of the care process for all healers at the point of care. The words of Thomas Jefferson provide direction: "In matter of style, swim with the current; in matters of principles, stand like a rock."

Self-Reflective Questions

1. If you are a decision-making leader at the table for any technology that will be used by clinicians, how can you best make sure the technology is appropriate?

2. What is your vision—and is it clear—as to what technology can do to transform practice at the point of care?

3. Are you co-leading the practice/technology polarity?

4. How can you implement technology to intentionally strengthen and transform your current state of practice?

5. Are you automating processes that engage your point of care providers in critical thinking and in advancing practice using a professional practice model? If not, why not?

6. What are the barriers being faced by clinicians in the delivery of their professional scope of practice?

7. How does the technology being used (or planned to be used) at the point-of-care bring evidence-based content to the fingertips of the clinicians?

8. How does the technology ensure an integrated, interdisciplinary, usable plan of care?

9. What are your unit-based partnership infrastructures to lead the transformation at the point of care?

10. How can you monitor the impact on practice and the clinical outcome improvement reached with each change implemented?

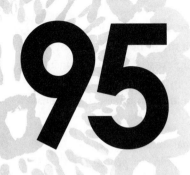

95

Theory and Practice:
Bringing Them Together at the Point of Care

"Theory is a powerful tool for explaining and predicting. It shapes questions and allows the systematic examination of a series of events."

—Patrica Benner

Mentor
Joy Gorzeman, MSN, RN, MBA
Former Senior Vice President
  Patient Care Services, and
  Chief Nursing Officer
Trinity Health
Novi, Michigan, USA
Interim Chief Nursing Officer
Tri-City Medical Center
Oceanside, California, USA

Mentee
Gay Landstrom, MS, RN
Senior Vice President Patient
  Care Services and Chief
  Nursing Officer
Trinity Health
Novi, Michigan, USA

One of the observations I (Joy) have made over the years with young nursing leaders is that they have a tendency to promote theory and evidence-based *clinical* practice, forgetting the need to ground their own *leadership* practice in theory and evidence. With graduate school completed and master's degrees obtained, nursing theorists too often become people no longer relevant to the young nursing leader. Yet, without theory as a firm foundation and available evidence in hand, how can the leader analyze problems, create solutions, make decisions, and lead change?

More specifically, without nursing theory, how can roles be defined or changed without risking the loss of the essence of the professional role of the nurse? Without systems theory, how can the complexity of health care institutions be understood? And without social psychology, organizational, and change theories, how will the leader determine the best actions to influence the behavior of others?

On a broad scale, I believe it is unfortunate that nurses are not more closely aligned in how we govern, practice, and educate within our profession. On a more personal level, a recent opportunity to merge theory into practice at the bedside was to implement the role of the clinical nurse leader (CNL) as the navigator of care in our journey to creating excellence in the care experience within the Trinity Health system. It took a while for others on the team to understand my vision of this role as the coordinator and integrator of the patient's experience and to facilitate communication and connection for the patient and family. Additionally, the education of the CNLs required a partnership with a university to help close the gap between academia and service.

We had the opportunity to develop a pilot program at one of our Trinity Health hospitals with the University of Detroit Mercy as our academic partner. This partnership made sense because this hospital and the university were already working together on several other educational initiatives and offerings.

We adapted the required curriculum to align with our philosophy. For example, Trinity Health had a strong commitment to diversity and was also using Lean as a process improvement tool, so both of these topics were added to the CNL curriculum.

The Challenges: Mentor

One of the challenges for nursing leaders is to envision the care models of the future and determine the roles needed to enable those models. It can be hard to think outside the box to look at scope of practice and "the way we have always done it" when thinking about new ways of being. It was complex work to align this project with the strategic needs of the health system's commitment to creating excellence in the care experience, while grounding the role in solid nursing theory and incorporating other relevant theories to optimize outcomes, and I saw this as an opportunity for a strong leader/performer in my department to develop this project.

I urged my mentee to explore nursing theory relevant to the CNL role, but also to explore other theories and conceptual models that should be applied to this role. We also needed to include other cultural initiatives, such as Lean

(Hadfield, Holmes, Fabr, Dudek, Williams, & White, 2006) process-improvement principles. Lean is a defined value analysis process that includes staff participation and is focused on eliminating waste and is being used in health care organizations to improve efficiency and patient flow. Diversity and inclusion training was also included as this was a priority for the health care system overall and would be integral to the CNL role. I also encouraged her to review several theorists to understand what motivates people to engage in such forward-thinking change and how to apply concepts they were learning into their everyday activities, or in other words, applying theory to practice.

The Challenges: Mentee

Although I had led many other changes in my career, I had never faced anything as big as designing an entirely new role for nurses. I needed my mentor to point me in the right direction. She shared her vision of what this role could be but did not give me the answers. Instead, she pointed me toward several theories upon which I could base my planning.

The work of constructing a model for the development, education, and implementation of a CNL role led me to look at a fundamental model of nursing. This resulted in the understanding that the CNL should be based upon a neomodern theory of nursing (Whall & Hicks, 2002): namely, one that incorporated the best of empirical evidence and measurement found in positivism, but also required the best of the nurse's post-modern "knowing" of patients: their environmental context and their needs.

Because this role needed to be a catalyst for process improvement and appreciation of diversity, those models needed examination. Additionally, this role would require significant change in how the nurse viewed herself, but also would require change in how the entire health care team operated.

Management professor John Kotter (1996) provided models about the need to create a sense of urgency for change. Bridges (2003) gave me theoretical understanding of how individuals change mental representations of their work and manage change transitions. Lastly, Rogers (2003) helped me to frame a theoretical understanding of how in large-scale changes, individuals can adopt change early or late in the process, depending upon many factors. With these theories understood, I gained the confidence that I needed to proceed with planning and implementing this large initiative.

Working with the university to address systems theory and incorporate these concepts into the curriculum has been a positive experience for our organization and the students. There has been a significant impact on how these students do their daily work based on their connection of theory to their daily practice. While this is a 3-year course, one of the most exciting outcomes so far was feedback from a program participant just 6 months into the program which was, "I am beginning to understand systems thinking, and I will never view my work the same."

Self-Reflective Questions

1. Have you, as a leader, identified a nursing theory that most closely aligns with your work philosophy?

2. How have you led your nursing/interdisciplinary leadership team through selecting a theory on which to build the foundation for the decision-making structure and caring model?

3. How flexible are you as to which nursing theory you support, depending upon the environment in which you are working?

4. How long has it been since you have interacted with patients and families and been on a nursing unit?

5. What experiences have you had with the health care system, and what is your philosophy regarding transformation of care?

6. How comfortable are you with change?

7. How have you successfully led and facilitated change?

8. Have you worked with an electronic health record? If so, how has that affected practice in your arena?

9. How can you best assess the need for transformation of care and then communicate that need to your executive team colleagues?

10. When you experience the synergy of knowing that the theory you believe in is being practiced at the bedside, how can you share that positive result to other stakeholders?

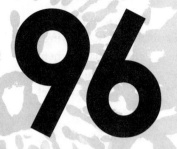

96

Time Management

"Concentrate on results, not on being busy."

—Author Unknown

Mentor
Ecaterina Gulie, RN, MS
President
Romanian Nursing
  Association
Bucharest, Romania

Mentee
Mirela Bidilič, RN
Director of Care
Central Military Hospital
Bucharest, Romania

Time management is defined by leadership capacity and the ability to achieve clearly defined objectives to increase efficiency and productivity. Good time management offers the possibility to waste less time doing the things we have to do so we have more time to do the things we want to do, making us more effective and able to deliver better care.

Nurse leaders and nurse managers have many demands on their limited time. Time is an important resource in nursing and for nurses, and finding time is a challenge even in the best situations. Great time management means being effective as well as efficient. To manage time effectively, achieve outcomes, and minimize stress, we need to define what the present activities are and what important activities are. The effective use of time-management skills thus becomes an even more important tool to achieve personal and professional goals. With good time-management skills, we are in control of our time, lives, stress levels, energy levels, and we make progress at work. We can maintain balance in our work, personal, and family lives, and have enough flexibility to respond to the new opportunities.

Time-management skills test our abilities to recognize and solve not only personal time management problems, but also problems in our organization. Thus, delegation skills are important for personal and organizational time management. Personal time management includes the knowing of self and depends upon self-awareness, self-assessment, and self-management. As for the skill of delegation, the nurse leader/manager must understand his or her role and the staff's abilities to effectively delegate. When the authority is delegated, the nurse leader/manager must set the limits of responsibility.

Good time managers combine a sense of purpose and flexibility, allowing them to react to the unpredictable while still getting routine tasks done in an efficient manner. Achieving this balance brings credibility to leadership. Managing time means managing yourself in relation to your time.

How Time Management Helped Me: Mentor

In my career, I have had to follow many objectives that I thought were important for my development as a nurse. Now I understand that every period of life is conducted by specific objectives, related to the knowledge and beliefs of the moment.

At the beginning of my career, I worked as a nurse in the surgical department in one of the biggest hospitals in my country. As a young nurse, I established short-term goals (as a young mentee, namely to have more knowledge and to have good skills). I worked with experienced colleagues, and I learned more from them.

After eight years, things were the same because I lived in the communist period, and I had few, if any, opportunities for something new. Because something was lacking in my career, and I felt that I was able to do more, I started to work with the students in nursing practice. I became a mentor for the clinical stage in the surgical department. Now, I must plan my activities both as a nurse and as a mentor, which meant that I had to have time-management skills.

As a mentor I helped students develop confidence and skills, including the ability for good communication with patients, collecting data, planning, and working collaboratively with clinical staff.

The Mentor as Mentee

In the second part of my career, more things changed. After the Romanian revolution, nurses had more opportunities to study and to develop their career. In 1990, I became a member of the Romanian Nursing Association (RNA). Here, I met Gabriela Bocec, president of RNA and director at the Center for Continuing Education. She was the new mentor, leader, and life model for me.

She introduced the nursing concept in Romania, and dedicated her life to education in the spirit of nursing, despite the resistance of some leaders from our country regarding the nursing process.

Gabriela had a democratic leadership style (participative) and engaged us in decision-making. She had trust in us and stimulated us to do more. It made us have trust in ourselves. She taught us not to abandon the fight, but instead, be consistent in supporting an idea. Gabriela also taught us not to lose time with negative things, to think positively, and to focus on what we do.

I appreciated her intelligence, dignity, commitment, creativity, professional, and personal qualities so much that I decided to follow the same way in my personal career.

In a short time, I became chief nurse in general surgery, and a mentor. In 2000, I became a member of the board of directors of the RNA. I enrolled in the first Romanian University education courses for nurses. It was a very hard period for me, both to plan my objectives and for accomplishing my goals.

My skills regarding time management had to adapt to my new life. For the first time, I planned objectives not only for the short term but for the long term, and I had to establish priorities—to stay in collaboration with nurse teachers from nursing school, to attend courses regarding nursing concepts, to establish objectives for students' modern education, and to find solutions regarding the practice of students in my department. Because of the large number of students, I had to work in the morning and afternoon. Despite all these difficulties, I solved problems using the knowledge of time management and leadership—I worked in the mentorship process with two nurse leaders.

Gabriela served as a role model for us. She organized workshops on collaboration between the nursing school and hospital, to reduce the gap between school and hospital. She invited mentors and teachers in nursing from all districts of the country to attend the workshops. Here, I learned about clinical teaching. It was an important progress for me. I applied clinical teaching in practice when I worked with the students. The students have gained more skills and more interest for nursing, and they were proud that they could learn more.

The Mentor Matures

I acquired new knowledge regarding the nursing process and began teaching this in practice. I graduated with a university education in nursing and in management of health services, and, together with a few colleagues and Gabriela Bocec, published nursing articles.

From October 2006, I have served as president of RNA. The time management interfered again. Together with board members, we established priorities, delegated activities, and assigned responsibilities. With good time-management and delegation skills, we were able to edit and publish many items, including a journal, a student manual, and a few books; organize and attend national and international conferences; develop a nursing research project; translate and publish NANDA International's *Nursing Diagnoses: Definitions & Classification, 2007–2008*, and collaborate with the Ministry of Education (MOE), universities, and other associations. We were also able to attend international meetings organized by ICN (International Council of Nurses), EFN (European Federation of Nursing Association), and EFNNMA (European Forum of National Nursing Midwives Association), and WHO.

In conclusion, I try to demonstrate that a nurse leader/manager can use time wisely to accomplish everything that is expected of her. But this takes planning, and time is one of the most important aspects to plan.

The Mentee Perspective

My name is Mirela Bidilic, and I work as director of care at the Central Military Hospital in Bucharest. I'm a member of the board of directors at RNA. From 2000–2004, I served as president of the RNA. I have had the opportunity to meet and work on the team with the great nurse from Romania, Gabriela Bocec, and with Ecaterina Gulie. After the death of Gabriela, Ecaterina became the president of RNA.

I appreciate Ecaterina's professional quality and her professional value as a leader/mentor/manager. She is a strong woman, she has vision, and she wants to introduce something new in our profession. She is also an example for us and for our profession. I'm amazed at how she finds time to solve the problems of our association. In the past two years, she has achieved significant goals. She has the power to accomplish many tasks. Her personality is marked by the following values: professionalism, commitment, good communication, sociability, tolerance, honesty, and awareness. She is able to build good relationships and maintain them, share knowledge and information, give advice and guide the students, love our profession, work on a team, be a good collaborator, and have fidelity to nursing.

Ecaterina inspired me in the area of professional and personal development and she was an example for me in developing my career. I identified my goals and became committed to achieving these goals. I decided to continue my education in nursing, and I enrolled in the Romanian University education courses for nurses. After finishing my university education, I became director of care in the hospital.

Self-Reflective Questions

1. What are your plans to change something in the nursing profession?

2. How often do you find yourself running out of time (hourly? daily? weekly?), and what are your plans to improve this?

3. What do you perceive as a gap between theory and practice in nursing?

4. Do you consider nursing to be a profession or an occupation, and why?

5. How do you define a mentor? As a facilitator of learning? As one who has a genuine interest in helping others to succeed?

6. How do you define a mentee? As an individual with a sense of responsibility and accountability for his/her own career development?

7. How do you feel that the mentoring experience has influenced clinical practice?

8. How do you define the complexity of delegation? Low? Medium? High?

9. How can you better actively seek solutions to improve practice?

10. What strategies do you propose to support continuous education?

Transforming Practice at the Point of Care

97

"It is very important for those who wish to create a new culture, a new society, a new state, first to understand themselves."

—Krishnamurti

Mentor

Bonnie Wesorick, RN, MSN, DPNAP, FAAN
Founder and Chair, Clinical Practice Model Resource Center
Grand Rapids, Michigan, USA

Mentee

Stacy Jepsen, RN, BS, CCRN
Critical Care Educator
Critical Care Nurse Clinician, Fairview Southdale Hospital
Edina, Minnesota, USA

Leading transformation of practice at the point of care is legacy work (Wesorick, 2008). This chapter looks at the lessons learned from leading members of the Clinical Practice Model Resource Center's (CPMRC) International Consortium of more than 240 rural, community, and university settings that are collectively engaged in practice transformation at the point of care. The focus here is narrowed to two fundamental components for success: first, the essence of the leader, and second, the leader's awareness of the work needed to transform practice.

The Essence of the Leader

Transformation starts with a new kind of leader, a leader who knows him- or herself and can live and be true to the very elements of transformation he or she is leading. These new leaders have a tacit awareness that transformation is not about them, but about the collective shared vision being pursued. Their integrity, courage, competency, and compassion are palpable. Other leaders of transformation speak about the nature of the work: Ben Franklin noted, "There are three things that are hard: steel, diamond, and to know oneself." Starting to know oneself is a commitment to do the personal work that Gandhi reminded us is essential if we really want to transform practice. That is, "Each of us needs to be the change we want to see in this world."

The consortium learned that transformation calls for leaders who are committed to serve those whom they are privileged to lead while knowing when they need to shift from leader to follower. We have found that this self-knowledge begins with leaders doing their own values clarification work coupled with their commitment to learn the deep values that sit in the hearts of those they serve.

Max DePree has written that the first accountability of a leader is to know reality (DePree, 1989). The CPMRC International Consortium delineated the second accountability. That is, to commit to the work necessary to bridge the gap between the daily reality and the desired reality.

The Look at Reality

John Naisbitt noted, "The seeds of the future are embedded in the truths of today's reality" (Naisbitt, 2006). Both those who give and those who receive care are issuing a deafening call to transform health care. Many of the quality and safety challenges are familiar:

- Stressful fast-paced cultures.
- Shortages.
- Task-driven versus evidence-based practice.
- Inadequate infrastructures to support integrated care across the continuum.
- Lack of infrastructures to sustain partnership across disciplines to end the silos, fragmentation of care, duplication, repetition, and omission.

And all of this is topped with the worst financial times in almost a century. In these seeds of reality, we can find clear direction.

From Clarity to Action

The International Consortium has learned great lessons about transformation at the point of care, the point where the hands of those who give and receive care meet. In almost three decades of work we've seen a clarity evolve concerning the fundamental elements that must be present to sustain the best places to give and receive care. Figure 1 shows the fundamental elements. The nature of transformation work is to ensure these elements are strong. We use a molecule as a metaphor because a molecule teaches us that if any one atom is missing from the molecule, it is no longer the same molecule. All atoms must be present. One is not more important than the other; they are integrated. The elements of the molecule are reflected in the national health care priorities (National Priorities Partnership, 2008; Daschle, 2008; Kohn et al. (Eds.), 2000; Institute of Medicine, 2001; Kenney, 2008).

Those who dare to lead must start with seeking an understanding of the whole of the health care system. Although we consider multiple factors, the lessons in the Consortium point to two fundamental factors essential for success: Use a practice framework to guide the work and combine Polarity Management with problem solving.

Why a Framework?

To prevent fragmented, reactionary, and ultimately doomed transformation interventions, the Clinical Practice Model/Framework (CPM) was developed to guide the transformation work. John Naisbitt, the world-renowned futurist, explained his often-uncanny ability to predict the future in a complex, noisy world when he said, "With a simple framework, we could begin to make sense of the world. And we could change the framework as the world itself changed" (Naisbitt, 2006). For almost three decades, CPM has been guiding transformation work (Wesorick, 1990; Wesorick, 1991a; Wesorick, 1991b).

Figure 2 shows the CPM framework. The base reflects the realization that it is essential to know "what matters most" for both those who give and those who receive care. The process to achieve this shared purpose is called a Core Belief Review (Wesorick, 2008). The early phases of this work showed the need for dialogue, Polarity Management, and partnership skills (Johnson, 1996; Wesorick et al., 1998; Senge, 1990; Wesorick & Shiparski, 1997).

Fundamental Elements for Point-of-Care Trasformation
Co-creating and sustaining the best places to give and receive care

: Shared Purpose
- Legacy work around what matters most.
- Unveils the capacity and connects souls.
- Shifts from doing to becoming.

olarities=mission and margin, medical are and whole person care, client and taff satisfaction, retention and recruitment

: Healthy Relationships
- Rooted in honor and respect.
- Helps one know self and others.
- Enhance leadership and followership skills.
- Requires forgiveness, compassion, vulnerability and trustworthiness.
- Live principles of partnership.

olarities=hierarchy and partnership, onditional and unconditional respect, roductivity and relationships

: Scope of Practice
- Honors each individual's choice to serve.
- Clarifies the uniqueness of accountabilities.
- First step in assuring competency.
- Helps prevent variability of practice.
- Focuses not just on tasks but professional accountability.

olarities=task and professional services, eatment and prevention services

:: Competency
- Reflects scope of practice.
- Is evidence-based.
- Requires standardization and individualization.

olarities=task and professional services, olicy/procedure and evidence based, ndividualized and standardized

;: Integrated Competency
- Individual competency is not enough.
- Competency must integrate with other disciplines.
- Know others scope of practice.
- Know how scope of practice impacts others.
- Know what you need from others to enhance services.
- Stops fragmentation, duplication, and repetition.

olarities=individual competency and ntegrated competency, safety, and eedom

D: Dialogue or Meaningful Conversation
- Advances thinking, practice and relationships—prevents dehumanization.
- Taps collective wisdom.
- Increases awareness of sacredness of words.
- Requires skills based on principles.
- Invites diversity and polarities which keep learning alive.
- Invites another's voice and wisdom.
- Generates new knowledge.

Polarities=hierarchy and partnership, conditional and unconditional respect, productivity and relationships

Healthy Work Culture

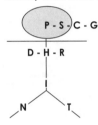

H: Hand-Off/Professional Exchange
- Standardizes processes.
- Honors the patient's story.
- Honors the team's contribution.
- Improves communication.
- Invites dialogue and healthy relationships with colleagues.
- Outcomes of care transparent.

Polarities=safety for patient and staff, plan and implement patient and staff outcomes, mutuality and priority

"No matter how large the corporation you work in, it is too small for one human soul."
David Whyte

I: Infrastructures
- Break silos, establish innovation.
- Provide resources and support.
- Show what is valued in organization.
- Enhance safety for those who give and receive care.
- Support efficient and effective processes.

Polarities=stability and change, relationships and resources

N: Networking (Partnership Councils)
- Break silos by connecting people across the system.
- Place to develop dialogue, partnership and polarity management skills.
- Taps wisdom of other disciplines, roles, departments, or settings.
- Helps create and sustain healthy relationships/partnerships.
- Helps manage problems and unsolvable problems or dilemmas/polarities.
- Stops dehumanization process.
- Foundation for integration and innovation.

Polarities=directive and participatory/decision making, centralized and decentralized

T: Tools and Resources
- Helps live what matters most.
- Support individual and integrated scope of practice delivery.
- Include patient's story, plan of care, documentation and education.
- Stimulate critical thinking, mutuality and enhances outcomes.
- Bring evidence-based knowledge to bedside to enhance critical thinking.
- Stop fragmentation, variability, duplication and repetition.
- Organize and advance all steps of process saving time, money, and lives.
- Meet legal, reimbursement and credentialing standards.
- Foundation for technology that supports transformation

Polarities=paper and automated, general content and evidence-based content

Figure 1   The fundamental elements and polarities related to point of care transformation work.

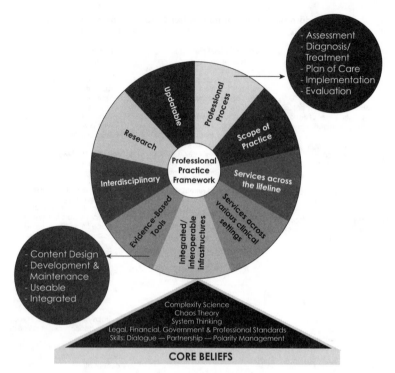

Figure 2   The components of the CPM Professional Practice Framework to guide Point of Care Transformation.

A guiding framework needed to be rooted in the understanding of legal, financial, governmental/credentialing and professional standards. In addition, it was critical to understand the theories of systems thinking, complexity, and chaos science (Senge, 1990; Waldrop, 1992; Wheatley, 2006). This theoretical foundation moves the wheel of progress toward a vision of the future because we ensure all the intentionally designed actions to transform the cultures must do the following:

- Integrate with the professional process.

- Support the scope of practice/services.

- Ensure that care is delivered with the intention to serve humanity from pre-birth to death and across multiple settings that are interdisciplinary, that care is integrated, and that care is driven by evidence-based tools continuously updated and based on research.

The framework helps leaders, and thus those who follow them, focus on priorities and action.

Why Polarity Management?

Barry Johnson, creator of Polarity Management™ (PM) helped clarify why so many good ideas and change efforts fail or are not sustainable (Johnson, 1996; Wesorick, 2002). Historically, pressing issues were seen as problems to solve. Yet, the Consortium learned that the common issues haunting leaders were not just problems to be solved, but also polarities to be managed. Problem solving is a decision-making model that comes from the context of either/or, black or white. It is a model designed to find the problem and fix it. In contrast, polarities are the presence of two or more values (called poles) that look different, appear as opposite or competitive, but are interdependent. Interdependent means they need each other; each represents half the truth, and one is not more important than the other. A dynamic tension exists between them.

A metaphor for PM is inhaling and exhaling. Both inhaling and exhaling are important, but because they are interdependent, without one or the other, you will die—a definite downside to avoid. Interdependence means it is never either/or but both/and. Polarities are not something to be solved, nor will they ever go away. Instead, we need the vigilance to strengthen each pole continuously. These statements are true for all polarities. We will encounter many problems to fix, but most are connected to polarities that have not been managed well. In Figure 1, some of the polarities that relate to each of the fundamental elements are listed.

Can you remember a time when these polarities of cost (margin) and quality (mission), staff and patient satisfaction, staff workload and patient needs, patient and staff safety, tasks and scope of practice, policy/procedure and evidence-based services, relationship and productivity, and so on, were not a concern? Again, we must realize that these polarities can never be solved or fixed. There needs to be a vigilance to take actions that support both poles In simplest terms, polarity management is about harnessing the tension that exists between opposite or competing values or forces and using it as a springboard to higher ground. For example if all effort is focused on patient satisfaction and staff satisfaction is ignored, patient satisfaction will not be achieved and therefore the higher purpose to have the best places to work and receive care will not be reached.

The CPM Consortium has learned many lessons while leading transformation at the point of care. The importance and value of the foundation shared in Figures 1 and 2 and the skill of PM become apparent through the following words of my mentee whose leadership and experience brings hope and deep insights for those who lead transformation.

Mentee: Transformation at the Point of Care during Financial Crisis

During our financial crisis, resulting in layoffs, I immediately saw the importance of our practice framework and the work we did in the hospital and on our unit to ensure each element of the Clinical Practice Framework was strong. When the financial stress hit us, we already had a partnership council in place that enhanced the trust and partnership among management, other disciplines, and staff. We had already developed trusting relations with our chief nurse officer, and we had a place to come to the table together to deal with the cold financial facts. We did not have to reinvent the wheel; we had the structures and elements of the framework in place and needed to use all our skills to address the serious issues at hand. We had a common understanding that we would not decrease the quality of our professional services and go back to task dominated–only practice. We already had the tools and resources to support us and the continuation of evidence-based practice.

Understanding PM was so important. It helped prevent the paralysis of fear that comes when people are losing jobs. We knew that all decisions would not be based on just cost, but also quality. We knew we needed to continue to be creative as an interdisciplinary team and come up with creative ideas to offset our financial situation.

A Continuing Journey

We have come to understand that the journey of transformation has no such thing as arriving. Instead, when transformation work removes barriers that interfere with healers living what they deeply value, when it enhances their ability to live their professional values, and when it provides the framework to support them, colleagues become inspired and in fact will continue the journey to continuously learn and improve care no matter what obstacles they meet. They will volunteer, be creative, and sacrifice to continue the work that sustains the best place to give and receive care. This work is the "finest of the fine arts."

Self-Reflective Questions

1. What are the deep values you hold that guide your role as leader related to practice at the point of care?

2. What values clarification have you done with nursing and interdisciplinary teams to solidify a shared purpose?

3. In what ways is transformation at the point of care being addressed within the organization?

4. What are the gaps between reality and the desired vision to practice in the best places to give and receive care?

5. How can you assess the strengths of each of the fundamental elements in your culture?

6. In what ways can you articulate to your peers the importance of a Clinical Practice Model/Framework to guide transformation at the point of care?

7. How can you differentiate between the problems to be solved and polarities to be managed?

8. What are the fundamental polarities that need to be managed in your culture for it to sustain the best places to give and receive care?

9. What steps can you take to measure if you have adequate resources to support transformation at the point of care?

10. In what ways can you measure the financial return on investment when the work to transform practice at the point of care is committed to by leadership?

Transitioning Novice Nurses Into Complex Health Care Environments

98

"Listen to your own voice; listen to what you're doing in your practice. Take it seriously, have the courage to be an innovator in your practice. Talk about what you do, in story form, and do not allow your practice to be silenced."

—Patricia Benner

Mentor
Charles Krozek, MN, RN, FAAN
President and Managing
  Director
Versant RN Residency
Los Angeles, California, USA

Mentee
Larissa Africa, BSN, RN
Director Process Integration
Versant RN Residency
Los Angeles, California, USA

The nursing shortage has made it challenging for hospitals to meet sufficient RN staffing numbers. Responding to this challenge, nursing schools nationwide expanded their capacity to educate new nurses. According to the American Association of Colleges of Nursing, there has been an increase in baccalaureate level enrollment over the past few years (American Association of Colleges of Nursing, 2008). Consequently, hospitals face the challenge of having novice nurses who struggle to transition successfully from a student to the professional role. The apparent "preparation gap" must be bridged if the novice nurse is to practice safe patient care independently.

The result of this difficult transition is illustrated in the July 2007 PricewaterhouseCoopers' Health Research Institute study that found the average turnover for first-year nurses was 27.1%.

Over time, the preparation gap continues to widen as acute health care environments become more complex. Thus, the once-adequate new graduate–orientation program traditionally used in hospitals has become increasingly ineffective in transitioning the new graduate RNs from a student to a competent and confident professional. A recent study showed that new graduate RNs are most vulnerable at the third month of practice; however, approximately 80 percent of current hospital-based transition programs are only 12 weeks or less in duration (Suling, 2007). Compounding this, stretched educational resources limit a hospital's capacity to build a comprehensive residency, which results in new graduate programs that typically have such limitations as:

- A fragmented and mostly unit-based program with little or no hospital-wide standardization.

- New-graduate transition programs too short in duration. The average 12-week program moves the new graduate to independent practice when most vulnerable.

- Sole use of skill checklists to validate competency. Variation in preceptor competency and practice can result in questionable reliability and accurate completion of new-graduate evaluation.

- Outdated content resulting from a rapidly changing health care environment.

- A "one size fits all" approach developed without the use of a proven role-analysis process.

- Little or no empirical outcome data to evaluate new-graduate performance or the integrity of the residency program.

- Little or no assistance from technology resulting in a resource-intensive/paper-based program.

- Lack of support systems designed to meet the new-graduate's emotional needs.

Using the Versant RN Residency

The Versant RN residency was established to provide health care organizations with the highest quality solutions to strategically develop and stabilize the RN workforce while maximizing its internal capabilities. The RN residency is a comprehensive education and training system designed specifically to transition newly graduated registered nurses from students to safe, competent professional practitioners. The components of the RN residency include a guided clinical experience, mentoring, debriefing/self-care sessions, and instructor-led curriculum. By providing new graduate nurses with the support and training clinically and professionally, the RN residency addresses the gap between the education system and clinical setting (Reinsvold, 2008). The Versant RN residency, which has been implemented in hospitals across the nation since 1999, is guided by several core principles:

- **Develop and implement a standardized system throughout a hospital or hospital system.** Nursing buy-in from the entire hospital and/or system is necessary for standardization to occur. Versant uses a system containing "core" curriculum—designed for all nurses, regardless of their specialty—and specialty curriculum dovetailed with the core.

- **Use a tested role analysis process to identify content appropriate for new graduate RNs.** Versant uses a process called DACUM (Develop A Curriculum), which is a competency-based analysis to identify duties, tasks, knowledge, skills, and traits of the new RNs (Norton, 1997). New graduate nurses attend core curriculum pertinent to all nurses as a basis for general nursing practice. In addition, each new graduate nurse attends specialty curricula such as neonatal intensive care and perioperative specialties applicable to the area they are hired into.

- **Provide adequate "protected time" with trained preceptor.** The new-graduate RN is most vulnerable between the third and sixth month of their new professional practice (Suling, 2007). High stress levels and low self-confidence increases risk for error and, ultimately because of low role satisfaction, a high probability for turnover (Halfer, 2006). Sufficient clinical practice time under a trained preceptor coupled with appropriate and focused experiences will accelerate the new graduate's development of confidence and competence, increase role satisfaction, and increase retention (Beecroft, Kunzman, & Krozek 2001).

- **Go beyond the traditional skills checklist.** The traditional skills checklist is not sufficient to reflect nurse competency in today's complex patient care environment. Significant variation exists for how preceptors assess and document competency with a traditional checklist. As a backup, or "safety net," the Slater Observation Nursing Competencies Rating Scale is used. The Slater Scale consists of items performed by nurses in the clinical setting such as actions directed toward meeting the psychosocial and physical needs of the patient (Wandelt and Stewart, 1975).

- **Continuous improvement.** The health care workplace and regulatory environment is a moving target. Residency content and processes must be consistently assessed for effectiveness and enhanced to meet the resident, patient, and organizational goals. Without continuous enhancement, content will become obsolete, thus reducing effectiveness of the program and increasing risk to the patient.

- **Integrate support systems appropriate to the new-graduate RN.** Formal support systems, integrated into the RN residency, can assist the new graduate in managing stress through this vulnerable period. Strategies such as debriefing groups, trained preceptors, and a formal mentor program contribute to the acceleration of new-graduate RNs in attaining confidence in their abilities, increasing satisfaction with their new employer, and a sense of commitment to the profession— all of which ultimately increase retention. The formal mentoring provides new graduate nurses with a sponsor into the profession of nursing. The mentor and mentee (new graduate nurse) identify key professional development goals and create plans towards achieving them. The mentor-mentee relationship is confidential in nature allowing the mentee to feel comfortable disclosing any concerns. Topics on professional development such as understanding the hospital's chain of command, nurse practice act, and the American Nurses Credentialing Center's Magnet Recognition Program are provided to assist the mentor in goal planning with the resident. The goal of the mentoring component is to help smooth the transition of new graduate nurses from student to a nursing professional.

- **Include all key stakeholders.** To be effective, buy-in and participation of key stakeholders from the RN staff member to the corporate chief executive officer is essential. The hospital's chief nursing officer (CNO) is an excellent choice as the residency champion, whose complete support and strong leadership is necessary for the development and integration of a comprehensive residency.

- **Customize for the unique needs of the new-graduate RN.** The residency's content, framework, and processes must be customized for effective learning and skill acquisition. New graduates who are given too much information and responsibility too fast will become over-whelmed and ultimately dissatisfied, and will leave the organization prematurely.

- **Integrate extensive empirical evaluation.** You can't manage what you don't measure. Accurate and current outcome data is essential to assess resident progress and effectiveness of the residency. The quantitative analyses of the residency allow hospitals to measure outcomes, demonstrate effectiveness, and identify weaknesses.

- **Integrate innovative technology.** A standardized, outcome-based RN residency system is very complex. To maintain program integrity, Voyager, a web-based suite of workforce development applications, was developed to help manage and update content and processes, collect data, and produce reports. Technology assists in consistent implementation over time, and is key to continued program success in meeting organizational goals.

Mentee's Perspective

As Charlie Krozek's mentee, I have learned to use these core principles to successfully implement and maintain the Versant RN residency in hospitals across the nation. I collaborate with hospital stakeholders in standardizing and aligning their existing new-graduate program with the Versant content, framework, and processes. The complexity of the RN residency requires the ability to transfer the information into processes that are understandable and clients can identify with easily. It is important that as a mentee, I understand the goals of the RN residency for the hospital by actively listening and observing how my mentor communicate the benefits of the RN residency with hospital leadership. The standardized implementation of the residency also requires customization at each facility based on their needs. By seeking feedback from my mentor on the successes and challenges I have experienced, I am able to continuously improve the implementation process.

The implementation of the core principles requires strong commitment, involvement, and leadership from key stakeholders, such as the CNO of the facility. These core principles need to be communicated to the CNO so that he or she may have a full understanding of the core principles that must be adopted for successful implementation of the residency. Curriculum delivery and support systems available at each facility are evaluated to ensure their alignment with the residency's core principles.

The novice-to-expert team precepting approach systematically introduces residents to more experienced preceptors as learning advances. Preceptors at the competent level concentrate on basic skills of being a new nurse, while expert preceptors concentrate on developing the resident's critical thinking skills. To complement the support given to residents in the clinical area, mentors and debriefing facilitators serve as additional resources. The mentor provides guidance in the resident's professional role development, and the debriefing facilitators provide residents with tools on coping with challenges of working with patients, families, and colleagues.

To validate the effectiveness of the residency in transitioning new graduates, residents complete measurement tools at various stages of the program. The results of these measurement tools are used by the facility to further develop the residency and enhance the environment affecting new-graduate transition. A key aspect of my role is to guide facilities in using their data to make informed decisions that affect the implementation of the residency.

To further create efficiency and enhance processes, Versant Voyager was created for on-going RN residency administration, implementation, evaluation, and refinement. Voyager enables key stakeholders within a facility to track documentation of resident's competency achievement, preceptor performance, and mentor and debriefer involvement. The integration of these core principles is the key to successful implementation of the Versant RN residency.

As mentioned earlier, dire staffing shortages can require the new-graduate RN to be pulled from orientation and start practice prematurely, thus creating a risk for patient safety and contributes to new-graduate dissatisfaction and high turnover with 30-65% leaving by the second year (Halfer, 2006). The solution requires an innovative approach to transitioning the new graduate— a comprehensive, outcome-based RN residency complete with content, framework, and processes focused on the unique needs of the novice nurse. A formal mentoring component is a key ingredient in supporting the smooth new graduate nurse transition to professional nursing by providing a confidential support system and guidance toward professional development.

Self-Reflective Questions

1. How can you best make sure that new RNs transition smoothly into the nursing workforce?

2. What can you do to improve retention rates at your hospital?

3. What can you do to assist your facility in improving your current new graduate orientation program?

4. How does your facility support the new graduate transition?

5. What components of a new graduate residency program are currently being implemented at your facility, if any?

6. How does your facility initiate a culture change?

7. Who are the key stakeholders in your facility who can champion the issue if you want to initiate a culture change?

8. What resources would you need at your facility if you want to restructure the nursing orientation?

9. What type of information do you need to collect in order to support the need for an RN residency at your facility?

10. How can preceptors and mentors be supported so that they may perform their role effectively in transitioning new graduate nurses?

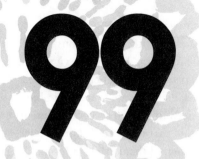

99

Truth and Honesty

"The quality of the nurse manager is the single most significant factor in promoting change and developing a professional standard of nursing practice."

—Joyce C. Clifford

Mentor
Mary J. Connaughton, MS, RN
Principal, Connaughton Consulting
Newton, Massachusetts, USA

Mentees
Melissa Joseph, MSN, RN
Nurse Manager, Faulkner Hospital
Boston, Massachusetts, USA

and

Sara Macchiano, MS/MBA, RN
Nursing Director, Massachusetts General Hospital
Boston, Massachusetts, USA

A colleague, Jim Hassinger, and I (Mary) present an advanced leadership development program called *The Practice of Wise Leadership*. The program is based on our collective 30-plus years of consulting experience and the cross-cultural research of Dr. Angeles Arrien (Arrien, 1993, 2005). In my consulting practice, I have the opportunity to coach both senior and novice nurse leaders to help them expand their leadership expertise. It was a privilege to teach and coach the talented nurse managers featured here.

According to Dr. Arrien's research, one of the universal character traits of leadership is honesty. Honesty involves two distinct steps: First, the ability and willingness to *see the truth* of a situation, and second, the ability and willingness to *speak the truth*.

This chapter illuminates the challenges that two remarkable novice nurse leaders face as they try to accurately assess and address difficult situations, using the wise leadership principles they learned in the program. In separate vignettes, the nurse leaders describe what they learned from situations that challenged their ability to both see and speak the truth. They demonstrate both admirable openness and courage to examine their own leadership, as well as a commitment to learn from their experiences. It is frequently said that we learn best from our mistakes, but many of us are too proud to admit them. I thank Melissa Joseph and Sara Macchiano for sharing their stories so that we can all learn from their ordinary yet extraordinary experiences.

Lessons Learned about Seeing the Truth

TRUTH: The ability and the willingness to see the essence of a situation clearly and objectively, without blind spots

Some nurse leaders see what they want in order to avoid the discomfort of addressing a difficult problem or admitting they need help. When we allow our fears or emotions to taint the picture of what is really happening, we develop blind spots. If we are unaware of our blind spots, or lack a mechanism to screen for them, we base our leadership actions on a distorted picture of the truth. It is like prescribing treatment for an inaccurate diagnosis: The real problem is not effectively addressed, and potential harm can come from the wrong leadership action. In the self-reflective checklist at the end of this chapter, a checklist of potential barriers to seeing clearly serves as a quick screen for blind spots. Knowing our tendencies makes it more likely that we can see situations just as they are.

Sara

This is what happened. The orientation of a new graduate nurse was complicated by her performance, the preceptor's approach, and my inability to see the truth of the situation. The new graduate deflected all critical feedback and implied the preceptor was the real problem. As a new manager, I had selected this preceptor who had been very supportive of me in my first managerial role. In reality both the orientee *and* the preceptor had performance issues.

This is why I was challenged to see the truth clearly. I struggled to see this situation clearly because of my blind spots of hope and denial. Hope because I desired success for the new graduate, the preceptor, and myself. Denial because I wanted there to be just one problem—the new graduate's shortcomings. I chose to believe my hand-picked preceptor was blameless. My blind spots prevented me from seeing the truth about the preceptor's performance.

This is the action that I took. As orientation progressed with no improvement, the new graduate was given a different preceptor. I did not address her concerns about the preceptor.

This is what resulted from my actions. The new graduate did not complete orientation. I concluded that her feedback about the first preceptor was baseless. Not until a different orientee (without performance issues) had the same concerns about the preceptor, did I see the preceptor's challenges clearly.

This is what I learned. I learned from this experience that I have a fear of conflict, particularly when a supportive relationship is involved. Therefore, I am at risk for minimizing/rationalizing poor performance to avoid dealing with it. I now know that I need to periodically reassess my truth of a situation. To support this, I rely on the input of my team whose perspectives add balance to the assessment.

Melissa

This is what happened. A popular internal patient care assistant applied to become a newly licensed nurse but gave a mediocre interview. I ignored my gut feeling—and the poor interview—and hired him anyway. Practice concerns emerged quickly during orientation, and he eventually resigned.

This is why I was challenged to see the truth clearly. I was challenged to see the truth because I was focused on two things: winning the approval of the staff and supporting the organizational culture to promote from within. I became overly optimistic that this nurse would succeed. My enthusiasm for wanting to promote from within and to please the staff blinded me to the reality that this individual could not be successful in our acute environment.

This is the action that I took. Although performance concerns were quickly noted by preceptor #1, the newly licensed nurse was transitioned to preceptor #2 with hope that his practice would improve.

This is what resulted from my actions. Although his performance improved briefly with preceptor #2, practice concerns persisted. Finally, a serious medication error occurred.

This is what I learned. I learned that I am capable of ignoring what I know to be true to please the staff, a practice I will guard against in the future. As a leader I must trust my observations and my intuition, regardless of the culture or common practice. I am learning to reassess situations routinely and involve others, especially my leadership team, to expand our collective understanding.

Lessons Learned About Speaking the Truth

HONESTY: The ability, the willingness, and the courage to speak the truth without blame or judgment

Sara

This is what happened. A staff nurse with 5 years' experience had received feedback from coworkers, a clinical nurse specialist (CNS), and me about not meeting expectations. Despite receiving the feedback well and promising to improve, the pattern of poor performance continued. The latest incident put a patient at risk, causing me to question her practice.

This is why I was challenged to speak honestly. I needed to address the practice concerns, but I did not want to come across as being punitive during a time when we are working to establish a blameless culture regarding errors. Also, I had been coaching the staff to give 1-to-1 feedback and did not want to undermine their efforts to hold each other accountable.

This is the action that I took. I presented the facts to the nurse supported with evidence from patient records. I kept an open mind that she might have a different version of the truth. I shared my assessment that she had a pattern of sloppy practice and that I believed she had the knowledge and capability to do better.

This is what resulted from my actions. The nurse agreed with my assessment. She also shared some personal issues she was dealing with, without using them as an excuse. This opened the door for our conversation about self-care, including asking for time off before things progress to a point where patients are put at risk.

This is what I learned. In the past I have mistakenly equated honesty with bluntness; therefore, I have a fear that if I am honest I am going to be perceived as blunt. From this experience I learned that I can be honest without being callous. Because I presented the facts without placing blame, our conversation was more productive, we avoided defensiveness, and we addressed the issues more quickly. Now I try to honestly frame difficult situations from my own perspective instead of analyzing the many possibilities that might or might not be contributing to the issue.

Melissa

This is what happened. An experienced nurse, who is a highly valued resource among her peers, demonstrated lack of depth and critical thinking in her practice. My assessment of her practice differed greatly from that of the staff.

This is why I was challenged to speak honestly. As a relatively new nurse manager I was hesitant to be honest with this nurse because I feared that she and the staff would challenge my assessment of her skills, leading to tension and divisiveness on the unit.

This is the action that I took. After a few weeks of avoiding the nurse, I found the courage to share my assessment with her. I was honest, giving her specific examples when she was unable to answer questions about her patients on rounds and when her nursing notes were incomplete and lacked depth.

This is what resulted from my actions. My honest discussion with this nurse created an opening for her to reflect on her practice, something she acknowledged she had not done in a long time. She appreciated the honest feedback presented in a factual, non-judgmental way, and agreed to work on practice goals.

This is what I learned. Despite my fear of being honest, I realized my avoidance could hinder her development. Though I have a strong desire to preserve the dignity of others, I also realize that being honest is a powerful way of demonstrating that I care. Now I reverse roles and ask myself, "How would I feel if I knew other people knew something about me but never shared it with me?" This inspires me to find the courage to tell the truth.

Some people reason that as long as they are not telling outright lies they are being honest. Wise leaders, however, recognize that honesty involves saying what we see, what we know, and what we don't know, regardless of the consequences. Nurse leaders might hesitate to give honest feedback for fear of hurting someone's feelings or other repercussions, or fear of getting it wrong. Playing it safe, keeping the peace, and providing comfort/reassurance to people who are struggling might feel good in the moment. However, many of us look back over our careers and are grateful for the mentor who challenged us to improve, or the brave and curious colleague who asked questions, or for the person who risked her job by taking a stand on a politically charged issue. Speaking the truth requires courage. When we develop habits of speaking honestly, we build a reservoir of courage for future challenging moments (Connaughton and Hassinger, 2007).

Self-Reflective Questions

Here is a diagnostic checklist for seeing the truth and screening for blind spots that prevent us from seeing clearly.

	YES	NO
1. Does your overly optimistic personality cause you to underestimate the true depth and scope of a problem?	☐	☐
2. Does your fear of conflict cause you to give too many chances to an under-performer?	☐	☐
3. Does your fear of hurting someone's feelings prevent you from speaking honestly?	☐	☐
4. Does your tendency to doubt yourself lead you to agree with the majority vs. trusting that your opposing view point is important?	☐	☐
5. Does your desire to look good cause you to ignore important facts?	☐	☐
6. Does your desire to appear to have it all together prevent you from asking questions and seeking help?	☐	☐
7. Does your need to do things your way blind you to new ideas or alternative approaches?	☐	☐
8. Does your emotional response to situations cloud your judgment about what really happened?	☐	☐
9. Does your desire to avoid more stress cause you to move into wishful-thinking mode that a problem will get better on its own?	☐	☐
10. Does your wish to be a good team player cause you to overlook dis-respectful behavior?	☐	☐

100

(Building) Unity Within the Nursing Profession

"If a leader stays on message, then others will hear the message."

—Angela Barron McBride

Mentor
Leana R. Uys, D Soc Sc, RN, RM
Professor
University of KwaZulu-Nata
Durban, South Africa

Mentee
Judith Bruce, PhD, RN, RM
Associate Professor
University of the Witwatersrand
Johannesburg, South Africa

In 2007 South Africa had 103,792 registered nurses and midwives living and working in 9 provinces (South African Nursing Council, 2008). Many of these nurses have specialist qualifications, such as nursing education or critical care nursing. The challenge for the profession has always been how to create national organizations in which nurses and midwives can come together to solve their practice problems, to get updated in their knowledge and skill, and to influence policy. Nurses are not the best-paid health workers, so they find travel to meetings and conferences expensive. In South Africa, they are also mainly women, so they are not only nurses, but also wives and mothers. These multiple roles make it difficult for them to be active nationally in voluntary professional organizations.

I (Leana) have been involved in national nursing organizations for many years. I was one of the nurse educators who launched the Nursing Education Association, which addressed the needs of nurse educators for many years. I was also involved for years in the Nursing Research

Association, which ran research mentor workshops all over the country. So, I had much experience in organizing nurses and midwives nationally.

But a new challenge emerged in 2000—three nurse leaders from South Africa and Botswana decided to start an at-large chapter of Sigma Theta Tau International (STTI), which would include all the university nursing schools in Africa. Now the challenge was no longer how to involve and unite the nurses of one country, but rather how to involve and unite the nurses of a continent! Africa is a continent with 57 countries. The majority of the countries have French as a major language, the largest surface area of the continent speaks English, and three countries speak Portuguese. To a large extent, the language determines the nursing and midwifery education and practice systems in the country because the language indicates the colonial system from which the current health and education systems developed. When nurses and midwives talk to each other, they often approach issues from very different frames of reference. So the challenge of creating a unified and active organization across the continent was daunting.

Challenges Unifying Large Nursing Organizations

You can sum up the challenges by pointing to a lack of resources. However, all associations have limited resources—sometimes *very* limited—and I would prefer to try to analyze what can be done within such an environment.

The first problem is marketing the organization to the people who belong in it. Face-to-face contact always works best. But how do you establish face-to-face contact from Cape to Cairo on a very limited budget?

The second major challenge is to keep contact with members. They need to be reminded often of what the organization is doing and how they can participate. Without such frequent contact, they begin to question their membership, and the organization loses contact with what they need and fails to harness their energy for the organization.

Another challenge is to manage the workload of such an organization when you have few resources and are busy with 101 other things. Ideally you can recruit a large, active, and reliable committee, and each member can take total responsibility for a portion of the. In my experience, however, most committee members do not know how to approach tasks on a continental basis, and they have difficulty in fitting these tasks into their daily work and personal schedule.

Lastly, the larger and more geographically dispersed the organization is, the more heterogeneous is its membership and the more diverse their needs and interests. How does a chapter work to the lived experience of a recent graduate in Ghana and also to a new head of a nursing school in Kenya? How do we address research, all practice areas, education, management, policy formulation, and all other areas in which it is important to give leadership?

Mentee

It is true that no organization comes without its challenges. What is important is that these challenges not become a deterrent to leading and leadership. Neither should these prevent you from learning—not only learning a skill set to lead successfully but also learning skills to identify and access resources in environments where these are limited. In working with Leana over a number of years, I learned about philanthropic receiving and giving. Giving of yourself and volunteering and sharing some of your own resources might be required. Reciprocity in leadership is not an expectation but a reward if it does happen. My experience with donors and social investors to support some of our chapter initiatives has broadened in the process of shadowing my mentor. I learned about the kinds of funding support available and what donors are prepared to fund and what they are not, how to draft a spending plan or budget and how to account for it. Most importantly, I learned from Leana that simply receiving money is not enough; you need sustainability measures. Many organizations and their projects fail because they do not plan for sustainability and self-perpetuation.

In resource-constrained environments the old adage "where there is a will there is a way" has become more of a reality for me. I recall our trip to Niger. Despite a shoestring budget, Leana secured meetings with key persons and organizations including the Minister of Health. Although we had to adapt our objectives for this visit, it was a great success. I believe that a persevering attitude in pursuit of organizational goals can help overcome some resource challenges.

Strategies for Leadership

I do not think any single strategy or even a group of strategies can make these challenges go away or solve all of them. However, the very fact that the Nursing Education Association is still going strong in South Africa and that the Tau Lambda-at-Large chapter of STTI is growing every year means that some things do work. I want to share with you what I think are the essentials.

The first lesson in leading a large organization is to manage yourself well. First, do not get into a leadership position in a nursing organization unless you are willing to work twice as hard as anybody else and to pick up all the tasks no one else wants to do, as well as those others drop. I believe in nursing organizations. I believe that they are a force for good and that they are the mechanisms by which nurses can address their own problems and those of the health care system and of the people. This belief drives me to ensure that the organizations I am involved in work. This belief enables me to be philosophical when people do not live up to their responsibilities and when sponsors pull out. I do not mind when my presidential duties include putting the tables out before the conference, registering participants, and opening the conference as president. I also know that keeping such large organizations going is very hard work. It does not take just a few minutes before a meeting or a day or two at a conference. It demands many hours of preparing documents, making contact with people, consulting, encouraging, assisting, going out of your way to visit institutions for face-to-face contact, getting to know the people, and many other activities.

Mentee

The idea that no single leadership strategy or a cookbook of strategies for leadership challenges exist resonates well with me. I think much lies in managing yourself and your inner resources and bringing these resources to bear in your daily work. My service ethic, instilled as a result of my personal and professional socialization, plays a big part in what I learn about leadership and how this translates into leadership action. After Leana led the Tau Lambda-at-Large chapter for a number of years, I took over as president. As a mentee, I learned from Leana that it is not about how big the shoes are that you have to or are expected to fill, but rather the nature of the print it leaves behind. The footprint gives direction and shape to the task ahead and gives the mentee the opportunity to bring new patterns and imprints to the leadership role. In a big, continent-wide organization, I believe this approach is important for the growth of "novice" leaders. It was important to me that Leana did not withdraw after her period in office, but remained involved to support my own leadership. In my view this is uniquely beneficial not only to me, but also to the executive and the members who over time have come to associate Leana with organizational success stories. Leana has a prodigious capacity for work and for service. This, I believe, is not just the product of her physical energy and mental determination, but comes from an inner strength that's not easily eroded. Topping up your inner resources deliberately and consistently is vital for service leadership.

Mentor

After you have made up your mind to lead an organization and have the right mindset, you can take on a leadership position such as on committees or boards.

I suggest that you organize this task as a project because project management provides a useful framework for such a long-term task. You can choose from many tools, such as network plans or software packages. The busier you are, the more systematic and thorough your planning should be to ensure that you and your committee remain on track.

Mentee

As a nurse, you learn to be organised, systematic, and thorough; these skills translate into virtually any position you may rise to in a nursing organization. Leana and I worked intimately during two international visits related to the work of Tau Lambda. In the process of shadowing her, I learned to re-order my work processes. In describing Ubuntu as an African management philosophy, Mbigi and Maree (1995) refer to the importance of collective education and rituals to lead organizations successfully. Developing, educating, building, and sharing within a (project) management framework have become important "rituals" in my leadership style. In re-ordering my system of work, I've learned to pause along the way and to take a step back every time I get ahead. During mentoring, I soon realised that leading a nursing organization such as Tau Lambda on the African content is about having the people *with you* and not *behind you*.

Mentor

The primary strategy for any organization is contact—and contact as direct as possible. Over the years we have used the following strategies for contact:

- An annual meeting that moves from centre to centre to allow as many members as possible to attend over the period of a few years. These meetings should allow for local input and should also introduce nurses from other countries to their local counterparts. In this way networks are formed, and those networks greatly strengthen the organization.

- Leaders should use every possible opportunity to visit local members. For example, when I visit Kenya for an unrelated conference, I offer to speak at the local universities if they invite their STTI members. This kind of serendipitous contact has been made famous by the international Rotary and Lions organizations. When you arrive in a town, you often see a board indicating where and when the local Rotarians meet so that visitors can join them. Because travel is so expensive, we should optimize the use of every visit. This kind of contact demands forward planning.

- Use electronic media to facilitate contact. We use telephone conferences for almost all our board and committee meetings. Such conferences are sometimes a challenge when you "lose" participants halfway through a meeting, but still, they have attended part of the meeting and feel connected. We also use e-mail extensively to circulate documents for comment and to circulate our newsletters.

- I believe the contact should be as personal as possible. We should also make provision for the social and not just the professional part of each member. For example, members want to know who gets promotions and who gets a new job. They want us to keep them updated on the professional network, and they want to keep the group updated on their own progress. Members also service the needs of other members. They send articles, distribute information about funding opportunities and conferences, invite members from other countries to act as examiners or as co-researchers, and create opportunities for further studies. In this way the organization becomes useful to all.

Mentee

Direct contact in large, geographically dispersed organizations is impractical. If attempted, direct contact can be costly and labour intensive for the people involved. In non-English speaking countries in particular, personal contact is key to building and sustaining an organization. I learned valuable lessons from Leana about an organizational buddying system for personal and professional networking. The buddy system works between entities or activities within the organization—whether that organization is a nursing school, an academic programme, or a research project—rather than the organization as a whole. Buddying is based on the principles of cooperation, solidarity, commonality of purpose, trust, mutual respect, and a collective conscience, which is derived from common experiences. Buddying is determined mainly by the development needs or advancement goals of a group within the organization and is often requested by the leader or an emerging leader. In many respects it is about "mentoring the mentor" in the buddying process. Most successful organizations globally have many strong leaders—not just one leader—working together to create success (Maxwell, 2005). This situation is the result of leaders equipping others by building capacity around them. In addition to the strategies discussed previously, personal contact with individuals such as Leana has made my leadership experience richer, more rewarding, and worthwhile. In the process I have learned that identifying and harnessing similarities rather than differences is important for unifying people in a continent-wide organization.

Learning Leadership

Leadership has many rewards, and it is a skill well worth learning. Start small and work with a mentor if you can. Or work in a team—convince a friend or colleague to join you in a committee, and learn together. You never know—you may also end up leading a very big organization to the benefit of many.

Self-Reflective Questions

Check off each statement that is true. The key for scoring your leadership potential is at the end of the chapter.

1. You want to have a leadership position because it looks good on your CV. ☐

2. You are willing to serve as a leader. ☐

3. You believe in the importance of nursing organizations. ☐

4. You are willing to be involved in an organization only when every member does his/her part. ☐

5. You are sometimes quite disorganized. ☐

6. With good planning, you can fit a leadership position into your life. ☐

7. It is the responsibility of members to keep contact with our organization. ☐

8. Electronic contact is as good as face-to-face contact with members. ☐

9. A project plan can be changed. ☐

10. Monitoring of implementation starts at the first deadline. ☐

Key to Self-Evaluation

You have potential as a leader if you checked 2, 3, 6, 9. You might have difficulty leading a large organization successfully if you checked 1, 4, 5, 7, 8, 10.

Values, Vision, and Driving the Mission

101

"If what shone afar so grand,
Turn to nothing in thy hand,
On again, the virtue lies
In the struggle, not the prize."

—R. M. Milnes

Mentor

Maggie Kirk, PhD, BSc Hons, RGN, DipN
Lead Professional Specialist (Nursing), NHS National Genetics Education and Development Centre
University of Glamorgan
Pontypridd, Wales, United Kingdom

Mentee

Paul Gill, PhD, BSc (Hons.), MSc (Oxon.) RN
Senior Post Doctoral Research Fellow, Faculty of Health, Sport and Science
University of Glamorgan
Pontypridd, Wales, United Kingdom

I (Maggie) found the short passage by Milnes in my mother's autograph book many years ago. It had been inscribed by my grandfather; words of advice for a daughter. The quotation seems apt to set the scene for this chapter in which we discuss the importance of vision, values, and mission in driving us to reach "what shone afar so grand."

Implicit in the text is that the reader has a vision, albeit one that might seem distant and difficult to reach. The vision is of something worth striving for, deserving of one's continuing efforts. It follows that focus and drive are personal qualities critical to success, where success is measured more by effort than the ultimate attainment of the goal itself. Milnes manages to convey both encouragement and a willingness to forgive. There is a gentleness to the message that says "it's OK if you fail, you can try again—and just keep trying" that resonated with me as a child and continued to do so throughout my career.

My professional journey began when I moved from genetics research to nursing. It became apparent that genetics was afforded little importance in nursing practice and education at a time of substantial investment in genetics research, where the potential benefits for health care, and the related ethical issues, were significant. The nursing profession was clearly unprepared for this quiet revolution, and I became passionate about bringing about change in practice for the benefit of patients and families affected by the issues of genetic health care. There is still a long way to go (Kirk et al. 2008a). Although our visions differ, I recognize the same "passion" in my mentee.

Vision

Mentor

A vision is an imagined possible future representing a better state of being. It may take many years to develop to the point where it can be clearly articulated, shaped by experience, and informed by research. Kakabadse et al. (2005) argue that the conviction to craft the future is one of the components of leadership, along with the ability to communicate the vision and engage others in realizing it, and the passion and determination to persist. There are two lessons to be learnt in this.

First, a "grand" vision can seldom be achieved single-handed, and a willingness to share is essential, although a strong sense of ownership can undermine this. However the communities formed through collaboration can evolve as powerful systems of influence, and so much more can be achieved. Identifying like-minded people is an important precursor to building networks from which communities can emerge.

Second, careful thought has to be given to those with whom you need to engage with your vision. Inevitably, this will involve communicating with people outside your network, perhaps using less familiar channels. You will encounter people who are indifferent to your vision, or even hostile. It is up to you to demonstrate its value, and that it is achievable.

Mentee

My professional journey began as a critical care nurse, where I developed an interest in organ transplantation, through caring for multi-organ donors and their families. Despite the significant implications of organ transplantation for nursing practice, nursing research in this area then was somewhat limited.

I wanted to help inform practice through education and research that would benefit transplant patients and their families. Consequently, my vision is to help develop an evidence base to guide clinical practice, ensuring transplant patients and their families receive the highest standards of treatment, care, and support. Given the complexity and dynamic nature of organ transplantation and health care, this vision is perhaps situated (at a particular point in time) and perpetual.

Mentorship has taught me that articulating and developing an achievable vision takes patience, time, guidance, and support. Mentorship can be, and in my experience has been, instrumental in facilitating this learning and development process (Gopee 2008). Working with an experienced mentor has allowed me to recognize the "bigger picture," address my sense of ownership, and realize that networking and collaboration are essential if this vision is to be achieved.

Mission

Mentor

Kakabadse et al. (2005) acknowledge the confusion around the terms "vision"' and "mission," and they themselves do not make a clear distinction. My *vision* is of a health service where the needs of patients and families with genetic health care issues are met by nurses who are sufficiently competent and confident in seeking specialist genetics support when appropriate. My *mission* is to engage with others in leading educational reform to promote nursing competence in genetics. The mission thus defines the purpose. Your role/mission must be based on an understanding of your strengths, what motivates you, and what values are important to you.

Mentee

My *mission* is to engage and, where appropriate, collaborate with others to develop an evidence base to inform practice. However, the mission should not be based solely on an understanding of strengths, but also on a recognition of weaknesses and how these may be addressed.

Mentorship should involve creating an enabling environment; a process that requires engagement in the mentee's own values, guidance in keeping with the principles of self directed learning, and the creation of awareness for opportunities that facilitate discovery and development (Hoffman et al 2008). This process should not involve seeking answers or solutions to problems. Instead, it should be about working closely with a mentor who questions and challenges ideas and provides encouragement and support.

Values

Mentor

Your values guide your actions that lead to the vision. Stanley (2008) talks of the importance of congruent leadership, where the actions of the leader are matched and driven by the leader's values and principles. He argues that it is on the basis of where the leader stands, rather than where he is going, that a leader acquires followers. Thus not only must you communicate your values, you also need an awareness of what is valued by those with whom you want to engage.

Mentee

Personal values are essential to any endeavor, but are not always shared with others. This can be problematic, particularly when dealing with more senior colleagues with whom you need to engage. It is therefore extremely important to establish what is valued by those with whom you want to engage and respect the visions and values of others.

The Struggles Along the Way

Mentor

Spitzer (2003) acknowledges that "without question there are and will be bumps along the road" (p. 4). She recommends that these be seen as challenges from which you learn new and innovative approaches to overcoming obstacles. Perhaps we can learn more from examining our struggles and failures than from celebrating the successes along the way.

One of the barriers is in overcoming negative (or neutral) attitudes, or working with people whose values may differ from your own. Goleman (2000) outlines the important components of emotional intelligence in addressing such issues, including self-awareness and dealing with conflict resolution.

Defining how the vision is to be realized presents a major challenge. Vision is often depicted as a shining light on the horizon, reached by a long and tortuous path with frequent intersections. In reality your vision does not come with a ready-prepared road map. It is up to you to find a path and to define your role in doing so. A strategic approach to translating your vision into action is essential, particularly where major change is a prerequisite to success. The NHS National Genetics Education and Development Centre nursing program is informed by change theory and this strategic framework has been invaluable (Kirk et al. 2008b). However, flexibility is essential, particularly in the dynamic environment of health care.

Mentee

A bend in the road is not the end of the road, unless you fail to make the turn (Anonymous). Personal and professional development is seldom a smooth process. Struggles are to be expected, particularly at the outset, and should be viewed as opportunities for learning. Personal struggles and mentorship have enabled me to appreciate the importance of being flexible and overcoming obstacles.

Reflection

Mentee

Preparing this chapter has been a valuable learning process through which I have realized that self-belief is essential to the achievement of a vision. If you do not believe in what you want to achieve, others almost certainly will not. Guidance, support, and constructive criticism from your mentor are crucial. This reflective process has also made me appreciate that, while achieving "what shone afar so grand" is a struggle, it is well worth creating a path toward it.

Self-Reflective Questions

1. Can you articulate your vision? What is it?

2. With whom have you shared your vision?

3. What are the steps to be taken to realize your vision?

4. What values guide your actions that lead to the vision?

5. What are the values of those with whom you need to engage?

6. Who are the people you want to journey with in realizing your vision?

7. How will you engage those people who are essential for the realization of your vision?

8. What skills do you have to deal with situations where there are competing values?

9. What's your role in realizing the vision?

10. Do you reflect on your struggles in order to learn from them?

102 Work-Life Balance for Self and Staff

"Before you can care for others well, in your personal or professional life, you must first know how to care for yourself."

—Diann B. Uustal

Mentor
Philip D. Authier, RN, BSN, MPH
Partner, Chief Operating Officer,
  Edgework Institute, Inc.
Rockford, Michigan, USA

Mentee
Kimberly N. Slaikeu, RN, PhD,
  APRN-BC
CEO & Founder, Relevan, LLC
Grand Rapids, Michigan, USA

The role of the nurse leader is filled with multiple challenges. On a daily basis, you are called upon to make critical decisions that impact the lives of patients and your staff. To be effective in your role, you must be committed to constant self-renewal and rejuvenation. Not allowing yourself these opportunities leads to burnout and increased stress, symptoms that are seen much too often in our profession. To say the least, maintaining a positive work-life balance is fundamental to being successful and sustainable in your role as a leader and in other areas of your life.

Do you have times where you are exhausted before the day even begins? Are your days filled with tasks that demand much of your time and energy, yet you wonder if they really matter in the end? Do you not like the person you have become at work and at home? If you answered yes to any of these questions, you could be at risk for professional burnout and even health issues. Now is the time for change! Work-life balance isn't easy and cannot happen on its own. It takes intent, focus, and effort on your part.

Determining What Matters to You

A key question to ask yourself is this: "What is my intent around work-life balance?" or, in other words, "What is most important to me?" Fortunately, no cookie cutter recipe to finding work-life balance exists. The beauty of work-life balance is that it can, and should, be tailored to meet your unique emotional, physical, and spiritual needs. In the book titled *Now What? 90 Days to a New Life Direction*, Laura Berman Fortgang (2004) identifies setting clear priorities as an important step in achieving balance. Thus, we recommend that you take some time to reflect on the following questions:

1. If my life could focus on one thing only, what would it be?

2. If I could add a second thing, what would it be?

3. A third thing?

By working through this exercise, you soon identify a list of your top priorities. This list might include your children, spouse, career, or self. Remember this is *your* list, not what you think others would identify as being important for you.

Finding the Time

Scheduling time for yourself is one way to ensure that you are successful in achieving balance. If it is on your schedule, it most likely gets done, unless something of higher priority bumps it. This concept was described using the metaphor of a rock in the book titled *First Things First; To Live, to Love, to Learn, to Leave a Legacy*, (Covey, S., Merrill, A.R., & Merrill, R.R., 1994). This metaphor suggests that we each think of high priorities as boulders and the lower priority items that seem to take up a lot of our time but yield less as the pebbles. If we put the boulders in first, the small stuff has to fit around them. The boulders are what we value most in our lives, those things that you identified as discussed previously, and they are always placed first to ensure they fit into our time. If we do all the small, unimportant stuff, those "pebbles" take up all the space and leave us feeling out of balance, dissatisfied, and disconnected from our life's purpose.

Caring for Self

We often hear nurses and other caregiver's state that self-care feels like a selfish act, so they resist doing it. However, this belief is not true and often leads to burnout. Caring for self is important in maintaining the balance needed to appropriately deal with the stress of our lives.

Once when I was getting a ride from the airport to a hotel, the taxi driver was very apologetic. After he picked me up, he stated, "I am sorry. I had another fare just before picking you up, and I didn't have time to stop for gas. If I don't pull in here and fill my taxi with gas, you will not get to where you are going." What a great metaphor for us. We, too, need to stop and fill our tanks with gas to be sustainable in the important work we are doing in all areas of our lives.

So, what fills your tank? Is it exercise? Reading? Meditating? Being with loved ones? Listening to your favorite music? Sleeping? The key is to be knowledgeable of what regenerates you so that you can consciously build in something you love to do each day. For me, balance previously meant free time for myself. But as my life filled with activities, I found I didn't have free time, so I changed my perception of balance. I looked at my days and found that every day was filled with activities, yet on some days I felt balanced, and on others I didn't. I found that I could divide activities into three categories: things I needed to do, things I liked to do, and things I loved to do— in other words, things that gave me energy and things I looked forward to doing. I found that the key for me was to build into each day time for something I loved to do, no matter how brief the experience.

Considering the importance of this idea, we invite you to consider what gives you energy and make a list of what you love to do. Thereafter, make sure to schedule something each day from your list.

Eliminating Unneccessary Distractions

After you identify the things that are most important to you, you might find that you are devoting a significant amount of time to things that didn't make your list. You need to eliminate activities that keep you away from the things that matter most to you. If you examine your behaviors carefully, you are going to find that you actually have more time available than you originally thought. For example, how much time do you spend doing activities such as vegging out in front of the television or surfing the Internet?

Seeking Help: An Accountability Partner

Very few things are more powerful than having an accountability partner. An accountability partner is an individual who can push you to continue taking care of yourself. I meet with my partner once every other week to provide an update on my status. We encourage you to find a trusted partner and exchange your goals regarding work-life balance. Having someone to report to can make a world of difference in your success!

Your Impact on Others

As a leader, you are a role model for your staff. If you pay attention, you are going to find that your staff learns to mimic your behaviors. In fact, what you do is watched very closely by those around you. Your staff notes your effort, or the lack thereof. For a balanced, healthy life, you must take the effort to balance your time and energy at work with your time and energy for the ones you love at home.

One CEO said to me that he expects his people to work hard all the time, like running a sprint, immediately followed by running another sprint, and on and on. I asked him if he knew any sprinters. Sprinters would, of course, take time to rest between races so that they could be their best when they sprinted again. They intentionally set periods of rest to allow the muscles to regenerate and the lactic acid to clear. No one can push at 120% forever without adequate periods of rest.

Benefits to Others

What are the outcomes and benefits of making this commitment to self-care? You are going to find many for you, the team you work with, your organization, and society at large. Personally, you have a better chance of sustaining your health. The American Institute of Stress associates stress and burnout with health issues, so consider this commitment a preventative measure. As a leader, you are going to become more effective and successful. As a human being you gain a sense of peace and ease as you share your talents and pursue the deeper purpose calling you.

As far as the team and the organization are concerned, your example and commitment can inspire many to find their own balance. Your actions can invite and evoke the best from others. The organization then sees increases in staff and patient satisfaction. Turnover decreases while positive contributions increase.

When considering society at large, we need to keep one question in all our minds—as health care providers and stewards, shouldn't we be role models for health and wellness? It is so powerful to know the struggles of our patients as our own and be able to personally speak to our commitment to health and balance. What would this world be like if each person took this self-care challenge seriously and opened up new possibilities of being and contributing to the needs of our society? We ask you to ponder these questions and take action today.

Lessons Learned: From Kimberly

Throughout my life, I have been fortunate to be surrounded by individuals who have challenged me to become the best version of myself. These individuals have shown up in both personal and professional relationships. Regardless of the overwhelming support, work-life balance continues to be a challenge for me. Thus, I am intentional about implementing strategies that enable me to be successful in this area.

On a quarterly basis, I revisit the goals that I've set regarding satisfying activities and those things that I find to be most important. I categorize my goals into several key areas of my life: spiritual, family, wellness, emotional, professional, and financial. If you are having trouble getting started with goal setting, two books that have been most influential for me in recent years are *Release Your Brilliance* (Bailey, 2008) and *The Dream Manager* (Kelly, 2007). Both resources were instrumental in guiding me through the creation of my own personal work-life balance "action plan."

I involve my accountability partners to keep me honest and receive objective feedback. If you do not currently have an accountability partner, I encourage you to identify an individual that can support you in this way. In addition, you might find that you want several accountability partners depending on the area that you're working on. For instance, Phil has served as one of my accountability partners relating to my own personal self-renewal. Being exposed to his expertise in self-care and rejuvenation has been invaluable because he reminds me of the goals that I've set and provides coaching if my current actions are not consistent with what I've identified as being most important to me. Overall, the presence of individuals in my life who are cheerleaders and can hold my "feet to fire" when needed has kept me on track and has been the biggest key to my success in my journey of finding balance in my life.

Self-Reflective Questions

1. In what ways have you taken time to find your focus?

2. What steps have you taken to identify what matters most to you?

3. How much of your time is spent on pebbles?

4. What fills your tank? If you don't know, how can you find out?

5. What unnecessary distractions do you need to eliminate?

6. Who can you contract with to be an accountability partner?

7. In what ways are you who you would like to be?

8. In what ways do you mentor your team on the importance of work-life balance?

9. How might colleagues consider you a role model for work-life balance?

10. How gentle are you with yourself and your team?

103 Writing for Professional Journals

"All nurses have the potential to contribute to the scientific body of knowledge in the nursing profession."

—Donna Hallas and Harriet Feldman

Mentor
Barbara J. Brown, EdD, RN, FAAN, FNAP, CNAA
Editor-Chief, Nursing Administration Quarterly
Tuscon, Arizona, USA

Mentee
Susan Hetzer, RN, BS, MSN, CCRN
Charge Nurse, Intensive Care Center, St. Mary's Hospital
Leonardtown, Maryland, USA

Being a nursing journal editor for more than 35 years has provided me (Barabara) with many insights into how powerful the written word is and how much impact what is published has on all stages of professional and personal lives. Developing new writers is essential in the long-term evolution of thought provoking and relevant manuscripts. Not only is the development of new writers important, but also encouraging new editors via issue editing is a rewarding opportunity. Gaining active participation from an editorial board and support by the publisher for annual board meetings enhances the vitality of a journal. Several elements of writing for professional journals you should consider include the following:

1. Guiding new writers in both academic and professional practice settings.

2. Active participation of professional journal editorial board members in the direction of the journal, especially

determining future issue topics, engaging in the peer review process, and serving as guest issue editors.

3. Sharing the review process and serving as a guest issue editor, involving press timetables, prioritization of content within a specified page count, and avoidance of inappropriate use of power, maintaining objectivity.

Many authors have a tendency to overwrite, resulting in wordy, imprecise prose and unnecessary lengthy explanations. Oftentimes an editor has a difficult task of editing out and reconnecting pertinent ideas or content. Techniques for effective communication apply to both the written and spoken word and can assist the author in producing simple but understandable and academically acceptable manuscripts for professional journals. The frequently espoused 10 Cs for skills in writing are as follows:

1. **Completeness**. Have you included all the information needed? Have you anticipated questions the reader might have and answered them?

2. **Clarity, clearness**. Do your written words express your thoughts as clearly as possible? Have you chosen words and developed sentences to emphasize the most significant ideas? Have you defined technical and professional terms? Have you avoided ambiguity caused by errors in punctuation or grammar?

3. **Conciseness**. Have you omitted commonly known facts and unnecessary words and phrases? Do the words you use transmit your thoughts to the reader?

4. **Correctness, certainty**. Have you checked all the facts? Have you double-checked dates and numbers, bibliographic references and quotations? Is every word spelled correctly and used correctly?

5. **Consideration, courtesy, compassion**. Is your manuscript an article directed toward a target audience, namely the intended readers of the journal? Have you avoided words that might antagonize (such as sexist or racist words)? Have you considered the peer review suggestions and taken the time to revise and rewrite? Does your writing reflect your personal professional values?

6. **Character**. How does your manuscript sound to another person when read aloud? Are ideas arranged in a logical sequence to bring the reader to the intended conclusion? Are sentences varied in structure and length? Have you used an active voice or passive one? A positive

or negative posture? Standard or unusual nouns and verbs, adjectives and adverbs? Does your writing reflect you?

7. **Cohesiveness**. Does your entire manuscript fit together? Are transitions smooth and connected sequentially? Have you avoided shifts in tense or person? Are paragraphs the units of composition, each starting with a topic sentence or a sentence of introduction or transition?

8. **Concreteness**. Whenever you could, have you used definite, specific language-terms your intended readers can relate to instead of abstract terms?

9. **Candor**. Is your manuscript written without unwanted opinions, prejudice, malice, dishonesty, and overstatement?

10. **Creativeness**. Have you used your imagination and creative insight to provide fresh insight and a unique perspective? Have you achieved the effect you want without eccentricity?

The most important consideration is to follow the author guidelines for the journal for which your manuscript is intended. When you submit the manuscript, you will be required to sign an author consent form before the article is considered for peer review. This release form indicates to the editor and publisher that you are not submitting and have not submitted this manuscript to another journal. Peer review, which comes next, can take awhile.

As a long-time professional journal editor, I was recently asked about the barriers to the revision of manuscripts. Probably the most frequent barrier is that manuscripts are too long, especially when authors try to convert a master's thesis or dissertation into an article. Another barrier is that authors are insensitive to the target audience and designated topic, if the journal is topically focused. Sometimes authors send manuscripts that have no relevance to the journal and its target audience. An author should review the journal for which the article is intended and become sensitive to what is being published and the style of writing and recognize that recommended revisions are based on the target audience and relevancy to the topic.

Cut to the chase to make your writing usable for people in the field to help them with a particular subject matter. Know your subject matter and what the journal you are submitting to, is looking for. When a manuscript that has no obvious fit is received by a journal, the editors at that journal return it. Whether the manuscript is research based or not, it should have practical conclusions that the reader can apply. Following revision suggestions is the author's prerogative, but usually a manuscript is not going to be published if the reviewer's critique is not followed.

When a manuscript is accepted, the author usually receives a castoff or galley to respond to before the article is ready for press. This document contains author queries (AQs) for the author to answer. If the author does not respond in a timely manner as indicated by the editorial director, the manuscript might not be published. Therefore, an author needs to respond to the queries in a timely way. The final editing process is for the integrity of both the journal and the author. Finally, if an error occurs in a manuscript, most editors and publishers publish a correction, called errata, that usually appears in the next issue.

The personal satisfaction of expressing, with passion and personal perspective, opinions about issues, sharing concerns about the nursing practice and academic environments, and being an advocate for nursing wherever and whenever possible has sustained my writing for so many years. As I look to the future, I see our professional lives as enriched by the increasing number of journals and manuscripts from around the world. So WRITE IT, BELIEVE IT, and DO IT.

Mentee Reply

So I Ask Myself, Why Should I Write for Publication?

Publications help to disseminate knowledge, to develop skills, to engage nurses, and share clinical insights, developments, and research. (Wollin and Fairweather, 2007). They engage nurses in the ongoing development of our profession. But what do I, as a bedside nurse, have to offer my profession? And how do I engage others? I truly believe that regardless of what position we are in as nurses, we can contribute to our profession.

As I conclude my journey in the completion of my master of science in nursing, I shall take the advice shared by Dr. Brown and others found in my research and set forth on a new journey—submitting my work for consideration to be published in professional journals. Recognizing that barriers to writing for publication can include lack of time, fear of rejection, writer's block, and not knowing how to write for publication, I must plan my endeavor (Oermann, 2002). As I prepare for my journey and to overcome the barriers to writing, I ask myself the following questions:

1. What is my topic, and what do I have to share with others to make a difference?

2. What is already known about my topic, and what else has been published?

3. Who is my audience?

4. What journal will I submit to?

5. Is my topic on the "wish list" of the journal?

6. What are the guidelines of the journal?

Dottie Roberts (2008), editor of *MedSurg Nursing*, explains that the selected topic should be a subject that reflects my nursing passion. My passion is the integration of evidence-based research into clinical practice. I played an integral role in the development and implementation of the clinical practice council in my organization. I realize that my homework is far from complete because I must further research and develop my topic. However, my goal is clear—to inspire other bedside nurses, I want to share my story so that they, too, realize that with clear guidance from leadership, bedside nurses can change the practices in their own facility and contribute to the profession of nursing.

Though we have shared many of the "dos" of publication so far, you can only achieve success if you also avoid the "don't"s. Barber (2008) warns not to:

1. Give up and become disheartened.

2. Disregard the steps to writing a well-planned and researched article.

3. Forget that life needs balance between work and home.

4. Forget to have your article reviewed by friends and colleagues.

5. Take comments by journal reviewers personally but instead to consider them on a professional level.

6. Forget thoughtful revision that maintains the integrity of the material in your article by carefully considering the comments of the reviewers.

Self-Reflective Questions

1. In what ways is your topic one that makes a difference to the profession of nursing?

2. What journal are you submitting to and who is that audience?

3. How is your topic an appropriate subject matter for the chosen publication?

4. When writing your article, in what ways did you follow the guidelines of the publication?

5. In what ways have you included all the necessary information and answered anticipated questions?

6. Is your article clearly written? What professional terminology and unambiguous language have you used?

7. What steps have you taken to make your article concise and free of unnecessary information and verbiage?

8. What friends and colleagues have you had review your article?

9. How have you carefully considered suggestions and critiques to ensure the integrity of your material while meeting the expectations of the reviewers?

10. What is your opening sentence? Do you feel it is strong enough? How does the initial paragraph lead the reader to the content? How forceful is your closing statement?

Index

J-K-L

Index by Author

Index by Country

Author Biographies

A

Sabah Abu-Zinadah, BSN, MSN, PhD

Sabah Abu-Zinadah founded the first nursing board in the Kingdom of Saudi Arabia in 2002, where she continues in her role as chairperson. She advocates for the establishment of a Saudi nursing society. She specialized in nursing administration when she received her PhD at George Mason University, Fairfax, Virginia. She has 26 years of nursing experience in administration, education, regulation, quality improvement, and accreditation for program and services. She has been appointed as the chairperson for an international steering committee for regulation, the anticipated vehicle for starting an international nursing regulation organization. In 2000, she became the first Saudi nurse to attend the Arab ministries meeting in Lebanon. Abu-Zinadah is the second Saudi national to receive her doctorate in nursing and is passionately involved in promoting the professional practice of nursing in her country.

Larissa Africa, BSN, RN

Larissa Africa has been with Versant Advantage since its inception in 2004. Africa was a graduate of the first RN Residency Program at Children's Hospital Los Angeles. Her clinical experience includes caring for children with renal, gastrointestinal, and cardiac diseases. She assisted in transitioning the RN Residency from a department-based program to a non-profit company and was instrumental in the initial development of the RN Residency Web Management System, Voyager™. Africa is currently pursuing a Master's degree in business administration with a concentration in health care management.

Stephanie Wilkie Ahmed, DNP, FNP-BC

Stephanie Wilkie Ahmed is an associate of The Institute for Nursing Healthcare Leadership and a nurse practitioner with clinical appointments at Brigham and Women's Hospital and Massachusetts General Hospital (MGH) in Boston, Massachusetts. A member of the inaugural doctoral in nursing practice (DNP) class at the MGH Institute of Health Professions, Ahmed received a DNP in administration in 2008. She completed her MS-N at the University of Massachusetts at Lowell in 1999. In 2006 she traveled to South Africa as the first nurse practitioner deployed through the Harvard Global Nurse project.

Amal Al Barnawi, RN, MSN

Amal Al Barnawi is the director of the Medical/Oncology Nursing Program at King Faisal Specialist Hospital & Research Centre, Riyadh, the Kingdom of Saudi Arabia. She specialized in nursing administration, and she has 17 years nursing experience in Medical Oncology. She is a Member on the Nursing Scientific Board at Saudi Commission for Health Specialists since 2004.

Rumay Alexander, EdD, RN

Rumay Alexander is professor at the University of North Carolina Chapel Hill, School of Nursing. She leads the nationally ranked University of North Carolina at Chapel Hill School of Nursing's intentional efforts to develop an environment where the proper understanding and judicious application of equality and multicultural concepts for its students, faculty, personnel, and the patients served by their graduates thrives. Courageous Dialogues is a model she has developed and uses to hold candid conversations about the multi-faceted nature of diversity and the issues that often surface when communities develop the courage to ask questions, share stories, and open up environments for discussion. She draws on her 25 years of public policy experience, her lived experience as the CEO of her own consulting firm, and her own experiences of being a minority student, nurse educator as a clinical professor, health care association executive, and corporate executive in a majority culture.

Cherilyn Ashlock, RN, MSN

Cherilyn Ashlock has been a nurse for nine years, focusing primarily on pediatric critical care and the emergency department. Ashlock completed a master's degree in nursing education at California State University, Los Angeles, in 2006. She is and remains involved in both the clinical and academic arenas of nursing education as an adjunct faculty member for adult and pediatric nursing at her alma mater, Georgia Baptist College of Nursing of Mercer University in Atlanta, Georgia. Her primary work is as an implementation specialist of the Versant RN Residency. This role allows her to serve as the primary consultant for the intensive start up and ongoing facilitation of the evidenced-based residency in client hospitals. Involvement in the residency has driven her nursing career passion to focus on recruitment, training, and retention of new graduate nurses. Ashlock speaks on the transition of new graduate nurses into the workforce.

Philip Authier, RN, BSN, MPH

Philip Authier is a partner in Edgework Institute of Grand Rapids, Michigan. He has more than 30 years of nursing leadership experience, bringing strengths from mentoring and leadership development to communication and consensus building. He is a trained group facilitator and coach, believing that each role is important to the success of the health care system. Authier has been involved with the Center for Nursing Leadership in an ongoing effort to bring new aspects of management, knowledge, and leadership to the nursing profession. He is a past-president of the American Organization of Nurse Executives.

B

Lame Gaolatlhe Bakwenabatsile, RN

Lame Gaolatlhe Bakwenabatsile earned a bachelor's degree in nursing science and is currently reading for her bachelor of finance at the University of Botswana. She has worked as a nurse in Princess Marina Hospital (PMH) and has worked as a nurse in the male orthopedic ward at PMH since 2007. She provides in-service lectures. Bakwenabatsile has under-

taken several short courses and workshops in the area of HIV and AIDS and is a member of the Nurses Association of Botswana. Outside of nursing, she presents a music program for Radio Botswana.

Sarah Basinger, MHI, RN

Sarah Basinger is a new graduate of the Innovations Program at Arizona State University and a nurse manager at a major medical center in Arizona. Basinger most wants to be known as a good leader and facilitator of innovation, guiding nurses and health professionals into a new way of practice for the 21st century.

Marta Lima Basto, PhD, MSN, RN, EANS

Marta Lima-Basto is a member of the scientific committee and coordinator of the doctoral program in nursing of the University of Lisboa, Portugal, started in 2004. Research projects are related to nurse-client interaction and change processes of nursing practice. She graduated from a Nursing College in Lisboa and obtained the diploma in advanced nursing science and a master's degree at Manchester University, United Kingdom, and her doctoral Degree in Lisboa. Her international experience includes a World Health Organization scholarship in the United States, international working parties, being a scholar of the European Academy of Nursing Science, and the national representative at the Workgroup of European Nurse Researchers. She has worked in hospital, community, and at the government level. For most of her career she has been the coordinating professor of nursing, having retired from the Escola Superior de Enfermagem de Lisboa, in 2000. Lima-Basto has held the first coordinator of the Nursing Research and Development Unit in Lisboa. She has collaborated with several universities and supervised master's dissertations and doctoral theses. She has published a book and 40 articles, two of them in foreign publications. She was the first Portuguese nurse to get a doctoral degree in Portugal (1995) and continues to be active in professional associations and supervises doctoral thesis.

Kate Becker, MN, RN, BN, NP

Kate Becker is a nurse practitioner in neurosurgery at Royal North Shore Hospital. She has worked in this capacity since her authorisation in 2003, making her one of the first two neurosurgical nurse practitioners in Australia. Becker completed her bachelor of nursing in 1996 at the University of Technology Sydney (UTS). She completed certificates of neurosurgical nursing at the College of Nursing, a graduate diploma in nursing management, and her master's in advanced practice nursing at UTS. Becker has worked as a clinical nurse specialist in neurosurgery and as a nurse manager in neurosurgery. She is currently the co-chair of the Greater Metropolitan Clinical Taskforce NSW for Neurosurgery. Becker lectures at the College of Nursing in New South Wales and at UTS.

May Bennett, CPA, NHA

May Bennett is a consultant with FTE Healthcare's Finance practice, working with health care organizations on productivity and financial improvements. She received a bachelor's of science degree in medical technology in 1975 from Middle Tennessee State University, a master's degree in allied health education from Central Michigan University, and a master's degree in accountancy from Belmont University. Her prior work experiences include serving as the senior vice president of operations for Saint Thomas Hospital in Nashville, Tennessee, chief operating officer for the senior campus of the Metropolitan Nashville Hospital Authority, and chief operating officer of the hospital division of Diversified Specialty Institutes. She serves as adjunct faculty at the Owen Graduate School at Belmont University. She sits on several governing boards, including for the Comprehensive Care Center, the Tennessee Healthcare Association, and for Senior Citizens, Inc.

Mirela Bidilič, RN

Mirela Bidilič registered nurse from Romania. She was educated in nursing in Romania. She finished nursing school in Bucharest and nursing school inside the university from the town Arad. She also has a degree in psychology from Bucharest. Bidilič worked as a nurse in the Central Military Hospital in Bucharest. After a few years, she was promoted to chief nurse in intensive therapy. Now, she is director of care for the Central Military Hospital in Bucharest. Bidilic was president of the Romanian Nursing Association (RNA) from 2000 until 2005 and is now on RNA's board of directors. She has

published in Romania and is a contributor to the textbook titled *Nursing Procedures*.

Jennifer Bishop, RN, BSN

Jennifer Bishop received her bachelor's of nursing from Jacksonville State University in Jacksonville Alabama, in 2007, where she was the recipient of a nursing scholarship. She is currently employed at St. Vincent's East Hospital in Birmingham, Alabama, where she works in the emergency department. Bishop also has experience in rehabilitation nursing. Her inspiration for becoming a nurse comes from her grandparents whose encouragement to "never stop learning" encouraged her. Bishop hopes to continue her education within nursing.

Joanne Booth

Joanne Booth is senior research fellow in the School of Nursing, Midwifery, and Community Health, Glasgow Caledonian University, Glasgow, Scotland. Prior to this, she gained extensive experience in a number of clinical roles working with older people, the most recent as consultant nurse for a National Health Service Health Board. She has practiced in acute, rehabilitation, continuing care, and community contexts across the United Kingdom; however, her main expertise lies in rehabilitation, particularly following stroke, which was the subject of her doctoral studies. She has a developing program of research focused on nursing management of lower urinary tract symptoms and promotion of urinary continence in the older population, particularly in those with stroke disease.

Anna Margherita Toldi Bork, MSN, MBA, RN

Anna Margherita Toldi Bork is vice president for quality and safety and chief nursing officer for Hospital Israelita Albert Einstein (HIAE) in São Paulo, Brazil. Bork has led the HIAE safety system since its conception in 2006. She graduated from Universidade de São Paulo (USP) with a bachelor's degree. She earned a master of science degree in evidence-based health practice from Universidade Federal de São Paulo (UNIFESP). She is a fellow of the Johnson & Johnson/Wharton Fellows Program in Management for Nurse Executives from the Wharton School of the University of Pennsylvania. Bork started working at Albert

Einstein Hospital as a novice nurse in the intensive care unit for 5 years. She has published two books on nursing in Brazil (Evidence Based Nursing and Nursing: From Vision to Action). She is a nationally recognized speaker in the area of patient safety and nursing.

Marina Boykova, RN, BSN, MSc

Marina Boykova received her nursing diploma from Medical School #1, Saint Petersburg, Russia, in 1989. She received her bachelor's and master's (health promotion) in nursing degrees from the University of Chester, United Kingdom. She has 19 years of experience in neonatal intensive care nursing (Children's Hospital #1, Russia). She is the regional liaison to the Council of International Neonatal Nurses. Boykova is pursuing her doctoral degree through the University of Oklahoma, Oklahoma, with a passionate desire to return to her home country of Russia and make a significant difference in the profession of nursing.

Michael Bratton, RN, MA

Michael Bratton is vice president and chief nursing officer at Middle Tennessee Medical Center in Murfreesboro, Tennessee. He is president of Healthcare Connection, a consulting company he founded which specializes in bridging administration with bedside clinical practice, and emphasizes the value of frontline caregivers and the need for exceptional leadership. Bratton has more than 30 years of experience in clinical and leadership roles. He has practiced in acute care, critical care, homecare, and rehabilitation as a staff nurse, nursing manager, nursing director, and hospital vice president and chief nursing officer. He is a speaker and writer on the topics of retention, healthy work environments, leadership, and bedside clinical practice. Originally educated in a hospital-based school of nursing, he also holds bachelor and master degrees in nursing. He served as a College of Nursing board member at Bryan LGH College of Health Sciences in Lincoln, Nebraska.

Barbara J. Brown, EdD, RN, FAAN, FNAP, CNAA

Barbara J. Brown is the founding editor of *Nursing Administration Quarterly*, and she has continuously given editorial direction to the journal for more 33 years. During the earlier years of editing, she held leadership positions in Wisconsin, Washington, and Saudi Arabia.

She earned BSN, MSN, and EdD degrees. She has been a Fellow in the American Academy of Nursing since 1977 and has served as a faculty member at the University of Wisconsin, Marquette University, Ohio State University, the University of Washington, Vanderbilt University, the University of St. Francis, and most recently, the University of Arizona College of Nursing. She has been involved in the International Academy of Nursing Editors (INANE) for more than 30 years. She is the longest-term nursing editor worldwide. In 2005, as Editor-in-Chief, she launched a new magazine for young nurses—*MODRN Nurse*. She has received numerous awards for her work, published extensively, and has presented globally on a variety of topics.

Judith C. Bruce, PhD, RN, RM

Judith C. Bruce is an associate professor and head of the department of nursing education at the University of the Witwatersrand in Johannesburg. She teaches nursing education at the postgraduate level and maintains her clinical interest in trauma and emergency nursing. She is actively involved in developing nursing scholarship and leadership on the African continent. Bruce serves as vice-chair of the Forum of University Nursing Deans in South Africa (FUNDISA).

David Byres, RN, BA, BScN, MSN

David Byres is vice president of clinical programs and chief of professional practice and nursing at Providence Health Care (PHC), Canada. Byres has more than 17 years of professional experience in the health-care field, including mental health and nursing practice. His portfolio includes responsibility as the chief nursing officer, spanning professional practice and education for nursing as well as the senior leader responsible for professional practice in all allied health disciplines. He is also responsible for the mental health, addictions, and clinical HIV/AIDS programs at PHC's urban health and aboriginal strategies. Byres is a registered nurse who received his bachelor of arts in psychology from the University of Victoria. He received his bachelor of science in nursing and master of science in nursing from the University of British Columbia. He is an adjunct professor at the University of British Columbia School of Nursing.

C

Jennifer Campbell, BSN, RN

Jennifer Campbell seeks the perfect balance in life. To this end, she has earned the titles of house painter, barista, English-as a Second-Language teacher, ski instructor, and outdoors educator until she finally found nursing. She has been a practicing RN for five years, which has taken her from Colorado to Africa to Wisconsin and from medical-surgical nursing to community health volunteer, to the intensive care unit. Until her recent move to the Pacific Northwest, she prided herself on fitting all her possessions in her car.

Rita M. Carty, PhD, RN, FAAN

Rita M. Carty is professor and dean emeritus of George Mason University, Fairfax, Virginia. She has held numerous leadership position in her career including, secretary general of the Global Network of World Health Collaborating Centres for Nursing and Midwifery Development and as president of the American Association of Colleges of Nursing. Throughout her career, mentoring young professionals has been a priority for her. Many young leaders in nursing recognize her as a mentor. She continues to mentor young professionals through her consulting roles in international nursing and health care.

Carmen Rumeu Casares, MSc, RN

Carmen Rumeu Casares graduated from the University of Navarre, Pamplona, Spain, in 1991. She specialized as a psychiatric nurse and graduated with a master's of science degree from the University of Manchester, United Kingdom, in 1996. She is the chief executive nurse (and board vice president) at Clínica Universidad de Navarra, in Pamplona. She is also an associate professor at the University of Navarra, School of Nursing. She worked for seven years as a staff nurse at the laboratory site and in the psychiatric unit at Clínica Universidad de Navarra. She was a nurse manager of the psychiatric unit and followed as a chief director of several units of the hospital until taking on her current post. She has had several publications related to her field of expertise. She has benefited from several grants and has carried out a research project funded by the local government. She is a fellow of the Johnson & Johnson/Wharton Fellows Program in Management for Nurse Executives from the Wharton School of the University of Pennsylvania.

Carmen W. H. Chan, RN, BSN, Mphi, PhD

Carmen W. H. Chan, as an experienced academic, plays an active role in the development and delivery of nursing research and education within Hong Kong and Asia. The focus of her research and publications is on the development and evaluation of complex nursing care. Her proficient use of mixed methods and a corresponding analysis of the impact on process are particularly valuable in advancing implications for practice. She also has extensive teaching experience in advanced practice in oncology nursing as well as leadership roles and management functions in nursing. As a link nurse of the International Society of Nurses in Cancer Care, she collects ideas and current knowledge and practice experiences from local nurses and shares with nurses from China and worldwide for advancing the development of the nursing profession.

Jessica Charles, MSN, RN

Jessica Charles currently serves as supervisor of the inpatient unit 5 West at the Mayo Clinic Hospital in Phoenix, Arizona. Unit 5 West is a 36-bed unit specializing in neurology, ear-nose-throat, plastics, medical-surgical, and telemetry. Charles has worked as a primary care registered nurse on 5 West and in the intensive care unit. Her experience includes working as a team lead on 5 West prior to accepting a supervisor position. Charles was nominated for the 2008 Michael B. O'Sullivan, M.D. Award for Excellence in Clinical Nursing. She was educated at Colorado State University-Pueblo where she received a bachelor of science in nursing. In January 2009, she received her master's of science in nursing from the University of Phoenix.

Chua Gek Choo, RN, BHSN, Grad. Dip

Chua Gek Choo is deputy director of nursing at Alexandra and Khoo Teck Puat Hospitals and is an adjunct lecturer at the Nanyang Polytechnic School of Health Sciences. She researches widely and works relentlessly to design a safe and conducive environment for patient care in Singapore. She holds a BHSN, Grad. Dip (Higher Education), certificate in intensive care, certificate in management, and RN degree. She is a lifelong learner and updates herself frequently with the latest developments in health care advancement to guide nurses to deliver quality nursing care. With a strong heart for community outreach, she has devoted her work to advancing nursing in Singapore. An illustrious President's Nursing Award winner, she believes people skills is key to leadership success and is a proven principle-centered leader who aims to walk the talk as she mentors her family of nurses to impact the world.

Greg Clancy, BA, BSN, RN, MSN

Greg Clancy is currently employed at Mercy Hospital in Iowa City as a project coordinator for strategic initiatives. His role is to identify and implement performance improvement initiatives that are aligned with the hospital's goal. Using evidence-based practice guidelines, Lean, or Six Sigma methodology, Clancy provides leadership to quality improvement teams. Prior to his current position, he managed the national registry for the American College of Cardiology's data registry in Washington D.C. His previous roles include quality improvement manager, intensive care unit nurse manger, and staff nurse. He graduated from the University of Iowa College of Nursing, Iowa City, Iowa, with a master's in nursing administration.

Thomas Clancy, MBA, PhD, RN

Thomas Clancy currently serves as a clinical professor at the University Of Minnesota School of Nursing, where he teaches, publishes, and presents on the interface between nursing practice and technology. Clancy has worked in the health care field for more 30 years and has served as staff nurse, chief nursing officer, and as a consultant for a variety of health care systems and companies. He conducts research in the area of complex adaptive systems and nursing in which he applies computational modeling and simulation to analyze and predict clinical and process outcomes. Clancy publishes a quarterly article in the *Journal of Nursing Administration* titled, "Managing Organizational Complexity."

Michelle Clark, BSc, DipN, RN

Michelle Clark is a ward sister on the neonatal unit at Doncaster and Bassetlaw Hospitals National Health Service (NHS) Foundation

Trust from South Yorkshire, England. She qualified as a registered nurse in 2004 where she gained the advanced diploma in nursing studies. In 2006, she gained the BMed Sci (hons) in clinical nursing studies with honours from Sheffield University. Her research has included concepts of care of the newborn, high dependency care of the newborn, and intensive care of the newborn. This led to further development in completing the enhanced neonatal nursing course at Manchester University.

Joyce C. Clifford, PhD, RN, FAAN

Joyce C. Clifford served as senior vice president and nurse-in-chief at Beth Israel Deaconess Medical Center in Boston, Massachusetts, for more than 25 years before establishing The Institute for Nursing Healthcare Leadership, Inc. (INHL), for which she now serves as the president and chief executive officer. A graduate of St. Anselm College, she received her master's in nursing from the University of Alabama and a doctorate in the field of health planning and policy analysis at the Heller School of Brandeis University. She became a fellow of the American Academy of Nursing in 1980, is a former president of the American Organization of Nurse Executives, and was a member of the board of trustees of the American Hospital Association from 1991 to 1994. She remains a member of multiple professional organizations, as well as a trustee for her alma mater, Saint Anselm College in New Hampshire.

Kathleen Collins-Ruiz, MSN, RN, CNA

Kathleen Collins-Ruiz is the associate director for nursing care at the United States Department of Veterans Affairs Caribbean Healthcare System, which provides primary, specialty, acute, long term, and home care to more than 66,000 veterans in Puerto Rico and the U.S. Virgin Islands. She has been instrumental in developing advance practice nursing in Puerto Rico, using collaborative agreements and distance learning for her own staff, and later providing preceptor practice for community nurse practitioner candidates. Collins-Ruiz studied nursing at the Bellevue School of Nursing in New York City and completed both her bachelor's and master's in nursing at the University of Puerto Rico. She is currently pursuing a doctor of nursing practice degree at the Medical College of Georgia School of Nursing, is a member of the Advisory Board of the School of Health Sciences at the University of Turabo, and has been both mentor and preceptor to Nurse Executive Career Field candidates through the Veterans Health Administration succession planning program.

Dania Comparcini, RN

Dania Comparcini is from Casine di Paterno, Ancona, Italy, and obtained her undergraduate (2005) and master's (2008) nursing degrees from the University Politecinica delle Marche Faculty of Medicine. Comparcini was a professional nurse at the Dipartimento di Salute Mentale, ASUR zona territoriale 7, Ancona, from 2005 to 2007. She was a professional nurse at the Geriatric Hospital of Ancona I.N.R.C.A. from 2007-2008. Currently, she is a professional nurse at the Hospital of Ancona's Azienda Ospedaliero Universitaria Ospedali Riuniti. Comparcini is a member of Gruppo Infiermieristico Di Ricerca del Dipartimento di Salute Mentale di Ancona.

Mary Connaughton, MS, RN

Mary Connaughton founded Connaughton Consulting in 1997 after 18 years in nursing leadership roles in academic health care settings in Boston, Massachusetts. She specializes in executive coaching, leadership development, and strategic planning. Connaughton brings a rich tradition of patient-centered care, professional nursing practice, value for interdisciplinary collaboration and mentoring, and development of individuals and teams to her consulting practice. Through her executive coaching practice, she has helped health care leaders make profound changes in their leadership and achieve new levels of effectiveness. Connaughton is a highly regarded facilitator and teacher. With colleague Jim Hassinger, she developed "The Practice of Wise Leadership" program. This unique program has received high praise for its immediate and sustained positive impact on participants of all roles and levels of practice.

Patti Crome, RN, MN, CAN, FACMPE

Patti Crome is currently a principal and senior partner in the Rona Consulting Group, specializing in Lean methodologies to support organizations in the transformation of health care and pursuit of perfection in patient safety and quality. She holds a master's in nursing from the University of Washington, a fellowship in the American College of Medical Practice Executives, and a certification in nursing administration. As a former senior vice president at Virginia Mason Medical Center in Seattle, Washington, she is certified in Lean with training by the Shingijutsu Corporation and has spent hundreds of hours applying the tools of the Toyota Management System in health care. Crome has served on the board of the American Organization of Nurse Executives, as president of the Northwest Organization of Nurse Executives and on various local and national committees.

Ashley Currier, RN, BSN

Ashley Currier is manager for a 30 bed inpatient surgical unit at Northwestern Memorial Hospital (NMH) in Chicago, Illinois. Currier received her bachelor's of science in nursing from the University of Iowa College of Nursing in 2004. During her first staff nurse position at NMH, Currier became involved in a number of endeavors at the unit, division, and hospital wide. She became a manager following the reorganization of the patient care areas in 2007. She is a former chair and currently sits on the Nursing Research and Evidence Based Practice Council, is an active member of Academy of Medical-Surgical Nurses, Society of Urologic Nurses and Associates, and Illinois Organization of Nurse Leaders. Currier has led and participated in several hospital initiatives to improve safety and quality of patient care. Her research interests include nursing workflow and process analysis, with a focus on patient safety outcomes. Her future plans include pursuing further education in nursing studies.

D

John Daly, RN, PhD, FRCNA

John Daly is dean and professor of nursing in the Faculty of Nursing, Midwifery, and Health, and head of the World Health Organization's Collaborating Centre for Nursing, Midwifery, and Health Development at the University of Technology Sydney, New South Wales, Australia. In addition, he is chair of the Council of Deans of Nursing and Midwifery (Australia and New Zealand), chair of the Global Alliance for Nursing Education and Scholarship, an appointed member of the Nurses and Midwives Board of New South Wales, and editor-in-chief of Collegian, the refereed journal of the Royal College of Nursing Australia. He has also served for a number of years on the Research and Scholarship Advisory Council of Sigma Theta Tau International. Daly has a research and publications track record that spans professional nursing issues, cardiovascular health, palliative and aged care, leadership, and health workforce issues. He is emeritus professor of Nursing at the University of Western Sydney, a title awarded for distinguished service.

Patricia Mary Davidson, RN, PhD, FRCNA

Patricia Mary Davidson is professor of cardiovascular and chronic care at Curtin University, is director of the Cardiovascular and Chronic Care Centre, and is professor of cardiovascular nursing research at St Vincent's Hospital, Sydney, Australia. Her clinical and research specialty focuses on chronic cardiovascular disease, focusing on heart failure, women's health, indigenous health, and models of care development to improve access to effective primary, secondary, and tertiary care services. Davidson is the president of the International Council on Women's Health Issues and is secretary of the International Network for Doctoral Education in Nursing. She is chair of the Cardiovascular Nursing College of the Cardiac Society of Australia and New Zealand and president of the Australasian Cardiovascular Nurses College. She plays an active role in cardiovascular health care policy in Australia.

Sandra Davidson, RN, MSN, CNE

Sandra Davidson is a clinical associate professor and director of the Master of Healthcare Innovation Program at Arizona State University (ASU) College of Nursing and Healthcare Innovation. She is currently completing her PhD in Leadership Studies from Gonzaga University in Spokane, Washington. Prior to coming to ASU four years ago, she was a practicing RN in Canada for 11 years and held various positions such as charge nurse, surgical educator, clinical nurse specialist, and clinical education coordinator. Her clinical specialties are gerontology and chronic disease management and prevention. She has taught nursing and health care leadership

across the spectrum from the associate degree to the doctoral level. Her research interests are interdisciplinary education, chronic disease management, and innovation in education and health care. Davidson recently returned to the clinical setting and is transitioning to a new position as clinical education and organizational development specialist with Cancer Treatment Centers of America in Goodyear, Arizona.

Débora Falleiros de Mello, RN, PhD

Débora Falleiros de Mello is a professor of nursing at the World Health Organization's Collaborating Center for Nursing Research Development at the University of São Paulo in Ribeirao Preto, Brazil. She is a specialist in child nursing with a focus on child-care follow up. Her research projects are related to child care in the context of family, integrated management of childhood illness, follow-up of preterm infants, and mothers' experiences in child care. She has a master's of science and a doctoral degree, and she is a member of the Network for Child Health Nursing, a network that includes members in every country in Latin America as well as in Spain and the United States.

María Mercedes de Villalobos, RN, MSC

María Mercedes de Villalobos is originally from Bogota, Colombia, and attended the Universidad Nacional de Colombia, Bogota, where she obtained a bachelor's degree in nursing. She worked as a clinical nurse and staff nurse in hospitals in Bogota, Columbia, and Boston, Massachusetts. De Villalobos received a master's degree in nursing sciences and a certificate on advances graduate studies from Boston University. In 1974, she became part of the faculty at the School of Nursing at Universidad Nacional (UN) where she served as chair of the Department of Administration, director of Undergraduate Studies, and dean, and between 1985 and 1990 she was vice president of Students of the University. She has been a consultant for the World Health Organization and the Pan American Health Organization, as well as for the W. K. Kellogg Foundation for Latin America. Currently, de Villalobos is a titular and emeritus professor and teacher to master and doctoral students in the University (UN). She has been an invited visitant professor to University of La Sabana,

Bogota, several universities in Mexico, Central America, and Argentina.

Anna Dermenchyan, RN, BSN, PHN

Anna Dermenchyan, RN, BSN, PHN, is a clinical nurse at Cardiothoracic ICU in the Ronald Reagan UCLA Medical Center, Los Angeles, California. Dermenchyan received her bachelor's of science in neuroscience from UCLA in June of 2004 and a nursing degree from Mount St. Mary's College in May of 2008. She is a member of numerous professional organizations, including American Heart Association, American Association of Critical-Care Nurses, Sigma Theta Tau International, Oncology Nursing Society, and the American Holistic Nurses Association. Dermenchyan volunteers her time in the community as a mentor for an Armenian youth organization, as a camp nurse for Camp Del Corazon, and as a health service member for the American Red Cross. Her interests include health policy, international nursing, and global health. She recently completed the 2009 Nurse in Washington Internship (NIWI) program that educated about the federal legislative process and health policy. She is the recipient of the Nursing Student Leadership Award, Sister Callista Roy Award, and Eugenie B. Hannon Nursing Award from Mount St. Mary's College.

Lorena Chaparro Diaz, RN, BSN

Lorena Chaparro Diaz was born in Bogota, Colombia, and received a bachelor degree in nursing at the Universidad Nacional de Colombia in Bogota. During her bachelor formation, she worked as an assistant student of research groups and academic projects. Diaz worked with projects of caring with family caregivers as a nurse assistant in research and clinical settings as a nurse. She will receive a doctoral nursing degree from Universidad Nacional de Colombia with a grant of the best student graduate of Universidad Nacional de Colombia (2006-2008). In 2007, she was a student visitant of Florida Atlantic University (FAU) with the Christine E. Lynn College of Nursing. Her research interests relate to caring for those with chronic illness and knowledge development in nursing. Currently she is a teacher with Universidad Nacional de Colombia in the bachelor and master in nursing programs, specializing in caring in chronic conditions, epistemology of nursing, and basics skills in nursing.

Gina C. Dobbs, RN, MSN, CRNP

Gina C. Dobbs is a 2008 graduate of the University of Alabama at Birmingham's Family Nurse Practitioner Program. She is employed by the University of Alabama at Birmingham 1917 Outpatient HIV/AIDS Clinic. Prior to assuming her duties as a nurse practitioner, Dobbs practiced as an infectious disease nurse at the 1917 clinic while attending graduate school from 2006-2008. As a staff liaison to the Patient Advisory Board, Dobbs presented patient education programs on tobacco cessation, HIV and hepatitis C virus co-infection, and self-administration of parenteral antiretroviral medication (Fuzeon). She spent her formative years in nursing as a traveling neuroscience critical care RN in Alabama, California, Massachusetts, Rhode Island, and Washington, D.C.

Barbara Dossey, PhD, RN, AHN-BC, FAAN

Barbara Dossey is internationally recognized as a pioneer in the holistic nursing movement. She is international co-director and board member of the Nightingale Initiative for Global Health (NIGH), Washington, D.C. and Ottawa, Ontario, Canada, and is the director of Holistic Nursing Consultants in Santa Fe, New Mexico. She is a Florence Nightingale scholar and an author or co-author of 23 books. Her most recent books include Holistic Nursing: A Handbook for Practice (5th ed., 2008), Being with Dying: Compassionate End-of-Life Care Training Guide (2007), Florence Nightingale Today: Healing, Leadership, Global Action (2005), and Florence Nightingale: Mystic, Visionary, Healer (2000; Commemorative Edition, 2010). She has received numerous awards, including being an eight-time recipient of the prestigious American Journal of Nursing award. Dossey's Theory of Integral Nursing (2008) is considered a grand theory that presents the science and art of nursing. It includes an integral process, integral worldview, and integral dialogues that is praxis—theory in action. Her collaborative global nursing project, the Nightingale Declaration Campaign (NDC), has developed two United Nations resolution proposals for adoption—2010: International Year of the Nurse and 2011-2020: United Nations Decade for a Healthy World.

Rebecca Dotson, RN, BSN

Rebecca Dotson is clinical nurse manager of a 22-bed medical-surgical unit and 15-bed neuro-surgical unit located at St. Joseph's Hospital in Parkersburg, West Virginia. Her responsibilities include scheduling, staff support, budgeting, maintaining staffing guidelines, and providing direct nursing care as needed. As a nurse manager, providing a positive work environment to the front line staff is a top priority. She works closely with senior management and the nursing unit's staff to ensure that work is efficient and excellent patient care is provided. As a member of the leadership team, other responsibilities have included studying the Toyota Management System and working closely with Rona Consulting to embed the Lean system into the hospital culture. Currently, Dobson is implementing the zero waste aspect of the Toyota System on the medical-surgical unit. These efforts include monitoring the patient fall rate and developing and implementing a program that provides for significant reduction and ultimately complete elimination of patient falls.

Jeff Doucette, MS, RN, CEN, FACHE, NEA-BC

Jeff Doucette is a health care executive, international presenter, and author. His engaging leadership style and passion for culture development led him to his current role as the administrative director of Nursing for Stafford Hospital Center in Stafford, Virginia. Prior nurse executive service included associate chief operating officer for Emergency Services at Duke University Hospital in Durham, North Carolina, and executive director and vice president of Patient Care Services for Lee Memorial Health System in Fort Myers, Florida. He is known for his ability to ignite and empower teams, and he has become a trusted mentor for numerous professionals in business and health care. Doucette serves on the editorial advisory board for the Journal of Men in Nursing and contributes to a variety of respected nursing publications. Passion for his profession and the ability to engage audiences make Doucette a respected professional speaker and thought-leader in nursing.

Christine Duffield, PhD, RN, MHP, FRCNA, FACHSE, FAICD

Christine Duffield is a professor of nursing and health services management at the University of Technology, Sydney (UTS) where she has been the foundation director in the Centre for Health Services Management since 2000. She completed her nursing program at the University of Western Ontario, graduating with a bachelor's of science in nursing. She has also completed a diploma in nursing education, a master's in health planning, and a PhD in health services management from the University of New South Wales. Prior to her appointment in an academic post, Duffield spent many years as a clinical nurse, educator, and manager in a variety of acute care hospitals in Canada, Australia, New Zealand, and the United Kingdom. Duffield is internationally recognized for her work in the field of nursing workforce and management. For many years, she has worked on projects at the state, national, and international levels with the International Council of Nurses (ICN) and the World Health Organization (WHO). In 2008, she was appointed as deputy director of the WHO Collaborating Centre for Nursing, Midwifery, and Health Development at UTS. She is also a director for UnitingCare Ageing, Sydney Region and deputy chair on of the board of War Memorial Hospital. Duffield is a fellow of the Institute of Company Directors, the College of Health Service Executives, and the Royal College of Nursing Australia.

Pamela Dugle, RN, MSN

Pamela Dugle currently works for the Veterans Affairs Administration in Florida. She has 15 years nursing in the emergency department, intensive care, telemetry, and private physician practice. Dugle is a member of the Emergency Nurses Association, Sigma Theta Tau International, and was inducted into the Phi Theta Kappa Society. She has presented in nursing venues, published, and is active in local and national professional committees committed to improving care for the nation's veterans.

Susan MacLeod Dyess, PhD, RN

Susan MacLeod Dyess is the project director for the Novice Nurse Leadership Institute in the Christine E. Lynn College of Nursing at Florida Atlantic University where she recently completed her doctoral degree. She received her BSN from the University of Iowa and her MSN and PhD from Florida Atlantic University. Dyess has worked in a variety of clinical practice settings, including critical care, oncology, and faith community nursing. More recently, she focused her professional energy within baccalaureate nursing education. Her area of research interest is caring for adults in the faith community setting as well as caring for novice nurses as they transition from education into nursing leadership mindsets. For her contributions to nursing in the community, Palm Healthcare Foundation recognized her with a Commitment to Community award in 2007.

E

Malka (Mally) Ehrenfeld, RN, PhD

Malka (Mally) Ehrenfeld is currently the head of the department of nursing, Tel-Aviv University, Israel, and an associate professor of nursing. Her fields of interest include nursing education, public health, and women's health with a focus on health promotion. She earned her RN at the Hadassah Henrietta Szold School of Nursing, followed by a BA and MPH at the Hebrew University in Israel. Her PhD is from the University of Toronto, Canada. Besides her clinical work as a nurse at the Hadassah University Hospital, Jerusalem, Israel, she also worked as an instructor and was involved as a founding member of the small group who opened the first generic program of nursing in Israel. She had later coordinated the generic program at the Tel Aviv University for the first six years, followed by the coordination of the master's and the PhD program. She later became the director of the Department of Nursing at the School of Health Professions in the Tel Aviv University. Among her international activities, Ehrenfeld serves as the national Israeli representative for the International Council of Nurses and Workgroup of European Nurse Researchers. She has published extensively and presented papers at national and international nursing conferences.

Jeanette Ives Erickson, RN, MS, FAAN

Jeanette Ives Erickson is senior vice president for Patient Care and chief nurse at Massachu-

setts General Hospital (MGH); instructor at Harvard Medical School; assistant professor at the MGH Institute of Health Professions; and senior associate at The Institute for Nursing Healthcare Leadership. She has authored articles and book chapters and serves on several community boards. In 1998, she was awarded an inaugural fellowship in the Robert Wood Johnson Executive Nurse Fellows Program. Erickson has a strong interest in global health, focusing on developing professional nursing models of care delivery. Her work includes a partnership with Project Hope to mentor the chief nurse of the Basrah Children's Hospital in Iraq and with University Hospital in Dubai using Magnet Hospital elements as a framework for developing and evaluating a newly-built nursing service and health care system. She serves on the Health and Human Services National Advisory Council on Nurse Education and Practice and is co-chair of the Sigma Theta Tau International Deans and Chief Nursing Officers Advisory Council.

F

Chad Fairfield, BSN, RN

Chad Fairfield is director at the Clinical Practice Model (CPM) Resource Center and co-leads the design and development of the CPM knowledge repository and team collaboration efforts. Previously, he was a nurse clinician at a large CPM consortium site implementing the CPM Framework. He was a leader in the implementation of the partnership council infrastructure and scholarly work related to the revisions and approvals around Clinical Practice Guidelines. Today he is an on-site professional resource for multiple clinical settings implementing Intentionally Designed Technology to support practice transformation at the point-of-care. Fairfield received his undergraduate degree from MacMurray College and is currently pursuing his MSN at Southern Illinois University in Edwardsville, Illinois.

Katie Flaherty, BSN, RN

Katie Flaherty is from Richmond, Kentucky. As the daughter of a lawyer and a nurse, she learned professionalism, service, and human empathy at an early age, eventually leading her to nursing practice. In 2002, she earned her bachelor's in nursing from Xavier University in Cincinnati, Ohio. Along Flaherty's college journey, she was offered a nursing internship in Aspen, Colorado. She quickly fell in love with the small mountain town and accepted a job at Aspen Valley Hospital in 2002. Flaherty spent more than two years in Aspen before she decided to move back to Kentucky to spend time with her family and expand her nursing knowledge base. She worked in an Open Heart Intensive Care Unit from 2004 to 2005. She missed the mountain lifestyle, though, and returned to Aspen in 2006. Since her return to Aspen, Flaherty has taken a nursing mission trip to Africa and continued her nursing at Aspen Valley Hospital. She currently works full-time in the intensive care unit in Aspen, Colorado.

Jacqueline Filkins

Jacqueline Filkins was born and educated in Switzerland where she trained as a nurse. After serving, along with her husband, as a missionary in Malawi and Madagascar, Filkins returned to the United Kingdom where she developed her nursing career and studied social sciences at Birmingham University. Her interest in nursing leadership and education allowed her to take on executive jobs in the field, culminating as dean of Faculty of Health and Social Care. As co-founder and honorary president of the European Nurse Directors Association and vice-president of the European Specialist Nurses Organization, she remains a frequent guest speaker and adviser at international events. She works as a non-executive director for the Cumbria Partnership NHS Foundation Trust where she is chair of Clinical Governance and is a trustee of Hospice at Home.

Valerie Fleming, RN, RM, MA, PhD

Valerie Fleming commenced nursing education in 1974 in Scotland, and after qualifying, continued studies in midwifery. Following periods of clinical nursing and midwifery positions, she worked in India for a year and Thailand for six months before settling in New Zealand. In her 16 years in New Zealand, while working in clinical and hospital management positions, Fleming studied part time towards her BA in social sciences and her MA in nursing. She then worked as an independent midwife and part-time academic while completing her doctoral studies. Since completing her PhD in 1994, Fleming has been employed as a midwife in academic institutions in New Zealand and Scotland. Additionally, she has carried out consultancies in many parts of the world for the World Health Organization (WHO) and other institutions where her work in curriculum development is held in high esteem. She is currently professor and head of the division of Women and Child Health at Glasgow Caledonian University, director of the World Health Organization Collaborating Centre for Nursing and Midwifery, and secretary general of the global network of WHO Collaborating Centres in Nursing and Midwifery. Her research interests are in midwifery education and women's recovery after childbirth, in which areas she has published widely. She has recently commenced a joint project with the Royal Scottish Academy of Music and Drama, examining the effects of music in the antenatal; period on infant behaviour in the first year of life.

Adriano Friganović, RN, BSN

Adriano Friganović is registered nurse and new president of the Croatian National Nurses Federation. He has 10 years of work experience as nurse. He was the first president of the Croatian Society of Nurses for Anesthesia, Reanimation, Intensive Care, and Transfusion. He graduated at high nursing school and gained his BsN degree. He organized numerous professional gatherings—congresses, symposiums, and so on—and currently works at the Clinical Hospital Centre in Zagreb as the chief nurse of unit for Anesthesiology, Reanimatology and Intensive Care of Cardiac Patients.

Leslie Furlow, PhD, RN, MSN, MPH

Leslie Furlow is president and founder of AchieveMentors, a health care consulting company specializing in operation and management improvement. She has worked with more than 100 clients, providing more than 200 engagements in the United States in which she developed and implemented strategies that achieved lasting results. She is a partner with Sharon Judkins in Hardiness-Mentors, LLC, a research based development process that increases personal hardiness in middle managers and shows proven decreases in stress and unplanned absences. Her educational preparation includes a doctorate in management and a master's degrees in public health and nursing. She is certified as a Family Nurse Practitioner (FNP), professional behavioral analyst, facilitator, and in Total Quality Management. She also received board certification in leadership from the Society for the Advancement of Consulting in 2006 in part due to her hardiness research.

G

Nancy Rollins Gantz, MSN, RN, PhD, MBA, NE-BC, MRCNA

Nancy Rollins Gantz, editor and lead author of this book, has held nursing executive positions nationally and internationally and is published on multiple topics, including critical care administration, leadership, mentoring, empowerment, and succession planning in the multicultural work team. The American Organization of Nurse Executives (AONE) 2005 Prism Award was presented to her for her contribution in cultural diversity and the multicultural work team for her program called Cultural Appreciation through Professional Practice and Synergy (CAPPS), which has become a major focus for her work. With 30 years of experience in health care administration, critical care, pediatrics, cultural diversity, and international nursing, Gantz has lectured extensively in more than 45 countries and continued her academic education in traditional and non-tradition venues. She is listed in Who's Who in America, Who's Who in American Nursing, and has received numerous other honors and awards, most recently International Leaders in Achievement and the Decree of International Letters for Cultural Achievement. Gantz is a fellow of the Johnson & Johnson/Wharton Fellows Program in Management for Nurse Executives from the Wharton School of the University of Pennsylvania. During the writing of this book, she lived in Sydney, Australia, and Mesa, Arizona.

Barbara Gebert

Barbara Gebert is a pedagogic nurse with extensive experience as a head nurse on a medical ward. From 1995 to 2002, she was an assistant professor at the University of Bremen, Department of Education and Nursing Research, in Germany. She helped establish the Department of Nursing Pedagogics at the University of Bremen, Germany. Her research interest is decision-making and reflection in nursing. Since 2002, she has been the principal of the School for Geriatric Nursing in Berlin.

Paul Gill, PhD, BSc (Hons), MSc (Oxon), RN

Paul Gill, RN, BSc (Hons), MSc (Oxon.), PhD, trained as a nurse at East Glamorgan General Hospital in South Wales, United Kingdom, and has a background in critical care nursing. He obtained his BSc (Hons) nursing studies degree in 1997 and subsequently obtained an MSc in social anthropology in 1999 from the University of Oxford. Gill's PhD explored donor and recipient experiences of live kidney transplantation, and he was awarded the Royal College of Nursing Marjorie Simpson New Researcher Award in 2006 for this research. He is currently a Research Capacity Building Collaboration (RCBC) Wales Post-Doctoral Research Fellow at the Faculty of Health, Sport and Science, University of Glamorgan, where he is currently undertaking a two year study, exploring participants' experiences of kidney transplant failure.

Leah Gillham, RN, BSN

Leah Gillham, of Cherokee descent, is a recent nursing graduate and currently employed as a public health nurse in Alaska. She has previous experience working as a certified nursing assistant (CAN). Her desire for nursing came after working with the developmentally disabled and elderly. She received her BSN in nursing from the University of Alaska Anchorage and was a Recruitment and Retention of Alaskan Natives into Nursing (RRANN) participant. Gillham is currently in the process of choosing a graduate program.

Joy Gorzeman, RN, MSN, MBA

Joy Gorzeman has been in the health care profession for over 30 years. She began her career by graduating from St. Joseph Mercy School of Nursing, Sioux City, Iowa, in 1972. She obtained her RN license, and then pursued advanced degrees while working full-time in a variety of health care settings. In 1983, she obtained a master's of science in nursing from the University of Texas, Arlington, and in 2004 obtained a master's in business administration from San Diego State University. She is also a graduate fellow of the Johnson & Johnson/ Wharton Fellows Program in Management for Nurse Executives from the Wharton School of the University of Pennsylvania. During her lengthy career, she has served in the capacity of staff nurse, manager, educator, director, chief nursing officer, and chief operating officer for a number of not-for-profit hospitals and health care systems across the United States. Gorzeman has co-authored a textbook, Decision Making in Medical-Surgical Nursing, and has written a number of articles for professional journals. She is on the editorial board of the Journal of Nursing Administration. Gorzeman is passionate about making a meaningful difference in the lives of patients, providers, and others who are touched by the patient care process throughout the continuum of care.

Ecaterina Gulie, RN, MS

Ecaterina Gulie has been a registered nurse in Romania since 1973 and is currently a nurse in the Clinic Physiotherapy, Medical Rehabilitation. She finished nursing school post high school in Craiova in 1973. She worked in the Clinical Hospital of Emergency from the town Craiova, in the Clinic General Surgery from 1973 until 2001. From 1996 until 2001, Gulie was chief nurse in the Clinic General Surgery III. She worked as a mentor with students in clinical practice, in surgery 1982-2001.In 2005, she finished nursing school inside the university from Sibiu. In 2007, she received a diploma of her master's in management of health services from Sibiu. In 2002, she studied and received a certificate for a three-month program at Georgetown University in professional development in nursing education, leadership, and management in international health. In 1998 she became member of the board of directors for the Romanian Nursing Association (RNA). She became president of RNA in 2006. Since 2007, she has been chief editor of Nursing, RNA's journal. Gulie represents RNA at the International meetings and lives in Bucharest. She has published a book about research in the Romanian language, and she has contributed to several more books.

H

Alžbeta Hanzlíková, PhD, RN

Alžbeta Hanzlíková is an associate professor of nursing at the Faculty of Health, Department of Nursing, Catholic University in Ružomberok, Slovakia, since 2003, and at the Health and Social Work Department, St. Elizabeth University, Bratislava, Slovakia, since 2005. From 1992 to 2000, she was head of the department of nursing, Jessenius Medical Faculty, Commenius University, Bratislava, Slovakia. In her work and study, she has specialized in community nursing, focusing on health promotion. Her research projects focus on the attitude to health among the adult population in Slovakia. She published her works in Slovak and German. She studied nursing in Slovakia and the Czech Republic. She received her doctoral degree at the Commenius University in Bratislava and her senior readership degree at the South Czech University in eské Bud jovice, the Czech Republic. Since 1997 she has been working with and for the Slovak Chamber of Nurses and Midwifery.

Susan Hassmiller, PhD, RN, FAAN

Susan Hassmiller is senior adviser for Nursing for the Robert Wood Johnson (RWJ) Foundation and director of the RWJ Initiative on the Future of Nursing at the Institute of Medicine (IOM). Previously, Hassmiller was with the Health Resources and Services Administration, where she was the executive director of the U.S. Public Health Service Primary Care Policy Fellowship and worked on other national and international primary care initiatives. She has also worked in public health settings at the local and state level and taught public health nursing at the University of Nebraska and George Mason University in Virginia. Hassmiller is a fellow in the American Academy of Nursing and a member of the Joint Commission National Nurse Advisory Council and the New York Academy of Medicine. She received a PhD in nursing administration and health policy from George Mason University in Fairfax, Virginia, master's degrees in health education from Florida State University and community health nursing from the University of Nebraska Medical Center, and a bachelor's degree in nursing from Florida State University. She is a 2007 outstanding alumnus for both George Mason University and University of Nebraska Medical Center and is the 2008

John P. McGovern Award recipient from the American Association of Colleges of Nursing.

Wendy Hein, RN, BSN

Wendy Hein was born in Alaska and grew up in a military family, allowing her to be a world traveler from an early age. Inspired to become a nurse when shown great kindness in the hospital with the birth of her first child, she wanted to impact someone else's life the way this nurse had impacted her. Starting her career as a Licensed Vocational Nurse, and while pursuing this at Weatherford Community College, she made the dean's list and received the Florence Nightingale award. Working in a skilled nursing facility after graduation, Hein was promoted into management, going from charge nurse to unit manager to assistant director of nurses to director of staff development, all within seven months. She received her associate of science degree from Excelsior College while working on a medical-surgical floor at a county hospital. Immediately after completion of her associate's, she began working on a BSN. With BSN in hand, she was given supervisory responsibility for the largest department at Baylor Medical Center Waxahachie—without a manager. Hein is presently the childbirth educator for Women's Health Services at Baylor Medical Center in Waxahachie, Texas.

Anna L. Herrin, RN, BSN

Anna L. Herrin is a 2008 graduate of the University of Alabama in Huntsville (UAH) where she earned her bachelor's of science in nursing. She is a staff nurse in the surgical suite with a focus on orthopedics and sports medicine surgery at St. Vincent's Health System in Birmingham, Alabama. Her goals include a focus on nursing leadership and informatics as she pursues graduate studies. Herrin is a member of the American Organization of Nurse Executives (AONE) and the Association of Peri-Operative Registered Nurses (AORN).

Donna M. Herrin, RN, BSN

Donna M. Herrin has served the profession in a number of leadership roles since beginning her professional practice in 1977. She holds a master's degree in nursing from Vanderbilt University and is dual credentialed as an advanced nurse executive and a health care executive. She is a member of Sigma Theta Tau International, the American Nurses Association, the American College of Healthcare Executives (ACHE), and the American Organization of Nurse Executives (AONE). In 2009, she served as national president of AONE. Additionally, she serves the profession as editorial board member for The Journal of Nursing Administration (JONA) and as consultant on international nursing systems development. Herrin is clinical associate professor at the University of Alabama Huntsville (UAH) and senior advisor with Methodist Le Bonheur Healthcare. Her professional experience includes roles as senior vice president, system chief nurse executive, chief nursing officer, associate administrator, and director of women's and children's services.

Susan Hetzer, RN, BS, MSN, CCRN

Susan Hetzer has been a nurse since 1998. Currently, she is a charge nurse in the intensive care center at St. Mary's Hospital in Leonardtown, Maryland. While working at St. Mary's Hospital, she has been involved in activities to improve nursing practices, including the implementation of the hospital's clinical practice council, and other quality improvement projects. Her educational background includes a bachelor's of science in biology from Frostburg State University, an associate's of science in nursing, and current enrollment in the master's of science in nursing at the University of Phoenix.

Karen Hodge, RN, BBA, MSN

Karen Hodge is chief nursing officer for St. Alphonsus Regional Medical Center in Boise, Idaho. She received her associate's degree in nursing from Boise State University in 1974 and her bachelor's in business administration in management in 1994. Hodge completed her MSN in 2009. She worked as a staff nurse in obstetrics and the intensive care unit for 10 years before experiencing other aspects of health care such as utilization/discharge management and managed care operations. Hodge served as service line and nursing director for women's and children's services for eight years and added oncology service for three years. Almost all of her experiences have been at St. Alphonsus Regional Medical Center in Boise, Idaho.

Beth Houlahan, MSN, RN

Beth Houlahan is the senior vice president, Nursing and Patient Care Services at Mercy Medical Center, Cedar Rapids, Iowa, a position she has held since January 2008. She was previously the vice president of Nursing Excellence at Mercy from June 2007 until December 2008, when she moved into her current role. She was hired by Mercy in anticipation of her moving into the senior vice president position as a planned succession strategy. Houlahan received her BSN from Mt. Mercy College, her MSN from the University of Iowa, and she completed a fellowship from the Wharton School at the University of Pennsylvania. Houlahan's predominate career focus has been in the development and management of women's and primary care outpatient practices—in both private and academic settings.

Marion Eulene Francis Howard, PhD, MSN, BA, SCM, SRN

Marion Eulene Francis Howard has been a lecturer of nursing and midwifery in the Faculty of Nursing, Barbados Community College since 1987. She specialized in maternal child nursing and research. She coordinated and lectured in the midwifery programme, as well as taught obstetrics in the general nursing programme in Barbados. Her research projects include a wide range of topics and focused on HIV/AIDS, nursing education, men in nursing, women in management, and continuous quality improvement. She was educated in general nursing in Barbados, midwifery in Scotland, United Kingdom, and Los Angeles, California, and has worked as a nurse/midwife in all of these countries. She received a bachelor's degree in natural and social science, a post graduate diploma of education, and educational administration in Barbados; a master's of science in nursing, and a doctoral degree in business administration in the USA. Howard is the first nurse commissioner, National HIV / AIDS Commission of Barbados in the office of the Prime Minister of Barbados; the first nurse member of the board of directors, Queen Elizabeth Hospital board in Barbados. Howard is a certified nurse leader and trainer, International Council of Nurses (ICN) in the Leadership for Change Training Programme for Health Professionals.

Thresanne Howland, MSc Midwifery, BSc (Midwifery), RM

Thresanne Howland is from Mtarfa, Malta, and graduated with a diploma in midwifery in 1995. Howland worked in various areas of maternity department, specialising in delivery suite. Since 1995, she has been coordinating a private antenatal/postnatal clinic together with an obstetrician. In 2002, Howland registered with the Nursing Midwifery Council in the United Kingdom, after working in the Ulster Hospital, Northern Ireland. Howland graduated with a BSc in midwifery from the Caledonian University in the United Kingdom and then immediately started work toward her MSc in midwifery. In 2007, she was elected as a member on the Maltese Council of Nurses and Midwives. Howland joined the Department of Nursing Services and Standards in late 2008 to formulate Midwifery Standards.

J

Stacy Jepsen, RN, BS, CCRN

Stacy Jepsen is the critical care nurse clinician at Fairview Southdale Hospital (FSH) in Edina, Minnesota. She has worked at FSH for the past 10 years, advancing from a respiratory therapist, to staff nurse in the intensive care unit to her current position of critical care nurse clinician. She received her bachelor's degree in Bismarck, North Dakota, as a respiratory therapist and her nursing degree in Bloomington, Minnesota. She is currently working on her master's of science at Mankato State University in Minnesota, as a clinical nurse specialist. She specializes in adult critical care, with a focus in hemodynamic monitoring and ventilation. She played a vital role in the development and success of the Rapid Response Team at FSH and is co-chair of the Code Blue Committee. The hospital currently has code blue rate of less than 1%.

Lisa Johnson-Ford, MSN, CRNP

Lisa Johnson-Ford is a board certified acute care nurse practitioner and adjunct professor at Drexel University in the College of Nursing and Health Professions. She earned her master's of science degree from the University of Massachusetts. She is currently a doctoral student at Drexel University in the doctor of nursing practice program. Her research interest is in understanding the factors that influence African-American families to withhold or withdraw life-sustaining therapies for their next-of-kin. She has worked in oncology, intensive care, bone marrow transplant, and gastroenterology.

Deloras Jones, MS, RN

Deloras Jones is the executive director for the California Institute for Nursing and Health Care (CINHC), a not-for-profit organization dedicated to addressing California statewide nursing issues that impact the health of California citizens. A major focus of CINHC is the nurse shortage. Pursuant to this, CINHC has embarked on the development of a strategically driven master plan for the nursing workforce. Ms. Jones formerly was the chief nurse executive for Kaiser Permanente, providing strategic and operational leadership for nursing for the California division. Prior to her corporate role, she served as the chief nursing officer for the San Francisco Kaiser Hospital. Jones has an extensive background in addressing nursing practice and workforce issues, serving on multiple state and national committees. She was the project leader for a national study on registered nurses sponsored by the American Organization of Nurse Executives (AONE) and *NurseWeek*, and served as president of the Association of California Nurse Leaders and as a board member for AONE. Jones received her diploma in nursing from the Kaiser Foundation School of Nursing, her BSN from Columbia Union College, and her master's in nursing from the University of California San Francisco.

Karien Jooste, PhD, RN

Karien Jooste is a professor in the Faculty of Health Sciences at the University of Johannesburg, focusing on leadership in health services management with 27 years of tertiary teaching experience. She was recently appointed as a full member of the South African Nursing Council where she's involved in professional conduct hearings. She has published several articles in national and international accredited journals and serves on national and international editorial boards of peer reviewed journals. She is the author of textbooks in nursing management and has presented at numerous international conferences. Jooste has acted as chairperson of the Leadership Succession Committee of the Tau Lamda Chapter of Sigma Theta Tau International and is a member of the research subcommittee of the International Council of Nurses (ICN). She has served on the international taskforce for leadership development of Sigma Theta Tau International in developing a worldwide curriculum on global leadership.

Elsa Jordaan, RN, BSN

Elsa Jordaan is a lecturer at George Hospital Training School. She is responsible for the subjects of ethos and professional practice, unit management, education, and pharmacology. She is a member of the South African Nursing Council, Democratic Nursing Association of South Africa, and a member of Tau Lamda Chapter of Sigma Theta Tau International. She is involved in quality assurance and serves as a change agent in the hospital. Her forte is "the developing of students to become the leaders of the future," as well as development of ethical standards within the hospital. She has published a book on home nursing and has co-authored three textbooks.

Melissa Joseph, MSN, RN

Melissa Joseph has been a nurse manager of a 36 bed medical-telemetry unit at Faulkner Hospital since 2006. She received her undergraduate degree from University of Miami and her graduate degree from Loyola University. After working in intensive care units for five years, she developed an interest in management and leadership and completed an administration fellowship. Her particular interests are to propel nurses to learn and pursue their quest within nursing while supporting them to provide excellent patient care. She enjoys mentoring staff nurses and strives to be an example like many nurse leaders who have mentored her. She hopes to permeate the nursing profession with the energy, commitment, dedication, and research it needs to help advance nursing.

Sandra Jost, MSN, RN

Sandra Jost is the associate chief nursing officer (ACNO) at the Hospital of the University of Pennsylvania (HUP), a 704-bed acute, quaternary-level hospital located in Philadelphia, Pennsylvania. In her role, Jost provides operational oversight for the 35 inpatient and procedural areas at HUP. She received a BSN from the University of Delaware in 1988 and earned an MSN in 2000 from the University of Pennsylvania in nursing administration.

Jost is an effective nursing leader with several years of health care operational and consulting experience. She started her career at HUP as a clinical nurse where she worked closely with internationally educated nurses and also cared for the culturally diverse patients that visit the hospital. Jost meets regularly with the internationally educated nurses (IENs) at HUP to learn their unique needs.

Maria Eulàlia Juvé, RN, MMSN, MNLM, QRD

Maria Eulàlia Juvé received her diploma in nursing in 1990, her master's in medical-surgical nursing (MMSN) in 1994, and a master's in nursing leadership and management in 2008 from Barcelona University, Barcelona, Spain. She began her career as a nurse in the internal medicine ward at Bellvitge University Hospital. In 2005, Juvé accepted the position of general nursing coordinator, Direction of Hospitals Division at Catalan Institute of Health. She is a teacher in various courses on research and clinical practice methodology. She has published several articles in her homeland of Spain.

K

Anna Kagure Karani, PhD, MA, RN, BScN

Anna Kagure Karani has been a nurse for more than 30 years, with wide experience in nursing education, general nursing, midwifery, and community health nursing. Karani has a PhD (2002) in nursing education and curriculum development from the University of Nairobi (UoN), an MA (Communication) from Wheaton, a BScN (AWU), DAN (UoN) RN/M/CHN. She was promoted to associate professor in 2008, senior lecturer in 2002, and was lecturer from 1996. From 1971, she worked in the National Hospital in different areas, including accident and emergency and intensive care. She has been involved in leadership, mentoring, developing curriculum, research, and community service. She is the lead trainer for the International Council of Nurses in Kenya, chief nursing officer for St John Ambulance in Kenya, and she is chairman of Kenya Nursing Journal and the Leadership for Change board and chapter in Kenya. She is a board member of Kenya

Research and Ethics Committee (KEMRI) and for Kenyatta National Hospital and University of Nairobi ERC. She is a fellow of the Johnson & Johnson/Wharton Fellows Program in Management for Nurse Executives from the Wharton School of the University of Pennsylvania (2008). She earned a Head of State Commendation in 2003 and a gold medal in 1987 during the All Africa Games for service as a first aider and for promoting continuing education for nurses. Karani has published many articles in peer reviewed journals, books, and has participated in research with international collaborators like St Luke's College of Nursing in Japan.

Zeina Ghaleb Kassem, RN

Zeina Ghaleb Kassem is a registered nurse (RN) at the American University of Beirut Medical Center (AUBMC) in Lebanon. Kassem has been working for the past six years in a medical oncology unit as an RN and incharge. She finished her master's in clinical nursing, focusing on the educational preparation of oncology nurses and was trained at MD Anderson Cancer Center. Kassem contributed extensively on enculturation of the concept of shared governance and Magnet at AUBMC. She is considered a clinical resource, a preceptor, and mentor, and is highly involved in activities that improve the quality of care and patient outcomes. She worked with colleagues on disseminating the concepts of evidence based practice and research. Kassem is so proud to be a member in the first Magnet designated hospital in the Middle East (nursing services).

Carole Kenner, DNS, RNC-NIC, FAAN

Carole Kenner is dean and professor at the University of Oklahoma College of Nursing. She received her bachelor's in nursing from the University of Cincinnati. She received both her master's (completing both the perinatal CNS and neonatal NP programs) and DNS in curriculum design and higher education from Indiana University. She has more than 25 years experience in higher education and has taught at all levels of nursing from the BSN through PhD programs. Kenner has presented on local, state, national, and international levels regarding neonatal/perinatal/genetics and nursing education related issues. She is president of Consultants with Confidence, Inc., and president and executive director of the Council of International Neonatal Nurses, Inc. She serves on the Nursing Advisory Board of the National March of Dimes. She represented the American Nurses Association; the Association of Women's Health Obstetrics, Gynecology, and Neonatal Nursing; and the National Association of Neonatal Nurses to the American Academy of Pediatrics Committee on Fetus and Newborn, which was responsible for the Perinatal Guidelines. She has also served on the Recommended Guidelines committee for the Neonatal Intensive Care Unit (NICU) Environment for 17 years. This group has set the recommendations worldwide for NICU designs. In addition, her research is in the area of transition from hospital to home for mothers and babies, fetal alcohol syndrome, and family context for clinical genetics, as well as her current project with families of newly diagnosed children with cancer. Dr. Kenner has published more than 100 articles and more than 15 textbooks covering topics related to neonatal care, genetics, and academic leadership. Her recent textbook, Teaching IOM: Implications of the IOM Reports for Nursing Education (2007) co-authored with Anita Finkelman, won the Society of Technical Communication Award for Excellence (2007-2008).

Karlene Kerfoot, PhD, RN, NEA-BC, FAAN

Karlene Kerfoot has held a variety of positions in nursing and patient care administration, clinical practice, academic positions in nursing, MHA and MBA programs, and health care. Currently, she is vice president and chief clinical officer for the Aurora Health Care System in Wisconsin. In this position, Kerfoot has responsibility for specific clinical areas and quality programs throughout the system. She has earned a doctorate in nursing from the University of Illinois, Chicago, a master's and BSN from the University of Iowa in Iowa City, and is a fellow of the Johnson & Johnson/Wharton Fellows Program in Management for Nurse Executives from the Wharton School of the University of Pennsylvania. Her honors include induction into the American Academy of Nursing, the Mary Tolle Wright Award for Excellence, and the Pioneering Spirit Award

from the American Association of Critical-Care Nurses.

Richard Kimball, Jr., RN, MSN, MPH

Richard Kimball, Jr., practices in the nurse-directed Outpatient Amyotrophic Lateral Sclerosis Clinic at Johns Hopkins Hospital in Baltimore, Maryland, where he has practiced for nine years in the fields of psychiatric, neurological, and community health nursing. He has completed his PhD coursework in Health Policy at the University of Maryland in Baltimore and is working on his dissertation. Mr. Kimball received his master's degrees in community health nursing and public health from Johns Hopkins University in 2001.

Maggie Kirk, PhD, BSc (Hons), DipN, RGN

Maggie Kirk is head of research in the Faculty of Health, Sport, and Science at the University of Glamorgan, South Wales, United Kingdom. She has particular responsibility for research across the Faculty, driving the strategic development of research and research capacity building. Raising the profile of genetics in the education of health professionals has been an important goal for her since she entered higher education in 1992. Prior to this, Kirk practised in the coronary care setting, having made a career move to nursing from the field of mammalian genetics. In 2004, Kirk commenced an additional role as programme lead for nursing professional groups at the National Health Services National Genetics Education and Development Centre. At the University of Glamorgan, Kirk is leader of the Genomics Policy Unit (GPU) which was established in 1996 to explore the impact of advances in new genetic technologies on health care, assessing the implications for professionals and public alike.

JoEllen Koerner, RN, PhD, FAAN

JoEllen Koerner works as a senior consultant for Dynamis Healthcare Advisors, providing support and resources for healthcare workforce development for underrepresented sectors of society. She graduated from South Dakota State University with an MSN in 1982 and lives in Sioux Falls, South Dakota. Koerner completed her PhD in human and organizational development at the Fielding Institute in Santa Barbara, California, in 1993. She has published and lectured extensively, as well as received numerous honors and awards. She currently holds an adjunct faculty position at Kansas University Medical Center while also offering on-line courses with several other educational institutions. Koerner also works in Manila, Philippines, on professional development for registered nurses. Her passion for health and healing is further supported by educational activities related to multi-cultural holistic health care practices.

Catherine Siow Lan Koh, RN, MSN

Catherine Siow Lan Koh is assistant director of nursing at the National University Hospital, member of the National University Health System, Singapore. Koh received her master's in science in nursing studies from Manchester University, United Kingdom, in 2005 and is currently reading her doctor of nursing practice at the University of Colorado. Her interests include clinical standards in nursing practice and nursing resource development. She is the recipient of the Ministry of Health (MOH) Nurses' Merit Award, MOH Health Management Development Program, National Health Group (NHG) Cluster Research Fund Small Innovative Grant, NHG Specialty Development Fund Fellowship Award, and the Public Service Commission Overseas Scholarship.

Yanika Kowitlawakul, PhD, RN

Yanika Kowitlawakul is originally from Thailand. She currently works as an assistant professor at the Nursing Education Department, The George Washington University, Washington, D.C. She received her bachelor's of science in nursing from Khon Kaen University, Thailand, in 1991, and master's of nursing administration from George Mason University in 2000. She has been interested in international nursing since she began her PhD at George Mason University in 2002. Kowitlawakul received her PhD in nursing in 2008. Her professional experiences have included critical care nursing and clinical teaching.

Charles Krozek, MN, RN, FAAN

Charles Krozek is founder, president, and managing director of Versant, with the vision of enhancing the profession of nursing by bringing outcome-based education to the workplace and thereby ensuring safe and competent care for patients. Krozek has more than 25 years of professional nursing experience. He specialized in education and research for the past 19 years, and has been involved in nursing advocacy efforts for many years. He has testified on numerous occasions before the California State Assembly and Senate committees on issues related to the nursing shortage. Additionally, Krozek served on the Los Angeles County Workforce Investment board and acted as chair of California's Economic Development's Statewide Health Occupations Advisory Committee. A graduate of Humboldt State University with a BA in biology and a BS in nursing, he completed his MN in nursing at the University of California, Los Angeles. He is an established author and speaker and has served on the editorial advisory boards of several nursing journals, including Journal of Nursing Staff Development. He has co-authored articles, include "RN Internship: Outcomes of a One-Year Pilot Program." Krozek also received the Association of California Nurse Leaders' 2005 award for Excellence in Advancement of Clinical Practice in recognition of his significant contribution to nursing education and research.

L

Vicki D. Lachman, PhD, APRN, MBE

Vicki D. Lachman joined the Drexel University faculty as a clinical associate professor in the College of Nursing and Health Professions in 2002. Her primary responsibility is teaching ethics in the DrNP and MSN nursing programs, as well as acting as the track coordinator for the "MSN in Innovation and Intra/Entrepreneurship in Advanced Nursing Practice" program. Prior to this, she was president of V. L. Associates, a consulting, training, and coaching firm specializing in the changing needs of the health care industry. She earned her master's from the University of Pennsylvania in psychiatric nursing and in bioethics. She also holds a PhD in education from Temple University, where her focus was on organizational development. She has published more than 100 articles in leading professional publications, as well as a book, Applied Ethics in Nursing. Her third book, Developing Your Moral Compass: A Guide for Healthcare Professionals, will be released in 2009.

Claudia Lai, PhD, RN

Claudia Lai is associate professor in the School of Nursing at The Hong Kong Polytechnic University. She obtained her master's degree from the University of Toronto and her doctoral degree from the University of Hong Kong. She has practiced nursing in Hong Kong, Canada, and England, and has worked briefly as a volunteer nurse in India. Her program of research focuses on various aspects of long-term care and, in particular, on the care of people suffering from dementia. She has volunteered her time at the Hong Kong Alzheimer's Disease Association for more than 13 years. She has published books, book chapters, and journal papers, both locally and internationally. She took second place in the 2003 International Psychogeriatric Association Research Awards in Psychogeriatrics and was selected as a 2004 recipient of the Sigma Theta Tau International Research Dissemination in Nursing Award for Region 1.

Peter Lai, MNurs, BN, RN, ET

Peter Lai received his professional training in the School of Nursing of the Queen Mary Hospital in 1992. After graduation, he worked in the field of critical care while furthering his study in different nursing specialties, including critical care and enterostomal therapy. In 2001, he underwent training in burn care in the United States. He obtained a masters degree in nursing from the University of Hong Kong in 2008. His clinical and research interests include critical care, burn care, wound, and stomal nursing. He is currently serving as an advanced practice nurse in an adult intensive care unit and is responsible for leading the wound team, burn team, and respiratory working group. He also actively participates in volunteer services of different professional associations, such as Hong Kong Enterostomal Therapists Association, Hong Kong Association of Critical Care Nurses, and the Norma N. Gill Foundation.

Winsome Lam, RN, APN, MN

Winsome Lam is an advanced practice nurse at the School of Nursing, The Hong Kong Polytechnic University. She specialized in community health nursing and renal nursing. She received her bachelor's and master's degrees in nursing in Hong Kong. Before joining The Hong Kong Polytechnic University in 2007, she worked as a renal nurse, community nurse, and honor clinical mentor in Hospital Authority, Hong Kong. She is now teaching the undergraduate program in community health nursing.

Sarah Lamkin, MSN, RN

Sarah Lamkin is a nurse and certified specialist in poison information (CSPI) at the Drug and Poison Information Center located at Cincinnati Children's Hospital Medical Center, Cincinnati, Ohio, where she provides poison/drug information, drug abuse services, and toxicology consultations to both health professionals and the local community. She graduated from the University of Cincinnati with a BSN in 2004. She pursued further educational opportunities and recently completed two master's programs at Xavier University in nursing and education. She holds an adjunct faculty position with Xavier University's College of Nursing. Lamkin plans to complete the pediatric nurse practitioner program at the University of Cincinnati by December 2011. She brings her passion for education and research to the Village Life Outreach Project and is currently creating outcome measures for several of the organization's signature projects in Tanzania.

Gay Landstrom, MS, RN

Gay Landstrom received her BS in nursing from Rush University in Chicago. While serving as a staff nurse and assistant head nurse at Rush, she completed her MS in nursing administration at the University of Illinois at Chicago, going on to be a nurse manager and director of nursing roles in the Chicago area. Landstrom returned to Michigan to join Trinity Health (formerly Mercy Health Services) as the chief nursing officer in two of the organization's facilities and now serves as the interim chief nursing officer for the system. Landstrom is currently attending the University of Michigan, working on completion of a PhD in nursing. Her research interests focus on cognitive representations, brain function, and therapeutic use of imagination to create change.

Diana T. F. Lee, PhD, RN

Diana T. F. Lee is chair and professor of nursing, director of the Nethersole School of Nursing, and assistant dean of the Faculty of Medicine at the Chinese University of Hong Kong. She is also a visiting professor of the

University of London in the United Kingdom (UK) and advisory professor of Fudan University and Guangzhou Medical College in China. Besides her teaching and administrative roles, Professor Lee has researched and published widely, especially in the area of gerontological nursing. She has successfully obtained more than HK$95 million from various competitive research grants and has just been honored with an excellent research award in health services research by the Hong Kong Government. Most of her research efforts are focused on promoting the health and well-being of elderly people in residential care homes and in the community. She has expertise in a range of research methodologies. She has also established international joint research work, especially in China and the UK, on elderly care. Lee has published more than 150 refereed journal articles, book chapters, and conference papers. Her latest publications include papers in the Journal of the American Geriatrics Society, the Gerontologist and Quality of Life Research. She is also the editor and reviewer for a number of international nursing and gerontological journals. Lee has been invited to deliver keynote addresses in numerous international and national conferences.

Siu Yin Lee, RN, MHS

Siu Yin Lee is director of nursing at the National University Hospital, member of the National University Health System, Singapore. Lee received her master's in health sciences from the University of Sydney in 2002. She is involved in numerous nursing committees, contributing to different facets of nursing related issues such as management, education, ethics, and so on. She is also associate professor at the Alice Lee Centre for Nursing Studies, National University of Singapore, lending her expertise in charting strategic direction for upgrading the skills and competencies of nurses through formal academic programs. She is the recipient of the prestigious President's Award for Nurses, and the Inaugural Outstanding Citizen Award from the National Health Group, Singapore.

Eunice Nah Swee Lin, MSc HRM, BHSN

Eunice Swee Lin Nah is currently a senior staff nurse at the SingHealth Polyclinics under the Singapore Health Services cluster. She has seen a tour of duty that includes medical-surgical nursing, oncology ambulatory treatment, community health care, human resource management in nursing and allied health administration, strategic management, and policy analysis at cluster level. With a passion for people development and improvement planning, she is also the chair of the information technology and research committee of the Singapore Global Network, American Society for Training & Development (2008-2010). In addition to master's and bachelor's degrees, she has an advanced diploma in nursing (community health), a diploma in human resource development, and a diploma in nursing.

Shirley K. L. Lo, RN, MSN, LL.B

Shirley K. L. Lo is a clinical associate with the School of Nursing (SN), The Hong Kong Polytechnic University since 2007. She obtained general nursing and midwifery training in Hong Kong, a bachelor's degree in laws from the University of London and a master's of nursing from the University of Western Sydney. She has worked as a nurse in Hong Kong and in Canada. She is interested in the holistic care and welfare of seniors. As a member of the Ageing and Health Research Group at SN, she leads a project team that develops domestic cordless phone for seniors. She is committed to activities related to increasing awareness of elder abuse and promotion of seniors' independent living in the community. Presently, she started writing on topics of her interest for publication in academic journals and has several manuscripts under review.

Yuen Jean Tak Alice Loke, RN, MN, PhD

Yuen Jean Tak Alice Loke is professor at the School of Nursing, The Hong Kong Polytechnic University. She has been teaching at university nursing programs since 1984. She specialized in community health with a focus on promotion of health among women and school age children. Her publications included topics on women's exposure to cigarette smoking, sexual health of adolescents, and health and lifestyle of school aged students. She received her baccalaureate degree and master's degree in the United States, and her PhD in community health from the Faculty of Medicine, The University of Hong Kong. She has held the position as the scheme coordinator for the Postgraduate Program in Health Care and Nursing. She is now leading the Family and Community Health Research Group and developing specialty program for nurses in advancing the community health specialty.

Maria dos Anjos Pereira Lopes, PhD, MSN, RN, EANS

Maria dos Anjos Pereira Lopes is coordinating professor of nursing with the Escola Superior de Enfermagem de Lisboa, Portugal, since 1986. She specialized in medical-surgical nursing. Her research projects are related to care of the elderly, with emphasis on experiential nursing knowledge developed through nurse-patient interactions. She has published 25 articles. She graduated as a nurse in Portugal, where she completed a master's degree and a doctoral degree in nursing sciences. Lopes worked for 14 years in a heart disease intensive care unit. She is a scholar of the European Academy of Nursing Science, a member of the Scientific Committee of the Doctoral Programme in Nursing of the University of Lisboa, since 2008, and a member of the coordinating committee of the Nursing Research and Development Unit in Lisboa, Portugal.

Cristiana Luciani, RN, MSN

Cristiana Luciani works in the quality and accreditation department at the Sant'Andrea Hospital ll Faculty of Medicine and Surgery Sapienza University of Rome in Rome, Italy. She graduated in nursing science cum laude and also holds a second-level master in engineering and management of quality at Sapienza University in Rome. She has training and experience in critical care, surgical assistance, and management. Luciani has taught from 1996 to the present at local universities and is the author of books, publications, and is a presenter at national and international conferences.

Sanduţa Ludmila

Sanduţa Ludmila was born in a Ciniseuti village, Rezina region, in the Republic of Moldova. She graduated from the City Medical School in Chisinau. She began her professional activity at Nr.1 Municipal Clinical Hospital as a surgery nurse. From 1988, she was chief nurse in Intensive Therapy and Reanimation ward of the same institution. Since 2008, she has been a nurse teacher at the Continuing Education Centre for Nurses in

Chisinau and also a national trainer in education for Health and Home Care. She attended a lot of professional courses and seminars that helped her to improve herself. Also, she elaborated a lot of works as materials for Training for Trainers course, materials for the Second Congress for family doctors in the Republic of Moldova. She is an honored member of the Nursing Association of Republic of Moldova.

M

Sara Macchiano, MS/MBA, RN

Sara Macchiano has been a nursing director of a 25-bed general medical unit at Massachusetts General Hospital since December 2006. She received her bachelor's of science in nursing from Wilkes University in 2003 and her master's in nursing with a focus on clinical nurse specialist adult health tract and a master's in business administration from Boston College in 2006. She was motivated to pursue a leadership position early in her career because of conversations with nurse leaders—each of these provided Macchiano with their time and encouragement to pursue her first formal leadership role in a management position. Most recently, she has served as co-chair for an organization wide cost reduction tiger team and as the chair for a medical visiting scholar program. She is also a member of American Organization of Nurse Executives, the Massachusetts Organization of Nurse Executives, and Sigma Theta Tau International.

Darlene MacKinnon, RN, BScN, MHA

Darlene MacKinnon is director of Clinical and Non Clinical Programs, Providence Legacy Projects, Providence Health Care. Prior to this, she spent several years in management positions in geriatric medicine/rehabilitation, family practice, ambulatory, and residential care. She also held positions in professional practice and quality improvement. She completed her BScN from Dalhousie University in Halifax, Nova Scotia and a master's in health administration from the University of British Columbia. She received certificates in critical care nursing and post anesthesia recovery nursing from the British Columbia Institute of Technology. Her clinical work included adult and pediatric cardiac surgery and step-down, adult ICU and Recovery Room and Cardiac Rehabilitation.

Karin Maechler

Karin Maechler received her nursing diploma in Switzerland, where she was born. Five years ago, she came to Germany and became a head nurse of a medical ward in the Protestant hospital Diakonisches Krankenhaus in Dresden, Germany. As a part-time student, she studies nursing science and nursing administration at the Protestant University of Applied Science in Dresden. Maechler introduced primary nursing to her team members and provides lectures about aromatherapy in nursing.

Kathy Malloch, PhD, MBA, RN, FAAN

Kathy Malloch is a recognized expert in leadership and the development of effective evidence-based processes and systems for patient care. She serves the health care community as a consultant, educator, and regulator. She has published five textbooks on leadership with Tim Porter-O'Grady. She served as the first program director for the Arizona State University, College of Nursing, masters in healthcare innovation program, an innovative, multidisciplinary leadership program. Currently, she is in her fourth term as president of the Arizona State Board of Nursing. At the national level, she co-created the Taxonomy of Error Root Cause Analysis Protocol (TER-CAP) with the National Council of State Boards of Nursing, a seminal contribution to the national error management effort. Most recently, Malloch assumed a clinical consultant role with API Healthcare, Inc., in Hartford, Wisconsin, to facilitate the implementation of a patient classification system.

Diane J. Mancino, EdD, RN, CAE

Diane J. Mancino serves as the executive director of the National Student Nurses Association (NSNA) and the Foundation of the NSNA. Her formal education includes a doctorate in nursing education from Teachers College Columbia University, New York; a master's of arts, New York University; and a bachelor's of science in nursing, State University of New York at Buffalo, New York. Mancino's doctoral dissertation, "The Role of the National Student Nurses' Association in Addressing Social and Political

Issues that Contributed to Student Unrest from 1960-1975," traced student and civil rights movements in nursing. She is executive producer of several award-winning videos including two documentaries: "To Advance We Must Unite! 100 Years of the American Nurses' Association 1896-1996," and "Not for Ourselves but for Others: 50 Year History of the National Student Nurses Association 1952-2002." The most recent video release, "Nursing—the Career of a Lifetime," inspires all nurses to advance their careers through formal education, credentialing, and involvement in professional organizations.

Mellon Nsingu Manyonga-Jordan, MSc, BA, RN

Mellon Nsingu Manyonga-Jordan, is considered a change agent and is passionate about issues of justice, fair play, inequality, and alleviating human suffering at every level in whatever form it presents itself. Her philosophy is to "do unto others as I would want them to do unto me." This passion led her to the noble profession of nursing as a second career. In 2004 to 2007, she undertook general nursing studies at the Barbados Community College, and was subsequently awarded an associate degree in general nursing. In June 2008 she became a registered nurse on the surgical ward, Queen Elizabeth Hospital, Barbados. Manyonga-Jordan is passionate about making a difference in Nursing.

Pamela Maraldo, PhD, RN

Pamela Maraldo is currently serving as executive director of Girls Inc. of New York City. She is also managing partner of PJM Associates, a strategy consulting company. Maraldo has consulted across the gamut of health care concerns, as well as several not-for-profits, including the National Cancer Institute, the NYC Health Department, several of the nation's pharmaceutical companies, integrated health systems and national membership organizations. Prior to establishing PJM Associates, Maraldo served as chief executive officer of two national organizations, Planned Parenthood Federation of America and The National League for Nursing, for which she led financial revitalizations, created strong marketing capabilities, and provided strategic direction in the public policy arena. She is a fellow in the American Academy of Nursing, as well as the New York Academy of Medicine. Maraldo serves on several boards of directors and is a frequent speaker and writer on a wide range of health care topics, including health policy issues, women's health, and the mind body connection.

Christina (Tina) Marczak, MSN, RN

Christina (Tina) Marczak is a registered nurse at the Hospital of the University of Pennsylvania in Philadelphia, Pennsylvania. She began her professional career in 1993. After two years of medical-surgical nursing, Tina shifted her focus to women's health and has practiced since 1995 in labor and delivery. During her tenure, she has served as childbirth educator, lactation consultant, fetal monitoring instructor, and nurse manager. In addition, Tina is certified in basic ultrasound, microscopy, and pelvic exams. Tina received her bachelor's of science in nursing from Villanova University in 1993, and her master's of science in nursing in 2009 from the University of Phoenix.

Nada Massode, BSN

Nada Massode is infection control coordinator for the Security Forces Hospital Program, Riyadh, Kingdom of Saudi Arabia. She specialized in infection control. She has 10 years nursing experience. She is a member of the Nursing Scientific Board at Saudi Commission for Health Specialist since 2004.

Penelope Minor, RN, BScN, MN

Penelope Minor is a manager of the Professional Practice Leader of Nursing program at Baycrest Geriatric Health Care System in Toronto, Canada, where she has worked for nearly nine years in a variety of leadership roles. These roles include unit director and clinical nurse specialist in gerontology with a specialty in working with individuals who suffer from dementia and related behaviours. She also holds a clinical appointment at the University of Toronto. Minor graduated from Lakehead University with a bachelor's of science in nursing and an interdisciplinary minor in gerontology from the Northern Educational Centre for Aging and Health in 1999, and a master's of nursing for the University of Toronto in 2003. Her particular interests, focus in the area of late life mental health, nursing leadership, and implementation of best practices in the care of the elderly.

Maria Mischo-Kelling

Maria Mischo-Kelling is a nurse with 15 years experience and is a doctoral candidate. Director in Hamburg, Germany, and now in Bozen, Italy, Mischo-Kelling is a well known author and has published books about primary nursing, nursing theory, nursing process, and two standard works about medical and surgical nursing. She offers lectures at various universities in Germany and does leadership coaching with CEOs in health care. Sanitaetsbetrieb Suedtirol is a large health care organization in the Health District of Bozen, Italy, with more than 2,000 employees where Mischo-Kelling, in her position as chief nursing officer, introduced a major changing process in staff development, by implementing primary nursing.

Cristina Satoko Mizoi, MSN, RN

Cristina Satoko Mizoi is a registered nurse who graduated at the Universidade de São Paulo. In 1988, she was hired at the Hospital Albert Einstein to work in an adult intensive care unit. In 1996, she was invited to work in a continuing education department, responsible for training the nursing team. In 2000, she was invited to be a member of the Shared Governance Group as a clinical nurse specialist. In 2004, she finished the master's degree course in adult health for the Universidade de São Paulo. In 2005, she started to work at the Albert Einstein Institute of Education and Research as coordinator of training, responsible for training for all the multi-professional team. She was working with new education strategy such as virtual education and simulation. Today, she is a manager of training, and she is also responsible for the Albert Einstein Realistic Simulation Center.

Kristine Mohr, MSN, RN

Kristine Mohr has held a number of professional roles in nursing, including a variety of direct-care experiences, house supervision, and patient care manager at Aurora Sinai Medical Center in Milwaukie, Wisconsin. As a direct care nurse, Mohr assumed the role of shared governance president for system shared governance structure representing Aurora Health Care's 6,000 nurses. She earned her master's of science in nursing in healthcare systems leadership from Marquette University in Milwaukee, Wisconsin, and is a member of Sigma Theta Tau International. She received her BSN from the University of Wisconsin-Oshkosh, in Oshkosh, Wisconsin.

Tshepo Rothi Monau, PhD, MS, BSc

Tshepo Rothi Monau has been a lecturer of pathophysiology and physiology with the School of Nursing, University of Botswana, since 2002. He specialized in physiology with an emphasis on the disease process. Research projects focus on perinatal adaptation to stress. He did his bachelor's degree in Botswana. He received his master's of science and doctoral degrees in California.

Wilson Cañon Montañez

Wilson Cañon Montañez is assistant professor of the nursing program of the University of Santander in Colombia. Montañez is a critical care nurse who has specialised in cardiology and shares his professional time in clinical practice, research, and epidemiology studies. Montañez is a founding member of the Colombian Committee of Critical Care Nurses (CECC-ANEC), since 2007, and a founding member of the Latin American Federation of Intensive Care Nurses (FLECI) in Lima, Peru, since 2006. In 2007, Montañez self funded a study program to live in Australia and learn English as well as develop his knowledge and understanding of health care systems and clinical practices and protocols. He is currently completing a master's degree in epidemiology and has published and presented his work in both English and Spanish.

Gladys Mouro, MSN, RN

Gladys Mouro is the chief nurse executive of the American University of Beirut Medical Center (AUBMC) in Lebanon. Mouro spearheaded the journey to Magnet excellence for the past six years, and in June 2009, AUBMC achieved Magnet designation—the first Magnet facility in the Middle East .AUBMC was also the first hospital to become an ANCC provider for continuing education in the Middle East. She initiated the first shared governance structure in the hospital in Lebanon, and she and her team initiated a study on shared governance using the Hess tool to determine the perception of shared governance among nurses in Lebanon and the region. This is an ongoing study that will identify the learning needs to create a shared governance environment and help improve patient

outcomes .AUBMC is a story of persistence and survival against all odds that begins from the inception of the civil war described in Mouro's book, An American Nurse Amidst all Chaos. Mouro insists that shared governance helps improve an environment toward better outcomes in spite of all the obstacles a facility can encounter.

Maria Munteanu

Maria Munteanu was born in a Galeshti village, Straseni region, Republic of Moldova. She graduated from the City Medical School in Chisinau. She began her professional activity at Nr.1 Municipal Clinical Hospital as nurse in the Intensive Therapy and Reanimation ward. From 1998, she was engaged as a teacher nurse at Family Medicine Department of Nicolae Testemitanu State University where she works; she is also the national trainer in education for health and home care. She attends a significant number of professional courses and seminars to improve herself as a nurse. She has elaborated works, such as the curriculum "Tuberculosis Control at Primary Medical Assistance Level" and "Reintegration of Old People in Society in Republic of Moldova." She is an honoured member of the Nursing Association of Republic of Moldova.

N

Susan Nardelli, RN, BSN, MSN/MHA

Susan Nardelli is a graduate from New England Baptist School of Nursing and continues to strive towards nursing excellence. She has a strong cardiac background in the acute care setting as well as home care and long-term care venues. Nardelli's passion is empowering clinicians to achieve a healthy work environment using ongoing learning. As a graduate from Daniel Webster College in Nashua, New Hampshire, she learned the value of seeking the business perspective in health care and being proactive with business changes. This perspective is invaluable as Nardelli achieved her BSN from Regis College in Weston, Massachusetts, and is a candidate for her MSN/MHA from the University of Phoenix. As director of Clinical Services, she is fortunate to be able to strengthen the nursing workforce using education to empower and to develop nurses' innate talents toward a high-reliability, collaborative, cost-effective, and safe environment for all.

Merav Ben Natan, PhD, RN

Merav Ben Natan is with the department of Nursing, Tel Aviv University, and has been since 1994. She specialized in nursing education and women's health, focusing on the geriatric field. Her research projects relate to elder abuse in institutions. She was educated in the Tel Hashomer School of Nursing and at the Department of Nursing, Tel Aviv University. She received her master's in nursing from the Department of Nursing, Tel Aviv University, followed by her PhD from Haifa University in Israel. She is working as a nurse educator at the Pat Matthews Academic School of Nursing, Hillel-Yaffe, Hadera, and serves as an instructor at the Department of Nursing School of Health Professions, Tel Aviv University.

Gladys Navarro

Gladys Navarro has been a nurse for 20 years with experience in medicine, surgery, maternity, geriatrics, hospice, and home care. Her primary focus is on geriatrics, extended care, and nursing administration. Navarro completed a master's in nursing administration at the University of Puerto Rico–Medical Science Campus in 2004. Her primary work is as associate chief nurse for Geriatrics and Extended Care at Veterans Administration Caribbean Health System. She provides executive leadership and assumes continuing and substantial responsibility for the coordination and evaluation of integrated programs that cross service and discipline lines. This role allows her to influence organizational mission, vision, values, and strategic priorities. She has a passion for organizational health, and this has led her to continue her professional growth through structured trainings regarding leadership. Navarro has received several awards for her outstanding contribution to education service.

Shabnam Noordin, RN, MSN

Shabnam Noordin is a registered nurse and clinical information analyst at Advocate Lutheran General Hospital, located in Park Ridge, Illinois. She received her bachelor's and master's (health systems management) of science degrees in nursing from Loyola University Chicago. Noordin's nursing background is in medical and cardiac intensive care. In her current role as a clinical information analyst, she participates in and leads informatics development projects related to the electronic health record; recommends plans of action; develops and maintains policies and procedures; communicates and trains department and hospital associates; and provides analytical, process, and problem resolution services. In 2006, Noordin was one of the 12 Advocate health care employees whose work was featured in an Advocate Healthcare campaign, in partnership with the local CBS network affiliate, to raise awareness of Advocate's highly skilled nursing professionals. Noordin is currently pursuing her certification in healthcare informatics.

Sharon Strutz Norton, RN, MSN

Sharon Strutz Norton, a lifelong Alaskan of Inupiaq Eskimo descent, is an independent contractor with the University of Fairbanks, Center for Alaska Native Health Research. Additionally, she has years of experience in acute care and as adjunct nurse faculty. Norton is an examination and skills testing administrator for the Alaska Board of Nursing. She is project director, completing the development and design of a web based interactive nurse suicide prevention course and informational website at www.akln.org. Norton received her associate's degree in nursing (ADN) at Anchorage Community College in Alaska and her bachelor's (BSN) and master's of science in nursing (MSN) degrees through the University of Phoenix. Currently, she is working toward earning her master's in suicidology through Griffith University in Sydney, Australia. Norton was honored to receive the Arctic Education Foundation Anagi Leadership Award for 2008, which will support her PhD and or DNP program of choice.

Liana Orsolini-Hain, PhD, RN

Liana Orsolini-Hain earned her PhD in nursing from the University of California, San Francisco. She has researched the influences on associate degree nurses who have not returned to school to pursue a more advanced degree in nursing. She served as a co-chair for the California Institute for Nursing and

Health Care's White Paper on Nursing Education Redesign for California's committee on nursing collaborative education models. She is currently working full-time as a nursing instructor for City College of San Francisco and is the coordinator of their California Community College Chancellor's grant on ADN-to-BSN and ADN-to-MSN Education Collaborative Model. She is also serving as the president of the California League for Nursing.

P

Paula Payne, RN, BSN

Paula Payne is a clinical practice manager for the Clinical Practice Model (CPM) Resource Center (CPMRC), a business unit of Elsevier. Her clinical background is in trauma, orthopedics, and spinal, where she practiced as a staff and charge nurse. Payne transitioned to a project manager position in a health care information technology company in 2004. Currently at the CPM Resource Center, she assists interdisciplinary teams within health care organizations to create healthy work cultures and advance clinical care with the CPM framework and Practice Transformation Services. These services include advancement of clinical partnerships, dialogue, evidence-based practice, partnership council development (shared governance), scope of practice, and clinical tools and technology. Payne brings great passion for working as an integrated team and the powerful difference this makes to transforming patient care. She has first-hand experience in advancing the engagement of staff and leadership as a member of the CPMRC Partnership Council, which is the shared governance structure for the CPM Resource center. In this effort, she has been instrumental in leading design and development of the CPM knowledge repository and team collaboration efforts.

Margarita Peya, RN, MMANS, MHCR

Margarita Peya received her nursing diploma at Nursing School University of Barcelona and did further work in paediatric nursing, occupational nursing, primary health care, and nursing management. She received her master's in administration and management in nursing services in 2005 from the University of Barcelona and her master's in research of

care from the University Compluyense of Madrid in 2007. Gascons has been a professor at the School of Nursing of the University of Barcelona since 1993. From 2005 to 2008, she was the president of the National Conference of Directors of Schools of Nursing in Spain. She is extensively published and is a well respected nurse leader in her country.

Gilda Pelusi, PhD, MS, RN

Gilda Pelusi is from Polverigi, Italy, and obtained her RN at the School of Nursing at Teramo in 1988. She eventually went on to the post of chief nurse of the School of Nursing S. Giovanni da Capestrano at Aquila in 1993. Pelusi received her master's (Modelli e Metodi della Tutorship, Laurea Specialistica in Scienze Infermieristiche ed Ostetriche University Politecnica delle Marche faculty of Medicine) cum laude in 2007. Pelusi practiced as a professional nurse at the Hospital of Ancona Azienda Ospedaliero-Universitaria Ospedali Riuniti, from 1989-2000; as chief nurse at the hospital of Ancona Azienda Ospedaliero-Universitaria Ospedali Riuniti, from 2000-2005; and as tutor at the School of Nursing University of Ancona Università Politecnica Regione Marche from 2005 to the present. She was also a teaching professor at the School of Nursing, Master di 1 Livello in Tecniche Manageriali per Coordinatori dell'Assistenza Infermieristica, from 2002-2003, and teaching professor at the School of Nursing University of Ancona, Università Politecnica Regione Marche, from 2007 to present.

Debra Pendergast, MSN, RN, NEA-BC

Debra Pendergast is the chair of the division of nursing services and an associate administrator at Mayo Clinic in Arizona (MCA). MCA is a three-shield (practice, education, research) focused organization that is composed of a 330-physician multi-specialty group practice (the southwestern group practice site of Mayo Clinic in Rochester, Minnesota). This practice includes a 244-bed acute care hospital. As the first chief nursing officer at the Arizona site, Pendergast was responsible for designing, developing, implementing, and integrating the nursing organization more than 10 years ago. She was instrumental in the startup of multiple complex subspecialty clinical programs. She spent 20 years in the Naval Reserve Nurse Corps, holding two national board-selected leadership positions. Pendergast has been the recipient of numerous awards and is an active adjunct faculty member. She was competitively selected as a Robert Wood Johnson Executive Nurse Fellow and is a fellow of the Johnson & Johnson/ Wharton Fellows Program in Management for Nurse Executives from the Wharton School of the University of Pennsylvania.

Gina Peragine, RN, BScN, MN

Gina Peragine is currently a program director at Baycrest Geriatric Health System in Toronto, Canada, where she has worked in progressive leadership positions for the past 10 years. She holds a BScN and master's degree in nursing from the University of Toronto. Her leadership mandate is to promote the integration of care, research, and education in order to enrich the elderly person's quality of life, promote best practice, and enhance the quality of work-life for staff. Her primary responsibilities include leading and managing organizational change and maintaining a dynamic environment that will transform aging and ensure the highest level of care among the residents at Baycrest. Peragine is also clinically cross appointed with the University of Toronto Faculty of Nursing and has published several articles in peer reviewed journals.

Chua Gek Phin, MN, BN, Grad. Dip (Onc), RN

Chua Gek Phin is director of nursing at the National Centre (Singapore) and is a major proponent of safe, evidence-based quality care. She is a World Health Organization fellow who has won three international scholarships since she joined nursing in 1975. Phin is the Singapore Tourism Board Ambassador for Healthcare and an illustrious winner of the National Commendation Medal for distinguished performance, efficiency, and devotion to duty as a nursing leader. In her passionate pursuit of quality improvement, research, and the advancement of oncology nursing, Phin co-chaired the 2008 International Conference on Cancer Nursing and has devoted much of her time to developing nursing talent in Singapore. She is a fellow of the Johnson & Johnson/Wharton Fellows Program in Management for Nurse Executives from the

Wharton School of the University of Pennsylvania.

Tim Porter-O'Grady, DM, EdD, APRN, FAAN

Tim Porter-O'Grady is senior partner for Tim Porter-O'Grady Associates Inc. and associate professor and leadership scholar in the Innovations Program at Arizona State University. He has consulted world-wide on issues of clinical systems, health leadership, shared governance, and organizational transformation. He has written 165 proctored journal articles and 19 books. Porter-O'Grady is known globally for his endless passion and contributions to the practice of nursing and the future of health care.

R

Angie Ramsey, RN, CPN

Angie Ramsey is a certified pediatric nurse and has worked on the pediatric medicine floor for nearly six years. Prior to becoming a nurse, Ramsey worked as a social worker and an emergency medical technician. Currently, she is the chair of the University of North Carolina (UNC) Hospital's Nursing Shared Governance Diversity Council and is enrolled in the RN-MSN program at UNC. Ramsey hopes to one day continue with her passion of working with children and their families as a clinical nurse leader.

Tebogo Rapaeye, BNS, RN

Tebogo Rapaeye is an assistant nursing officer in one of the tertiary hospitals in Botswana. He graduated with a second class first division (2:1) in his bachelor of science in nursing degree in 2007. He is currently pursuing a finance degree part-time with the University of Botswana to enhance his entrepreneurial skills in nursing. He is also interested in research and has been a research assistant for both the qualitative and quantitative research done in the School of Nursing.

James Luther Raper, DSN, CRNP, JD, FAANP

James Luther Raper is a nationally recognized expert in clinical advanced practice nursing policy development and regulation. His clinical and research interest is related to HIV/

AIDS. He is the past president of the Alabama Board of Nursing, serves on the National Council of State Boards of Nursing Advanced Practice Registered Nurse committee and is the president of the American Assembly for Men in Nursing. He has authored or co-authored 40 published manuscripts and 9 book chapters. He is the principle investigator on several Health Resources and Services Administration grants that support the delivery of primary health care to HIV-infected adults. Raper is nationally, regionally and locally involved in a variety of HIV-related projects and associations. He currently serves on the steering committee of the HIV Medicine Association Ryan White Medical Providers Coalition and the Nurse Practitioner Association of Alabama. He is an associate professor of Medicine and Nursing and the director of the 1917 HIV Outpatient, Research, and Dental Clinics at the University of Alabama at Birmingham.

Maria Aurora Rebultan-Suarez, BSN, RN, CCRN

Maria Aurora Rebultan-Suarez has been a registered nurse in California for 12 years. She worked as a critical care nurse for five years before she became the nurse educator at Citrus Valley Medical Center in Covina in 2004. Rebultan-Suarez is an American Association of Critical-Care Nurses (AACN) Certified Critical Care Registered Nurse (CCRN). She received her bachelor of science in nursing at the University of Santo Tomas in Manila, Philippines, and is currently working on her master of science as a clinical nurse specialist at Azusa Pacific University in Azusa, California.

Charles Reed, MSN, RN, CNRN

Charles Reed has served as the patient care coordinator for the Surgical Trauma Intensive Care Unit for University Hospital in San Antonio, Texas, since 1998. He is co-chair of the Nursing Research Committee and is active in the study of glycemic control, patient communication, and pressure ulcers. He has been the principal investigator or co-investigator on several glycemic research studies. His work on tight glycemic control and reduction in ICU mortality was published in 2007 in the Journal of the American College of Surgeons. He has presented his work on glycemic control at the Society of Critical Care Medicine (SCCM) Congress, the American Association of Critical

Care Nurses National Teaching Institute, and the American Association for Clinical Chemistry Conference. In 2008, he won the SCCM Administrative Award for "Improving Tight Glycemic Control With the Adjunct Use of a Data Management Software Program."

Jennifer Reich, MA, MS, RN, ANP-BC, ACHPN

Jennifer Reich is an adult nurse practitioner certified in hospice and palliative care. Currently, she is a doctoral student and graduate research associate at the University of Arizona College of Nursing, as well as a National Center for Complementary and Alternative Medicine Fellow in the Arizona Complementary and Alternative Medicine Training Program in the Department of Family and Community Medicine at The University of Arizona. Her background includes degrees in exercise science, English, and theatre. She has training and practice in mind-body stress reduction, Reiki, health appraisal, and meditation. She uses this diverse experience to design wellness programs and teach self-care strategies to nurses throughout the country. Her passion is exploring healing through poetry, story, and reflection.

Carol Reineck, PhD, FAAN, NEA-BC

Carol Reineck is chair and associate professor of the Department of Acute Nursing Care and the Amy Shelton and V.H. McNutt Professor, University of Texas Health Science Center (UTHSCSA). She graduated from the Intercollegiate Center for Nursing Education (BSN), Pepperdine University (MAEd), UTHSCSA (MSN), and the University of Maryland at Baltimore (PhD). Rising from private to colonel, from nurse manager to nurse executive, Reineck transitioned from 31 years of military service. Her final military position was chief nurse executive, U.S. Army Medical Command world-wide. She is a fellow of the Johnson & Johnson/Wharton Fellows Program in Management for Nurse Executives from the Wharton School of the University of Pennsylvania and is a fellow of the American Academy of Nursing. Reineck is an advocate for linking nursing education with practice and she was principal investigator on a study that resolved the heparin-saline debate and directed congressional studies on readiness.

Victoria L. Rich, PhD, RN, FAAN

Victoria L. Rich is the chief nurse executive for the University of Pennsylvania Medical Center, associate executive director for the Hospital of the University of Pennsylvania, and associate professor for nursing administration for the University of Pennsylvania School of Nursing. Rich is recognized for her leadership in health care, business, and nursing education. She is most known for her pioneering work in patient safety and cultural diversity. She has developed numerous patient safety initiatives for health care systems both nationally and internationally. Her experiential knowledge allowed her to develop a model for creating a risk reduction culture in health care through the process of systemic mindfulness. She is an acknowledged expert in root cause analysis and in the development of corrective action plans for hospitals and state and federal agencies. Since 1997, Rich has provided nationwide consultation to provide expert witness and testimony in malpractice cases involving nursing care. A cofounder of Rich and Rich Consultants, her expertise is sought by health care executives world-wide to improve programs and initiatives for patient safety.

Joy Richards, RN, BScN, MN, PhD

Joy Richards is vice president of Collaborative Practice and Quality and chief nursing executive at Baycrest Geriatric Health Care System in Toronto, Canada. She is also the president of the Academy of Canadian Executive Nurses and holds clinical appointments at the University of Toronto Faculty of Nursing, York University Faculty of Nursing, and Humber College. Richards graduated from the University of Toronto with a bachelor's of science in nursing in 1981 and a master's degree in nursing in 2000. She holds a master's of arts in human and organizational systems and a PhD in human and organizational development from Fielding Graduate University in Santa Barbara, California. She is also a graduate of the Queen's University Executive Program and is a fellow of the Johnson & Johnson/Wharton Fellows Program in Management for Nurse Executives from the Wharton School of the University of Pennsylvania. Her dissertation focused on exploring and understanding the development and practice of feminine courage in leadership.

Kim Richards, RN

Kim Richards has almost 20 years of experience in the nursing management and recruitment industry. She was hired by the Association of Perioperative Nurses (AORN) to evaluate and re-launch their interim management and consultation department. As the general manager of AORN Management Solutions, Richards led the business to significant growth through targeted marketing, development of strategic partnerships, and relationship building. After three years, she left AORN to restart her own executive search firm, Kim Richards and Associates, Inc., which specializes in national recruitment of top nursing talent. The company has been successful in providing interim, permanent, and consultative services for hospitals around the country. As a nurse and an executive recruiter, Richards became increasingly aware of the "revolving door" of nurses in acute care facilities. After participating in nursing conferences and interviewing hundreds of nurses, a common theme clearly emerged to her: Nurses were expressing signs and symptoms of compassion fatigue, a debilitating phenomenon caused by years of built up emotional residue. By combining her nursing, business, and extensive fitness background, Richards created the components of NurseFit®, the first comprehensive program dedicated to improving retention of engaged nurses by addressing their unique mental, emotional, and physical needs.

Phil Robertson

Phil Robertson qualified as a registered mental health nurse in 1982. Following qualification, he worked in a range of clinical roles in acute psychiatry for eight years. In 1990, he moved into a management post and played a significant role in the closure of a large institution in the North East of England. During the 1990s, he worked in a range of clinical management roles in the North East which included mental health, learning disability, drug and alcohol, district nursing, health visiting, and child protection services. In 2001, he was appointed as director of Mental Health in North Cumbria, prior to taking up the post of director of Nursing. Robertson's special interests include user/carer involvement and Total Quality Management development.

Catherine Robinson-Walker, MBA

Catherine Robinson-Walker is president of The Leadership Studio, an Oakland, California firm that has specialized in coaching nursing leaders and their teams since 2000. Robinson-Walker has extensive health care executive experience—she is a trained and seasoned executive coach, consultant, training facilitator, speaker, and author. In the 1980s she co-created and directed the Institute for Patient Care Executives, a week long national program for nurse leaders sponsored by 15 universities and held annually at the University of California, Berkeley. In 1985, Robinson-Walker was invited to launch the leadership program that led to the construction of the Florence Nightingale Museum of Nursing in London. In the mid-1990s, she directed the development and delivery of that program's replacement, the Center for Nursing Leadership, a joint venture with the American Organization of Nurse Executives. She has received considerable recognition throughout her career, including being named the "2006 Friend of Nursing" by the Association of California Nurse Leaders and "Woman of the Year" by Women Healthcare Executives of Northern California. Robinson-Walker's book, Women and Leadership in Health Care: The Journey to Authenticity and Power, is a Jossey-Bass health series bestseller. She is the author of "The Coaching Forum," an ongoing column published in Nurse Leader, the official journal of the American Organization of Nurse Executives/American Hospital Association.

S

Lourdes Casao Salandanan, MSN, RN-BC, FNP

Lourdes Casao Salandanan is director of the education department at Citrus Valley Medical Center in Covina, California, where she is responsible for corporate wide strategic planning, implementation, and evaluation of staff development and competency. Her projects focus on the development of a pipeline of well-prepared clinical nurses. She plans to extend the pipeline to nurse educators and nurse leaders. Salandanan earned her bachelor's degree in nursing at the University of the Philippines College of Nursing in Manila and her master's degree in nursing as a family nurse practitioner at Azusa Pacific University, in Azusa, California. She is the president of the Iota Sigma Chapter of Sigma Theta Tau International (STTI) and has recently been selected as STTI's international ambassador to the Philippines.

Marla E. Salmon, ScD, RN, FAAN

Marla E. Salmon is the Robert G. and Jean A. Reid Endowed Dean in Nursing and professor in the School of Nursing at the University of Washington (UW). She is also a professor in UW's Department of Global Health. Past experiences include directing the Division of Nursing for the U.S. Department of Health and Human Services, chairing the Global Advisory Group on Nursing and Midwifery for The World Health Organization, the National Advisory Committee on Nursing Education and Practice, serving on the White House Taskforce on Healthcare Reform, and as a delegate to the World Health Assembly. She founded and directed The Lillian Carter Center for International Nursing, is a director on the Robert Wood Johnson Foundation Board of Trustees, is a member of the National Advisory Council for Nursing Research, and is a director for the Institute for the International Education of Students (IES). Salmon's scholarship is focused on global and domestic health workforce policy and leadership. She consults with governments as well as regional and global organizations.

Leticia San Martín-Rodríguez, PhD, MSc, RN

Leticia San Martín-Rodríguez has a master's in nursing administration and a PhD in nursing from the University of Montreal, Canada. She graduated as a nurse from the University of Navarre and is a nurse manager at the Nursing Development Area at Clínica Universidad de Navarra, in Pamplona, Spain. She is also an associate professor at the University Of Navarra School Of Nursing. She worked for four years as a staff nurse in a medical unit. She is a member of the Consultative Committee of the Nursing Research Coordination and Development Unit (Ministry of Health), and is a member of the committee for allocation of health research funding of Carlos III Health Institute. San Martin-Rodriguez is a journal reviewer for

Evidence Based Nursing (Spanish edition) and Enfermería Clínica. Her research field is the organization of health services and inter-professional collaboration, and she has several publications related to these topics. She has benefited from several grants and awards related to her area of research and expertise.

Jenna Sanders

Jenna Sanders is a recent BSN graduate of the University of Saint Francis, in Fort Wayne, Indiana. Sanders spent three-and-a-half years of her undergraduate education involved in the local, state, and national levels of the National Student Nurses Association (NSNA). Her participation culminated with a year as president of the NSNA (2008-2009). Sander's experiences through NSNA opened up a world of opportunities and ignited her passion for health policy work. She is now pursuing a master's in nursing business and health systems with a health policy focus at the University of Michigan in Ann Arbor, Michigan.

Julita Sansoni, RN, MNS

Julita Sansoni holds the position of associate professor at the University La Sapienza in Rome, Italy. She holds a Dr. (doctor in pedagogy, post doctor education in adult education-1e2) and has held numerous leadership positions in abilitation, neurology, and neurosurgery. She is involved with ongoing doctoral studies (PhD) in Nursing Science Universita di Tampere (Finlandia). She is the author of numerous books and publications as well as scientific presentations at national and international conferences. The involvement of Sansoni for the development of nursing science and discipline is constant, and her engagement has been quite significant in her country. She is propelling and sustaining nursing development through education and political involvement in Italy.

Katherine Scarlett, BSN

Katherine Scarlett graduated in 2009 with her bachelor's of nursing from Charles Darwin University, Darwin, Australia. Prior to commencing nursing studies, Scarlett worked as a patient care attendant and has continued to work as a ward clerk at Royal Darwin Hospital while studying full time to be a registered nurse. She is the eldest daughter of Ged Williams, her mentor.

Nicole M. Schaefer

Nicole M. Schaefer graduated with a bachelor of science in nursing from Wright State University (Dayton, Ohio) in 1995. Following graduation, she spent two years as a charge nurse in an adult oncology unit at Miami Valley Hospital in Dayton, Ohio. She then went to Cincinnati Children's Hospital Medical Center and spent seven years working in the pediatric bone marrow transplant, hematology/oncology, and blood diseases unit. She also spent time working in the post anesthesia care unit. She spent much of that time as a charge nurse or a preceptor for new grads and nursing students. She developed a program for orientation to pediatric bone marrow transplant, was chair of the research council, guest lectured on pain, sickle cell anemia, and immune deficiency patient care management, and participated in the development and expansion of a new pediatric cancer center at Cincinnati Children's. Schaefer has been working at Stanford University's Lucile Packard Children's Hospital since 2004 as a nurse manager in the pediatric cancer center and as a staff nurse in the post anesthesia care unit/ perioperative area. She received her master's of science in nursing administration from San Francisco State University in 2009. She has received numerous recognition awards which have included the Cincinnati Tri-State area Florence Nightingale award and two hospital-wide outstanding nurse practice awards. She is an active member of the Association of California Nurse Leaders and The Association of Pediatric Hematology and Oncology Nursing. While in Cincinnati, she was one of the four primary nurses involved in the four-year process of the filming of "A Lion in the House," a PBS documentary on families dealing with acutely ill children.

Naomi Mmapelo Seboni, PhD, RN, RM

Naomi Mmapelo Seboni is the head of the School of Nursing in the Faculty of Health Sciences at the University of Botswana. She is also a director of the World Health Organization (WHO) Collaborating Centre for Nursing and Midwifery Development for the WHO African Region. She completed her bachelor's degree in nursing at the University of Botswana, her master's degree at Colombia University, and her PhD at the University of California, San Francisco. Her research and publications focus on adolescent sexual heath and rights, adolescent sexual risk behaviors, and HIV and AIDS. She teaches adolescent health and development, adult health, research, and nursing theory. Seboni has served as the president of Botswana Family Welfare Association (BOFWA), an International Planned Parenthood Federation (IPPF) affiliate; of the Nurses Association of Botswana; and of the Tau Lambda-at-Large chapter of Sigma Theta Tau International. Currently she serves as the honorary treasurer of IPPF.

Esther Salang Seloilwe, PhD, RN, RM

Esther Salang Seloilwe obtained a diploma in general nursing and midwifery in 1975 and 1976 from the then National Health Institute, Gaborone; a bachelor's of education from the University of Botswana and Swaziland in 1982; a master's and PhD from the University of California, San Francisco, in 1985 and 1997, respectively, specializing in mental health. She joined the University of Botswana as a staff development fellow in 1982 and became a full professor/lecturer in 1985 in the Department of Nursing Education. She was appointed head of the Department of Nursing Education for six years and currently is HIV and AIDS Coordinator for the University of Botswana and founding chair for the Centre for the study of HIV and AIDS. Seloilwe's area of research focuses on family care giving of mentally ill persons and HIV/AIDS. She also publishes on nursing issues, particularly regulation.

Franklin A. Shaffer, EdD, RN, FAAN

Franklin A. Shaffer is the executive vice president of Cross Country Healthcare and chief nursing officer of Cross Country Staffing in Boca Raton, Florida. He is the founder of Cross Country University and continues to serve as the chief learning officer, integrating learning and achievement of the enterprise's mission. He is responsible for developing standards, methods, and programs for ensuring Cross Country's health care professionals meet professional and regulatory agency requirements while providing career enhancement opportunities and collaborative arrangements with learning partners. He earned his doctorate in nursing administration and nursing education from Columbia University, New York. Shaffer was awarded an honorary doctorate of science for his contributions

at Cedar Crest College, Pennsylvania. He has authored or edited six books, as well as numerous chapters, and serves on several leading professional journal editorial boards. He has 40 years of progressive and varied nursing experience including administration, education, clinical, and research. Shaffer is the co-chair of the American Academy of Nursing's public relations and communications committee. He is a frequent speaker at domestic conferences and conventions. He has provided consultation and lectured in the Netherlands, the United Kingdom, Germany, Brazil, Japan, and Korea. He is a fellow of the American Academy of Nursing and is a recipient of the most distinguished R. Louise McManus Medal from Columbia University for his contributions to the profession.

Jesmond Sharples, MBA, M.Mus. (Comp.) (Lond.), BSc (Hons) (Nursing), Dip. Ger., FLCM

Jesmond Sharples is from Rabat, Malta. He qualified as a state registered nurse in 1988. Sharples worked in various settings and disciplines with the health care setting. He was appointed nursing officer in 1999 and was registrar to the Council for Nurses and Midwives (2000-2002). Since 2002, Sharples has occupied the position of director of Nursing Services. He attended various local and international scholarly events, some of which he was invited to as an expert speaker. In 2008, when the Department of Nursing Services Standards was originated, Sharples was given the responsibility to set up the department within the Public Health Regulation Division for the drafting of care standards and implementation and monitoring thereof.

Rose Sherman, EdD, RN, NEA-BC

Rose Sherman is the director of the Nursing Leadership Institute in the Florida Atlantic University (FAU) Christine E. Lynn College of Nursing where she is also an associate professor and program director of the Nursing Administration and new Clinical Nurse Leader tracks in the graduate nursing program. Prior to joining the faculty at FAU, Sherman had a 25 year nursing leadership career with the Department of Veterans Affairs. Her work has been published in Nurse Leader, Nursing Administration Quarterly, Leadership in Health Services, American Nurse Today, Journal of Nursing Administration, Journal of Nursing Education, Nursing Management, Online Journal of Nursing Issues, and Nursing Economics. In 2005, she was named Florida Nurse Leader of the Year by the Florida Organization of Nurse Executives for the work that she has done in the state to develop nursing leaders. In 2006, she was one of 20 nursing leaders nationally selected for a three-year Robert Wood Johnson Nurse Executive Fellowship.

Jean Shinners PhD, MSN, RN, CCRN

Jean Shinners has served as director for Collaborative Learning at Cross Country University since October 2004. In this role, she is responsible for assessing and maintaining competency and fostering professional growth of health care professionals by providing opportunities for career development and life long learning. Prior to joining Cross Country Healthcare, Shinners spent many years in the nursing world as a care provider (specializing in adult critical care and emergency department), an educator, and in various management positions. She continues to practice bedside nursing in the cardiovascular intensive care unit (CVICU) at Martin Memorial Health Center in Stuart, Florida. Shinners is active in professional organizations such as the American Association of Critical Care Nurses, as a continuing education panel review member, and is on the CCRN Exam Development Committee and is an appraiser and Accreditation Review Committee (ARC) member for the American Nurses Credentialing Center.

Laurie Shiparski, RN, BSN, MS

Laurie Shiparski is president of Edgework Institute, Inc., an organization dedicated to working with people to move through transitions and re-energize their work and lives. She has more than 30 years experience in health care, including critical care, hospital management, executive, consultant, and corporate business executive in a health care technology company. This includes experience at the CPM Resource Center in Grand Rapids, Michigan, where she supported health care organizations in advancing; staff engagement, interdisciplinary care, evidence-based practice, and automated clinical documentation. She is currently offering leadership and staff coaching, education, and consulting services through the Edgework Institute. Shiparski also shares expertise through her books, articles, workshops, and speaking engagements. She has authored numerous articles and books, including Change is Life, Riding the Waves of Change, Turning Points, Alive With Passion, and a poetry/music CD. She co-authored Can the Human Being Thrive in the Workplace and The Partnership Council Field Book.

Dragica Šimunec, RN

Dragica Šimunec is registered nurse and currently president of the Croatian Nursing Council, the self regulatory body for nursing in the Republic of Croatia. She has 20 years of experience as a surgical and cardiology nurse. She has worked as a nurse in the United Kingdom and Australia. For 10 years, she has held the position as Government Nurse at the Ministry of Health. In 1992, she was the founder of the Croatian Nursing Association and Editor in Chief of the affiliated Nursing Magazine. She also worked with the World Health Organization, the International Council of Nurses, and at present she is a board member of the European Council of Nursing Regulators.

Hiliary Siurna, RN, BSN, MSNc

Hiliary Siurna, BSN, RN, is a nursing practice leader at Toronto East General Hospital in Toronto, Ontario. She is currently pursuing her primary health care nurse practitioner master's of nursing degree at York University, Toronto, Ontario. Siurna has a range of clinical experiences across the lifespan. She began her nursing career as a perinatal nurse and is currently developing a program to enhance care of older adults hospital-wide as part of an interdisciplinary team. It is through this work and her work on the hospital's evidence-based falls prevention program that she learned the valuable impact of interdisciplinary partnerships. She received her undergraduate education at the University of Toronto and also holds a degree in life sciences from Queen's University, Kingston, Ontario, Canada.

Arna Skúladóttir, MS, BSN, RN

Arna Skúladóttir is a clinical nurse specialist, paediatric unit in Landspítala at the University Hospital, Iceland. She leads services for families with children with sleep problems. Her research activities are focused on testing interventions for children's' sleep problems and the well-being of their parents and, on evaluation, of an educational program for families with a child discharged from the NICU and maternity ward. She was educated in nursing in Iceland and received a BS and an MS degree from the University of Iceland, Faculty of Nursing. She has worked as paediatric nurse since 1978; for six years in a rural area of the country and for 21 years with the Landspítala University Hospital. She holds a post of clinical assistant professor and is a licensed advanced practice nurse in the management of children's sleep problems.

Kimberly Slaikeu, PhD, RN, APRN-BC

Kimberly Slaikeu is the chief executive officer and founder of Relevan, LLC, a consulting company committed to tangible transformation of clinical microsystems—where the patient and health care provider meet. With 14 years of nursing experience, she has served in several leadership roles, including director of nursing practice and magnet coordinator for Saint Mary's Health Care (Grand Rapids, Michigan), adult nurse practitioner, assistant professor, and various mid-level management roles. The diversification of her professional experience has led to the development of several areas of expertise, including the design and implementation of outcome-based onboarding (orientation) programs for mid-level health care leaders, the translation of evidence-based practice to the bedside, care of underserved and minority populations, and the creation and implementation of innovative teaching methods and strategies. She has received numerous awards for her professional practice and leadership throughout the years from state and national organizations. She has a special affection for mentoring youth and young adults.

Carolyn Hope Smeltzer, RN, EdD, FAAN, FACHE

Carolyn Hope Smeltzer from the patient bedside to the executive board room of Advocate Healthcare, Sister of Charity of Leavenworth Health System, Council of Regents, Loyola University Chicago, and the Journal of Nursing Quality Care, Smeltzer has enjoyed playing a part in all aspects of her nursing career. Her diploma is from Evanston Hospital School of Nursing, her BSN from Purdue University, and her MSN and EdD

from Loyola University Chicago. She has been a vice president for nursing at both the University of Arizona and the University of Chicago. She is currently a partner at PricewaterhouseCoopers. Smeltzer is a national lecturer and author and believes the stories of nurses have to be told. She has co authored two award winning books focused on nurse's stories: Ordinary People, Extraordinary Lives, the Stories of Nurses and the Chicago Nurse Parade.

Susan Smith, DBA, MBA, BSc Hons, RN, RM, RHV, FWT

Susan Smith has 38 years experience in health and social care in the United Kingdom. Her experience includes roles as nurse, clinical leader, midwife, health visitor, manager, director and latterly academic with the University of Leeds. She led one of the largest leadership programmes offered to front line staff in the National Health Service in England called "Leading and Empowering Organisation." Smith is now director and owner of Choice Dynamic International Private Limited Company. She supports individuals and organisations to increase their choices, through improvement in relationships and individual thinking. Recently, she has written leadership programmes for safeguarding children and articles and book chapters that highlight the importance of effective team working and coaching. Her conference presentations on the subject of leadership and empowerment reflects a scholarly approach to change. She has presented in the United States, Germany, Italy, Cyprus, Austria, England, and Scotland.

Roxane B. Spitzer, PhD, MBA, RN, FAAN

Roxane B. Spitzer is retired from the position of chief executive officer of the Metropolitan Nashville Hospital Authority, which included a university teaching hospital, a 500-bed long term care facility, a clinic for abused children, and multiple primary care and specialty clinics. She earned her PhD in executive management, under the mentorship of Peter Drucker, majoring in strategic management. Her expertise and focus is in strategic management, and she has successful conducted both the process and the content for multiple non-profit organizations and hospitals. She is a management consultant for Executive Service Corps, editor-in-chief of Nurse Leader magazine, and she continues to speak at various seminars on leadership, strategy, and health care finance. She is a fellow of the American Academy of Nursing and served on the boards of the Girl Scouts of Middle Tennessee, the Nashville Opera Association, Alive Hospice, and the Tennessee Hospital Association. Spitzer has been a nursing leader in the United States for numerous years and has influenced the positive progress of the practice of nursing.

Elena Stempovscaia, PhD

Elena Stempovscaia was born in a Zastinca, Soroca, Republic of Moldova. She graduated from School Medicine in Soroca. She began her professional activity at the Republican Clinical Hospital for Children as a nurse in the infant surgeon ward. From 1978, she was transferred to Nr.4 Municipal Clinical Hospital in Chisinau where she still works as chief nurse. She is also a graduate of Ion Creanga State Pedagogical University. In 2001, she asserted her scientific thesis of doctor in psycho-pedagogical sciences. In 2000, she graduated from the International Nursing Institute in the United States. With a teaching degree, she was able to work within the National College of Pharmacy and Medicine, the School of Specialization and Improvement of Middle Medical Personnel, and within the International Management Institute of Health Services and Social Assistance. For Special Virtues in Work, she was mentioned with Honorific title "Civical Merit" and "Eminent of Health Care."

Sandy Summers, RN, MSN, MPH

Sandy Summers is the founder and executive director of The Truth About Nursing, an international not-for-profit organization based in Baltimore, Maryland, that seeks to change how the public thinks about nursing, primarily through more accurate media portrayals of nurses. She is co-author of Saving Lives: Why the Media's Portrayal of Nurses Puts Us All at Risk (Kaplan Publishing). From 2001-2008, she served as executive director of the Center for Nursing Advocacy. In 2002, Summers earned master's degrees in community health nursing and public health from Johns Hopkins University.

T

Renate Tewes, PhD

Renate Tewes is a nurse, diploma psychologist, and leadership coach. As a professor for nursing science and nursing administration, her specialties are nursing theories and nursing research. Her fields of research include responsibility in nursing, leadership competencies, spirituality as a source for nurses, self-concept, and organizational culture in health care. As a coach, Tewes runs her own company, called Crown Coaching Germany, and offers leadership coaching for individuals and groups of leaders in Germany, Switzerland, Austria, and the United Kingdom. She is the author of the book, You Can Learn Leadership Competence with Springer Publishing in Berlin, Germany. Her mission is helping leaders to be successful and happy in decision making, including a well balanced work life.

Anu Thomas, RN, BSN

Anu Thomas is a registered nurse from India with more than five years of experience in health care education and nursing. She has a BSN and is enrolled in the MSN in Administration and Leadership program at the University of Pittsburgh. Thomas started her health care career in India as a nurse and nursing educator, preparing international nurses for U.S. nursing qualifying examinations. Over the past three years, she has been working in Pittsburgh, Pennsylvania, at the University of Pittsburgh Medical Center (UPMC) Presbyterian as an RN in the trauma and general surgery unit. Thomas is a member of the professional practice committee at UPMC Presbyterian, the planning and budget committee at the University of Pittsburgh, and the American Nurses Association. She is a recipient of the Cameos of Caring 2008 Scholarship. In 2003, she was featured on CNN's Lou Dobbs Show as a Nursing Educator for Indian nurses aspiring to work in the United States health care system.

Marga Thome, PhD, MS, RN, RNM

Marga Thome has been a professor of nursing/midwifery with the Faculty of Nursing, University of Iceland since 1977. She specialized in maternal child nursing with a focus on promotion of perinatal and infant mental health. Research projects are related to promotion of breastfeeding; promotion of post-partum maternal and infant mental health and experience of parenthood. Her publications are in English, Icelandic, and German. She was educated in nursing in Germany, in mid-wifery in Switzerland, in nursing education in Germany, and she received a diploma of advanced nursing studies, a master of science, and a doctoral degree in the United Kingdom. She has worked as a nurse/midwife in all of these countries. She held the first chair in Nursing Science with the University of Iceland and became the first dean of the Faculty of Nursing from 2000-2003.

Debra Thoms, RN, RM, BA

Debra Thoms completed her general nursing education at Prince Henry/Prince of Wales Hospitals, Sydney, and her midwifery education at the Royal Darwin Hospital, Northern Territory. She holds a bachelor of arts in economics and psychology and a master's of nursing administration. In addition, she holds a graduate certificate in bioethics and an advanced diploma in arts in history. Thoms has worked in metropolitan, rural, and remote health settings in New South Wales, the Northern Territory, and South Australia, in both acute and community health services. She has also held senior management positions as a chief executive officer and executive director. She commenced as the chief nursing and midwifery officer for the New South Wales Department of Health in May 2006. The chief nursing and midwifery officer has a leadership role for the approximately 40,000 nurses and midwives that work within the public health system. Prior to this, Thoms was the chief nursing officer in South Australia. Thoms was made an adjunct professor of nursing at the University of Technology, Sydney, in 2003, and at The University of Sydney in 2009. She is a Fellow of the College of Nursing and the Royal College of Nursing, Australia, and an Honorary Fellow of the Australian College of Health Service Executives. In 2005, she became a fellow of the Johnson & Johnson/Wharton Fellows Program in Management for Nurse Executives from the Wharton School of the University of Pennsylvania.

Gloria Thupayagale-Tshweneagae, RN, MSN

Gloria Thupayagale-Tshweneagae, a lecturer at the University of Botswana in the School of Nursing holds a master's of science in nursing with a major in psychiatric mental health nursing and a minor in health care management. She is currently pursuing her doctoral degree, which she hopes to finish in 2010. She has been head of psychiatric mental health nursing with the Government of Botswana and has been chair of the professional ethics and disciplinary committee of the Nursing and Midwifery Council of Botswana. She has published in the area of mental health, regulation, and nursing issues such as migration of nurses.

Agnes Tiwari, PhD, RN, MSc, DN, RNT, RCNT, MCMI

Agnes Tiwari is associate professor of the Department of Nursing Studies and assistant dean of the Li Ka Shing Faculty of Medicine, the University of Hong Kong. She has been a nurse educator for more than 25 years, working with undergraduate and graduate students as well as mentoring clinical nurses. She has conducted numerous educational research projects in pursuit of the best evidence to enhance teaching and learning and published the results in international journals and book chapters. Her more notable achievements include the validation of the Chinese version of the California Critical Thinking Disposition Inventory and the use of a randomized controlled trial to evaluate the effect of problem-based learning on students' critical thinking. In recognition of her commitment and expertise in education, she was awarded the Faculty Teaching Medal in 2004 and the Inaugural Outstanding Teaching Award of the University of Hong Kong in 2008.

Debbie Tolson

Debbie Tolson is currently head of research within the School of Nursing, Midwifery, and Community Health at Glasgow Caledonian University. Her early career began in London where she completed her BSc in nursing studies (Honors, First Class) and her master's in nursing science. Her commitment to advancing the nursing care of older people began as a hospital staff nurse and continued as she moved through the clinical ranks to become a senior charge nurse within an English teaching hospital. She then moved north to Scotland, changing to an academic career. In 1999, she was awarded Professor Merit by Glasgow Caledonian University for her research contributions to gerontological nursing. The Caledonian team was honored by Sigma Theta Tau International, receiving the Best of Worldviews on Evidence-Based Practice Award in 2007.

Debra Townsend, RN

Debra Townsend has dedicated her personal and professional life to the service of others. She has been acknowledged as one of the most dynamic and dazzling professional speakers in the country, igniting audiences with her grace and eloquent style. Her presentation savvy gleans from more than three decades as an international keynote speaker and institute leader. A respected health care executive and pioneer for women in business, Townsend is the chief executive officer (CEO) and president of four companies. She consults for a variety of organizations, assisting them with culture development and establishing a more healthy work environment. Her contributions as a professional nurse, leadership consultant, platform/career coach, and distinguished author are many. She takes pride in being an eloquent and trusted mentor, bringing to the world messages of inspiration, hope, and healing. To celebrate her 40 years in nursing, Townsend continues her legacy work as the CEO and president of The National Center for Compassionate Care, a center dedicated to patient, family, and caregiver advocacy.

Carol Tuttas, MSN, RN, CAN, BC

Carol Tuttas serves in the role of clinical liaison and interview services manager for Cross Country Staffing in Boca Raton, Florida, where she has been employed since 2006. She has also served as professional services educator at Cross Country. Tuttas's career history includes nurse manager/director roles in South Florida acute care hospital settings from 1995 through 2006. Her clinical forte has been cardiac telemetry and, in more recent years, skilled nursing and long-term care settings where she works as a direct care provider several times a month. Tuttas received her initial nursing training at Mohawk College in Hamilton, Ontario, Canada. After relocating to South Florida, she received

her baccalaureate degree in nursing at Lynn University in Boca Raton, Florida, and her master's degree in nursing (administration) at Florida Atlantic University in Boca Raton, Florida. Tuttas has been accepted to the Medical University of South Carolina where she is studying to earn her PhD in nursing.

U

Leana R. Uys, D Soc Sc, RN, RM

Leana R. Uys is currently the deputy vice chancellor and head of the College of Health Sciences of the University of KwaZulu-Natal. She has published more than 90 peer reviewed articles and has been involved as author and/or editor in the publication of 27 books. She has been active in a range of general and specialist nursing organization in South Africa and internationally. She has led numerous educational development and research projects in Africa and received the Mary Tolle Wright Founders Award for Excellence in Leadership from Sigma Theta Tau International in 2007.

V

Drahomíra Vatehová, PhD, RN, MSN

Drahomíra Vatehová has been a teacher of vocational subjects at Secondary Nursing School in Svidnik since 2002 and a part-time lecturer at the Institute of Health and Social sciences of Blessed P.P.Gojdic in Prešov of St.Elizabeth University of Health and Social Sciences in Bratislava since 2008. She ended her secondary school studies in Humenné in 1994. From 1994 to 1997 she worked as a nurse at the department of anaesthesiology and intensive medicine at The Hospital with policlinics in Svidnik. From 1997 to 2002, she studied nursing at Jessenius Medical Faculty of Commenius University in Martin, where she was awarded a master's degree in nursing. In 2004, she obtained pedagogical qualification for educational activities at the Faculty of Pedagogy of Commenius University. Currently, she is a part time doctoral student at the Institute of Health and Social Sciences of Blessed P.P.Gojdic in Prešov of St. Elizabeth University of Health and Social Sciences in Bratislava, Slovak Republic.

Maria De La Ó Ramallo Veríssimo, RN, PhD

Maria De La Ó Ramallo Veríssimo has been a professor of nursing at the University of São Paulo, Brazil, since 1987. She is a specialist in child nursing with a focus on child health and promotion of child development. She received her master's and doctoral degrees from the University of São Paulo in Brazil. She has conducted research projects related to health promotion and integrated management of childhood illnesses in child care centers and in primary care health services. She participated in the International Nursing Leadership Institute at the University of Alabama in Birmingham in January 2008, where she developed a collaborative research project with Dr. Lynda Wilson.

James F. (Jim) Veronesi, RN, MSN, CNAA-BC, CHE

James F. (Jim) Veronesi is currently a director and faculty member of the Advisory Board Academies, a division of The Advisory Board Company in Washington, D.C. With more than 22 years of professional nursing experience, Veronesi's current role is to teach classes, conduct workshops, and assist with development of leadership curriculum for leading hospitals in the United States. Prior to joining the Advisory Board, he held a variety of nursing leadership positions, including chief nurse executive. He is active in professional nursing and health care leadership organizations and currently serves as past president of the Pennsylvania Organization of Nurse Executives. In addition, he is active in nursing publications, authoring more than 50 articles and book contributions, including a bi-monthly column in Home Health Care Management & Practice. Veronesi serves on the editorial board of both RN and Home Health Care Management & Practice.

Frances R. (Fran) Vlasses, RN, PhD, NEA-BC

Frances R. (Fran) Vlasses received a BSN from Villanova University in 1972 and an MSN in community mental health from Ohio State University in 1974. She received a PhD in nursing from Loyola, with distinction, in 1997. Her thesis was titled "Too Familiar for Words: An Analysis of Invisible Nursing Work." Prior to pursuing her doctorate, Vlasses had extensive experience in nursing service administration, project management, hospital nursing staff professional development, clinical and classroom instruction, and nursing and health care consulting. She is currently an assistant professor at the Niehoff School of Nursing, Loyola University Chicago and nursing research facilitator for Northwestern Memorial Hospital, Chicago, Illinois. Since coming to Loyola, Vlasses has taught graduate level courses for accelerated BSN students. In 2003, she co-developed an interprofessional seminar with the Stritch School of Medicine that has become a permanent component of the medical school and nursing curriculum. She was recently appointed a Nurse Educator Fellow by the Illinois Board of Higher Education. She continues to publish and speak on issues related to the quality of nursing work life and creative strategies for health care leadership. Her first book, Ordinary People, Extraordinary Lives: The Stories of Nurses, with Carolyn H. Smeltzer, EdD, has been a best seller and was honored with a Media Award, Honorable Mention, from the American Academy of Nursing and Best of Books for the Biennium (2005) from Sigma Theta Tau International. Her second book, The Chicago Nurse Parade: Images of America, (Smeltzer, C. H, Vlasses, F. R, Robinson, C, Arcadia Press) was released in Spring 2005. The book received the American Academy of Nursing Media Award in 2005. These projects represent Vlasses' creative initiatives to affirm the work of nursing and to educate the public about the importance of the caring professions. Her research interests include topics related to creating a healthy work environment and innovative models of care delivery.

W

Patrick Kimani Wairiri, MA, BScN

Patrick Kimani Wairiri has an MA (2008) from Kenya Methodist University and a BScN (1999) from the University of Nairobi. He worked at Aga Khan Hospital Kenya in the Paediatric Department, after which he was teaching at Kenya Methodist University in community health, nursing education, and he coordinated clinical supervision, placements, and assessments for all the BScN students in all areas. He was a member of St John Ambulance and had leadership roles in

Nairobi Nurses Association as secretary of Nairobi Branch among other activities. He has recently taken a nursing position in Texas. He is a nurse who likes challenges.

Shao Ling Wang, RN, BSN

Shao Ling Wang is currently a PhD student at the School of Nursing, Hong Kong Polytechnic University. She obtained a certificate in nursing from Guangzhou Health School in Mainland China and worked in The First Affiliated Hospital of Guangzhou Medical College as a staff nurse and then a head nurse of the respiratory intensive care unit for six years. In 1988, she successfully passed the stringent selection criteria and was admitted to the Hong Kong Polytechnic for the post-registration diploma in the health care education (nursing) program. She returned to mainland China in 1990 as a tutor of Guangzhou Medical College and an associate head of the nursing department in the college affiliated hospital. She immigrated to Hong Kong in 2000 and received her BSN with distinction from the Hong Kong Polytechnic University in 2004. After graduation, she worked as a part-time tutor for a collaboration BSN program between the Hong Kong Polytechnic University and Zhejiang University, China, until she started her postgraduate study in Hong Kong Polytechnic University in 2006.

Deborah Washington, RN, MS

Deborah Washington has been a nurse at Massachusetts General Hospital since 1986 and director of Diversity for Patient Care Services since 1995. She is a graduate of the Boston University School of Nursing and a 1993 graduate of the Boston College School of Nursing with a master's in adult mental health. Presently, Washington is a doctoral student at the Boston College School of Nursing where her research interest is the impact of bias on clinical decision-making. She presents locally and nationally on topics such as teamwork, managing a multicultural workforce, conflict resolution, cross-cultural communication, and cultural competence. She is a frequent consultant to organizations interested in supporting a focus on mentorship programs for their multicultural students or employees. She has produced two videos exploring the professional experiences of the Black nurse and the cultural positives of living in a minority community.

Carol Watson, PhD, RN, CENP

Carol Watson has been a nurse for more than 38 years and has held positions as staff nurse, nurse educator, nurse manager, and nurse executive. She is currently a professor with the University of Iowa College of Nursing, teaching in the masters and doctoral nursing programs. Her previous position was as the senior vice president of Clinical Services and chief nurse executive at Mercy Medical Center, Cedar Rapids, Iowa, a position she held for 21 years before leaving in December 2008. In that position, she had responsibility for all nursing departments, as well as several clinical support departments. Mercy is a stand-alone community hospital with 445 beds and a full continuum of services. She is the past president for the American Organization of Nurse Executives. She is certified through the American Organization of Nurse Executives as a Certified Executive in Nursing Practice (CENP). She is a member of the Editorial Review Board for the Journal of Nursing Administration and Applied Nursing Research. In 2004, she was appointed as the first nurse executive member of the Iowa Hospital Association Board of Trustees. The Iowa Organization of Nurse Executives recognized her as the Outstanding Nurse Executive in 1992.

K.T. Waxman, DNP, MBA, RN, CNL

K.T. Waxman has more than 25 years of experience as a nurse leader in California. She currently is the program director for the Bay Area Simulation Collaborative (BASC) and the California Simulation Alliance (CSA) for the California Institute for Nursing & Health Care (CINHC). She is also president of KT Waxman & Associates, a health care consulting firm. Waxman began her career as an RN at UCLA Medical Center in the medical-surgical division. A nationally known speaker, Waxman addresses such topics as leadership development, health care finance, networking, and communication. Waxman holds an RN degree from Napa Valley College, a bachelor's degree in Healthcare Administration, an MBA from the University of La Verne, and a doctorate in nursing practice (DNP) from the University of San Francisco with a concentration in health systems leadership, with an emphasis on simulation. She is now a part-time faculty member and teaches masters students in USF's nursing program.

Bonnie Wesorick, RN, MSN, DRNAP, FAAN

Bonnie Wesorick is the founder and president of the Clinical Practice Model Resource Center (CPMRC) and the chairperson of the CPMRC International Consortium. Her innovative work around CPMRC's mission to co-create and sustain the best places to practice and the best places to receive care has brought health care providers together from across the continent. Over the past two decades she has partnered with thousands of interdisciplinary practitioners from rural, community, and university settings who have formed an International Consortium to carry out the work necessary to create healthy, healing practice cultures and a patient centered, integrated health care system. Her leadership in the development and implementation of an interdisciplinary professional practice framework with evidence-based tools and resources has revolutionized practice and automation. Wesorick led the first practice-technology partnership between a technology company, Eclipsys Corporation, and a professional resource center, CPMRC. This unprecedented and entrepreneurial partnership brought the first automated, preconfigured, evidence-based interdisciplinary documentation system to the health care arena. She has shared her expertise and learned from the expertise of others from more than 1,000 diverse clinical settings and professional organizations, both within and beyond the health care arena. She is an internationally known speaker, storyteller, author, and visionary who has authored many books, articles, videos, CDs, and audiotapes. Wesorick connects with the hearts and minds of others and brings a sense of direction and hope in the midst of chaos in today's health care arena.

Gerald Francis (Ged) Williams, MHA, RN, FAAN, FRCNA, FCHCE

Gerald Francis (Ged) Williams is executive director of Nursing and Midwifery, Gold Coast Health Service District and professor of Nursing, Griffith University, Queensland, Australia. He has held numerous senior nursing leadership posts in various parts of Australia, including principal nurse consultant for the Northern Territory from 2000-2003. Williams has postgraduate qualifications in midwifery, critical care nursing, health administration, public sector management, company governance, and law. He is a fellow of the Royal College of Nursing Australia, Australian College of Health Care Executives, and the American Academy of Nursing, He is the founding president of the Australian College of Critical Care Nurses; a life member, founding chair, and president of the World Federation of Critical Care Nurses; and a director with the World Federation of Societies of Intensive Care and Critical Care Medicine. William's research and publication interests are broad and include workforce planning, clinical practice, education and training program development; and other management and leadership issues in nursing and health. He has more than 30 peer-reviewed publications and is regularly involved in strategic nursing activities at the state, national, and international level. He is a fellow of the Johnson & Johnson/Wharton Fellows Program in Management for Nurse Executives from the Wharton School of the University of Pennsylvania

Lynda Law Wilson, RN, PhD

Lynda Law Wilson is professor of Nursing, assistant dean for International Programs, and deputy director of the Pan American Health Organization/World Health Organization Collaborating Center on International Nursing at the University of Alabama at Birmingham (UAB). She was prepared as a pediatric nurse practitioner and has conducted extensive funded research to evaluate the effects of touch and massage on premature infants in the neonatal intensive care unit, promoting positive family relationships, and evaluating community-based interventions for immigrant Latino families in the United States. She has also conducted collaborative research with international partners in Brazil, Chile, and Honduras. Wilson is fluent in Spanish and currently serves as vice coordinator of the Network for Child Health Nursing, a network that includes coordinators in every country in Latin America as well as in Spain and the United States. Wilson coordinates an International Nursing Leadership Institute every other year at UAB.

Gail Wolf, RN, DNS, FAAN

Gail Wolf is a professor at the University of Pittsburgh where she is responsible for the master's and doctoral programs in Nursing Leadership. Prior to this appointment Wolf spent 23 years at the University of Pittsburgh Health Care System in a variety of senior leadership roles, including 10 years as the chief nursing officer for the system and its 19 hospitals. Wolf received her baccalaureate in nursing from West Virginia University, her master's in nursing from the University of Kentucky, and her doctorate in nursing administration from Indiana University in Indianapolis, Indiana. She is a fellow of the Johnson & Johnson/Wharton Fellows Program in Management for Nurse Executives from the Wharton School of the University of Pennsylvania, and she currently serves as chair of the Magnet Commission. She has published numerous articles and lectured extensively throughout the United States, Australia, Italy, Japan, Canada, and Finland on issues relating to leadership of patient care.

Frances Kam Yuet Wong, RN, PhD

Frances Kam Yuet Wong obtained her bachelor's of science in nursing at St. Olaf College, Minnesota, with Departmental Distinction. She earned her MA (education) and PhD (sociology) at the Chinese University of Hong Kong. She has extensive clinical experience in the intensive care unit, renal care, and general medicine. Her research work and publications are in the areas of advanced nursing practice, transitional care, and nursing education. She has published more than 70 papers and chapters in internationally refereed journals and reviewed books. She has been invited to speak at many local and international conferences. She serves on the editorial boards and review panels for a number of international journals. She is a visiting professor and external examiner at a number of universities within and outside Hong Kong. She acts as an advisor to a number of committees for health care agencies. She has served as president of the Pi Iota Chapter of Sigma Theta Tau International. She is now the chairperson of the Hong Kong Society for Nursing Education, the vice-president of the preparatory group for the Hong Kong Academy of Nursing, and an elected member of the Core Steering Group of the Advanced Nursing Practice Network, International Council for Nurses.

Z

Teja Zaksek, RM, MSc Midwifery, BSc (rad)

Teja Zaksek entered midwifery education in 1996 when—after 15 years of closure—the school for direct entry midwifery was re-opened. After graduation, she commenced with a master's study in midwifery in Glasgow Caledonian University, which she finished in 2006. She was nominated by the International Confederation of Midwives as one of the five young midwifery leaders globally. During this time, Slovenia has had the difficult experience of facing professional opposition from colleagues and leaders in nursing and midwifery. In her efforts to implement change, she has learned to build resilience identify support systems, utilize the Young Midwifery Leaders' network of colleagues, handle wounded personal pride, and persist with an issue under difficult situations in the face of opposition. Her mentor, Valerie Fleming, has been a support and confidante who has not only guided her in how to approach situations but also gave psychological support, helping Zaksek maintain good mental health practices. She was appointed as chief midwife in one of the community centers and has been offered the post of chief nurse in one of the regions of Slovenia. She has literally fought her way to achieving policy- and decision-making positions. Now she is working in University of Ljubljana, midwifery department, where she disseminates her knowledge to prospective midwives.

Alison Zecchin, RN

Alison Zecchin is the director of Nursing and Midwifery at Royal North Shore Hospital, Sydney, Australia, since November 2008. Zecchin has a varied career that spans surgical nursing, managing in a variety of units such as surgery, roster office, women s health, and drug and alcohol. She had also spent time working as a consultant with a computer software company. It has been through these experiences that she has gained a broad and varied understanding of nursing and management. She is a registered general nurse, has an acute care certificate, a personnel management certificate, and a master's of management.

References

1: Academic and Service Partnership

References

Cronenwett, L. R. (2004). A present-day academic perspective on the Carolina nursing experience: Building on the past, shaping the future. *Journal of Professional Nursing, 20*(5), 304-307.

Additional Resources

Collaborative Leadership Training Tools: http://www.collaborativeleadership.org/pages/tools.html

2: Aging Nursing Workforce

References

Annie E. Casey Foundation. (2005). Population resource center population matters. Retrieved 6 October 2009 from http://www.prcdc.org/

Caron, V. F. (2004). *The nursing shortage in the United States of America: What can be done to solve the crisis?* Kingston, RI: University of Rhode Island. Retrieved 6 October 2009 from http://www.uri.edu/research/lrc/research/papers/Caron_Nurse_Shortage.pdf

Dovlo, D. (2001). *Issues affecting the mobility and retention of health workers in commonwealth African states, London.* Report prepared for commonwealth states, London.

Klein. W.C. (2007). Redefining retirement years: Productive engagement of the older workforce, a qualitative study of employers and employees in Connecticut. Hartford, CT: Connecticut Commission on Aging. Retrieved 6 October 2009 from http://www.cga.ct.gov/coa/PDFs/Reports/report%20final%2011-2-07%20_2_.pdf

Thupayagale-Tshweneagae, G. (2007). Migration of nurses: Is there any other option? *International Nursing Review 54(1);* 107-109.

Tlou, S. D. (2005). HIV/AIDS in sub-Saharan Africa. *Dermatologic Clinics 24*(4), 421-429.

United States Department of Health and Human Services. (2007). *The registered nurse population: Findings from the 2004 national sample survey of registered nurses.* Retrieved 6 October 2009 from http://bhpr.hrsa.gov/healthworkforce/rnsurvey04/

Additional Resources

Bower, F. B., & Sadler, W. (2009). *Why retire: Career strategies for third age nurses.* Indianapolis, IN: Sigma Theta Tau International.

Dochterman, J. M., & Grace, H. E. (2001). *Current issues in nursing.* London: Mosby, Inc.

Motlaleng, K. (2005). The impact of HIV and AIDS on the nursing workforce. *Botswana society*: 12(6), 116-120.

Okumele, M. A. (2007). *Effective nursing management.* Johannesburg: Brooks/Cole Publishing Company.

Rick, M. (2003). Aging workforce: the reality of the impact of older workers and eldercare in the workplace. Alexandria, VA: *H.R Magazine.* Retrieved 6 October 2009 from http://findarticles.com/p/articles/mi_m3495/is_7_50/ai_n14814505/

3: The Art of Nursing

References

Dossey, B. M., Selanders, L. C., Beck, D. M., & Attewell, A. (2005). *Florence Nightingale today: Healing, leadership, global action.* Washington, D.C.: American Nurses Association.

Dossey, B. M. (2010). *Florence Nightingale: Mystic, visionary, healer* (2nd ed.). Philadelphia: F.A. Davis.

Dossey, B. M. (2008). Integral and holistic nursing. In Dossey, B. M., & Keegan, L. *Holistic nursing: A handbook for practice*, (5th ed.). Sudbury, MA: Jones & Bartlett, 23-36.

Nightingale, F. (1868). Una and the lion. *Good Words*, June; p. 362.

Additional Resources

American Holistic Nurses Association: http://www.ahna.org

Borysenko, J. & Dveirin, G. (2007). *Your soul's compass: What is spiritual guidance.* Carlsbad, CA: Hay House.

Burkhardt, M. A. & Najai-Jacobson, M. G. (2008). Spirituality and healing. In Dossey, B. M. & Keegan, L. *Holistic nursing: A handbook for practice* (5th ed.). Sudbury, MA: Jones & Bartlett.

Campbell, D. (2008). *Sound spirit: pathway to faith.* Carlsbad, CA: Hay House.

Curley, M.A. (2007). *Synergy: The unique relationship between nurses and patients.* Indianapolis, IN: Sigma Theta Tau International.

Freshwater, D., Taylor, B., & Sherwood, G. (2008). *International textbook of reflective practice in nursing.* Oxford: Wiley-Blackwell.

Halifax, J. (2008). *Being with dying: Cultivating compassion and fearlessness in the presence of death.* Boston: Shambhala.

Houser, B. P., & Player, K. N. (2008). *Pivotal moments in nursing: Leaders who changed the path of a profession*, vol. 2. Indianapolis, IN: Sigma Theta Tau International.

Koerner, J. E. (2007). *Nursing presence. The essence of nursing.* New York: Springer.

Nightingale Declaration: http://www.nightingaledeclaration.net

4: Autonomy

References

American Association of Nurse Attorneys. (Sept. 23, 2004). Position paper on expert testimony in nursing malpractice actions. Retrieved 6 October 2009 from https://listserv.temple.edu/cgi-bin/wa?A2=ind0607&L=net-gold&P=52480

Buresh, B., & Gordon, S. (2006). *From silence to voice: What nurses know and must communicate to the public.* New York: ILR Press.

California Board of Registered Nursing. (1997). An explanation of the scope of RN practice including standardized procedures. Retrieved 6 October 2009 from http://www.rn.ca.gov/pdfs/regulations/npr-b-03.pdf

General Laws of Massachusetts. (n.d.). Chapter 112: Registration of certain professions and occupations; Registration of nurses. Nursing practice: Advanced practice; licensed practical nurses. Section 80B.

International Council of Nurses. (2005). The ICN code of ethics for nurses. Retrieved 6 October 2009 from http://www.icn.ch/icncode.pdf

Mathes, M. (2005). On nursing, moral autonomy, and moral responsibility. *MedSurg Nursing*, December. Retrieved 6 October 2009 from http://findarticles.com/p/articles/mi_m0FSS/is_6_14/ai_n17211626/?tag=content;col1

Murphy, E. K. (2004). Judicial recognition of nursing as a unique profession. *Association of periOperative Registered Nurses Journal*, November. Retrieved 6 October 2009 from http://findarticles.com/p/articles/mi_m0FSL/is_5_80/ai_n6365100/

Pankratz, L., & Pankratz, D. (1974). Nursing autonomy and patients' rights: Development of a nursing attitude scale. *Journal of Health and Social Behavior*, Vol. 15, No. 3, pp. 211-216. Retrieved 6 October 2009 from http://www.jstor.org/stable/2137021

Rosenstein, A. H. (2002). Nurse-physician relationships: Impact on nurse satisfaction and retention. *American Journal of Nursing*, *102* (6), 26–34.

Sullivan v. Edward Hospital, 806 N.E.2d 645, 653-61 [Ill. 2004]). Retrieved 6 October 2009 from http://www.state.il.us/court/Opinions/SupremeCourt/2004/February/Opinions/Html/95409.htm

Summers, H. J. (2006). Q: Are you sure nurses are autonomous? Based on what I've seen, it sure looks like physicians are calling the shots. The Truth About Nursing. Accessed August 21, 2009 at http://www.truthaboutnursing.org/faq/autonomy.html

Texas Legislature. (n.d.) Occupations code; Subtitle E; Regulation of nursing; Chapter 301. Nurses; Subchapter A; General provisions. Medical Practice Act. Texas Occ. Code Ann. § 301.002.

Thornton, L. (n.d.). What is holistic nursing? American Holistic Nurses Association. Retrieved 6 October 2009 from http://www.ahna.org/AboutUs/WhatisHolisticNursing/tabid/1165/Default.aspx

Truth About Nursing. (n.d.). Codes of ethics for nurses. Retrieved 6 October 2009 from http://www.truthaboutnursing.org/research/codes_of_ethics.html

Additional Resources

Carey, L. & Jones, M.. (October 2000). Autonomy in Practice Is it A Reality? *Practice Nursing*, Elsevier Health Sciences. Accessed October 5, 2009 from http://books.google.com/books?id=Ke0iFGnUws0C&pg=PA290&lpg=PA290&dq=autonomy+nightingale&source=bl&ots=y5JWIhdXl0&sig=9rdm9NSOy2ryzaVGnuFGv6n0nUo&hl=en&ei=RQZ7SrKUE4faNfbDkNkC&sa=X&oi=book_result&ct=result&resnum=10#v=onepage&q=autonomy%20nightingale&f=false

State of California, Legislative Council. (n.d.). Business and professions code Section 2725-2742. Retrieved 5 October 2009 from http://www.leginfo.ca.gov/cgi-bin/waisgate?WAISdocID=754895497+1+0+0&WAISaction=retrieve

State of California. (2009). California nurse practice act. Retrieved 5 October 2009 from http://www.rn.ca.gov/regulations/npa.shtml

5: Business Acumen and Impeccable Ethics

References

Barnum, B. S. (1996). *Spirituality in nursing: From tradition to new age* (2nd ed.). New York: Springer.

Berwick, D. (2004). *Escape fire*. Hoboken, New Jersey: John Wiley and Sons.

Clark, P. A., Leddy, K., Drain, M., & Kaldenberg, D. (2007). State nursing shortages and patient satisfaction: More RNs—Better Patient Experiences. *Journal of Nursing Care Quality*, 22(2): 119-127.

Hirschhorn, L., & Gilmore, T. (2004). *Ideas in philanthropic field building: Where they come from and how they are translated into actions*. New York: The Foundation Center. Retrieved 5 October 2009 from http://www.foundationcenter.org/gainknowledge/research/pdf/practice-matters_06_paper.pdf

Institute of Medicine. (2006). *Crossing the quality chasm*. Washington, D.C.: The National Academies.

Additional Resources

Applying business acumen: http://www.makingstories.net/Gargiulo_ISPI_2006_All_Materials.pdf

Forbes, S. (2007). Open heart surgery—90% off. Retrieved 6 October 2009 from http://members.forbes.com/forbes/2007/0813/021.html

Millenson, M. (2003). Silence. *Health Affairs, 22*(2): 103-112.

Recognizing business acumen: http://www.businessknowhow.com/growth/businessacumen.htm

6: C-Suite Savvy

References

Judkins, S., Massey, C., & Huff, B. (2006). Hardiness, stress and use of ill–time among nurse managers: Is there a connection? *Nursing Economics, 24*(4), July/Aug, 187-92. www.nursingeconomics.net.

Kobasa, S. C, (1979). Stressful life events, personality, and health: An inquiry into hardiness. *Journal of Personality and Social Psychology, 37*(1): pp. 1-11.

Maddi, S. R. & Kobasa, S. C. (1984). *The hardy executive: Health under stress.* Homeward, IL. Dow-Jones-Irwin.

Rich, V. L. & Rich, A. R. (1987). Personality hardiness and burnout in female staff nurses. *Image, 19*(2), pp. 63-69.

Additional Resources

Collins, J. (2001). *Good to great in the social sector.* New York: Harper-Collins.

George, B. (2003). *Authentic leadership: Rediscovering the secrets to creating lasting value.* San Francisco: Jossey Bass.

Golman D., Boyatziz, R., & McKee, A. (2002). *Primal leadership: Realizing the power of emotional intelligence.* Boston: Harvard Business School Press.

Kriteck, P. (2002). *Negotiating at the uneven table.* San Francisco: Jossey-Bass.

Porter-O'Grady, T. (2007). *Quantum leadership: A resource for health care innovations.* Sudbury, MA: Jones and Bartlett.

Schaffner, J. W. (2007). *Cs of change in the c-suite,* JONA, *37*(12), 523-576.

Sqazzo, J.D. (2007). *Becoming a leader in the c-suite: How to develop necessary skills. Healthcare Executive, 22*(6), pp. 17-22.

Stone, D., Patton, B., & Heen, S. (1999). *Difficult conversations.* New York: Viking.

Whitworth, L., Kimsey-House, H., & Sandahl, P. (1998). *Co-active coaching.* Palo Alto, CA: Davies-Black Publishing.

7: Capacities

Reference

Colliére , M. F. (1989). *Promover a vida.* Lisboa: Sindicato dos Enfermeiros Portugueses. (Translated from the original French.)

Additional Resources

Argyris, C., & Schon, D. (1974). *Theory in practice: Increasing professional effectiveness.* San Francisco: Jossey-Bass.

Buresh, B., & Gordon, S. (2006). *From silence to voice: What nurses know and must communicate to the public.* New York: ILR Press.

Collière, M. F. (1982). *Promouvoir la vie.* Paris: InterEditions. (Original French ed.)

Cronen, V. (1995). Practical theory and the tasks ahead for social approaches to communication. In Leeds-Hurwitz, W. (Ed.), *Social Approaches to Communication.* New York: Guilford Press.

Ford, P., & Walsh, M. (1995). *New rituals for old: Nursing through the looking glass*. Oxford: Butterworth-Heinemann Ltd.

Landeweerd, J. A., & Boumans, N. (1994). The effect of work dimensions and need for autonomy on nurses' work satisfaction and health. *Journal of Occupational and Organizational Psychology*, 67: 207–217.

Smith, M. K. (2001). Chris Argyris: Theories of action, double-loop learning, and organizational learning. *The Encyclopedia of Informal Education*. Retrieved 6 October 2009 from www.infed.org/thinkers/argyris.htm

8: Caring

References
Hesselbein, F., & Cohen, P. M. (Eds.). (1999). *Leader to leader: Enduring insights on leadership from the Drucker Foundations' award-winning journal*. San Francisco: Jossey-Bass.

Additional Resources
Babcock, L., & Laschever, S. (2003). *Women don't ask: Negotiation and the gender divide*. Princeton, NJ: Princeton University Press.

Boykin, A., & Scheonhofer, S. O. (2001). *Nursing as caring: A model for transforming practice*. Sudbury, MA: Jones and Bartlett Publishers.

Dickenson-Hazard, N. (2008). *Ready, set, go lead!* Indianapolis, IN: Sigma Theta Tau International.

Family Support Network of North Carolina: Mentorship Program. Retrieved 6 October 2009 from http://www.fsnnc.org/Services/Mentor/whatismentorship.htm

Freeman, M. J. (Ed.). (2002). *Leadership knowledge base: Mentorship*. Retrieved 6 October 2009 from http://www.sonic.net/~mfreeman

Houser, B. P., & Player, K. N. (2008). *Words of wisdom from pivotal nurse leaders*. Indianapolis, IN: Sigma Theta Tau International.

Mackoff, B., & Wenet, G. (2001). *The inner work of leaders*. New York: American Management Association.

McKinley, M. G. (2004). A mentor gap in nursing? *Critical Care Nurse, 24*(2), 8011. Retrieved 6 October 2009 from http://ccn.aacnjournals.org/cgi/content/full/24/2/8

Pace, T. (2007). *Mentor: The kid & the CEO*. Edmond, OK: Mentor Hope Publishing.

Porter-O'Grady, T., & Malloch, K. (2007). *Quantum leadership: A resource for health care innovation* (2nd ed.). Sudbury, MA: Jones & Bartlett Publishers.

Reh, J. F. (2008). *Mentors and mentoring: Finding a mentor*. (Part 2 of the Series). Retrieved 6 October 2009 from http://management.about.com/cs/people/a/FindMentor.htm

Watson, J. (2008). Theory of human caring. Retrieved 6 October 2009 from http://www.nursing.ucdenver.edu/faculty/caring.htm

9: Celebrating

Additional Resources
Bridges, W. (1980). *Transitions: Strategies for coping with the difficult, painful, and confusing times in your life*. Cambridge, MA: Perseus Books.

Siebert, A. (2005). *The resiliency advantage*. San Francisco: Berrett-Koehler Publishers.

Sinetar, M. (1998). *The mentor's spirit: life lessons on leadership and the art of encouragement*. New York: St. Martin's Griffin.

10: Change Management

References

Malloch, K., & Porter-O'Grady, T. (2009). *The quantum leader: Applications for a new world of work.* Jones & Bartlett; Boston.

Porter-O'Grady, T., & Malloch, K. (2007). *Quantum leadership: A resource for healthcare innovation.* Jones & Bartlett; Boston.

Additional Resources

Greenleaf, R. (2002). *Servant leadership: A journey into the nature of legitimate power.* New York. Paulist Press.

Kelly, T. & Littman, J. (2005). *The ten faces of innovation.* New York: Doubleday.

Malloch, K. & Porter-O'Grady, T. (2006). *Introduction into evidence-based practice in nursing and healthcare.* Boston: Jones & Bartlett.

11: Changing the Future One Mentorship at a Time

References

Drucker, P. (2001). *The essential Drucker.* Collins Business Essential.

Rogers, C. R. (1961). *On becoming a person.* Boston: Houghton-Mifflin.

Strasen, L. (1992). *The image of professional nursing.* Philadelphia: Lippincott, Williams & Wilkins.

Additional Resources

Johnson, W. B., & Ridley, C. R. (2004). *The elements of mentoring.* New York: Palgrave Macmillan.

Top mentor publications: www.mentors.ca/topmenbks.html

Urban, R. (2006). *Choices that change lives.* New York: Simon & Schuster Publishing.

12: Coaching as an Essential Skill

Additional Resources

Crane, T. G. (1998, 1993). *The heart of coaching: Using transformational coaching to create a high performance culture.* FTA Press, San Diego, CA.

Goldsmith, M., Lyons, L., Freas, A., & Witherspoon, R. (2000). *Coaching for leadership.* San Francisco: Jossey-Bass/Pfeiffer.

Hargrove, R. A. (1995). *Masterful coaching.* San Francisco: Jossey-Bass/Pfeiffer.

Mauer, R. (1996). *Beyond the wall of resistance: Unconventional strategies that build support for change.* Bard Press, Austin, Texas.

Robinson-Walker, C., & Detmer, S. (2004–2007). *Coaching: The new nursing leadership skill.* NurseWeek Continuing Education Course #3020. NurseWeek.

Ting, S. & Scisco, P. (2006). *The center for creative leadership handbook of coaching: A guide for the leader coach.* San Francisco: Jossey-Bass.

Vail, Peter (1996). *Learning as a way of being.* San Francisco: Jossey-Bass.

Whitworth, Laura, et al. (2007). *Co-active coaching: New skills for coaching people toward success in work and life* (2nd ed.). Boston: Davies-Black.

Zachery, Lois J. (2000). *The mentor's guide.* San Francisco: Jossey-Bass.

13: Collaboration

References

California Institute for Nursing and Health Care (n.d.). *Optimizing the health of Californians through nursing excellence.* Retrieved 6 October 2009 from http://www.cinhc.org

Jones, D., Patterson, B., & Jackson, S. (2009). *Pathway to sustainability: A development guide 2008-2013.* California Institute for Nursing and Health Care.

Sigma Theta Tau International. (2006). *A daybook for nurse leaders and mentors.* Indianapolis, IN. Author.

Additional Resources

Collins, J. (2001). *Good to great: Why some companies make the leap and others don't.* New York, New York: HarperCollins Publishers.

Huston, C. (2008). Preparing nurse leaders for 2020. *Journal of Nursing Management,* (16), 905-911.

Potempa, K. (2002). Finding the courage to lead: The Oregon experience. *Nursing Administration Quarterly, 26*(4), 9-15.

14: Communication

References

Bryman, A. (1996). *Leadership in organizations.* In S. Clegg, C. Hardy, & W. Nord. Handbook of organizations studies, 276-290. London: Sage Publications.

Cardona, P. (2000). Transcendental leadership. *The Leadership & Organization Development Journal, 21*(4), 201-206.

Cardona, P., & Rey, C. (2008). *Dirección por misiones.* Barcelona: Deusto.

Duluc, A. (2000). *Leadership et confiance.* Paris: Dunod.

Ferguson-Paré, M. (1998). Respective: The world, your work, and you! *Canadian Journal of Nursing Administration 11*(4), 57-63.

Manning, G., & Curtis, K. (1988). *Communication: The Miracle of Dialogue.* Cincinnati: South-Western Publishing.

McKee, A., Boyatzis, R., & Johnston, F. (2008). *Becoming a resonant leader.* Boston: Harvard Business Press.

Mehrabian, A. (1968). Communication without words. *Psychology Today, 2*(9), 52-55.

Pérez-López, J.A. (1991). *Fundamentos de la dirección de empresas.* Madrid: Rialp.

Russell, R. F., & Stone, A. G. (2002). A review of servant leadership attributes: Developing a practical model. *Leadership & Organization Development Journal, 23*(3), 145-157.

Upenieks, V. V. (2002). What constitutes successful leadership: A qualitative approach utilizing Kanter's theory of organizational behaviour. *Journal of Nursing Administration, 32*(12), 622-632.

Additional Resources

Chambers Clark, C (2008) *Creative nursing leadership and management.* Jones and Bartlett Publishers. MA. USA.

Robinson-Walker, C (2007). The challenges of being new. *Nurse Leader, 5*(1): pp. 8-9.

15: Community

References

Curato, C. D., Jiongco, K. O, & Koerner, J. E. (2008). Migration. In Weinstein, S. M., & Brooks, A. M. T., (Eds.), *Nursing without borders*. Indianapolis, IN: Sigma Theta Tau International.

Additional Resources

Village Life Outreach Project: http://www.villagelifeoutreach.org/sitepages/ABOUT_home. html

16: Competency

References

Benner, P. (1984). *From novice to expert: Excellence and power in clinical nursing practice*. Menlo Park, CA: Addison-Wesley Publishing Company.

Choudhry, N. K., Fletcher, R. H., & Soumerai, S. B. (2005). Systematic review: the relationship between clinical experience and quality of health care. *Annals of Internal Medicine, 142*: 260-273.

Juvé M. E., Huguet, M., Monterde, D., & Sanmartín, M. J. (2007a). Theoretical and conceptual framework for hospital nurses'competency definition and evaluation. (Marco teórico y conceptual para la definición y evaluación de competencias del profesional de enfermería en el ámbito hospitalario.) *Nursing* (Spanish Edition) *25*(4): 56-61.

Juvé, M.E., Muñoz, S. F., & Calvo, C. M. (2007b). How do hospital nurses explain their clinical competences? (¿Como definen los profesionales de enfermería hospitalarios sus competencias asistenciales?). *Nursing* (Spanish edition) *25*(7): 62-73.

Juvé, M.E., Muñoz, S. F., Monterde, D., Sevillano Lalinde, M., Ollé, C. O., García, A. C. et al. (2008). Expertise threshold required for nursing competent performance. (Umbral de pericia requerido para la ejecución competencial). *Metas de Enfermería 11*(10): 8-15.

McConell, E.A. (2001). Competence vs. competency. *Nursing Management 32*(5): 14-15.

McMullan, M., Endacott, R., Gray, M., Jasper, M., Miller, C., Scholes, J., et.al. (2003). Portfolios and assessment of competence: A review of the literature. *Journal of Advanced Nursing, 41*(3), 283-294.

Ordre des infirmières de Quebec. (1985). *Normes et critères de compétance pour les infermrières*. Quebec OIQ.

Sociedad Española de Enfermería Oncológica. (1997). *Estándares de la práctica de la enfermería oncológica*. Madrid SEEO.

Teixidor, M. et al. (2003). Marc de referència professional per a la funció de supervisor d'infermeria. BCN EUI Santa Madrona- Fundació la Caixa.

Winskill, R. (2000). Is competency based training education useful for workplace training? *Contemporary Nurse 9*(2): 115-119.

Additional Resources

American Nurses Association. (1991). *Standards of clinical nursing practice*. Washington D.C.: ANA.

Dunn, S.V. (2000). The development of competency standards for specialist critical care nurses. *Journal Advanced Nursing, 31*(2): 339-346.

17: Confidence

References
Dubnichi, C., Sloan, S. (1991). Excellence in nursing management Competency-based selection and development. *Journal of Nursing Administration, 21*(6), 40–45.

Jeffers, S. (1987). *Feel the fear and do it anyway*. New York: Ballentine Books.

Kowalski, K., Yoder-Wise, P. (2003). Five Cs of Leadership. *Nurse Leader, 1*(5), 26–31.

Murthy, D. (2008). *Confidence*. Mysore, India: Thoughtfocus Technologies.

Vestal, K. (2005). Confidence: A key ingredient for success. *Nurse Leader, 3*(2), 12–13.

Additional Resources
Barrow, I. (1982). *Know your strengths and be confident: How to achieve confidence through positive thinking, self-acceptance, and self-esteem*. Auckland: Heinemann.

Johnson, R., & Swindley, D. (1994). *Creating confidence: the secrets of self-esteem*. Shaftesbury, Dorset; Rockport, M.A.: Element.

Mind Tools. Ltd. (2009). *Building self-confidence*. London: Author. Retrieved 6 October 2009 from http://www.mindtools.com/selfconf.html

Quan, K. (2006). *The everything new nurse book: Gain confidence, manage your schedule, and deal with the unexpected*. Cincinnati, OH: Adams Media.

Stevens, T.G. (2005). *4:self-confidence*. Retrieved 6 October 2009 from http://www.csulb.edu/~tstevens/h54confi.htm

18: Conflict

References
Anderson, E. W. (2005). A B C of conflict and disorder: Approaches to conflict resolution. *BMJ, 331*, 344-346.

Kantek, F., Kavla, I. (2007). Nurse-nurse manager conflict: How do nurse managers manage it? *The Health Care Manager, 26*(2), 147-151.

Kelly, J. (2006). An overview of conflict. *Dimensions of Critical Care Nursing, 25*(1), 22-28.

Montoro-Rodrigues, J. & Small, J. A. (2006). The role of conflict resolution styles on nursing staff morale, burnout, and job satisfaction in long-term care. *Journal of Aging Health, 18*:385-406.

Saltman, D. C., O'dea, N. A., & Kidd, M. R. (2006). Conflict management: a primer for doctors in training. *Post Graduate Medical Journal, 82*:9-12.

Schilling, D. (n.d.). Managing conflict by using strategies of obliging, getting help, and using humor. Retrieved 6 October 2009 from http://www.womensmedia.com/new/conflict-management-3.shtml

Siu, H., Lschinger, H. K., Finegan, J. (2008). Nursing professional practice environments: Setting the stage for constructive conflict resolution and work effectiveness. *The Journal of Nursing Administration, 38*(5), 250-257.

Tappen, R. M. (2001). Nursing leadership and management: Concepts and practice (4th ed.). Philadelphia: F A Davis Company.

Teambuilding, Inc. (2007). Motivation/relationship problems: Team conflict. Retrieved 6 October 2009 from http://www.teambuildinginc.com/tps/031a.htm

Van de Vliert, E. (1998). Conflict and conflict management. In Drenth, J. H., Thiery, H., & DeWolff C. J. (Eds.). *Handbook of work and organizational psychology* (2nd ed.). London: Psychology Press.

Williamson, G. M., & Schultz, R. (1993). Coping with specific stressors in Alzheimer's disease caregiving. *The Gerontologist, 33*, 747-755.

Winter, F. D., Cherrier, M. I. (2008). Conflict resolution in a different culture. Baylor University Medical Centre Proceedings, *21*(3), 300-303.

Additional Resources:

Conflict resolution: http://www.mindtools.com/pages/article/newLDR_81.htm

Conflict resolution tools: http://www.conflictresolution.com/

19: Creativity

References

Amabile, T. M., & Khaire, M. (2008). Creativity and the role of the leader. *Harvard Business Review*, *86*(10), 101-109.

Smeltzer, C. H., & Vlasses, F. R. (Eds.). (2003). *Ordinary people, extraordinary lives: The stories of nurses*. Indianapolis, IN: Sigma Theta Tau International.

Additional Resources

Amabile, T. M. (1998). How to kill creativity. *Harvard Business Review*, 76(5), 77-87.

Clark, C. C. (2008). *Creative nursing leadership & management*. Boston, MA: Jones and Bartlett Publishers.

Kerfoot, K. (1998). Leading change is leading creativity. *Nursing Economics*, *16*(2), 98-99.

Maxwell, J. C. (2005). *The 360 leader*. Nashville, TN: Thomas Nelson Inc.

Tharp, T. (2003). The Creative Habit: learn it and use it for life. New York: Simon & Schuster.

20: Credibility

References

Anderson, P. (Ed.) (1989). *Great quotes from great leaders*. Lombard.

Carroll, T. L. (2005). Leadership skills and attributes of women and nurse executives: Challenges for the 21st century. *Nursing Administration Quarterly*, *29*(2), 146-153.

Chase, L. (1994). Nurse manager competencies. *Journal of Nursing Administration*, *24*(48), 56-64.

Hader, R. (2005). How do you measure workforce integrity? *Nursing Management*, *36*(9), 32-37.

Kouzes, J. M. & Posner, B. Z. (2002). *The leadership challenge: The most trusted source on becoming a better Leader* (3rd ed.). San Francisco: Jossey-Bass.

Kouzes, J. M. & Posner, B. Z. (2003). *Credibility: How leaders gain and lose it, why people demand it* (rev. ed.). San Francisco: Jossey-Bass.

Petrick, J. & Quinn, J. (2000). The integrity capacity construct and moral progress in business. *Journal of Business Ethics, January*(23), 3-18.

Strubblefield, A. (2005). *The Baptist Healthcare journey to excellence*. Hoboken: John Wiley & Sons.

Additional Resources

Covey, S. R. (2003). *Principle-centered leadership*, New York: Free Press.

Porrini, P., Hiris, L., & Poncini, G. (2009). *How ethical CEOs create honest corporations*. Columbus, OH: McGraw-Hill.

21: Critical Thinking

References

American Philosophical Association (1990). *Critical thinking: A statement of expert consensus for purposes of educational assessment and instruction.* Recommendations prepared for the Committee on Pre-College Philosophy. (ERIC Doc. ED 315 423).

Brookfield, S. D., & Preskill, S. (1999). *Discussion as a way of teaching. Tools and techniques for university teachers.* London: The Society for Research into Higher Education and Open University Press.

Facione, N. C., & Facione, P. A. (1997). *Critical thinking assessment in nursing education programs: An aggregate data analysis.* Millbrae, CA: The California Academic Press.

Facione, P. A., & Facione, N. C. (1994). *The holistic critical thinking scoring rubric.* Millbrae, CA: The California Academic Press.

Facione, P. A., Facione, N. C., Tiwari, A., & Yuen, F. (2009). Chinese and American perspectives on the pervasive human phenomenon of critical thinking. *Journal of Peking University (Philosophy and Social Sciences), 46*(1), pp. 55-62.

Gabrenya, W. K. Jr., & Hwang, K. K. (1996). Chinese social interaction: Harmony and hierarchy on the good earth. In: M.H. Bond (Ed.). *The Handbook of Chinese Psychology.* Hong Kong: Oxford University Press. Pp. 309–321.

Paul, R. W., & Elder, L. (2002). *Critical thinking: Tools for taking charge of your professional and personal life.* NJ: Financial Times Prentice Hall.

Salili, F., Fu, H. Y., Tong, Y. Y., Tabatabai, D. (2001). Motivation and self-regulation: A cross-cultural comparison of the effect of culture and context of learning on student motivation and self-regulation. In: C. Y. Chiu, F. Salili, Y. Y. Hong. (Eds.). *Multiple competencies and self-regulated learning: Implications for multicultural education.* Greenwich, CT: Information Age Publishing.

Titler, M. G. (2004). Overview of the U.S. invitational conference "Advancing Quality Care through Translation Research." *Worldviews on Evidence-based Nursing,* Third Quarter (Suppl.): S1-S5.

Tiwari, A., Lai, P., So, M., & Yuen, K. H. (2006). A comparison of the effects of problem-based learning and lecturing on the development of students' critical thinking. *Medical Education* 40, 547-554.

Additional Resources

Critical thinking development and measurement: http://www.insightassessment.com/

Critical thinking: A statement of expert consensus for purposes of educational assessment and instruction. Executive Summary. http://www.insightassessment.com/pdf_files/DEXadobe.PDF

22: Cultural Diversity

References

Dick, L. (2009). It takes a village to raise a nurse: "Dance Professor Dance" poem. *Transforming nursing education: The culturally inclusive environment.* Springer Publishing Company, 345-346.

Rogers, M. (1997b). Canadian nursing in 2020: Five scenarios. Ottawa: Canadian Nurses Association.

Van Manen, M. (1990). *Researching lived experience: Human science for an action sensitive pedagogy.* Albany, New York: State University of New York Press.

Additional References

Bower, F. (2000). *Nurses taking the lead: Personal qualities of effective leadership*. Philadelphia: W. B. Saunders, Company.

Freire, P. (1970). *Pedagogy of the oppressed*. New York: Herder and Herder.

Wheatley, M. J. (2002). *Turning to one another: Simple conversations to restore hope to the future*. San Francisco: Berrett-Koehler Publishers.

23: Customer Focused

Additional Resources

Blankenbaker, S. E. (2005). Mentor training in a military nurse corps. *Journal for Nurses in Staff Development: 21*(3); 120-125.

Centers for Medicare and Medicaid. HCAHPS Fact Sheet. Accessed October 2, 2009 from http:www.cms.hhs.gov/HospitalQualityInits/Downloads/HospitalHCAHPSFact-Sheet200807.pdf

Customer focus and community engagement. http://www.improvementnetwork.gov.uk/imp/core/page.do?pageId=1068196

Dey, P. K.; Hariharan, S.; & Ho, W. (2009). Innovations in healthcare services: A customer-focused approach. *International Journal of Innovation and Learning*, 6(4), March 27, 2009, pp. 387-405(19).

Lampton, B. (2003). Show and tell: The Ritz-Carlton Hotel part 3. Retrieved 6 October 2009 from http://www.expertmagazine.com/artman/publish/printer_392.shtml

24: Data Collection

References

Hendrich, A., Chow, M., Skierczynski, B., & Zhenqiang, L. (2008). A 36-hospital time and motion study: How do medical-surgical nurses spend their time? *The Permanente Journal, 12*(3), 25-34.

Institute For Healthcare Improvement. (2008). TCAB improvements double nurse time at the bedside: An interview with IHI's Pat Rutherford. *The Business of Caring, July/August 2008*. Retrieved 5 October 2009 from http://www.ihi.org/NR/rdonlyres/0FF90B6F-2AA8-4981-96EE-53608A177F0E/0/RutherfordTCABImprovementsinterview_HFMABusinessof-CaringAug08.pdf

Rutherford, P., Lee, B., & Grelner, A. (2004). *Transforming care at the bedside*. Cambridge, MA: Institute for Health Care Improvement

Additional Resources

Institute for Health Care Improvement. (2008). Transforming care at the bedside framework. Retrieved 5 October 2009, from http://www.ihi.org/NR/rdonlyres/37FDB5E8-52ED-4CC2-8E43-E2C22DA53AFE/0/VisioTCABframework4908.pdf

Kohn L. T., Corrigan, J. M., Donaldson, M. S., (Eds.). (1999). *To err is human: Building a safer health care system*. Committee on Quality of Health Care in America, Institute of Medicine. Washington, D.C.: National Academies Press.

25: Decision Making and Leadership

References

Bandman, E., & Bandman, B. (1988). *Critical thinking nursing*. New York: McGraw-Hill/Appleton & Lange.

Blegen, M. A., Goode, C., Johnson, M., Maas, M., Chen, L., & Moorhead, S. (1993) Preferences for decision-making autonomy. *IMAGE: Journal of Nursing Scholarship* 25(4): 339-344.

Carroll, J. S., & Johnson, E. J. (1990). Decision research. A field guide. *Applied Social Research Methods*, Vol. 22.

Curtin, L. (1996). Why good people do bad things. *Nursing Management*, 27(7): 63-66.

Dijksterhuis, A. (2007). Intuition will gut überlegt sein. *Harvard Business Manager*, 2: 22-23.

Dijksterhuis, A., & Nordgren, L. (2006). A theory of unconscious thought. *Perspectives on Psychological Science*, 1(2): 95-109.

Easen, P., & Wilcockson, J. (1996). Intuition and rational decision making in professional thinking: A false dichotomy? *Journal of Advanced Nursing*, 24: 667-673.

Grohar-Murray, M. E. & DiCroce, H. R. (1997). Leadership and management in nursing. Stamford, Connecticut: Appleton & Lange.

Kramer, M., Schmalenberg, C.E (2003). Magnet hospital staff nurses describe clinical autonomy. *Nursing Outlook.* 51(1): 13-9.

Laschinger, H., Shamian, J., & Thomson, D. (2001). Impact of magnet hospitals characteristics on nurses' perceptions of trust, burnout, quality of care, and work satisfaction. *Nursing Economics*, 19(5): 2009-2219.

Lennik, D., & Kiel, F. (2005). Moral intelligence: Enhancing business performance and leadership success. Philadelphia: Wharton School Publishing.

Manthey, M. (1980). The Practice of Primary Nursing. Minneapolis, MN: Creative Nursing Management.

Mrayyan, M. (2003). Nurse autonomy, nurse job satisfaction, and client satisfaction with nursing care: Their place in nursing data sets. *Nursing Leadership*, 16(2): 74-82.

Nash, L. (1990). Good intention aside: A manager's guide to resolving ethical problems. Boston: Harvard Business School Press.

Taylor, F. (2005). A comparative study examining the decision-making process of medical and nursing staff in weaning patients from mechanical ventilation. *Intensive and Critical Care Nursing*, 22(5): 253-263.

Tewes, R. (2008). Fuehrungskompetenz ist lernbar. Praxiswissen für Fuerhungskraefte in Gesundheitsfachberufen. Berlin: Springer.

Additional Resources

Kaspar, R. W., & Wills, C. E.; Kaspar, B. K. (2009). Gene therapy and informed consent decision making: Nursing research directions. *Biological Research for Nursing*. 11 (1): 98-107.

King, A. J., & Cowlishaw, G (2009). Leaders, followers, and group decision-making. *Communicative & Integrative Biology*. 2(2): 147-50.

Schlairet, M. C. (2009). Bioethics mediation: The role and importance of nursing advocacy. *Nursing Outlook*, 57(4); pp. 185-93.

Shirey, M. R. (2009). Authentic leadership, organizational culture, and healthy work environments. *Critical Care Nursing Quarterly*. 32 (3): 189-98.

Tewes, R. (2009). Entscheidungen treffen (decision making). In Tewes: *Fuehrungskompetenz ist lernbar*. Pp.107-124. Berlin: Springer.

26: Delegation

References

Barrera, L., Pinto, N., & Sánchez, B. (2006). Cuidando a los cuidadores: Un programa de apoyo a familiares de personas con enfermedad crónica. *Index de Enfermería*, 15(52-53): 54-58.

Barter, M. (2002). Follow the team leader. *Nursing Management*, 33(1), 54-57.

Cohen, S. (2001). Pass it on? *Nursing Management, 31*(8), 24-25.

Cohen, S. (2004). Delegating versus dumping: Teach the difference. *Nursing Management, 35*(10), 14-18.

Feltner, A., Mitchell, B., Norris, E., & Wollfle, C. (2008). Nurses' views on the characteristics of an effective leader. *AORN Journal, 87*(2), 363-372.

Fisher, M. (1999). Do your nurses delegate effectively? *Nursing Management, 30*(5), 23-25.

National Council of State Boards of Nursing (1995). Delegation: Concepts and decision-making process. National Council Position Paper. Retrieved 5 October 2009 from https://www.ncsbn.org/323.htm

Sherman, R., Bishop, M., Eggenberger, T. & Karden, R. (2007). Development of a leadership competency model. *Journal of Nursing Administration, 37*(2), 85-94.

Sullivan, J., Bretschneider, J., & McCausland, M. (2003). Designing a leadership development program for nurses' managers. *Journal of Nursing Administration, 33*(10), 544-549.

Valiga, T & Grossman, S. (2007). Leadership and followership. In *Nursing leadership and management: Theories, process, and practice*. R. Patronis (Ed.), pp. 3-12. Philadelphia: Davis Company.

Additional Resources

Hudson, T. (2008). Delegation: Building a foundation for our future nurse leaders. *MedSurg Nursing*. Retrieved 5 October 2009 from http://findarticles.com/p/articles/mi_m0FSS/is_6_17/ai_n31297752/?tag=content;col1

Huber, D. (2006). *Leadership and nursing care management* (3rd ed.). Philadelphia: Elsevier Health Sciences.

Thomas, S., & Hume, G. (1998). Delegation competencies: Beginning practitioners' reflections. *Nurse Educator*. 23(1), pp 38-41.

27: Diversity

References

Benner, P. (1984). *From novice to expert: Excellence and power in clinical nursing practice*. Menlo Park, CA: Addison-Wesley Publishing Company.

Dreyfus, H. L., Dreyfus, S. E., & Athanasiou, T. (1986). *Mind over machine*. New York: The Free Press.

Institute of Medicine (2004). *In the nation's compelling interest: Ensuring diversity in the health care workforce*. Washington, D.C.: The National Academies Board on Health Sciences Policy.

Sullivan Commission (2004). Missing persons: Minorities in the health professions. Retrieved 6 October 2009 from http://www.kaisernetwork.org/health_cast/hcast_index.cfm?display=detail&hc=1141

Additional Resources

Center for Cross-Cultural Health (CCCH). The mission is to integrate the role of culture in improving health to ensure diverse populations receive culturally competent and sensitive health care. http://www.crosshealth.com/

Office of Minority Health Resource Center (OMHRC). Established by the United States Department of Health and Human Resources (DHHS), the OMHRC serves as a national resource and referral service on minority health issues. http://www.omhrc.gov

Provider's Guide to Quality and Culture. This is a joint project of Management Sciences for Health (MSH), United States Department of Health and Human Resources, Health Resources and Services Administration, and the Bureau of Primary Health Care. This site is designed to assist health care organizations in providing high quality, culturally competent services to multi-ethnic populations. http://erc.msh.org/mainpage.cfm?file=1.0.htm&module=provider&language=English&ggroup=&mgroup=

28: Empowerment

References
Allison, P., & Laschinger, H. K. S. (2005). The effect of structural empowerment and perceived organizational support on middle level nurse managers' role satisfaction. *Journal of Nursing Management*, 14, 13-22.

Anderson, E. F. F. (2000). *Empowerment, job satisfaction and professional governance of nurses in hospital with and without shared governance.* New Orleans, LA: Louisiana State University Medical Center School of Nursing.

Bass, B. M. (1985). *Leadership and performance: Beyond expectation.* New York: Free Press.

Breisch, R.L. (1999). Motivate! *Nursing Management*, 30(3), 27-30.

Conger, J.A., & Kanungo, R.N. (1988). The empowerment process: Integrating theory and practice. *Academy of Management Review, 13*(3), 471-482.

French, J., Raven, B. (1968), The basis of social power. In Cartwright, D., & Zander, A. (Eds.) *Group dynamics, research, and theory* (3rd ed.). New York: Harper & Row.

Huber, D. (2000). *Leadership and nursing care management,* (2nd ed.) Philadelphia: Saunders.

Kanter, R. (1993). *Men and woman of the corporation,* (2nd ed.) New York: Basic Books.

Kuokkanen, L., Suominen, T., Rankinen, S., Kukkurainen, M. L., Savikko, N., & Doran, D. (2007). Organizational change and work-related empowerment. *Journal of Nursing Management, 15*(5), 500-507.

Lancaster, J. (1985). Creating a climate for excellence. *Journal of Nursing Administration, 15*(1), 16-19.

Laschinger, H.K.S., Finegan, J., & Shamian, J. (2001). Promoting nurses' health: Effect of empowerment on job strain and work satisfaction. *Nursing Economics, 19*(2), 42-52.

Manojlovich, M., & Laschinger, H. K. S. (2002).The relation of empowerment and selected personality characteristics to nursing job satisfaction. *Journal of Nursing Administration, 32*(11), 586-595.

Welford, C. (2002). Transformational leadership in nursing. *Nursing management, 9*(4), 7-11.

Additional Resources
Curtin, L. (2000). The first ten principles for the ethical administration of nursing services. *Nursing Administration Quarterly, 25*(1), 7-13.

Lucas, V., Laschinger H. K., & Wong, C. A. (2008). The impact of emotional intelligent leadership on staff nurse empowerment: The moderating effect of span of control. *Journal of Nursing Management, 16*, 964-973.

29: Energy

References
Daily, T. (2008). *Four gateways coaching: Evoking soul wisdom.* Boulder, CO: Living Arts Publishing.

Gordon, J. (2006). *The 10-minute energy solution.* New York: Penguin Putnam.

Johnson, B. (1996). *Polarity management: Identifying and managing unsolvable problems.* Amherst, MA: HRD Press.

Wesorick, B. & Shiparski, L. (1997). *Can the human being thrive in the work place? Dialogue as a strategy of hope.* Grand Rapids, MI: Practice Field Publishing.

Additional Resources
Buckingham, M., & Clifton, D. (2001). *Now, discover your strengths.* New York: The Free Press.

Emerald, D. (2006). *The Power of TED: The Empowerment Dynamic.* Bainbridge Island, WA: Polaris Publishing.

Hicks, E. & Hicks, J. (2006). *The law of attraction*. Australia: Hay House Inc.

Plotkin, B. (2008). *Nature and the human soul*. Novato, CA: New World Library.

Senge, P. (2008). *The necessary revolution*. New York: Doubleday Publishing.

Tolle, E. (2005) *A new earth: Awakening to your life's purpose*. New York: Penguin Putnam.

Williamson, M. (2004). *The gift of change*. New York: Harper Collins.

30: Environment

References

Analects. (n.d.). Retrieved 5 October 2009 from http://chinese.dsturgeon.net/text. pl?node=1088&if=en

Andersen, R. M., & Davidson, P. L. (2001). Improving access to care in America: Individual and contextual indicators. In Andersen, R. M., Rice, T. H., & Kominski, G. F. *Changing the U.S. health care system: Key issues in health services, policy, and management*. San Francisco: Jossey-Bass, 3–30.

Blumenthal, D., & Hsiao, W. (2005). Privatization and its discontents: The evolving Chinese health care system. *The New England Journal of Medicine*, 353: 1165–1170.

Brooten, D., Naylor, M. D., & York, R. (2002). Lessons learned from testing the quality cost model of advanced practice nursing (APN) transitional care. *Journal of Nursing Scholarship*, 34(4): 369–375.

Fung, H., Tse, N., & Yeoh, E. K. (1999). Health care reform and societal values. *Journal of Medicine and Philosophy*, 24: 638–652.

Gao, J., Tang, S., Tolhurst, R., Rao, K. (2001). Changing access to health services in urban China: Implications for equity. *Health Policy and Planning*, 16: 302–312.

Harvard Team. (1999). *Improving Hong Kong's health care system: Why and for whom?* (Main report and special reports). Hong Kong SAR Government.

Hong Kong SAR Government. (2008). *Health reform consultation document*. Hong Kong: Author.

Liu, X. P., et al. (2002). A discussion about the referral management with the conception of patient focus. *Chinese General Practice*, 5: 369–370.

Miller, A. (1984). *Salesman in Beijing*. New York: The Viking Press.

Naylor, M. D., Brooten, D., Campbell, R., Jacobsen, B. S., Mezey, M. D., Pauly, M. V. et al. (1999). Comprehensive discharge planning and home follow-up of hospitalized elders. *Journal of the American Medical Association*, 281: 613–620.

World Bank (1997). *Financing health care: China 2020 Series*. Washington D.C.: The World Bank.

Additional Resources

Ministry of Health of the People's Republic of China: http://www.moh.gov.cn/publicfiles//business/htmlfiles/wsb/index.htm

World Health Organization: http://www.who.int/en/

31: Evolving Leadership

References

Caramanica, L., Maljanian, R., McDonald, P., Taylor, J., MacRae & Beland, D. (2002). Evidence-based nursing practice, part 2: Building skills through research roundtables. *Journal of Nursing Administration*, 32, 85-90.

Caramanica, L., & Roy, J. (2006). Evidence-based practice: Creating the environment for practice excellence. *Nurse Leader*, 4(6)), 38-41.

Chiokfoong-Loke, J. (2001). Leadership behaviours: Effects on job satisfaction, productivity, and organizational commitment. *Journal of Nursing Management, 9*(4), 191-204.

Cullen, L., & Titler, M. G. (2004). Promoting evidence-based practice: An internship for staff nurses. *Worldviews Evidence-Based Nursing, 1*(4), 215-223

Graham, I. (2003). Leading the development of nursing within a nursing development unit: The perspectives of leadership by the team leader and a professor of nursing. *International Journal of Nursing Practice, 9*(4), 213-222.

Heller, B. R., Oros, M. T., & Durney-Crowley, J. (2005). The future of nursing education: 10 Trends to Watch. *Nursing and Health Care Perspectives, 21*(1), 9-13.

King, G. (2001). Perception of intentional wrongdoing and peer reporting behavior among registered nurses. *Journal of Business Ethics, 34*, 1-13.

Medland, J., Howard-Ruben, J., & Whitaker, E. (2004). Fostering psychosocial wellness in oncology nurses: Addressing burnout and social support in the workplace. *Oncology Nursing Forum, 31*(1), 47-54.

Perednia, D. A., & Allen, A. (1995). Telemedicine technology and clinical applications. *Journal of the American Medical Association, 273*, 483-488.

Scott-Cawiezell, J., Schenkman, M., Moore, L., Vojir, C., Connolly, R., Pratt, M., & Palmer, L. (2004). Exploring nursing home staff's perceptions of communication and leadership to facilitate quality improvement. *Journal of Nursing Care Quality, 19*(3), 242-252.

Street, M. D., Robertson, C., & Geiger, S. W. (1997). Ethical decision making: The effect of escalating commitment. *Journal of Business Ethics, 16*, 1153-1161.

Tabak, N., Reches, R., & Wagner, N. (1995). *Whistle blowing: Attitudes of Israeli nurses.* Tel Aviv University, Department of Nursing.

Upenieks, V. (2003). Nurse leaders' perceptions of what compromises successful leadership in today's acute inpatient environment. *Nursing Administration Quarterly, 27*(2), 140-152.

32: Excellent Care

References
Peters, T. & Waterman, R. (2004). *In search of excellence: Lessons from America's best-run companies.* London: HarperCollins Business.

Waitley, D. (1988). *Seeds of greatness: The best kept secrets of total success.* New York: Pocket Books.

Additional Resources
Austin, N. & Peters, T. (1989). *A passion for excellence: The leadership difference.* New York: Grand Central Publishing.

Byrne, R. (2006). *The secret.* New York: Beyond Words Publishing.

33: Facility Design

References
Advisory Board. (February 21, 2003). *Benefits of private hospital rooms: Literature review.* Washington, D.C.: Author.

Bilchik, G. S. (2002). A better place to heal. *Health Forum Journal, 45*(4), 10-15.

Hamilton, D. K. (2000). *Design for patient units.* Retrieved 5 October 2009 from http://muhc-healing.mcgill.ca/english/Speakers/hamilton_p2.html

Hendrich, A. L., Fay, J. & Sorrells, A. K. (2004). Effects of acuity-adaptable rooms on flow of patients and delivery of care. *American Journal of Critical Care, 13*(1), 35-45.

Lowers, J. (1999). Improving quality through the built environment. *The Quality Letter, 11*(8), 2-9.

Marberry, S. O. (Ed.). (2006). *Improving healthcare with better building design*. Chicago: Health Administration Press.

NOP World-Technology. (2001). *Wireless LANS benefits study*. Retrieved 5 October 2009 from www.sparcotech.com/Cisco%20WLAN%20Benefits%20Study.pdf

Reid, P. P., Compton, W. D., Grossman, J. H., & Fanjiang, G. (Eds). (2005). *Building a better delivery system: A new engineering/health care partnership*. Washington, D.C.: National Academies Press.

Ulrich, R., Quan, X., Zimring, C., Joseph, A., & Choudhary, R. (2004). *The role of the physical environment in the hospital of the 21st century: A once-in-a-lifetime opportunity*. Robert Wood Johnson Foundation and The Center for Healthcare Design. Retrieved 5 October 2009 from http://www.rwjf.org/pr/product.jsp?id=21022

Watson, C. A. (2005). Integration of technology and facility design: Implications for nursing administration. *Journal of Nursing Administration, 35*(5), 217-219.

Additional Resources

Agency for Healthcare Research and Quality. (2007). *Transforming hospitals: Designing for safety and quality*. (AHRQ Publication No. 07-0076-01). Rockville, MD: Author.

American Institute of Architects. (2006). *Guidelines for design and construction of health care facilities*. Washington, D.C.: Author.

American of Organization of Nurse Executives. (2009). *Guiding principles for creating the hospital of the future*. Washington, D.C.: Author.

Center for Health Design. A research and advocacy organization for health care and design professionals who are leading the quest to improve the quality of health care through building architecture and design: www.healthdesign.org

McCullough, C. (2009). *Evidence-based design for healthcare facilities*. Indianapolis, IN: Sigma Theta Tau International.

Robert Wood Johnson Foundation. (2007). *Designing the 21st century hospital*. Princeton, NJ: Author.

34: Financial Management

References

National Coalition on Health Care. (n.d.) *Health insurance costs*. Retrieved 5 October 2009 from www.nchc.org/facts/cost.shtml

United States Department of Health and Human Services Centers for Medicare and Medicaid Services. (n.d.). *2006 national health care expenditures data*. Retrieved 5 October 2009 from http://www.cms.hhs.gov/NationalHealthExpendData/02_NationalHealthAccountsHistorical.asp

Waxman, KT. (2008). *A practical guide to finance and budgeting: Skills for nurse managers* (2nd ed.). Marblehead, MA: HCPro, Inc.

Additional Resources

Finkler, S., & Kovner, C. T. (2000). *Financial management for nurse managers and executives* (2nd ed.). Philadelphia: W.B. Saunders.

Marelli, T. M. (2004). *The nurse manager's survival guide* (3rd ed.). St. Louis: Mosby.

35: First 100 Days

References
Kouzes, J. M. & Posner, B. Z. (2003). *Encouraging the heart: A leader's guide to rewarding and recognizing others.* San Francisco: Jossey-Bass.

Secretan, L.H.K. (2004). *Inspire! What great leaders do.* NJ: John Wiley & Sons, Inc.

Additional Resources
Anderson, M. (2007). *You can't send a duck to eagle school.* Naperville, IL: Simple Truths.

Asch, S. (2007). *Excellence at work: The six keys to inspire passion in the workplace.* Scottsdale, AZ: WorldatWork Press.

Bradt, G. B., Check, J. A. & Pedraza, J. E. (2006). *The new leader's 100-day action plan: How to take charge, build your team, and get immediate results.* Hoboken, NJ: John Wiley & Sons.

Fitz, M. (2008). *The truth about getting things done.* Harlow, UK: Pearson Education.

Koch. R. (2008). *Living the 80/20 way.* London: Nicholas Brealey Publishing.

Lustberg, A. (2008). *How to sell yourself: Using leadership, likability, and luck to succeed.* Franklin Lakes, NJ: Career Press.

Maxwell, J. C. (2007). *The 17 indisputable laws of teamwork: Embrace them and empower your team.* Nashville, TN: Thomas Nelson Publishers.

Rath, T. (2006). *Vital Friends: The people you can't afford to live without.* New York: Gallup Press.

Zaffron, S. & Logan, D. (2009). *The three laws of performance: Rewriting the future of your organization and your life.* San Francisco: Jossey-Bass.

36: Gifts

Additional Resources
Covey, S. (2006). *The speed of trust.* New York: Simon & Schuster.

Maxwell, J. (2008). *Leadership gold.* Nashville, TN: Thomas Nelson, Inc.

Peters, T. (2005). *Leadership: Inspire, liberate, achieve.* New York: DK Publishing, Inc.

37: Global Nursing at Its Best

References
Buchan, J. (2006). Impact of global nursing migration on health services delivery. *Policy, Politics, and Nursing Practice,* 7(3): 16–25.

Connell, J., Zurn, P., Stilwell, B., Awases, M. & Braichet J. (2007). Sub-Saharan Africa: Beyond the health worker migration crisis? *Social Science & Medicine,* 64(9), 1876-1891.

Cowen, P. S. & Moorhead, S. (2006). Nursing: A global view. In Cowen, P. S., & Moorhead, S. (Eds.), *Current Issues in Nursing* (7th ed.). Mosby Elsevier: 784–787.

Daly, H. E. (1999). Globalization versus internationalization implication. Economics 31, 31–37.

International Council of Nurses. (2005). *The global nursing shortage: Priority areas for prevention.* Report from ICN/FNIF.

Kingma, M. (2006). Nurses on the move: Migration and the global health care economy. Ithaca, NY: ILR, an imprint of Cornell University Press.

Schober, M. & Affarwa, F. (2006). Advanced nursing practice. Blackwell Publishers, Koramangala.

Seloilwe, E. (2004). Globalization and nursing. Guest Editorial. *Journal of Advanced Nursing,* 50(6): 571.

Tshweneagae, G. (2006). *Migration of nurses in Botswana*. BIDPA and Nurses Association of Botswana.

Upvall, M. J. (2006). International graduate nursing education. In Cowen, P. S., & Moorhead, S. (Eds.), *Current Issues in Nursing* (7th ed.). Mosby Elsevier: 86–92.

Additional Resources

Cowen, P. S., & Moorhead, S. (2006). *Current issues in nursing* (7th ed.). Mosby Elsevier.

International Council of Nurses, the Global Nursing Review Initiative: Policy options and solutions. Retrieved 5 October 2009 from http://www.icn.ch/global

38: Global Perspective

References

Cañon, W., Agudelo, N., Manosalva, J., Rincon, F., Rivera, L. N., Para, M. et al. (2008). Critical care nursing in Colombia: The formation of a new critical care nursing association. *CONNECT*, 6(3), pp. 51–53.

Williams G., Chaboyer, W., Alberto, L., Thornsteindóttir, R., Schmollgruber, S., Fulbrook, P. et al. (2007). Critical care nursing organisations and activities—a second worldwide review. *International Nursing Review*, 54, pp. 151–159.

Williams G., Chaboyer, W., Thornsteindóttir, R., Fulbrook, P., Shelton, C., Chan, D. et al. (2001). World wide overview of critical care nursing organisations and their activities. *International Nursing Review*, 48(Dec): 208–217.

Additional Resources

Colombian Committee of Critical Care Nurses: http://www.obolog.com/users/acecc

CONNECT: The World of Critical Care: www.connectpublishing.com/

International Council of Nurses: www.icn.ch

Medecins Sans Frontieres: www.msf.org/

Sigma Theta Tau International Institute: www.nursingsociety.org/default.aspx

World Federation of Critical Care Nurses. Retrieved 5 October 2009 from www.fccn.org/

39: Goal Setting

References

Adair, J. (1983). *Effective leadership*. London: Panmacmillan.

Australian Institute of Health and Welfare. (2008). *Australia's health 2008*. Cat no. AUS 99, Canberra: AIHW.

Covey, S. (1999). *First things first*. New York: Simon & Schuster.

Musker. M. (2004). Leading, motivating, and enthusing. In Crowther A. *Nurse Managers: A Guide to Practice* (Crowther, A., Ed.). Melbourne: Ausmed Publications.

Williams. G., Chaboyer, W., & Schluter, P. (2002). Assault-related admissions to hospital in central Australia. *Medical Journal of Australia*, 177: 300–304.

Additional Resources

Covey, S. (2004). *The 7 habits of highly effective people*. New York: Free Press.

40: Grants

References

Booth, J., Kumlien, S., Zang, Y., Gustafsson, B., & Tolson, D. (2009). Rehabilitation nurses practices in relation to urinary incontinence following stroke: A cross-cultural comparison. *Journal of Clinical Nursing*. 18 1049-1058.

Tolson, D., Booth, J., & Lowndes, A. (2008). Achieving evidence-based nursing practice: Impact of the Caledonian Development Model. *Journal of Nursing Management*, 16: 682–691.

Tolson, D., Irene, S., Booth, J., Kelly, T. B., & James, L. (2006). Constructing a new approach to developing evidence-based practice with nurses and older people. *World Views on Evidence-Based Nursing*, 3(2): 62–72.

Tolson, D., Schofield, I., Booth, J., & Kelly, T. B. (2007). Partnerships in best practice: Advancing gerontological care in Scotland. In Nolan, M., Hanson, E., & Grant, G. (Eds.), *User participation in health and social care research: Voices, values, and evaluation.* . Open University Press.

Additional Resources

Holtzclaw, B. (2008). *Grant writing handbook for nurses* (2nd ed.) Sudbury, MA: Jones & Bartlett.

Systematic Review Libraries: http://www.joannabriggs.edu.au/pubs/systematic_reviews.php and www.cochrane.org/reviews/

41: Groups and Individuals

References

Boykin, A., & Schoenhofer, S. (2001a). *Nursing as caring: A model for transforming practice*. Sudbury, MA: Harper Perennial.

Boykin, A., & Schoenhofer, S. (2001b). The role of nursing leadership in creating caring environments in healthcare delivery systems. *Nursing Administration Quarterly*, 25(3): 17.

Covey, S. (2004). *The 7 habits of highly effective people*. New York: Free Press

Koloroutis, M. (Ed.) (2004). *Relationship-based care: A model for transforming practice*. Minneapolis: Creative Health Care Management.

Newman, M. A. (1994). *Health as expanding consciousness* (2nd ed.). Boston: Jones and Bartlett.

Newman, M. A. (2008). *Transforming presence: The difference that nursing makes*. Philadelphia, PA: F. A. Davis Company.

Newman, M. A., Smith, M. C., Pharris, M. D., Jones, D. (2008). The focus of the discipline revisited. *Advances in Nursing Science*, 31(1): E16–E27.

Ray, M., Turkel, M., & Marino, F. (2002). Transformative process for nursing in workforce redevelopment. *Nursing Administration Quarterly*, 26(2): 1–14.

Sherman, R. (2006). Leading a multigenerational workforce: Issues, challenges, and strategies. *The Online Journal of Issues in Nursing*, 11(2): Manuscript 2. Accessed at http://www.nursingworld.org/MainMenuCategories/ANAMarketplace/ANAPeriodicals/OJIN/TableofContents/Volume112006/No2May06/tpc30_216074.aspx

Additional Resources

Chambers-Clark, C. (Ed.). (2009). *Creative nursing leadership and management*. Boston: Jones and Bartlett.

Fagin, C. M. (2000). *Essays on nursing leadership*. New York: Springer Publishing.

Feldman, H. (Ed,). (2008). *Nursing leadership: A concise encyclopedia*. New York: Springer Publishing.

42: Growing Through Lifelong Learning

References

Zinn-Kabat, J. (2005). *Coming to our senses: Healing ourselves and the world through mindfulness;* New York: Hyperion.

Additional Resources

Childre, B., & Cryer, B. (2000). *From chaos to coherence: The power to change performance.* Boulder Creek, CA: Planetary Publications.

43: Healing

References

American Holistic Nurses Association and American Nurses Association (2007). *Holistic nursing: Scope and standards of practice.* Silver Spring, MD: NurseBooks.org.

Dossey, B. M. (2008). Integral and holistic nursing. In Dossey, B. M., & Keegan, L. *Holistic nursing: A handbook for practice* (5th ed.). Sudbury, MA: Jones & Bartlett.

Dossey, B. M. (2010). *Florence Nightingale: Mystic, visionary, healer* (2nd ed.). Philadelphia: F.A. Davis.

Dossey, B. M., Selanders, L. C., Beck, D.-M. (2005). *Florence Nightingale today: Healing, leadership, global action.* Washington, D.C.: NurseBooks.Org.

Additional Resources

American Holistic Nurses Association: http://www.ahna.org/Home/tabid/1231/Default.aspx

Nightingale Declaration: http://www.nightingaledeclaration.net

44: Image

Additional Resources

World Health Organization. Nursing and midwifery at WHO: http://www.who.int/hrh/nursing_midwifery/en/

45: Influence

Additional Resources

Izzo, J. & Withers. P. (2000). *Values shift.* Vancouver: Fair Winds Press.

Marriner-Tomey, A. (1993). *Transformational leadership in nursing.* St. Louis: Mosby Year Book.

Quinn, F. (1995). *The principles and practice of nurse education.* London: Chapman & Hall.

Royal College of Nursing (2004). *Helping students get the best from their practice placements.* UK: RCN Publication.

46: Information Technology

References

Clancy, T. R. (2008). Fractals: Nature's formula for managing hospital performance metrics. *Journal of Nursing Administration,* 38(12), pp. 510–513.

Clancy, T. R. & Delaney, C. (2005). Complex nursing systems. *Journal of Nursing Management,* 13(3), pp. 192–201.

George, G. L. (2003). *Lean six sigma for service.* New York: McGraw Hill.

Institute of Medicine. (1996). *Crossing the quality chasm.* Washington, D.C.: National Academies Press.

Kurzweil, R. (2005). *The singularity is near: When humans transcend biology.* New York: Viking Press.

Skyttner, L. (2001). *General systems theory: Ideas and applications.* Singapore: World Scientific.

Webster's Online Dictionary. (n.d.) Retrieved 5 October 2009 from http://www.websters-online-dictionary.org/definition/elegant

Additional Resources
Joint Commission: http://www.jointcommission.org/PatientSafety/

47: Innovating

Additional Resources
Berkun, S. (2007). *The myths of innovation.* Sebastopol, CA: O'Reilly.

Fonseca, J. (2002). *Complexity and innovation in organizations.* New York: Routledge.

Kelley, T. (2005). *The ten faces of innovation.* New York: Doubleday.

Malloch, K., & Porter-O'Grady, T. (2005). *The quantum leader: Applications for the new world of work.* Sudbury, MA: Jones & Bartlett.

Palmer, P. J. (2000). *Let your life speak: Listening for the voice of vocation.* San Francisco: Jossey-Bass.

Porter-O'Grady, T. & Malloch, K. (2007). *Quantum leadership: A resource for healthcare innovation.* Sudbury, MA: Jones & Bartlett.

Senge, P. M.; Scharmer, C. O.; Jaworski, J.; & Flowers, B. (2006). *Presence: An exploration of profound change in people, organizations, and society.* New York: Currency.

48: Jobless

Additional Resources
Drain, P. (1992). *Hire me!* New York: PSS Adult.

Templar, R. (2005). *The rules of work.* London: FT Press.

49: Leadership Models

References
Evans, W. J., Honemann, D. H., Robert, H. M., Balch, T. J. (2000). *Robert's rules of order* (Newly rev., 10th ed.), Cambridge, MA: Da Capo Press.

Mancino, D. J. (2002). *50 years of the national student nurses' association.* New York: National Student Nurses Association.

Additional Resources
Code of Conduct for NSNA Meetings. (2006). National Student Nurses' Association. http://www.nsna.org/meetings/code_of_conduct_members.asp.

Code of Professional Conduct (1999). National Student Nurses' Association. http://www.nsna.org/pubs/resources/professional_conduct.asp

Mancino, D. J. (Producer). (2005). *Mentoring—the experience of a lifetime* (DVD). New York: National Student Nurses Association.

Mancino, D. J., (Producer). (2009). *Nursing—the career for a lifetime* (DVD). New York: National Student Nurses Association.

National Student Nurses Association. (2008). *NSNA code of professional conduct for the board of directors*. New York: Author.

Vance, C. & Olson, R. (1998). *The mentor connection in nursing*. New York: Springer Publishing Company.

50: Leading Interdisciplinary Partnership at the Point of Care

References

Johnson, B. (1996). *Polarity management: Identifying and managing unsolvable problems*. Amherst, Massachusetts: HRD Press Inc.

Wesorick, B. (1995). *The closing and opening of a millennium: A journey from old to new thinking*. Wisdom from the Field Nursing Series, Book 1. Grand Rapids, MI: Practice Field Publishing.

Wesorick, B. (1996). *The closing and opening of a millennium: A journey from old to new relationships in the work setting*. Wisdom from the Field Nursing Series, Book 2. Grand Rapids, MI: Practice Field Publishing.

Wesorick, B. (2002). 21st century leadership challenge: Creating and sustaining healthy, healing work cultures and integrated service at the point of care. *Nursing Administration Quarterly*, 26(5): 18–32.

Wesorick, B. (2008). Live a legacy or live a lie. *Nurse Administration Quarterly*, 32(2): 142–158.

Wesorick, B., Shiparski, L., Wyngarden, K., & Troseth, M. (1998). *Partnership council field book—strategies and tools for co-creating a healthy work place*. Grand Rapids, MI: Practice Field Publishing.

Zaiss, C. (2002). *True partnership: Thinking about relating to others*. San Francisco: Berret-Koehler Publishers.

Additional Resources

CPRM Resource Center: www.cpmrc.com

Hock, D. (2005) *One from many: VISA and the rise of chaordic organization*, San Francisco: Berrett-Koehler Publishers.

Institute of Medicine. (2004). *Keeping patients safe: Transforming the work environment of nurses*. Washington D.C.: Author.

Shiparski, L., (2005). Engaging in shared decision making: Leveraging staff and management expertise. *Nurse Leader*, 3(1). Pp 36-41.

Technology Informatics Guiding Education Reform (TIGER). (2007). *Evidence and Informatics Transforming Nursing: 3-Year Action Steps toward a 10-Year Vision*. The TIGER Initiative (2007): 1-15. Retrieved 5 October 2009 from http://www.aacn.nche.edu/Education/pdf/TIGER.pdf

Walker, P., & Newbold, S. (2007). TIGER on the move: Vision, action, collaboration. *Nursing Outlook*, 55(6). Pp. 327-328.

51: Listening

References

Encarta. (n.d.). Retrieved 5 October 5, 2009 from http://encarta.msn.com/encnet/refpages/search.aspx?q=listening

Pier 9. (2006). *Women who changed the world: Fifty inspirational women who shaped history*. London: Murdoch Books.

Additional Resources

Cloud, H. (2006). *9 things a leader must do*. Nashville, TN: Thomas Nelson.

George, B. (2003). *Authentic leadership: Rediscovering the secrets to creating lasting value*. San Francisco: Jossey-Bass.

Jaques, E., & Clement, S. (2006). *Executive leadership: A practical guide to managing complexity*. Malden, MA: Blackwell Publishing.

Maxwell, J. (2008). *Leadership gold: Lessons I've learned from a lifetime of leading*. Nashville, TN: Thomas Nelson.

McKee, A., Boyatzis, R., & Johnson, F. (2008). *Becoming a resonant leader: Develop your emotional intelligence, renew your relationships, sustain your effectiveness*. Boston, MA: Harvard Business Press.

Morgan, M., Levitt, R., & Malek, W. (2007). *Executing your strategy: How to break it down and get it done*. Boston, MA: Harvard Business School Press.

Nambisan, S., & Sawhney, M. (2008). *The global brain*. Upper Saddle River, NJ: Wharton School Publishing.

Tabrizi, B. (2007). *Rapid transformation*. Boston, MA: Harvard Business School Press.

Wageman, R., Nunes, D., Burruss, J., & Hackman, J. (2008). *Senior leadership teams: What it takes to make them great*. Boston, MA: Harvard Business School Press.

52: Meeting Management

References

Hansten, R. & Washburn, M. (1994). *The nurse manager's answer book*. Aspen Publishers, Gaithersburg, MD: 125–127.

Additional Resources

Osuagwu, C. & Osuagwu, G. (2006). *From staff nurse to manager: A guide to successful role transition*. A FalconQuest Production USA: 18–20.

Pepper, G. (2001). *Conducting effective meetings—Strategies, tactics for successful meetings*. Louisville, KY: Brown Herron.

Public Policy and Consensus Building Institute. (2003). *Managing effective meetings*. Retrieved 6 October 2009 from http://cnrep.org/documents/tools/Managing%20Effective%20Meetings.pdf

Reh, J. (n.d.). *Meeting management*. Retrieved 6 October 2009 from http://management.about.com/cs/people/a/MeetingMgt0601.htm

53: Moral Courage

References

Aristotle. (1954). *Nichomachean Ethics*, Book 3. Ross, D (Trans.) London, England: Oxford University Press.

Dossey, B. M. (Ed.). (2004). *Florence Nightingale today: Healing, leadership, global action*. Silver Spring, MD: American Nurses Association.

Einstein, A. (n.d.). International Albert Schweitzer Association. Retrieved October 5, 2009 from http://www.schweitzer.org/english/aseind.htm

Lachman, V.D. (2007). Moral courage: A virtue in need of development? *MedSurg Nursing*, 16(2): 131–133.

Nightingale strength still needed today. (2007). *Nursing Standard*, 22(1): 11.

Roosevelt, Eleanor. E-Knowledge. Retrieved October 5, 2008, from http://www.e-knowledge.ca/quotes.php?topic=Courage.

Stanford Encyclopedia of Philosophy. (2007). Plato's ethics: An overview. Retrieved October 5, 2008, from http://plato.stanford.edu/entries/plato-ethics/.

Additional Resources

Lee, G., & Elliott-Lee, D (2006). *Courage: The backbone of leadership*. San Francisco: Jossey-Bass.

Keefe, S. (2006). Best nurse leaders: The greater New York/New Jersey metro area. *Advance for Nurses*. Retrieved 5 October 2008, from http://nursing.advanceweb.com/Article/Best-Nurse=Leaders.aspx?CP=8

Kidder, R. (2005). *Moral courage*. New York: HarperCollins.

Rhode, D. L. (2006). (Ed.) *Moral leadership: The theory and practice of power, judgment and policy*. San Francisco: Jossey-Bass.

54: Management

Additional Resources

Armstrong, S., Appelbaum, M. (2003). *Stress-free performance appraisals: Turn your most painful management duty into a powerful motivational tool*. Franklin Lakes, N.J.: Career Press.

Girvin, J. (1996). Leadership and nursing part four: motivation. *Nursing Management*, 3(5): 16–18.

Goleman, D., Boyatzis, R., & McKee, A. (2002). The motivation to change. In *The New Leaders: Transforming the Art of Leadership into the Science of Results* (pp. 113-138). Great Britain: Little, Brown.

Grohar-Murray, M. E., & DiCroce, H. R. (2003). *Motivation in the work setting. In Leadership and Management in Nursing* (3rd Ed.) (pp.199–214). New Jersey: Prentice Hall.

Henderson, M. C. (1995). Nurse executives: Leadership motivation and leadership effectiveness. *Journal of Nursing Administration*, 25(4): 45–51.

Hiam, A. (2003). *Motivational management: Inspiring your people for maximum performance*. New York: AMACOM, American Management Association.

Sellgren, S., Ekvall, G., & Tomson, G. (2006). Leadership styles in nursing management: Preferred and perceived. *Journal of Nursing Management*, 14: 348–355.

Stapleton, P., Henderson, A., Creedy, D. K., Cooke, M., Patterson, E., Alexander, H. et al. (2007). Boosting morale and improving performance in the nursing setting. *Journal of Nursing Management*, 15: 811–816.

55: Multi-System, Organization-Wide Mentoring

References

Tutu, D. (2007) *Believe*. Boulder, CO: Blue Mountain Arts, Inc.

Additional Resources

Block, P. (1993) *Stewardship. Choosing service over self-interest*. San Francisco: Berrett-Koehler Publishers.

Heifetz, R. A. (1994) *Leadership without easy answers*. Cambridge, MA: Belknap Press.

Senge, P. (2006) *The fifth discipline*. New York: Bantum Dell

56: Needs Assessment

References

Benner, P. (1984). *From novice to expert: Excellence and power in clinical nursing practice*. Menlo Park, CA: Addison-Wesley Publishing Company.

Benner, P. (2001). *From Novice to expert: Excellence and power in clinical nursing practice* (Commemorative ed.). Upper Saddle River, New Jersey: Prentice-Hall.

Nightingale, F. (1914). *Florence Nightingale to her nurses: A selection from Miss Nightingale's addresses to probationers and nurses of the Nightingale School at St. Thomas's hospital.* London: Macmillan and Co.

Additional Resources

Gupta, K. (2007). *A practical guide to needs assessment.* San Francisco: Jossey-Bass/Pfeiffer.

57: Needs-Based Resource Development and Allocation

References

Canadian Nurses Association (2000). Working with limited resources: Nurses' moral constraints. *Ethics in Practice*, (9)1-4. Retrieved 5 October 2009 from http://www.cna-nurses.ca/CNA/practice/ethics/inpractice/default_e.aspx

Canadian Nurses Association (2008). *Code of ethics for registered nurses. Centennial edition.* Ottawa, ON: Canadian Nurses Association. Retrieved 5 October 2009 from http://www.cna-nurses.ca/CNA/practice/ethics/code/default_e.aspx

Foreldraskóli [School for Parents]. Accessed 5 October 2009 from http://www.foreldraskoli.is

ICN International Nurse Practitioner/Advanced Practice Network. *Frequently asked questions.* Retrieved 6 October 2009 from http://icn-apnetwork.org

Landspítali University Hospital [LUH] (2006). *Treaty of collaboration between the University Hospital and the University of Iceland.* Retrieved 5 October 2009 from http://landspitali.is/

Marcé Society. Retrieved 5 October 2009 from http://www.marcesociety.com

Ministry of Health (2003). *Reglugerd um veitingu sérfraedileyfa í hjúkrun* [Regulation of Advanced Practice Nurses]. Retrieved 5 October 2009 from http://eng.heilbrigdisraduneyti.is/laws-and-regulations and http://www.heilbrigdisraduneyti.is/starfsleyfi//nr/2561

Papousek, M., Schieche, M. & Wurmser, H. (Eds.) (2007). *Disorders of behavioural and emotional regulation in the firs years of life: early risks and intervention in the developing parent-infant relationship.* Washington D.C.: Zero to Three.

Skuladottir, A. (2006). *Draumaland [Dreamland].* Reykjavik: Sögur.

Skuladottir, A. & Thome, M. (2003). Changes in infant sleep problems after a family centered intervention. *Pediatric Nursing, 29*(5), 375-378.

Skuladottir, A., Thome, M. & Ramel, A. (2005).Improving day and night sleep problems in infants by changing day time sleep rhythm: a single group before and after study. *International Journal of Nursing Studies, 42*, 843-850.

Society for Reproductive and Infant Psychology (SRIP). Retrieved 5 October 2009 from http://www.srip.ac.uk

Thome, M. & Alder, B. (1999). A telephone intervention to reduce fatigue and symptom distress in mothers with difficult infants in the community. *Journal of Advanced Nursing, 29*(1), 128-137.

Thome, M. & Skuladottir, A. (2005a). Evaluating a family-centred intervention for infant sleep problems. *Journal of Advanced Nursing, 50*(1), 5-11.

Thome, M. & Skuladottir, A. (2005b). Changes in sleep problems, parents distress and impact of sleep problems from infancy to preschool age for referred and unreferred children. *Scandinavian Journal of Caring Sciences, 19*, 86-94.

University of Iceland, School of Health Science, Faculty of Nursing. Accessed 18.11.2008 from http://www.hi.is/en/school_of_health_sciences_departments/faculty_of_nursing/main_menu/home

World Association for Infant Mental Health (WAIMH). Retrieved 5 October 2000 at http://www.waimh.org/

Wright, L.M. & Leahey, M. (1994). *Nurses and families. A guide to family assessment and intervention*. Philadelphia, PA: F.A. Davis.

58: Negotiation: Principles and Practices

References

Fisher, R, Ury, W., & Patton, B. (1991). *Getting to yes: Negotiating agreement without giving in*. New York: Penguin Publishers.

Shendell-Falik, N. (2002). *The art of negotiation*. Professional Case Management Vol. 7 (6): 228. Philadelphia: Lippincott, Williams & Wilkins.

Additional Resources

Hiltrop, J. M., & Udall, S. (1995). *The essence of negotiations*. Europe: Prentice Hall.

Hindle, T. (1998). *Negotiating skills*. New York: DK Publishing, Inc.

Stone, D., Patton, B., Heen, S., & Fisher, R. (1991). *Difficult conversations: How to discuss what matters most*. New York: Penguin Publishers.

Watkins, M. (2003). *Negotiation*. Boston, MA: Harvard Business School Publishing Corp.

Zabreskie, K. (2009). *Negotiation power skills: how to get what you want without being a jerk*. Port Tobacco, MD: Business Training Works, Inc.

59: Negotiation: Strategies

References

Fisher, R., & Ury, W. (1981). *Getting to yes: Negotiating agreement without giving in*. New York: Penguin Books, 1981: 104.

Additional Resources

Gosselin, T. (2007). *Practical negotiating: Tools, tactics and techniques*. Hoboken, NJ: John Wiley & Sons, Inc.

Spangler, B. (2003). Best alternative to a negotiated agreement (BATNA). Conflict Research Consortium, University of Colorado Boulder. Retrieved 5 October 2009 from http://www.beyondintractability.org/essay/batna/

Thomas, J. (2005). *Negotiate to win: The 21 rules for successful negotiation*. New York: Harper Collins.

Williams, S. (2007). Negotiation skills for minority nurses. *Minority Nurse*.

60: Novice to Expert

References

Conger, J. A., & Kanugo, R. N. (1988). The empowerment process: integrating theory and practice. *Academy of Management Review*, 13(3): 471482.

Falk-Rafael, A. R. (2001). Empowerment as a process of evolving consciousness: a model of empowered caring. *Advances in Nursing Science*, 24(1): 1–16

Faugier, J., & Woolnough, H. (2002). Blazing a trail. *Nursing Times*, 98 (50): 23–28

Kanter, R. M. (1993). *Men and women of the corporation*. New York: Basic Books.

Laschinger, H. K., Wong, C., McMahon, L., & Kaufmann, C. (1999). Leader behaviour impact on staff nurse empowerment, job tension, and work effectiveness. *Journal of Nursing Administration*, 29(5): 28–39.

Manojlovich, M., & Laschinger, H. K. (2002). The relationship of empowerment and selected personality characteristics of nursing job satisfaction. *Journal of Nursing Administration,* 32(11): 586–995.

Rock, D. (2006). *Quiet leadership.* Six Steps to transforming performance at work New York: HarperCollins.

Schon, D. A. (1983). *The reflective practitioner: How professionals think in action.* London: Temple Smith.

Stogdill, R. M. (1948). Personal factors associated with leadership. *Journal of Psychology,* 25: 37–71.

Webb, J. (1980). *The harmonious circle: The lives and work of G. I. Gurdjieff, P. D. Ouspensky, and their followers.* New York: G. P. Putnam's Sons.

Additional Resources

Dreyfus, H. L., & Dreyfus, S. E. (1986). *Mind over machine: The power of human intuition and expertise in the era of the computer.* Oxford: Basil Blackwell.

Enneagramme. George Ivanovitch Gurdjieff. http://eng.gurdjieff.es/content/view/30/134/

Fineman, S., Sims, D., & Gabriel, Y. (2005). *Organising and organizations (3rd ed.)* London: Sage Publications.

National Health Service Institute for Innovation and Improvement, Productive Ward. www.institute.nhs.uk

Smith, S., & Edmonstone, J. (2001). Learning to lead. *Nursing Management,* 8(3):10–13.

61: Nursing Process

References

Aggleton, F., & Chalmers, H. (2000). *Nursing Models and Nursing Practice.* London: MacMillan Press LTD. p. 210.

George, J.B. (Ed.) (1985). *Nursing theories: The base for professional nursing* (2nd ed.). Englewood Cliffts, N.J.: Prentice-Hall.

Grohar-Murray, M.E., & DiCroce, H.R. (2003). *Zásady vedení a ízení v oblasti ošet t ovatelské pé e.* Praha: Grada Publishing. P 20.

Kozierová, B. et al. (1995). *Ošetrovate stvo 1.* Martin, Vydavate stvo Osveta. 836.

Royal College of Nursing (2003). 20 Cavendish Square London WIG ORN 020 7409 33 33 Code of publication 001 983.

WHO Regional Office for Europe. (1997). *Nursing in Europe: A resource for better health.* Copenhagen: (WHO Regional Publications, European Series, No 74).

Závodná, V. (2005). *Pedagogika vošetrovate stve.* Martin: Vydavate stvo Osveta, spol. S r. o., 86.

Additional Resources

Kay, D., & Hinds, R. (2005). *A practical guide to mentoring.* Oxford, UK: How-to-Books.

Marquis, B., & Huston, C. (2009). *Leadership roles and management functions in nursing: Theory and application* (6th ed.) New Philadelphia: Wolters Kluwer.

Morton-Cooper, A., & Palmer, A. (2000). *Mentoring, preceptorship and clinical supervision: A guide to professional support roles in clinical practice* (2nd ed.). Oxford, UK: Blackwell Science.

Oliver, R., & Endersby, C. (1994) *Teaching and assessing nurses: A handbook for preceptors.* London, UK: Bailliere Tindall.

Shaw, S. (2007). International Council of Nurses: *Nursing Leadership,* March 2007, Wiley-Blackwell.

62: Organizational Development

Additional Resources

ukljek S. (2005). Basic of nursing care. Zagreb, University of Applied Health Studies.

Healthcare Occupation and Higher Education Act (2007). Amendments. Narodne novine; (46): 16.

Kalauz S., Orli Šumi , M., & Šimunec, D. (2008). Nurses in Croatia, past, present, future. *Croatian Medical Journal, 49*: 298-306.

Nursing Act. (2003). Croatian Nurses Council.

Santri V. (1990). Basic trends and problems in the process of creating a professional occupation: The case of nursing. Revija za sociologiju, Udruga sociologa Hrvatske, 21: 311-39.

University of Applied Health Studies (2005). The students guide. Zagreb, University of Applied Study.

University of Applied Health Studies (2005). The students guide for specialisation studies. Zagreb, University of Applied Study.

63: Outcomes

References

Donabedian, A. (1986). Criteria and standards for quality assessment and monitoring. *Quality Review Bulletin, 14*(3): 99-108.

Donabedian, A. (1990). The seven pillars of quality. *Archives of Pathology and Laboratory Medicine*, 114: 1115-1118.

Waltz, C.F., & Strickland, L.O. (1988). *Measurement of Nursing Outcomes.* New York: Springer Publishing Company.

Additional Resources

Redefining Health Care: http://www.hbs.edu/rhc/

Value-Driven Health Care: http://www.hhs.gov/valuedriven/

64: Paradoxical Role Models

References

Richards, J. (2008). The Development and practice of courageous leadership: A phenomenological inquiry of female leadership within the Canadian health care system. (Doctoral dissertation, Fielding Graduate University, 2008). Dissertation Abstracts International.

Rilke, R. M. (1993). *Letters to a young poet.* (M. D. H. Norton, Trans.). New York: W. W. Norton & Co. (Original work published 1934)

Additional Resources

Aisenberg, N. (1994). *Ordinary Heroines.* New York: Continuum Publishing.

Belenky, M. F., Clinchy, B. M., Goldberger, N. R., & Tarule, J. M. (1997). *Women's ways of knowing: The development of self, voice, and mind.* New York: Basic Books. (Original work published 1986)

Burns, J. (1978). *Leadership.* New York: Harper and Row.

Cook, B. W. (1992). *Eleanor Roosevelt.* New York: Penguin Books.

Frankl, V.E. (1984). *Man's search for meaning: An introduction to logotherapy* (3rd ed.). (I. Lasch & G. W. Allport, Trans.). New York: Simon and Schuster. (Original work published 1959)

Fraser, A. (2003). *The warrior queens.* London: Phoenix Press.

Gandhi, M. (1927). *The story of my experiments with truth (Vol. I)*. (M. Desai, Trans.). Ahmedabad: Navajivan.

Gandhi, M. (1928). *The story of my experiments with truth (Vol. II)*. (M. Desai, Trans.). Ahmedabad: Navajivan.

Gardner, H. (1993). *Creating minds: An anatomy of creativity seen through the lives of Freud, Einstein, Picasso, Stravinsky, Eliot, Graham, and Gandhi*. New York: Basic Books.

Gardner, H. (1999). *Intelligence reframed: Multiple intelligences for the 21st century*. New York: Basic Books.

Gilligan, C. (1993). *In a different voice: Psychological theory and women's development*. Cambridge, MA: Harvard University Press.

Kennedy, J. F. (1961). *Profiles in courage*. New York: Harper & Brothers. (Original work published 1955)

Lao Tzu. (1963). *Tao te ching* (D. C. Lau, Trans.). London: Penguin Group. (Original work published n.d.).

65: Patient Safety

References
Frankel, L. M., Simmons, T., & Vega, K. (2004). *Achieving safe and reliable healthcare: Strategies and solutions*. Chicago, IL: Health Administration Press.

Kohn, L. T., Donaldson, M.S., & Corrigan, J.M. (2000). *To err is human: Building a safer health system*. Washington D.C.: National Academy Press.

Reason, J. T. (1997). *Managing the risks of organizational accidents*. Brookfield, VT: Aldershot, Hants, England.

Reason, J. T. (1998). Achieving a safe culture: Theory and practice. *Work and Stress, 12*: 293-306.

Turner, B. A., & Pidgeon, N.F. (1997). *Man-made disasters* (2nd ed.). Boston: Butterworth.

Additional Resources
American Organization of Nurse Executives: *Role of the nurse executive in patient safety guiding principles toolkit*. Retrieved 5 October 2009 from www.aone.org/aone/resource/home.html

Liker, J. K. (2004). *The Toyota way*. New York: McGraw-Hill.

National Patient Safety Foundation: www.npsf.org

McKesson Corporation. (2005). *Nursing Leadership Congress, Building Bridges: Medication Safety*.

Rona, J. M. (2007). American health care system: A wasteland of opportunity. *The Journal of Competitive Lean Thinking*.

Turney, S. (2005). Quality patient care is a team effort. *MGMA Connexion*, p. 5-6.

White, P., Tregunno, D., O'Connor, P., Nicklin, W., Mass, H., Jeffs, L., et al. (2004). Patient safety culture and leadership within Canada's academic health science centres: Toward the development of a collaborative position paper. *Nursing Leadership, 22-34*.

Yellman, T. W. (2006). Eight safety-related definitions. *Journal of System Safety*.

66: Peer-to-Peer Mentoring

References
Byrne, M. W., & Keefe, M. R. (2002). Building research competence in nursing through mentoring. *Journal of Nursing Scholarship, 34*(4), 391-396.

Cumbie, S., Weinert, C., Luparell, S., Conley, V., & Smith, J. (2005). Developing a scholarship community. *Journal of Nursing Scholarship, 37*(3), 289-293.

World Health Organization. (2007). Integrated management of childhood illnesses. Retrieved 5 October 2009 from http://www.who.int/child-adolescent-health/integr.htm

Additional Resources

Bally, J. M. G. (2007). The role of nursing leadership in creating a mentoring culture in acute care environments. *Nursing Economics, 25(3)*, 143-148.

Campbell, C. (2007). Mentoring in nursing: Commitment with results. *American Academy of Ambulatory Care Nursing Viewpoint*. Retrieved 5 October 2009 from http://findarticles.com/p/articles/mi_qa4022/is_200711/ai_n21280025/

Grossman, S. M. (2007). *Mentoring in nursing: A dynamic and collaborative process*. New York: Springer.

67: People Skills

References

Collins, F. L. (1967). *The FBI in peace and war*. New York: G.P. Putnam.

Maslow, A. H. (1970). *Motivation and personality* (2nd ed.). New York: Harper and Row.

Additional Resources

Asch, S. (2007). *Excellence at work: The six keys to inspire passion in the workplace*. Scottsdale, AZ: WorldatWork Press.

Benson, S. G., & Dundis, S. P. (2003). Understanding and motivating health care employees: Integrating Maslow's hierarchy of needs, training, and technology. *Journal of Nursing Management. 11(5)*, 315-320.

Buckingham, M., & Clifton, D. O. (2001). Now discover your strengths: How to develop your talents and those of the people you manage. London: Simon & Schuster UK Ltd.

Covey, S. M. R., & Merrill, R. R. (2006). *The speed of trust: The one thing that changes everything*. New York: Free Press.

Hopkins, L. (2005). People skills: Eight essential people skills. Retrieved 5 October 2009 from http://ezinearticles.com/?People-Skills:-Eight-Essential-People-Skills&id=12294

Hyde, J. & Cook, M. J. (2004). Managing and supporting people in healthcare: Six steps to effective management series. Oxford: Elsevier Health Sciences.

Kouzes, J. M. & Posner, B. Z. (2003). Encouraging the heart: A leader's guide to rewarding and recognizing others. San Francisco: Jossey-Bass.

Liew, M. L. (2008). *Building people*. Singapore: John Wiley & Sons (Asia) Pte. Ltd.

Maxwell, J. C. (2005). *The 3600 leader*. Nashville, TN: Thomas Nelson Books.

Self test: How good are your people skills? Retrieved 5 October 2009 from http://www.3smartcubes.com/pages/tests/peopleskills/peopleskills_instructions.asp

68: Performance and Improvement

References

American Nurses Association. (2001). Standards of clinical nurses practice. Washington, D.C.: Author.

Marquis, B. L., & Huston, C. J. (2003). *Leadership roles and management functions in nursing: Theory and application* (4th ed.) Philadelphia: Lippincott, Williams & Wilkins.

Plunkett, W. R., Attner, R. F., & Allen, G. S. (2005). *Management meeting and exceeding customer expectations* (8th ed.) Mason, OH: Thomson South-Western.

Queen Elizabeth Hospital. (2006). Terms and conditions of service. Barbados.

Vestal, K. W. (1995). *Nursing management concepts and issues* (2nd ed.) Philadelphia: Lippincott, Williams & Wilkins.

69: Perseverence

References

Hesselbein, F., Goldsmith, M., & Beckhard, R. (1996). *The Drucker foundation: The leader of the future.* San Francisco: Jossey-Bass.

Osho (1999). *Courage: The joy of living dangerously.* New York: St. Martin's Griffin.

Additional Resources

Bennis, W., & Goldsmith, J. (1997). *Learning to lead: A workbook on becoming a leader.* Reading, MA. Addison-Wesley.

Covey, S. (1989). *The seven habits of highly effective people (restoring the character ethic).* New York: Simon and Schuster.

Gilley, K. (1997). *Leading from the heart: Choosing courage over fear in the workplace.* Boston: Butterworth-Heinemann.

Porter-O'Grady, T. & Malloch, K. (2002), *Quantum leadership: A textbook of new leadership.* Gaithersburg, Maryland: Aspen Publishers.

70: Person-Centered Model of Care

References

Allen, D., & Vitale-Nolen, R. (2005). Patient care delivery model improves nurse job satisfaction. *The Journal of Continuing Education in Nursing, 36*(6), 277-282. Retrieved December 11, 2008, from EBSCOhost database.

Boynton, D., & Rothman, L. (1995). Stage managing change: Supporting new patient care models. *Nursing Economics, 13*(3): 166-173.

Joynt, J., & Kimball, B. (2008). Innovative care delivery models: Identifying new models that effectively leverage nurses. *White paper submitted to The Robert Wood Johnson Foundation by Health Workforce Solutions, LLC.* Retrieved 5 October 2009 from http://www.innovativecaremodels.com/docs/HWS-RWJF-CDM-White-Paper.pdf

Spotswood, S. (2006). U.S. medicine information central. VA working to change culture of care in veteran nursing homes. December 2006.

Additional Resources

American Association of Colleges of Nursing: http://www.aacn.nche.edu

American Nurses Association: http://nursingworld.org

Innovative Care Models: http://www.innovativecaremodels.com

Pontin, D. (1999). Primary nursing: A mode of care or a philosophy of nursing? *Journal of Advanced Nursing, 29*(3): 584-591.

Robert Wood Johnson Foundation: http://www.rwjf.org

71: Philosophy

References

Richards, J. (2008). *The Development and practice of courageous leadership: A phenomenological inquiry of female leadership within the Canadian health care system.* (Doctoral dissertation, Fielding Graduate University, 2008). Dissertation Abstracts International.

Additional Resources

Becker, E. (1973). *The denial of death.* New York: Free Press.

Bell, D. (2002). *Ethical ambition: Living a life of meaning and worth.* Vancouver, BC: Raincoast Books.

Chicago, J. (2006). *Through the flower: My struggle as a woman artist.* New York: Author's Choice Press.

Daly, M. (2005). *Amazon grace: Re-calling the courage to sin big.* New York: Palgrave MacMillan.

de Beauvoir, S. (1989). *The second sex.* New York: Random House. (Original work published 1952)

Homer. (1961). *Iliad.* (R. Lattimore, Trans.). Chicago: Phoenix Books.

Kidder, R. M. (2005). *Moral courage: Taking action when your values are put to the test.* New York: HarperCollins Publishers.

Lorde, A. (1984). *Sister outsider.* Trumansburg, New York: The Cross Press.

Maslow, A. H. (1971). *The farther reaches of human nature.* New York: Viking Press.

May, R. (1975). *The courage to create.* New York: W. W. Norton & Company.

Palmer, P. J. (1998). *The courage to teach: Exploring the inner landscape of a teacher's life.* San Francisco: Jossey-Bass.

Parks, R. (1994). *Quiet strength.* Grand Rapids, MI: Zondervan Publishing House.

Sparks, H. (1997). Dissident citizenship: Democratic theory, political courage, and activist women. *Hypatia, 12*(4), 74-110.

72: Presentation

References

Miller, J. (2007). Are You the Invisible Employee? *MSN Careers.* Retrieved 5 October 2009 from http://msn.careerbuilder.com/Article/MSN-647-Workplace-Issues-Are-You-the-Invisible-Employee/?sc_extcmp=JS_647_advice&SiteId=cbmsn4647

Additional Resources

Avillion, A. (2009). Core curriculum for staff development (3rd ed.) Pensacola, FL: NNSDO.

Puetz, B.E., & Aucoin, J.W. (2002). *Conversations in nursing professional development.* Pensacola, Florida: Pohl.

73: Program Project Management

References

European Union. (2005). Mutual recognition of health professionals' education. Brussels: DIRECTIVE 2005/36/EC.

Fleming, V. & Holmes, A. (2005). Basic nursing and midwifery education programmes in Europe. Copenhagen: World Health Organization EUR/05/5049082.

Miller, S., Hickson, D., & Wilson, D. (2008). From strategy to action: Involvement and influence in top level decisions. *Long Range Planning, 42*(6), 606-628.

Additional Resources

Basic nursing and midwifery education programmes in Europe: http://www.euro.who.int/document/e86582.pdf

Official Journal of the European Union: http://eur-lex.europa.eu/LexUriServ/LexUriServ.do?uri=OJ:L:2005:255:0022:0142:EN:PDF

74: Public Policy

Additional Resources

American Academy of Nurse Practitioners. http://www.aanp.org/AANPCMS2

Carroll, D. (Ed.). (1859). *Notes on nursing* (Commemorative ed., Rev.). Philadelphia: Lippincott, Williams & Wilkins.

Institute for Nursing Healthcare Leadership: www.inhl.org

Mitchell, C. C., Ashley, Z. W., Zinner, M. J. & Moore, F.D. (2007). Predicting future staffing needs at teaching hospitals. *Archives of Surgery*, 142, 329-334.

Schwartz, M.D., Basco, W.T., Grey, M. R., Elmore, J. G. & Rubenstein, A. (2005). Rekindling student interest in generalist careers. *Annals of Internal Medicine*, 142, 715-724.

75: Qualities of Leadership

Additional Resources

Feldman H. R., Greenberg M. J. (2005). *Educating nurses for leadership.* New York: Springer Publishing Company.

Marquis B. L., & Huston C. J. (2008). *Leadership roles and management functions in nursing: Theory and application* (6th ed.). Philadelphia: Lippincott, Williams & Wilkins.

76: Quality Outcomes

References

Girard, N. (2009). Dissemination of findings: The final step of investigation. *Perioperative Nursing Clinics*, 4(2009), 297-306.

Malesker, M., Foral, P., McPhillips, A., Christensen, K., Chang, J., & Hilleman, D. An efficiency evaluation of protocols for tight glycemic control in intensive care units. (2007). *American Journal of Critical Care*, 16(6), 589–598.

Moghissi, E. S., Korytkowski, M. T., DiNardo, M., Einhorn, D., Hellman, R., & Hirsch, I. B., et al. American Association of Clinical Endocrinologists and American Diabetes Association Consensus statement on inpatient glycemic control. (2009). *Diabetes Care*, 32(6), 1119-1131.

Rohman, C. (2008). Modifying organizational structure and processes to enhance patient outcomes. *Nurse Leader*, 6(4), 50–52.

Solylemez W. R., Wiender, D., Larson, R. J. (2008). Benefits and risks of tight glucose control in critically ill adults. *Journal of the American Medical Association*, 300(8), 933-944.

Additional Resources

Academic Center for Evidence-Based Practice: http://www.acestar.uthscsa.edu

Agency for Healthcare Research and Quality: http://ahrq.gov/clinic/outcomix.htm

American Organization of Nurse Executives: http://www.aone.org

Anderson, M. D.: http://www.mdanderson.org/education-and-research/resources-for-professionals/clinical-tools-and-resources/clinical-safety-and-effectiveness-educational-program/index.html

Institute for Healthcare Improvement: http://www.ihi.org

Joint Commission: http://www.jointcommission.org

National Patient Safety Foundation: http://www.npsf.org

National Quality Forum: http://www.qualityforum.org/nursing/

Robert Wood Johnson Foundation: http://www.rwjf.org

University of Texas Health Science Center at San Antonio, Educating for quality and safety program: http://www.uthscsa.edu/cpshp/equips.aspx

Wolf, L. (2008). The use of human patient simulation in E.D. triage training can improve nursing confidence and patient outcomes. *Journal of Emergency Nursing, 34*(2), 169–171.

77: Reciprocal and Supportive Mentoring

References

Cummings, G., Lee, H., MacGregor, T., Davey, M., Wong, C., & Paul, L. (2008). Factors contributing to nursing leadership: A systematic review. *Journal of Health Services Research & Policy, 13*(4), 240-248.

Daly, J., Speedy, S., & Jackson, D. (Eds.) (2004). *Nursing leadership.* Sydney: Churchill Livingstone.

Davidson, P. M., Elliott, D., & Daly, J. (2006). Clinical leadership in contemporary clinical practice: Implications for nursing in Australia. *Journal of Nursing Management,* 14, 180-187.

Firth-Cozens, J., & Mowbray, D. (2001). Leadership and quality of care. *Quality in Healthcare, 10*(Supplement), ii3-ii7.

Heifetz, R.A. (1994). *Leadership without easy answers.* Cambridge: Belknap Press.

Kouzes, J. M., & Posner, B.Z. (2002). *The leadership challenge* (3rd ed.). San Francisco: Jossey-Bass.

Additional References

Kouzes, J. M. & Posner, B. Z. (2003). *The leadership challenge workbook.* Hoboken, New Jersey: Pfeiffer.

Kouzes, J. M. & Posner, B. Z. (2008). *The leadership challenge* (4th ed.). San Francisco: Jossey-Bass.

78: Regulating Advanced Practice Nursing

References

APRN Consensus Work Group & the National Council of State Boards of Nursing APRN Advisory Committee. (2008). *Consensus model for APRN regulation: licensure, accreditation, certification & education.* Retrieved 5 October 2009 from http://www.aacn.nche.edu/Education/pdf/APRNReport.pdf

International Council of Nurses. (2005). *Nursing regulation: A future perspective.* Retrieved 5 October 2009 from http://icn.ch/ps_icn_who_regulation.pdf

Ketefian, S., Redman, R.W., Hanucharurnkul, S., Masterson, A., & Neves, E.P. (2001). The development of advance practice roles in the international nursing community. *International Council Review, 48,* 152-63.

O'Connor, T. (2008). The challenges of regulating nursing. *Kai Tiaki: Nursing New Zealand, 14*(9), 11.

Poe, L. (2008). Nursing regulation, the nurse licensure compact, and nurse administrators, working together for patient safety. *Nursing Administrative Quarterly, 32*(4), 267-72.

Robinson, M. (2008). Closing perspectives; nursing regulation not stagnation. *Alberta RN, 68*(8), 38.

Safriet, B. J. (1994). Impediments to progress in health care workforce policy: license and practice laws. *Inquire, 31*(3), 310-317.

Sheer, B. & Wong, F. K. Y. (2008). The development of advanced nursing practice globally. *Journal of Nursing Scholarship, 40*(3), 204-211.

Additional Resources

APRN Consensus Work Group & the National Council of State Boards of Nursing APRN Advisory Committee. (2008). *Consensus model for APRN regulation: licensure, accreditation, certification & education.* Retrieved July 8, 2008, from American Association of Colleges of Nursing Web site: http://www.aacn.nche.edu/Education/pdf/APRNReport.pdf.

Stanley, J. M. (2009). Reaching consensus on a regulatory model: What does this mean for APRNs? *Journal for Nurse Practitioners 11 May 2009.* Retrieved 5 October 2009 from http://acp.duhs.duke.edu/wysiwyg/downloads/APRN.pdf

79: Regulatory and Organizational Standards

References

Brown Jr., H. J. (1991). *Life's little instruction book: 511 suggestions, observations, and reminders on how to live a happy and rewarding life.* Nashville, TN: Rutledge Hill Press.

Carrier-Walker, L. (2008). New specialist on regulation and licensure joins ICN staff. Retrieved 5 October 2009 from http://www.icn.ch/PR19_08.htm

Directorate Nursing Standards Services (DNSS). (2009). Ministry of Social Policy. http://www.sahha.gov.mt/pages.aspx?page=37

Hakala, D. (2008). The top ten leadership qualities. *HR World.* Retrieved 5 October 2009 from http://www.hrworld.com/features/top-10-leadership-qualities-031908/

International Council of Nurses (ICN). (1989). Guidelines for national nurses' associations: Development of standards for nursing education and practice. Geneva: ICN.

Reddy, J. N. (2008). A word to the wise: Memorable sayings. http://helium.com/items/347866-a-word-to-the-wise-memorable-sayings

Schnurr, S. (2008). Surviving in a man's world with a sense of humour: An analysis of women leaders' use of humour at work. *Leadership. 4*(3), 299-319.

World Health Organization (WHO). (2002). Nursing and midwifery: A guide to professional regulation. Cairo: Alzahraa Printing.

Additional Reading

Goleman, D. (1999). Working with emotional intelligence. New York: Bantam Books.

Gobillot, E. (2008). The connected leader: Creating agile organizations for people, performance, and profit. London: Kogan Page.

Johnson, M., Stewart, H., Langdon, R., Kelly, P., & Yong, L. (2003). Women-centered care and caseload models of midwifery. *Journal of the Royal College of Nursing Australia. 10*(1), 30-34.

Kareseras, H. (2006). *From new recruit to high flyer. No-nonsense advise on how to fast track your career.* London: Kogan Page.

80: Retention Starts With Recruitment

Additional Resources

Butler, M. R. (2006). Tool kit for the staff mentor: Strategies for improving retention. *The Journal of Continuing Education in Nursing, 37*(5).

Grossman, S. C. (2007). *Mentoring in nursing: A dynamic and collaborative process.* New York: Springer Publishing Inc.

Price, S. L. (2009). Becoming a nurse: a meta-study of early professional socialization and career choice in nursing. *Journal of Advanced Nursing, 65*(1), 11-19.

81: Risk Management

References

Brennan, T. A., Leape, L. L, Laird, N. M., Hebert, L., Localio, A. R., Lawthers, A. G., et al. (1991). Incidence of adverse events and negligence in hospitalized patients. *New England Journal of Medicine*, 324(6), 377-384.

Cousins, D. (1998). *Medication use: A systems approach to reducing errors.* Oakbrook Terrace, IL: Joint Commission on Accreditation of Healthcare Organizations.

Reason, J. T. (2001). Understanding adverse events: the human factor. In Vincent, C. (Ed.). *Clinical Risk Management.* (pp. 9-30). London: BMJ Books.

Additional Resources

Buerhaus, P. I. (2007). Is Hospital Patient Care Becoming Safer? A conversation with Lucian Leape. *Health Affairs, 26*(6), 687- 696.

Dickinson, G. (1995). Principles of risk management. *Quality in Healthcare, 4*(2), 75-79.

Hammond, J. (2004). Simulation in critical care and trauma education and training. *Current Opinion in Critical Care, 10*(5), 325 -329.

Jha, A. K., Duncan, B. W., & Bates, D. W. (2001). *Simulator-based Training and Patient Safety.* Rockville, MD: Agency of Healthcare Research and Quality (AHRQ) Publications.

Towbridge, R. & Weingarten, S. (2001). Educational techniques used in changing provider behavior. Rockville MD: Agency of Healthcare Research and Quality (AHRQ) Publications.

82: Self Leadership

References

Elloy, D. F. (2008). The relationship between self-leadership behaviors and organization variables in a self-managed work team environment, *Management Research News*, 31(11): 801–810.

Georgianna, S. (2007). Self-leadership: a cross-cultural perspective. *Journal of Managerial Psychology*, 22(6): 569–589.

Holcomb, P. (2005). Leadership is congruent self expression that creates value. 21st Century Leadership. *This Week.* April Newsletter: 1–2. (An excerpt from a newsletter authored by Phil Holcomb.)

Jooste, K. (Ed.) (2009). *Leadership in health services management.* 2nd Edition. Kenwyn: Juta.

Politis, J. D. (2006). Self-leadership behavioural-focused strategies and team performance. *Leadership and Organization Development Journal*, 27(3): 203–216.

Additional Resources

Oshagbemi, T. & Gill, R. (2004). Differences in leadership styles and behaviour across hierarchical levels in UK organizations. *The Leadership and Organization Development Journal*, 25(1): 93–106.

Quick MBA. (n.d.) SWOT (Strengths, Weaknesses, Opportunities, and Threats). Retrieved 5 October 2009 from http://www.quickmba.com/strategy/swot/

83: Self Recovery and Renewal

References

Stanney, B. (2004). *Secrets of six figure women: Surprising strategies to up your earnings and change your life.* New York: Harper Paperbacks.

Additional Resources
Compassion Fatigue Awareness Project: http://compassionfatigue.org

Figley, Charles books: http://sites.google.com/site/charlesfigley

Kollak, I. (2008). *Yoga for nurses*. New York: Springer Publishing, LLC

Nurse Fit: http://www.nursefit.com/articles.htm

Sherbun, M. A. (2005). *Caring for the caregiver: Eight truths to prolong your career.* Sudbury, MA: Jones and Bartlett Publishers.

84: Self Image and Self Esteem

References
Buresh, B., & Gordon, S. (2006). *From silence to voice: What nurses know and must communicate to the public.* New York: ILR Press.

Covey, S. 1992. *Principle-centered leadership*. London: Simon and Schuster.

Goleman, G. 1998. *Working with emotional intelligence*. New York: Bantam Books.

Yoder-Wise, P. S. & Kowalski, K. E. 2006. *Beyond leading and managing. Nursing administration for the future.* St. Louis, MO: Mosby Elsevier.

Additional Resources
Leadership Challenge: www.leadershipchallenge.com

Kouzes, J., & Posner, B. 2008. *The leadership challenge* (4th ed.). San Francisco: Jossey-Bass.

85: Shared Governance: Looking Back and Looking Forward

References
CPMRC Partnership (2008) *CPMRC partnership council workbook*. Grand Rapids, MI: CPM Resource Center/Elsevier.

Institute of Medicine. (2001). *Crossing the quality chasm: A new health system for the 21st century.* Washington D.C.: National Academies Press.

Shiparski, L. (2005). Engaging in shared decision making: Leveraging staff and management expertise. *AONE Nurse Leader*, 3(1): 36-41.

Shiparski, L., Troseth, M., Wesorick, B., & Wyngarden, K. (1997). Partnership council field book: Strategies and tools for co-creating a healthy work place. Grand Rapids, MI: Practice Field Publishing.

Additional Resources
Porter O'Grady, T., (Ed.) (1992) *Implementing shared governance*. St. Louis: Mosby Books.

Porter O'Grady, T., (Ed.) & Tornabeni, J. (1993). Outcomes of shared governance: Impact on the organization. Seminars for Nurse Managers.

Porter O'Grady, T., Minors, P., & White, J. (1996). Assessing shared governance: An example of instrument development in a hospital setting. *Current Topics in Management*, 1.

Wesorick, B., & Shiparski, L. (1997). *Can the human being thrive in the work place? Dialogue as a strategy of hope.* Grand Rapids, MI: Practice Field Publishing.

Wesorick, B. (2002). 21st century leadership challenge: Creating and sustaining healthy, healing work cultures and integrated service at the point of care. *Nursing Administration Quarterly*, 26(5): 18-32.

86: Staffing and Workforce Management: Is It a Numbers or Body Game?

References

Alvarez & Marsal (22 April 2008). *More than half of U.S. hospitals are now technically insolvent or at risk of insolvency*. New York: Author. Retrieved 6 October 2009 from http://www.alvarezandmarsal.com/en/news/article.aspx?article=6093

Bureau of Labor Statistics, U.S. Department of Labor, (2008-09 ed.) *Occupational outlook handbook: Registered nurses*. Retrieved 6 October 2009 from http://www.bls.gov/oco/ocos083.htm

McFarland, P. (12 March 2008). California study offers new perspective on relationship between staffing ratios and patient safety. Sacramento, CA: Collaborative Alliance for Nursing Outcomes.

Additional Resources

Buerhaus, P. I., Staiger, D. O., Auerbach, D. I. (2008). Future of the nursing workforce in the United States: Data, implications, and future trends. Sudbury, MA: Jones & Bartlett.

Tallier, P. (2008). *Nurse staffing ratios and patient outcomes: A critical look at nurse staffing ratios and the impact on patient outcomes*. Saarbrücken, Germany: VDM Verlag.

87: (Taking One) Step at a Time (or You Cannot Do Everything at Once, But You Can Do Something)

References

Alpert, P. T., Fjone, A., & Candela, L. (2002). Nurse practitioner: Reflecting on the future. *Nursing Administration Quarterly, 26*(5), 79-89.

Australian Nurse Practitioners Association (2008). A potted history of Nurse Practitioner movement. Retrieved 13th February 2009 from http://www.nursepractitioners.org.au/History/

Chyna, J. T. (2000). Climbing the ladder: what it takes to succeed in healthcare management. *Healthcare Executive, 15*(6), 12-17.

Cross, S. (2009). Nurse practitioner/advanced practice network: Network history. International Council of Nurses. Retrieved 6 October 2009 from http://66.219.50.180/INP%20APN%20Network/About%20INPAPNN/Network%20History.asp

Duffield, C. M., Moran, P., Beutel, J., Bunt, S., Thornton, A., Wills, J. et al. (2001). Profile of first-line managers in NSW, Australia in the 1990s, *Journal of Advanced Nursing*, vol. 36 (6), pp. 785-793.

Furlong, E., & Smith, R. (2005). Advanced nursing practice: policy, education, and role development. *Journal of Clinical Nursing, 14*(9), 1059-1066.

Hill, C., & Pickup, M. (1998). Nurse practitioners and Canadian healthcare: Toward quality and cost effectiveness. Retrieved 6 October 2009 from http://www.cwf.ca/V2/files/199809.pdf

Hyde, P., McBride, A., Walshe, K., & Young, R. (2004). A catalyst for change? The national evaluation of the changing workforce programme. Manchester, UK: National Health System. Retrieved 6 October 2009 from http://www.healthcareworkforce.nhs.uk/working_time_directive/planners_mcr/changing_workforce_national_evaluation.html

Hyde, P., McBride, A., Young, R., & Walshe, K. (2005). Role redesign: new ways of working in the NHS. Bingley, United Kingdom: Emerald Group Publishing Limited.

Johnstone, P.L. (2003). Nurse manager turnover in New South Wales during the 1990s. *Collegian, 10*(1), 8-16.

Kleinpell, R. M. (2005). Acute care nurse practitioner practice: Results of a 5-year longitudinal study. *American Journal of Critical Care, 14*(3), 211-219; quiz 220-211.

Moran, P., Duffield, C., Beutel, J., Bunt, S., Thornton, A., Wills, J. et al. (2002). Nurse managers in Australia: Mentoring, leadership, and career progression. *Canadian Journal of Nursing Leadership, 15*(2), 14-20.

Pelletier, D., & Duffield, C. (1994). Is there enough mentoring in Australian nursing circles? *Australian Journal of Advanced Nursing, 11*(4), 6-12.

Royal Australian College of General Practitioners (1999). Position Statement: Nurse Practitioners. South Melbourne.

Tobin, M. J. (2004). Mentoring: seven roles and some specifics. *American Journal of Respiratory & Critical Care Medicine, 170*(2), 114-117.

Additional Resources

Australian Council and Midwifery Council. (n.d.). *Competency standards for nurse practitioners.* Retrieved 6 October 2009 from http://www.anmc.org.au/userfiles/file/competency_standards/Competency%20Standards%20for%20the%20Nurse%20Practitioner.pdf

Gardner, G., Chang, A., & Duffield, C. (2007). Making nursing work: Breaking through the role confusion of advanced practice nursing. *Journal of Advanced Nursing, 57*(4), 382-391.

Jones, M. L. (2005). Role development and effective practice in specialist and advanced practice roles in acute hospital settings: systematic review and meta-synthesis. *Journal of Advanced Nursing, 49*(2), 191-209.

Nurses and Midwives Board of New South Wales. (n.d.). Nurse practitioners. Retrieved 6 October 2009 from www.nmb.nsw.gov.au/**Nurse-Practitioners**/default.aspx

Reay, T., Golden-Biddle, K., & Germann, K. (2003). Challenges and leadership strategies for managers of nurse practitioners. *Journal of Nursing Management, 11*(6), 396-403.

88: Strategic Management

References

Bose, P. (2003). *Alexander the great's art of strategy.* New York: Gotham/Penguin Group USA, Inc.: New York, New York, p. 63.

Kaplan, R., & Norton, D. (1996). *The balanced scorecard: Translating strategy into action.* Boston, MA: Harvard Business School Press.

Spitzer, R. (1994). *Strategic responses of hospitals to the changing reimbursement environment.* Doctoral dissertation for Claremont Graduate University.

Sun-Tzu. (1994). *The art of war.* Ralph D. Sawyer, trans. Boulder, Colorado: Westview Press.

Additional Resources

Bryson, J. M. (2004). Strategic planning for public and non-profit organizations: A guide to strengthening and sustain organizational achievement (3rd ed.). San Francisco: Jossey-Bass.

Online integrated library on Strategic Planning (Profit and Non-Profit Organizations). http://managementhelp.org/plan_dec/str_plan/str_plan.htm

89: Stress Management: Starting a New Chapter in a Professional Nursing Life

Additional Resources

Driscoll, L. G., Parkes, K. A., Tilley-Lubbs, G. A., Brill, J.M., & Pitts Bannister, V.R. (2009). Navigating the lonely sea: Peer mentoring and collaboration among aspiring women scholars. *Mentoring & Tutoring: Partnership in Learning,* 17(1): 5-21.

Leidman MB (2006) Utilizing role theory and mentoring to minimize stress for new faculty. Paper prepared for the Eastern Communications Association Annual Convention.

Olsen D. (1993) Work satisfaction and stress in the first and third year of academic appoint-ment. *The Journal of Higher Education*, 64(4):453-471.

Sorcinelli, M.D., Yun, J. (2007). From mentor to mentoring networks: Mentoring in the new academy. *Change: The Magazine of Higher Learning*, 39(6): 58-61.

90: Student Mentoring at the International Doctoral Level

References
Carty, M. R., Moss, M. M., Al-Zayyer, W., Kowitlawakul, Y., & Arietti, L. (2007). Predictors of success for Saudi Arabian students enrolled in an accelerated baccalaureate degree program in nursing in the United States. *Journal of Professional Nursing*, 23(5): 301–308.

Hunt, J. (2003). Coach? Mentor? Leader? Manager? Coaching connection. Retrieved 6 Octo-ber 2009 from http://www.managers-gestionnaires.gc.ca/coaching/documents/coach_mentor_leader_manager-eng.asp

Wellington, S., & Spence, B. (2001). *Be your own mentor*. New York: Random House.

Additional Resources
Grossman, S. C. (2007). *Mentoring in nursing: A dynamic and collaborative process*. New York: Springer Publisher.

Harvard Business Essentials. (2004). *Coaching and mentoring: How to develop the top talent and achieve stronger performance*. Boston, MA: Harvard Business School Press.

Peddy, S. (2001). *The art of mentoring: Lead, follow and get out of the way*. Corps Christi, Texas: Bullion Books.

Stoddard, D. A. & Tamasy, R. (2003). *The heart of mentoring: Ten proven principles for developing people to their fullest potential*. Colorado Springs, CO: NAV Press.

91: Succession Planning

Additional Resources
Canadian Nurses Association. (2003). *Succession planning for nursing leadership*. Retrieved 6 October 2009 from http://www.cna-aiic.ca/CNA/documents/pdf/publications/succession_planning_e.pdf

Dion, K. W., Everett, L. Q., Morin, K. H., Yurdin, D. B. (n.d.). *Developing tomorrow's nurse leaders: Bridging the gap through succession planning and leadership development*. Retrieved 6 October 2009 from http://www.decisioncritical.com/documents/DTNL.pdf

Heathfield, S. M. (n.d.) Succession planning: http://humanresources.about.com/od/glossarys/g/successionplan.htm

Wandel, J. C. (n.d.). *The legacy of leadership: Succession planning in nursing*. Retrieved 6 October 2009 from http://www.nursingspectrum.com/CareerManagement/Articles/Legacy_pw2005.html

92: Synergy and Win-Win: The Goals of Effective Leadership

References
Goleman, D. (1998). *Working with emotional intelligence*. London: Bloomsbury Publishing.

Graham, H., & Bennett, R. (1998). *Human resources management* (9th ed.). Essex: Pearson Education Limited.

House, R. (1971). A path-goal model of leader effectiveness. *Administrative Science Quarterly*, 16, 321-323.

House, R. & Baetz, M. (1979). Leadership: Some empirical generalizations and new directions. *Research in Organization Behavior*, 1, 385-386.

Jones, G. R. (2007). *Organizational theory, design and change*. New Jersey: Pearson Education LTD.

National Health Service. (2006). Leadership qualities framework. Retrieved 6 October 2009 from http://www.nhsleadershipqualities.nhs.uk

Taylor, R., & Taylor, S. (Eds.) (1994). *The AUPHA manual of health services management*. Gaithersburg, MD: Aspen Publishers, Inc.

Additional Resources

Goleman, D. (2006). *Emotional Intelligence: 10th Anniversary Edition: Why It Can Matter More Than IQ*. New York: Bantam.

Shortell, S. M. & Kaluzny, A. D. (2006). *Health Care Management: Organizational Design and Behavior* (5th ed.). New York: Thomson Delmar Learning.

93: Teams, Team Players, and Team Building

References

Blanchard, K., & Bowles, S. (2000). *High five! The magic of working together*. New York: William Morrow.

Additional Resources

Bennis, W. G. (1997). *Organizing genius: the secret of creative collaboration*. New York: Perseus Books.

Condit, P. (1997). *Working together in the 21st century* at the Frontiers of Engineering meeting, The Boeing Company, National Academy of Engineering. Retrieved 6 October 2009 from http://www.boeing.com/news/speeches/1997/970918.html

Katzenbach, J. R. (2001). *The discipline of teams: A mindbook-workbook for delivering small group performance*. Hoboken, NJ: John Wiley & Sons.

LaFasto, F., & Larson, C. (2001). *When teams work best: 7,000 team members and leaders tell what it takes to succeed*. Thousand Oaks, CA: Sage Publications.

Maxwell, J. C. (2001). *The 17 indisputable laws of teamwork*. Nashville, TN: Thomas Nelson, Inc.

Strauss, David. (2002). *How to make collaboration work: powerful ways to build consensus, solve problems, and make decisions*. San Francisco: Berrett-Koehler Publishers.

94: Technology to Transform Practice at the Point-of-Care

References

Belmont, C., Wesorick, B., Jesse, H., Troseth, M., & Brown, D. (2003). Clinical documentation. *Health Care Technology: Innovating Clinical Care Through Technology*. San Francisco: Montgomery Research, Inc.

Doebbeling, B., Chou, A., & Tierney, W. (2006). Priorities and strategies for the implementation of integrated informatics and communications technology to improve evidence-based practice. *Journal of General Medicine*, 21, S50-57.

Eden, S., Wheatley, B., McNeil, B., & Sox, H. (2008). *Knowing what works in health care: A road map for the nation*. Washington, D.C.: National Academies Press.

Gillean, J., Shaha, S. H., & Sampanes, E. (2006). The search for the "holy grail" of health care: A correlation between quality and profitability. *Healthcare Financial Management*, Dec.: 114-121.

Hanson, D., Hoss, B. L., & Wesorick, B. (2008). Evaluating the evidence: Guidelines. *AORN J; 88*(2), 184-196.

Institute of Medicine. (2004). *Keeping patients safe: Transforming the work environment of nurses.* Washington, D.C.: National Academies Press.

Johnson, B. (1996). *Polarity management: Identifying and managing unsolvable problems.* Amherst, MA: HRD Press, Inc.

Troseth, M. (2009, 23 February). Technology: A gift for nursing. *Reflections on Nursing Leadership, 35*(1). Retrieved 6 October 2009 from http://www.reflectionsonnursingleadership.org/Pages/Vol35_1_Troseth.aspx#

Wesorick, B. (2008). Live a legacy or live a lie. *Nursing Administration Quarterly, (32)*2, 142-158.

Wesorick, B., Troseth, M., & Cato, J. (2004). Intentionally designed automation creates the best places to work and receive care. *Health Care Technology: Innovating Care through Technology, 2.* San Francisco: Montgomery Research, Inc., pp. 3-7.

Additional Resources

National Priorities Partnership. (2008). National priorities and goals: Aligning our efforts to transform America's healthcare. Washington, D.C.: National Quality Forum.

Weaver, C., Carr, R., Delaney, C, & Weber, P. (in press) Nursing and Informatics for the 21st Century: an international look at practice, trends, and the future (2nd ed.) HIMSS Publications.

95: Theory and Practice: Bringing Them Together at the Point of Care

References

Bridges, W. (2003). *Managing transitions* (2nd ed.). Cambridge, MA: Da Capo Press.

Hadfield, D., Holmes, S., Fabr, T., Dudek, E., Williams, J., & White, H. (2006). *Lean healthcare: 5 keys for improving the workplace environment.* Chelsea, MI: MCS Media, Inc.

Kotter, J.P. (1996). *Leading change.* Boston, MA: Harvard Business School Press.

Rogers, E.M. (2003). *Diffusion of innovations* (5th ed.). New York: Free Press.

Whall, A. (2005). "Lest we forget": An issue concerning the doctorate in nursing practice (DNP). *Nursing Outlook, 53,* 1.

Whall, A. & Hicks, F. (2002). The unrecognized paradigm shift within nursing: Implications, problems, and possibilities. *Nursing Outlook, 50,* 72-76.

Additional Resources

Benner, P. (2001). *From novice to expert: Excellence and power in clinical nursing practice.* New Jersey: Prentice Hall Health.

Koerner, J.G. (2007). *Healing presence: The essence of nursing.* New York: Springer Publishing Company.

Koloroutis, M. (Ed.) (2004). *Relationship-based care: A model for transforming practice.* Minneapolis, MN: Creative Health Care Management, Inc.

Reed, P., Shearer, N., & Nicoll, L. (2004). *Perspectives on nursing theory* (4th ed.). Philadelphia: Lippincott, Williams, & Wilkins.

96: Time Management

References
Bocec, G., & Gulie, E. (2003). *Leadership and management in nursing*. M.G.C. –Top S.R.L. Bucharest, Romania.

Yoder-Wise, P.S. (2003). *Leading and managing in nursing* (3rd ed.). St. Louis, MO. Mosby.

Sullivan, E. J., & Decker, P. J. (1992). *Effective management in nursing* (3rd ed.), 1992, Redwood City, CA: Addison-Wesley.

Additional Resources
Personal Time Management Guide at http://www.time-management-guide.com

Time Management by Randy Pausch at http://video.google.com/videoplay?docid=-5784740380335567758

Time Management by MindTools at http://www.mindtools.com/pages/main/newMN_HTE.htm

97: Transforming Practice at the Point of Care

References
Daschle, T. (2008). *Critical: What we can do about the health-care crisis.* New York: Thomas Dunne Books.

DePree, M. (1989). *Leadership is an art.* New York: Doubleday.

Institute of Medicine. (2001). *Crossing the quality chasm: A new health system for the 21st century.* Washington, D.C.: National Academy Press.

Johnson, B. (1996). *Polarity management: Identifying and managing unsolvable problems.* Amherst, Mass: HRD Press Inc.

Kenney, Charles. (2008). *The best practice: How the new quality movement is transforming medicine.* New York: Public Affairs.

Kohn, L. T., Corrigan, J. M., & Donaldson, M. S. (Ed.) (2000). *To err is human: Building a safer health system.* Washington, D.C.: National Academy Press.

Naisbitt, J. (2006). *Mind set! Reset your thinking and see the future.* New York: HarperCollins Publishers.

National Priorities Partnership. (2008). *National priorities and goals: Aligning our efforts to transform America's healthcare.* Washington, D.C.: National Quality Forum.

Senge, P. (1990). *The fifth discipline: The art & practice of the learning organization.* New York: Currency Doubleday.

Waldrop, M. (1992). *Complexity: The emerging science at the edge of order and chaos.* New York: Simon and Schuster.

Wesorick, B. (1990). *Standards of nursing care: A model for clinical practice.* Philadelphia: Lippincott, Williams & Wilkins.

Wesorick, B. (1991a). Creating an environment in the hospital setting that supports caring via a clinical practice model (CPM). In *Caring: The compassionate healer.* Gaut, D., & Leininger, M. (Eds.). New York: National League for Nursing Press.

Wesorick, B. (1991b). Nursing standards for professional practice: The Wesorick model. In *Approaches to nursing standards.* Schroeder, P. (Ed.) Gaithersburg, Maryland: Aspen Publishers.

Wesorick, B. (2002). 21st century leadership challenge: Creating and sustaining healthy, healing work cultures and integrated service at the point of care. *Nursing Administration Quarterly, 26*(5): 18–32.

Wesorick, B. (2008). Live a legacy or live a lie. *Nursing Administration Quarterly, 32*(2): 142–158.

Wesorick, B., & Shiparski, L. (1997). *Can the human being thrive in the work place? Dialogue as a strategy of hope.* Grand Rapids, MI: Practice Field Publishing.

Wesorick, B., Shiparski, L., Troseth, M., & Wyngarden, K. (1998). *Partnership council field book: Strategies and tools for co-creating a healthy work place.* Grand Rapids, MI: Practice Field Publishing.

Wheatley, M. (2006). *Leadership and the new science: Discovering order in a chaotic world.* San Francisco: Berrett-Koehler Publishers.

98: Transitioning Novice Nurses into Complex Health Care Environments

References

American Association of Colleges of Nursing (AACN). (26 February). AACN press release: Despite surge of interest in nursing careers, new AACN data confirm that too few nurses are entering the healthcare workforce. Retrieved 6 October 2009 from http://www.aacn.nche.edu/media/NewsReleases/2009/workforcedata.html

Beecroft, P.C., Kunzman, L., & Krozek, C. (2001). RN internship: Outcomes of a one-year pilot program. *Journal of Nursing Administration, 31*(12), 575-582.

Halfer D., Graf, E. (2006). Graduate nurse perceptions of work experience. *Nurse Economics 24*(3): 150-155.

Norton R. (1997). DACUM handbook (2nd ed.). Columbus, OH: The Ohio State University.

PriceWaterHouseCoopers. (2007). What works: Healing the healthcare staffing shortage. Retrieved 6 October 2009 from http://www.pwc.com/us/en/healthcare/publications/what-works-healing-the-healthcare-staffing-shortage.jhtml

Reinsvold, S. (Dec 2008). Nursing residency: Reversing the cycle of new graduate RN turnover. *Nurse Leader 6*(6): 46-48.

Suling, L. (7 June 2007). *The impact of transition experience on practice of newly licensed registered nurses.* National Council of State Boards of Nursing. Retrieved 6 October 2009 from https://www.ncsbn.org/Suling.ppt

Wandelt, M. A., & Stewart, D. S. (1975). Slater nursing competencies rating scale. New York: Appleton-Century-Croft.

Additional Resources

Beecroft, P. C., Dorey, F., & Wenten, M. (2007). Turnover intention in new graduate nurses: a multivariate analysis. *Journal of Advanced Nursing. 62*(1). 41-52.

Krozek, C. (Oct. 2008). The new graduate RN residency: Win/win/win for nurses, hospitals, and patients. *Nurse Leader.* 41-44.

99: Truth and Honesty

References

Arrien, A. (1993). *The four-fold way: Walking the paths of the warrior, teacher, healer, and visionary.* New York: HarperCollins Publishers.

Arrien, A. (2005). *The second half of life: Opening the eight gates of wisdom.* Boulder, CO: Sounds True, Inc.

Connaughton, M., & Hassinger, J. (2007). Leadership character: Antidote to organizational fatigue. *Journal of Nursing Administration, 37:* 464–470.

Additional Resources

Buckingham M. & Coffman, C. (1999). *First, break all the rules: What the world's greatest managers do differently.* New York: Simon & Schuster.

Patterson, K., Grenny, J., McMillan, R., & Switzler, A. (2002). *Crucial conversations: Tools for talking when stakes are high.* New York: McGraw-Hill.

Young, D. (2007). *Save the first dance for you: The complete nurse's guide to serving your profession, your patients, and yourself.* Norfolk, VA: Young Publications.

100: Unity Within the Nursing Profession (Building)

References
Maxwell, J. C. (2005). *The 4 pillars of leadership.* Nashville, TN: Thomas Nelson, Inc.

Mbigi, L. & Maree, J. (1995). *Ubuntu: The spirit of African transformation management.* Pretoria: Sigma Press (Pty) Ltd.

South African Nursing Council (SANC). (2008). *Growth in the registers and rolls: 1998 to 2008.* Retrieved 6 October 2009 from http://www.sanc.co.za/stats.htm

Additional Resources
Reh, F. J. (2008). *How to manage a project.* Retrieved 6 October 2009 from http://management.about.com/od/projectmanagement/ht/ProjMgtSteps.htm

101: Values, Vision, and Driving the Mission

References
Goleman, D. (2000). Leadership that gets results. *Harvard Business Review*, March-April: 79–90.

Gopee, N. (2008). *Mentoring and supervision in healthcare.* London: Sage Publications.

Hoffman, S. J., Harris, A., & Rosenfield, F. (2008). Why mentorship matters: Students, staff, and sustainability in interprofessional education. *Journal of Interprofessional Care*, 22(1): 103–105.

Kakabadse, N., Kakabadse A., & Lee-Davies L. (2005). Visioning the pathway: A leadership process model. *European Management Journal*, 23(2): 237–246.

Kirk, M., Lea, D., & Skirton, H. (2008a). Genomic healthcare: Is the future now? *Nursing and Health Sciences, 10*(2) 85–92.

Kirk, M., Tonkin, E., & Burke, S. (2008b). Engaging nurses in genetics: The strategic approach of the NHS National Genetics Education and Development Centre. *Journal of Genetic Counseling*, 17(2): 180–188.

Spitzer, R. (2003). Keeping the mission in sight helps smooth bumps along the road. *Nurse Leader*, 46(4).

Stanley, D. (2008). Congruent leadership: Values in action. *Journal of Nursing Management*, 16: 519–524.

Additional Reading
Bally, J. (2007). The role of nursing leadership in creating a mentoring culture in acute care environments. *Nursing Economics*, 25(3): 143–148.

Mockett, L., Horsfall, J., & O'Callaghan, W. (2006). Education leadership in the clinical health care setting: A framework for nursing education development. *Nurse Education in Practice*, 6: 404–410.

102: Work-Life Balance for Self and Staff

References
American Institute of Stress. *America's #1 health problem.* Retrieved 6 October 2009 from http://www.stress.org/americas.htm?AIS=bdb3eb21b038a5420c1a6d655676b97f

Bailey, S. T. (2008). *Release your brilliance: The 4 steps to transforming your life and revealing your genius to the world.* New York: HarperCollins.

Berman, F. L. (2004). *Now what? 90 days to a new life direction.* New York: Jeremy P. Tarcher/Penguin.

Covey, S., Merrill, A. R., & Merrill, R. R. (1994). *First things first: To live, to love, to learn, to leave a legacy.* New York: Simon and Schuster.

Kelly, M. (2007). *The dream manager.* New York: Beacon Publishing.

Additional Resources

Blanchard, K., Blanchard, M., & Edinton, D. (1999). *The one minute manager balances work and life.* New York: Harper Paperbacks.

Johnson, S. (1998). *One minute for yourself: A simple strategy for a better life.* New York: Quill Publishing.

Swenson, R. A. (1998). *The overload syndrome: Learning to live within your limits.* Colorado Springs, CO: NavPress.

Swenson, R. A. (2004). *Margin: Restoring emotional, physical, financial, and time.* Colorado Springs, CO: NavPress.

Travis, J., & Ryan, R. (2004). *Wellness workbook: How to achieve enduring health and vitality.* Berkeley, CA: Celestial Arts.

Tubesing, D., & Tubesing, N. (1991). *Seeking your healthy balance: A do-it-yourself guide to whole person well-being.* Duluth, MN: Whole Person Associates.

103: Writing for Professional Journals

References

Barber, C. (2008). The dos and don'ts of writing for publication. *British Journal of Healthcare Assistants,* 2(7): 359–360.

Hallas, D., & Feldman, H. (2006). A guide to scholarly writing in nursing. *NSNA IMPRINT* (September/October); 80-83.

Oermann, M. (2002). *Writing for publication in nursing.* Philadelphia: Lippincott, Williams & Wilkins.

Roberts, D. (2008). Publication: A mark of professionalism. *MedSurg Nursing,* 17(1): 8.

Wollin, J., & Fairweather, C. (2007). Finding your voice: Key elements to consider when writing for publication. *British Journal of Nursing (BJN),* 16(22): 1418–1421.

Additional Resources

Jaarsma, T. (2005). Writing a publication on cardiac nursing: Just do it! *European Journal of Cardiovascular Nursing,* 4(4), 265-266.

Manion, J. (1998). *From management to leadership: Interpersonal skills for success in health care.* Chicago, IL: AHA Press.

Richardson, S. (2008). It's all about making a difference. *Kai Tiaki Nursing New Zealand, 14*(1), 15-16.